To Dr E. E. Wallach,
In appreciation of
the excellent training received
at Pennsylvania Hospital.
Lawrence S. Borow, MD

Atlas of GYNECOLOGIC LAPAROSCOPY and HYSTEROSCOPY

By

K. SEMM, Prof. Dr. Med.

Director of the Gynecological Clinic of
the Kiel Obstetrical Institute

Introduction by

Prof. Dr. RAOUL PALMER, Paris

Translated by

ALLAN LAKE RICE, Ph. D.

Edited by

LAWRENCE STEPHEN BOROW, M.D.

Division of Obstetrics and Gynecology,
Lankenau Hospital, Philadelphia, Pennsylvania

1977 W. B. SAUNDERS COMPANY Philadelphia / London / Toronto

W. B. Saunders Company: West Washington Square
Philadelphia, PA 19105

1 St. Anne's Road
Eastbourne, East Sussex BN21 3UN, England

1 Goldthorne Avenue
Toronto, Ontario M8Z 5T9, Canada

Atlas of Gynecologic Laparoscopy and Hysteroscopy ISBN 0-7216-8063-1

Typesetting, printing and binding: W. B. Saunders Company, Philadelphia and W. F. May, Miesbach, Obt. Germany.

Last digit is the print number: 9 8 7 6 5 4 3 2 1

Editor's Foreword

Kurt Semm's *Atlas of Gynecologic Laparoscopy and Hysteroscopy* provides the English language reader with the most complete text available on this subject. It represents a distillation of experience acquired from thousands of cases over more than a decade. The present state of the art, both as a diagnostic and surgical tool, is presented in light of all known indications and contraindications. This is followed by a discussion of precise technique which enables achieving the objective with maximum safety. The colored line drawings illustrating the text plus the superb laparoscopic photographs comprising the Atlas make this an easily understood primer for the novice and a graduate refresher course for the more experienced laparoscopist.

In this English language edition of Semm's Atlas unfamiliar German terminology has been anglicized for more ready understanding. The compendious bibliography retains the original language for the reference titles for easier retrieval by the reader.

I wish to thank George Vilk and John Dyson of W. B. Saunders for their help in bringing this Atlas to the English-speaking audience, and my wife Suzy and son Todd for their support and encouragement while editing this valuable textbook.

Lawrence S. Borow, M.D.

Introduction

Semm's Atlas of Gyecologic Laparoscopy is far more than a mere atlas. It represents the sum total of present day knowledge of gynecologic laparoscopy in general. It can serve as a *reference work* as well as an *atlas for basic instruction*, and is highly informative on all facets of the subject.

Semm is at great pains to differentiate between *laparoscopy* and *pelvoscopy*.* The technical term "laparoscopy" he confines to endoscopic procedures in the upper abdomen, performed by gastroenterologists and hepatologists, as a rule under local anesthesia, with a very low accident rate. *Pelvoscopy*, on the other hand, normally requires complete narcosis, involving numerous risk factors. This demands unfailing precautionary measures and even fully automatic monitoring apparatus to hold these risks to a minimum.

In my own initiation to pelvoscopy, at a time when no teacher was available to me, experience in performing a large part of the surgical measures under local anesthesia stood me in good stead. I could not have popularized this method without presenting it as of equivalent value with exploratory laparotomy while involving much less dangerous consequences. All my pelvoscopies in the years 1943 to 1951 were performed under *local anesthesia*. This made it paramount to defer constantly to the patient's comfort, being mindful of the effects upon her of the Trendelenburg position, the intra-abdominal pressure and the manipulations with the intrauterine probe. The exploratory pelvoscopies were not *invariably* definitive. However, the patients were left with unfavorable memories of the ordeal, so that if after the initial operation a pelvoscopic follow-up was suggested, they invariably demanded general anesthesia the second time.

For these reasons, and especially also in order to be able to perform by pelvoscopy *operative procedures* such as biopsies and lysis of adhesions, and, since 1958, also sterilizations, I switched, from 1952 on, to general anesthesia, benefiting, of course, from the experience gained since 1943 on the importance of constant monitoring of intra-abdominal pressure during the course of the pelvoscopy.

It is obvious that Semm shows genius in his development of apparatus calculated to enhance the patient's *safety* and the *dexterity* of the practitioner. Many of these pieces of equipment which seem indispensable even to experienced pelvoscopists enable the novice to carry out certain manipulations more readily and more safely. Certainly use of the Semm Insufflator (CO_2-Pneu-Automatic) affords all members of the operating room team, especially the anesthesiologist, a greater measure of confidence during the celioscopy.

The same "*safety-first*" principle led Semm to wage a veritable crusade against the use of high-frequency electricity in pelvoscopy. Although he has performed

*Although Dr. Semm holds strong views on this distinction in terminology, in the Text and Atlas sections of this English-language edition we have chosen to follow the usage most familiar to our readers: "laparoscopy"—*not* "pelvoscopy."

over a thousand electrosurgical pelvoscopic procedures using high-frequency current with forceps, diathermy hooks and spot-coagulators without primary or secondary accident, I was as concerned as he at the large number of reports of accidents arising, especially at the hands of novices and even some seasoned practitioners. Semm's argument on this point was especially cogent to me, all the more so since he offered a well developed substitute solution to the problem of thermocoagulation, namely, absolutely minimum coagulation of the tissue grasped by forceps whose jaws are heated by a low-voltage current under complete control. All risk of remote burns was thus completely obviated.

I think, however, that my own suggestions of 1962 on tubal sterilization are still valid: only double coagulation and severance of the isthmic section of the tube can assure 99.9 per cent success.

In conclusion, we have Semm to thank for having made pelvoscopy a safe procedure at the hands of practically all practitioners.

RAOUL PALMER

Paris, August 1975

Preface

The introduction and proliferation of endoscopic procedures in gynecology and obstetrics have gone hand in hand with the technologic development of the necessary instrumentarium. Gynecologic laparoscopy and hysteroscopy made the severest demands. It came therefore as no surprise that these procedures were the last, after colposcopy and amnioscopy, to win their rightful place among clinical routines. Even though gynecologic laparoscopy and hysteroscopy were already subjects of scientific publication in past decades, their clinical importance remained of little more than theoretic value. The decisive break-through for gynecologic laparoscopy came at the end of the 1960s when the standardization of instruments and operative techniques rendered this procedure subject to rigid monitoring. Upon widespread application of the method it became evident that laparoscopy was bringing about decisive changes in our earlier concepts of gynecologic practice, contributing to the welfare of the patients entrusted to our care.

The rapid proliferation of a surgical technique—from the United States come statistics of more than 200,000 laparoscopies performed since 1970—pointed up the need for a reference work in which, over and above the operative procedure, visually diagnosable conditions could be extensively presented. This textbook and atlas in its present form is intended to stimulate even experienced practitioners to further progress as well as to aid novices in grasping the fundamentals. May this atlas, the record of my own ten year photographic pursuit of normal variants and pathologic conditions in the female pelvis, arouse and enhance in physicians, even nongynecologists, an understanding from picture to picture of the female reproductive organs and of the diseases to which they are subject. The extraordinary pictorial talents of our artist, Mrs. M. Rabe, have made it possible to supplant the usual black-and-white photos with didactically valuable sketches. The frequently confusing enalrged monocular laparoscopic views have been transformed, thanks to her lucid line drawings, into a readily intelligible anatomic picture. Numerals permit easy indentification of anatomic landmarks. By virtue of the gracious generosity of the F. K. Schattauer publishing house, who did not stint with regard to color reproduction, an exhaustive series of illustrations has become possible, and textual matter has been held to a minimum, serving largely to supplement the illustrations.

KURT SEMM

Kiel, November 1975

Contents

A

Pelvic Laparoscopy

I
Introduction*

The urge to bring the internal female genitalia within range of the physician's eye is a very ancient one. In the Talmud (completed about 500 A.D. after several centuries of both oral and written tradition) there is a reference to a *siphopherot,* apparently a tube made of lead. With its aid the external cervical os was rendered visible through dilation of the vagina. This reference is probably the oldest in the history of gynecologic endoscopy.

Steps began in the mid-19th century toward a deeper visual exploration into the biologic processes within the vagina and the uterine cavity. Thus, Aubinais in 1864 and Pantaleoni in 1868 told of their initial attempts to inspect the human uterine cavity with the naked eye. However, these and other similar studies in experimental hysteroscopy achieved only theoretic value and had no clinical significance. Achievements in the field were meager, both because of technologic insufficiency in the instruments employed and because of surgical difficulties in gaining access for the instruments.

It is only since the beginning of the present decade that techniques have begun to catch up with requirements and make possible practical, reproducible hysteroscopy. Until the middle of this century it was not customary, except by laparotomy, to explore those internal female genital organs not visually accessible through the vaginal canal.

Palmer (1947) was the first gynecologist to make clinical use of gynecologic laparoscopy; this procedure already was known and had been described in detail by Boesch in 1935, who used 40 to 50 degrees of pelvic elevation even in the presence of abdominal adhesions; but until then the procedure had been employed almost exclusively in the diagnosis of hepatic disease. However, the transabdominal route at first was not attractive for routine use because of technical difficulties and problems with the apparatus then available. For this reason, Decker (1946) suggested the vaginal route, which was more appropriate for the gynecologist.

This transvaginal procedure is known as *culdoscopy,* and the instrumentarium required has been standardized. The patient is positioned on her knees and elbows, or in extreme pelvic elevation (Figs. 45 and 46). Almost no variations are possible in operative technique. The point of entry, the vault of the vagina, determines the nature of the procedure. However, this endoscopic approach permits only limited exploration of the internal female genitalia, which severely restricts the clinical efficacy of the procedure in diagnosis and therapy. The technique itself, therefore, is not widely used and has few adherents in Europe and North America today.

In Germany after 1958, Frangenheim made great strides in endoscopy of the pelvis, as well as in the field of instrumental techniques and further development, and made an early choice in favor of the transabdominal route. Nonetheless, the

*In order to foster continuity in this Atlas, bibliographic references have been largely omitted in the description of techniques, methods, and diagnoses. However, for completeness, a compendious list of references can be found at the end of the book.

transabdominal laparoscopic technique for exploration of the internal female genitalia achieved only limited acceptance before the early 1960s, for the following reasons.

(1) The initial insertion, i.e., the blind puncture of the abdominal wall and the insufflation of air by hand-pump into the pneumoperitoneum, seemed too hazardous to the anesthetized patient.

(2) The insertion of a thumb-thick trocar, which introduced the lens into the abdomen, where pressures could not be monitored, was considered to entail greater risk than exploratory laparotomy.

(3) The close-range heat of the light bulb threatened burns in the likely event of contact with the bowel. Such intestinal contact can hardly be avoided in endoscopy of the lower abdomen, unlike the upper (as in examination of the liver).

(4) The optical quality of the image was poor. This, together with the 90-degree field of view (see Fig. 40), resulted in orientation problems in the pelvis.

(5) Anesthesia presented problems, especially in view of the lack of control over pressures in the pneumoperitoneum.

(6) Introduction of atmospheric air into the pneumoperitoneum always involved the risk of deadly air emboli.

In addition, the multiplicity of newly-coined terms for the procedure, ranging from abdominoscopy to ventroscopy, suggested a certain vagueness about this proposed operative technique.

Especially as a result of valuable contributions by Kalk (1929, etc.), an optimal instrumentarium for transabdominal endoscopic exploration of the upper abdomen has become available, and a standard operative technique has been worked out that is reproducible at any time under local anesthesia. Both of these achievements are of several decades' standing.

Until recently, however, no such perfected technique and standardized instrumentarium was available for gynecologic endoscopy of the lower abdomen. Reports exist of thousands of laparoscopies in internal medicine using local anesthesia without serious mishap, but statistics for gynecologic endoscopy in the lower abdomen record severe complications.

The chief difference lies in the fact that gynecologic endoscopy requires general anesthesia because it is painful, involving as it does displacement of the uterus. Only with a specific procedure, as for example in sterilization of the fallopian tubes by coagulation, is local anesthesia acceptable in gynecologic endoscopy.

If the trocar is inserted into the upper abdomen and aimed toward the liver, there is very little risk of injury to any vital organ. However, the situation is very different when the trocar is inserted into the pelvis and aimed toward the uterus, for here there are many possibilities that the tip of the trocar may cause damage to vital organs or blood vessels, resulting in fatal complications.

Another stumbling block to general acceptance of endoscopy of the lower abdomen has been the fact that usually both the instrumentarium (developed specifically for endoscopy of the upper abdomen) and the manual techniques for producing a pneumoperitoneum with air were foreign to this procedure. The unanesthetized patient can consciously follow all the surgeon's manipulations in the upper abdomen, and a running interrogation of the patient provides the operator with supplementary diagnostic information that is not possible with a patient under general anesthesia for endoscopy of the lower abdomen. The surgeon in the latter case is totally dependent on his own resources and skills. In the matter of the blind puncture, for example, the operator is unable to monitor by palpation the exact place the insufflation needle has reached, and cannot "feel" the possible puncture of an intestinal loop that may be adhering to the abdominal wall.

In upper abdominal laparoscopy, previous gallbladder surgery and the like are standard contraindications for the endoscopic approach. However, a prior operation on the lower abdomen is one of the chief *indications* for gynecologic endoscopy. If we were to limit the endoscopic technique only to abdomens that had not previously undergone laparotomy, the number of cases in which the technique is applicable would decrease by 80 per cent.

The possibility of inspecting the internal female genitalia without resorting to laparotomy, and thus of obtaining important diagnostic data in the course of an extremely brief hospitalization, constitutes a real breakthrough in gynecology. Both in diagnosis and therapy, routine endoscopy alters significantly earlier gynecologic thinking and techniques. To this end, it is necessary that a new diagnostic and therapeutic line in exploration of the lower abdomen be so fully perfected that it can be pursued with the same safety as exploratory laparotomy.

One benefit accruing to the patient is that some complaints can be discounted diagnostically as not of a gynecologic nature, or recognized as either characteristic or uncommon abdominal disorders for which appropriate therapy can be instituted. The long periods of observation and hospitalization without any real diagnostic success are becoming entirely a thing of the past as a result of the purposeful and routine introduction of endoscopy.

Gynecologic endoscopy, because of the confusion in nomenclature, has been until very recently the scapegoat for an incidence of complications and deaths that in the future no longer will be tolerated. In the last decade we have made a study of all the factors leading to such complications, and have attempted to eradicate them by introducing appropriate safety measures and refinements in the apparatus and instrumentarium.

If we are to work in the future with a standardized technique that excludes all possible accidents and complications, this undertaking must be identified by a specific, characteristic name.*

The recent reintroduction into endoscopy of low-voltage or "galvanic" current has succeeded in eliminating risks inherent in the use of high-frequency electricity. Likewise, modern lenses, gas control, cold light, and electronics have made revolutionary changes in the techniques of laparoscopy and have led to their simplification and improvement. Laparoscopy today is a standard procedure without which gynecology would be much the poorer.

Accordingly, the present atlas presents a selection of color photos from gynecologic endoscopic scans, taken from my own collection of slides, representing nearly a decade of experience. The atlas makes no claim to completeness nor to the inclusion of all possible pathologic changes in the internal female genitalia. Although laparoscopy, by its very nature, also envisages scanning of the entire abdomen, pathologic findings outside the confines of the pelvis have not been included; for these the reader is referred to other atlases.

Since line drawings, which can emphasize certain details, are often clearer than black-and-white photographs, the former have been chosen for the present atlas. Opposite each color photo stands a matching line drawing from which the

---

*Editor's Note: Dr. Semm strongly prefers the use of the term, "pelvoscopy" (in German, "Pelviskopie"), but in this English-language edition we have conformed to terminology that will be familiar to our readers.

topography of the various organs in the female pelvis can be clearly understood. The fold-out at the back of the book, with its numbered catalog of organs, affords ready orientation.*

*The technologic development of endoscopes in the past decade has brought important innovations. This atlas shows the most modern achievements of this technology at the time of compilation, but does not pretend to include the makes of all manufacturers. To do so would lead to constant repetition and confusion. The technologically optimal border values mentioned in the text are intended to encourage each prospective purchaser to test and compare the possibilities and capacities of the instruments offered before making an expensive purchase.

II
Historical Survey

Even today, in this age of laboratory diagnoses, exploration—direct visual study of the patient—is doubtless the most important means of medical diagnosis. Along with the time-honored examination methods of palpation, percussion, and auscultation, the physician has always been interested in the possibility of going beyond mere external observation to look inside the patient. Thus, the chief representative of the Kos school, Hippocrates II (460–375 B.C.), wrote as follows about examination of the rectum: "Then lay the patient backwards and look with the rectal speculum to see where the rectum is affected. . ." The Babylonian Talmud refers to a *siphopherot* made of lead, bent inward at its tip, where there is a *mechul* (wooden mandrin) to ease penetration into the vagina. This instrument, described in the treatise *Niddah,* folio 65b, and intended for distinguishing between vaginal and uterine bleeding, probably represents the oldest form of vaginal speculum, and therefore the earliest instance of endoscopy in gynecologic annals.

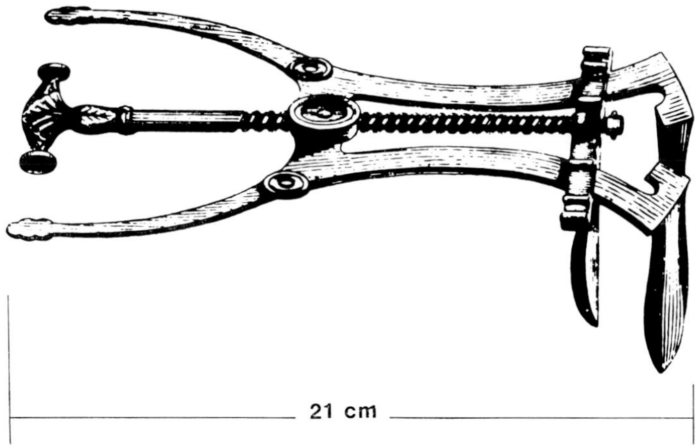

Figure 1

In Pompeii, which was destroyed in 70 A.D., a technically quite well developed three-bladed vaginal speculum was found (Fig. 1), with which a colposcopic examination in the modern sense must have been quite possible. To what a high degree even then the shape of the speculum and (most important in endoscopy) the light were described and discussed is made clear in the writings of Archigenes of Apamea in Syria, who practiced in Rome from 95 to 117 A.D. Aëtius reports on the preserved fragments of the very vaginal speculum fashioned by Archigenes, which he himself called a "thing to look through." Archigenes described the position of the woman's body and the station to be assumed by the physician, and was the first to mention the matter of illumination for endoscopic purposes in saying, "by that good bright light from the south." He also recommends selecting the speculum according to the age of the patient, and tries to render the dilation of the vagina as painless as possible by wrapping the blades of the speculum in wool.

Soranus of Ephesus, also active as an obstetrician in Rome from 98 to 108 A.D., described the vaginal speculum in similar fashion.

The first genuine instance of the use of a mirror, according to Avicenna (980–1037 A.D.), is to be ascribed to the Arabs. Abulkasim (912–1013 A.D.) held a glass mirror before the dilated vulva, and in this way reflected light into the vaginal cavity. He was thus the first to use reflected light for purposes of illumination and observation of the interior of the body.

The first endoscopic light must be credited to Tulio Caesare Aranzi, who in 1587 wrote of using the camera obscura for medical purposes. This had been invented by a Benedictine monk named Don Panuce, was mentioned by Leonardo da Vinci in 1519, and was first described under that name by Porta in 1589. Solar rays entering through a hole in a window-shutter were brought to a focus through a spherical glass flask filled with water and projected into the nasal cavity. When the sky was overcast, he recommended use of artificial light.

In the 16th century, double- and triple-bladed screw-specula of many sizes for anal, vaginal, and uterine dilation (Figs. 2 and 3) were described and depicted. The inventive genius of physicians and the increasing technologic skills of instrument-makers seem to have been concentrated on this field. In the 17th century the concave mirror was introduced by Peter Borell of Castres.

For the first lamp for endoscopic use, we have to thank the 18th century gynecologist Arnaud, who adapted for use in medicine the small lanterns then employed by burglars.

The birth of modern endoscopy came with Bozzini (1805), who invented a very complex apparatus that became the first light transmitter. This consisted of a device that conveyed rays of light into the inner cavities of the living body and out

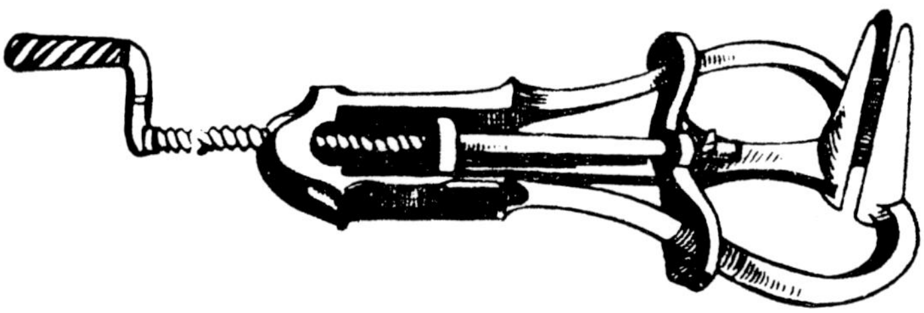

Figure 2

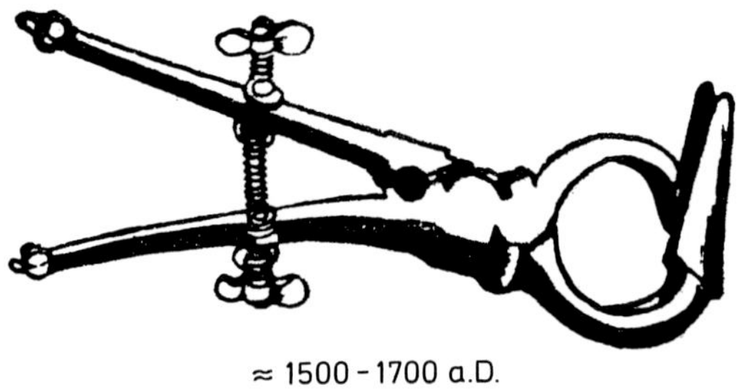

Figure 3

again to the eye of the observer. Its components were a lamp-housing (*A*, Fig. 4), and a light-transmitter in the form of a tube (*B*) carrying the light into the body cavities and of a reflex transmitter or tube (*C*) that brought it out again to the eye.

This lamp was followed by the first effective endoscope of Desormeaux (1843) (Fig. 5), who has been regarded as the father of endoscopy.

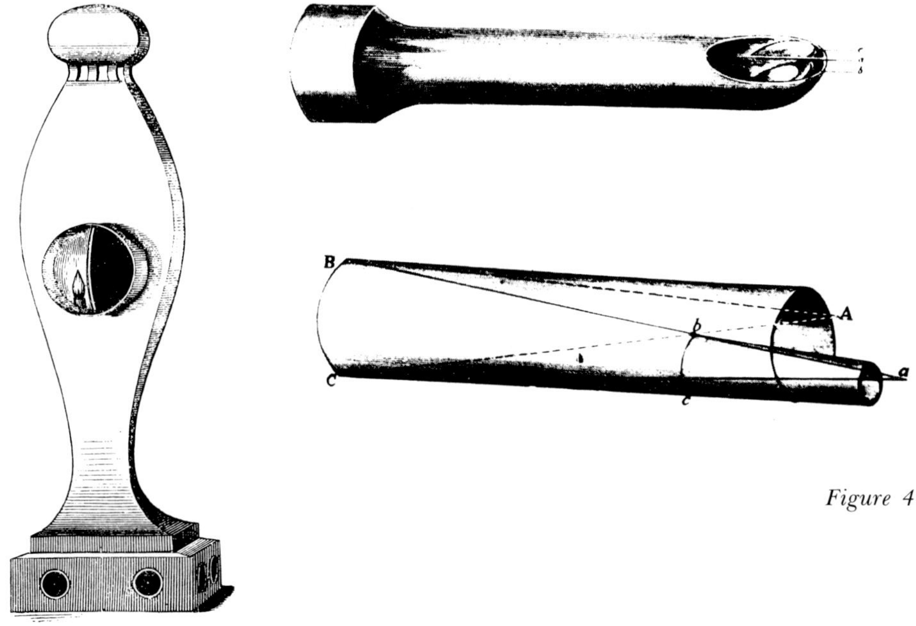

Figure 4

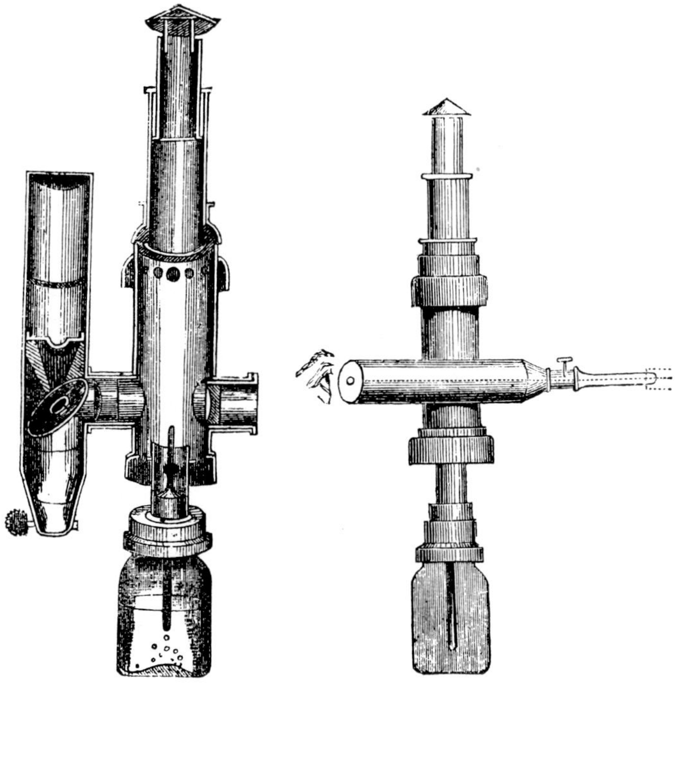

Figure 5

Meanwhile, a number of independent investigators had been undertaking experiments toward making the body cavities accessible to the eye. After Desormeaux, a separate development began in each medical specialty, in the course of which three basic types of light-source appeared, depending on which organ was to be explored. This was an exclusively endoscopic apparatus in which: (1) the enclosed light-source, reflector, and endoscopic probe were all integral; (2) the light-source was separate, but the reflector and endoscopic probe were interconnected; and (3) the light-source, reflector, and endoscopic probe all operated independently.

The difficulties encountered by the inventors of such endoscopes (Fig. 6) are illustrated in a remark by Fürstenheim, who reports that among any ten German physicians in 1863 to whom Desormeaux demonstrated stones in the bladder and inflammation and strictures in the male urethra with his apparatus there were always three or four who insisted they saw nothing!

The need for photographic documentation also became clear. Stein (Frankfurt), emphasizing the disadvantages of Desormeaux' and Fürstenheim's endoscopes, recommended in 1874 the "photoendoscope" that he had developed (Fig. 7).

Although gynecology was godfather to the original development of the endoscope, from that time in the mid-19th century on, when the first practical devices for observing living internal human organs appeared and first acquired their specific designation, "endoscope," gynecology and obstetrics no longer had this field of development to themselves.

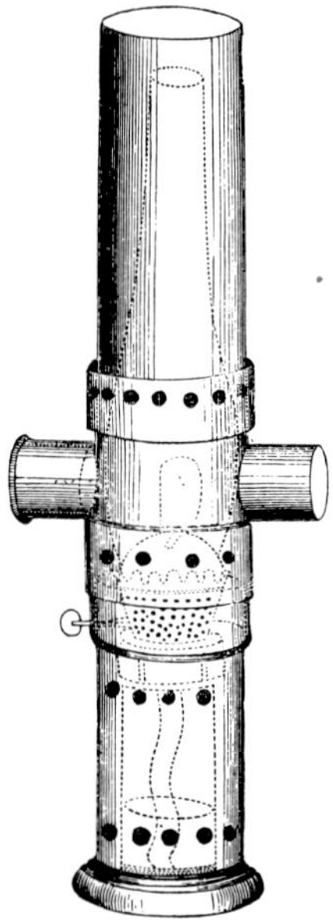

Figure 6

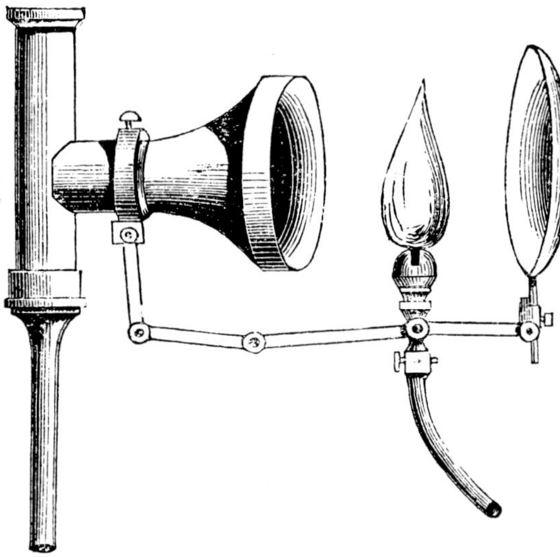

Figure 7

Just as Desormeaux recommended his endoscope for examination of the vagina and uterus, so also Brunton (1861) hoped that his otoscope (Fig. 8) would find vaginal, uterine, and other exploratory applications. This endoscope competed with Langlebert's urethroscope (Fig. 9).

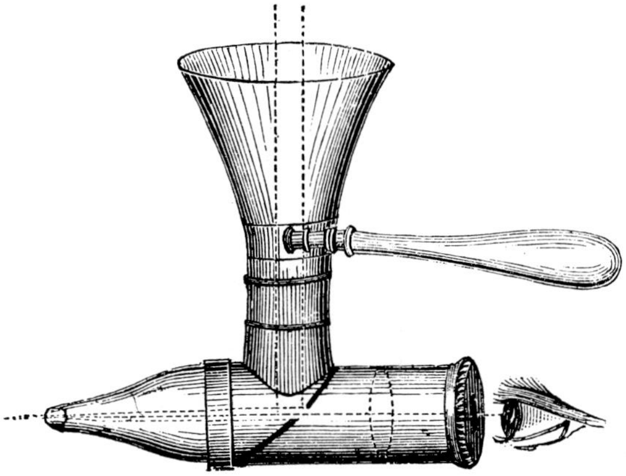

Figure 8

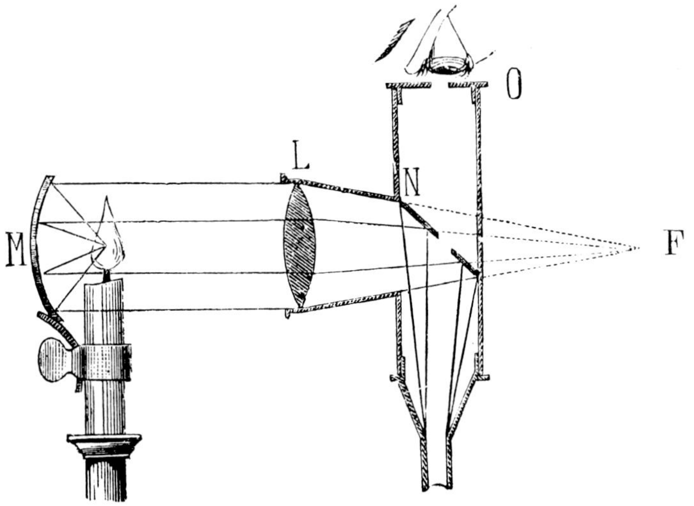

Figure 9

And so Desormeaux (1853), Aubinais (1864), and Pantaleoni (1868) pursued the idea of inspecting the interior of the uterus with the early endoscopes then at their disposal. All their efforts in the assault on body cavities as difficult to inspect as the endometrial cavity remained more or less theoretic attempts without practical value. This pioneer work in the field of gynecologic endoscopy, especially with reference to laparoscopy and hysteroscopy, has been recorded in numerous monographs and manuals in recent decades.

Perhaps the elaborate technologic requirements for cystoscopy may best be illustrated by Fig. 10, which affords a detailed insight into the cystoscope developed by Nitze.

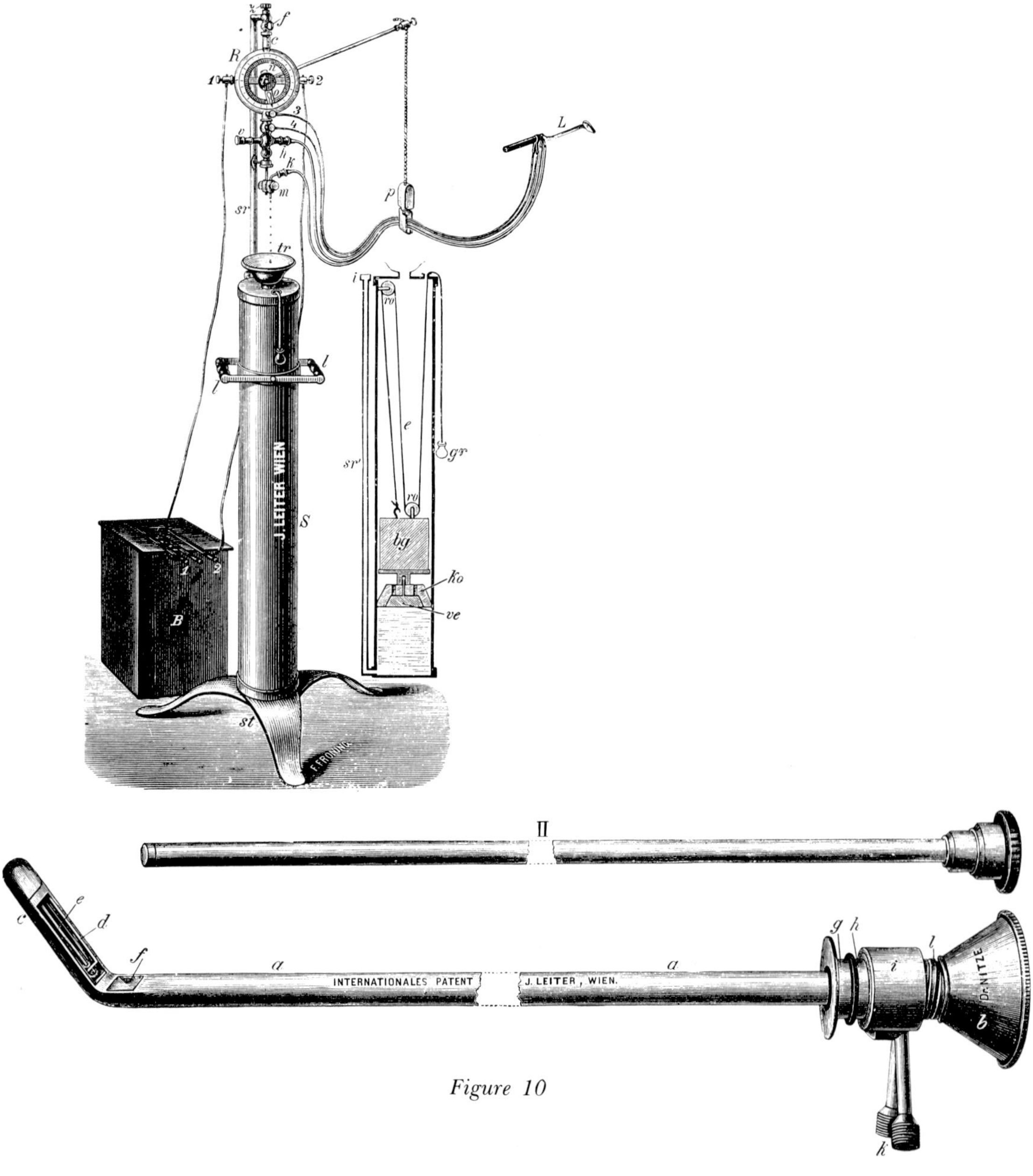

Figure 10

Pelvic laparoscopy today is a specialized form of general laparoscopy for gynecologic purposes. After the first endoscopic observation of the abdominal organs in an air-filled mammalian (canine) abdomen by Kelling in 1901, the first practical application of this new method to humans was done in Sweden by Jacobaeus in 1910. The method was ostensibly rediscovered twice, by the American Steiner in 1924 as "abdominoscopy" and by the Italian Redi in 1925 as "splanchnoscopy." The first textbook with an atlas of laparo- and thoracoscopy appeared in 1927 from Korbsch in Munich. Intra-abdominal adhesions were first severed by means of the coagulation probe of a ureterocystoscope by Fervers in 1933.

In his report on laparoscopy, Boesch (1935) in Aarau, Switzerland, spoke of "wonderful views of the normal female genital organs" and of how he had rendered visible hitherto hidden organs (for example, the ovaries) by means of an elevator. He goes on: "Finally, by means of the laparoscope, we are achieving a way of performing tubal sterilization, when indicated, without laparotomy. Using endoscopic procedures fully monitored by the eye, the tubes are coagulated at several places in three to five seconds by means of suitably insulated coagulation-clips. . ." (For independent discovery of the same technique in America by Power and Barnes in 1941, see p. 54). That report might be regarded as the dawn of modern laparoscopy, just as Goetze laid the cornerstone of safe puncture and gas-insufflation of the abdomen through his development in 1918 of the automatic needle (Fig. 11*).

*Original legend: Automatic needle. *a*—outer cannula, *b*—guide ear on the outer cannula, *c*—inner cannula, *d*—tension spring.

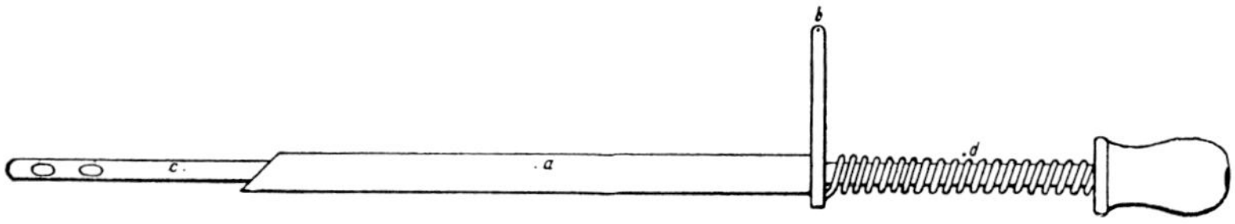

Figure 11

As the technique developed, some authors made contributions in the field of transabdominal observation of the internal female genitalia; others via the vault of the vagina. Decker made use of the instrumentarium of laparoscopy for the second route of exploration, namely, through the vault of the vagina. However, as explained in Chapter I, the simple transfer of techniques from upper abdominal inspection (performed under local anesthesia) to lower abdominal exploration (under general anesthesia) was not a happy one.

The extensive dissemination of gynecologic laparoscopy since the introduction of cold-light endoscopy and of the automatic insufflation of the pneumoperitoneum (Semm, 1963) underscores the fact that gynecology must use an endoscopic technique of its own and an instrumentarium created especially for lower abdominal endoscopy. This becomes more and more necessary as laparoscopy assumes its significant new role today on a large scale in the service of family planning. Purely for purposes of sterilization, perfectly healthy women are undergoing a procedure that must not involve the slightest risk. Here for the first time the physician is deviating from his traditional field of activity, that of detecting and treating disease.

Since 1965 the cold-light endoscope (Fig. 50) has met the requirements in optical quality (e.g., Lumina, Hopkins, et al.) for motion pictures and television. Like the "needlescope" (Fig. 12) with an outside diameter of 1.2 mm (e.g., for transabdominal amnioscopy or amniocentesis), it expands the scope for use, and soon there will be no limitation on our obstetric and gynecologic needs.

To what extent flexible endoscopes (Fig. 44) are introducing advances in laparoscopy over the earlier rigid scopes will be fully realized only as the importance of endoscopy in diagnosis and therapy in gynecology becomes apparent.

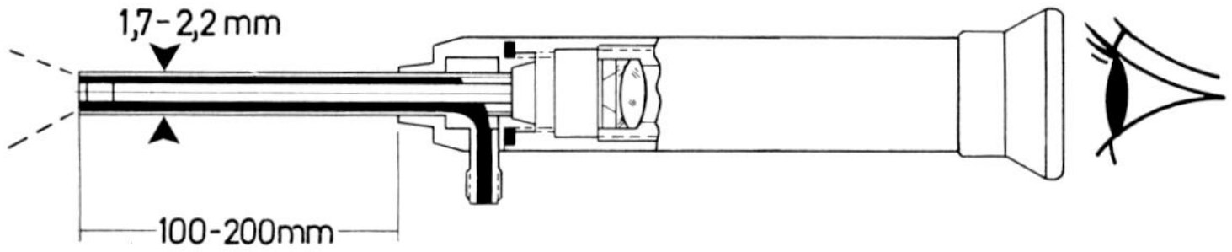

Figure 12

III
Risks and Dangers in Laparoscopy

In the bimanual exploratory technique (see Fig. 131) for the internal female genitalia, inaugurated by B. S. Schultze of Jena (1827–1919), the fingers inserted into the vagina served as the "eye of the gynecologist." If a diagnosis could not be made through such palpation, there was recourse to examination under anesthesia—and after that to exploratory laparotomy. Any decision to open the abdominal cavity for diagnostic purposes alone was rendered more difficult by the possibility of postoperative complications hardly less severe than those following a laparotomy done for therapeutic reasons.

Today, laparoscopy makes possible direct vision of the internal female genitalia without the serious effects of abdominal surgery and without the routine postoperative care required after laparotomy.

The essential distinction between exploratory laparotomy and laparoscopy of the pelvis lies in the instrumentarium and its use. Every surgeon is familiar from the very start of his training with the use of scalpel and forceps. The endoscopic instrumentarium demands, in addition, a high degree of technical knowledge, and its manipulation is far more difficult than that of the scalpel. Further, the recognition of the internal female genital organs through a monocular tube requires a greater familiarity with the anatomy of the pelvis than is needed in binocular observation from the vantage point of an incision at laparotomy.

Thus, laparoscopy is among the most difficult of procedures in gynecology, since the technique presupposes a gynecologic surgeon and diagnostician already trained. The monocular picture, impossible to render stereoscopically, demands an eye with years of training, both for orientation and recognition, and one entirely familiar with pelvic structures. Finally, the endoscopic operator must be capable of making his own repairs in case of injury. Another vital distinction between this and upper abdominal laparoscopy is that orientation is far more difficult in the lower abdomen, especially when adhesions are present. *Laparoscopy of the pelvis, therefore, must be the final step in training for specialization in gynecology.*

The risks and dangers lie first of all in failure to realize the basic difference between upper abdominal and pelvic laparoscopy, and secondly in the possibility that the operator may not have brought himself to that level of technical skill essential for the manipulation of endoscopic instruments. For this reason, until the end of the 1960s, pelvic laparoscopy was largely shunned by gynecologists. The chief sources of danger are listed below. The manner in which these can be eliminated safely will be dealt with later in the chapter on laparoscopic technique.

1. THE BLIND PUNCTURE

The blind puncture of the abdominal wall presents the greatest risk in laparoscopy. In order to establish the pneumoperitoneum, it is essential to perforate all layers of the abdominal wall so that a gaseous medium may be insufflated into the abdomen. Only in the bubble of gas thus produced can the optical inspection be carried out. No matter which topographic region of the abdomen the insufflation needle is inserted into, the following *false* placements are to be avoided.

(1) The needle may not be inserted far enough, i.e., its tip may not perforate all layers of the abdominal wall: skin; fat; muscle; fascia; and peritoneum (Fig. 13). When the gas is insufflated a preperitoneal emphysema results, which may

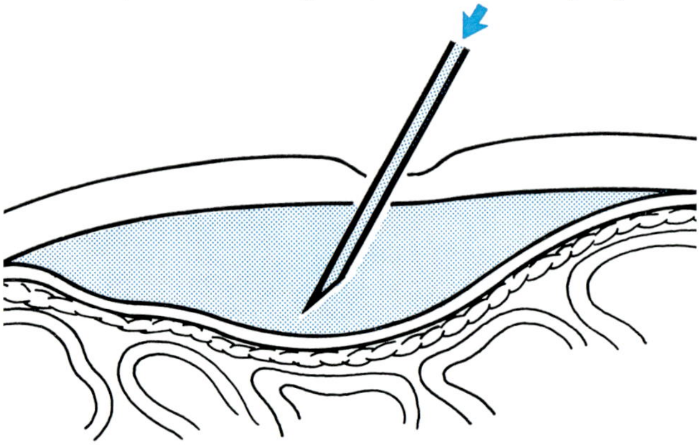

Figure 13

separate the peritoneum from its adjacent tissues and cause it to bulge into the abdominal cavity, making visualization of the pelvis impossible.

(2) An intestinal loop adhering to the abdominal wall as a consequence of a prior operation may be directly pierced after perforation of the peritoneum. The tip of the needle is then in a lumen of the intestine, and subsequent insufflation will inflate the intestine with gas (Fig. 14).

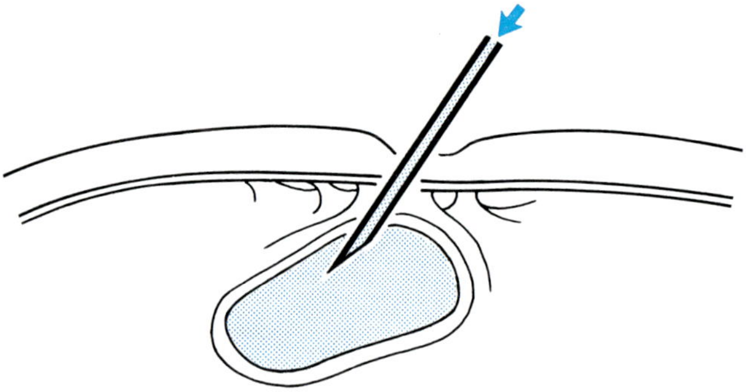

Figure 14

(3) The stomach may have become inflated inadvertently because of hyperventilation in the course of anesthesia before intubation is achieved. The stomach, which is tightly distended, is consequently displaced caudally and lies adjacent to the peritoneum in such a way that the stomach wall is likewise perforated by the inserted insufflation needle (Fig. 15). In any case, subsequent gas insufflation will inflate the intestinal tract as described under (2) above.

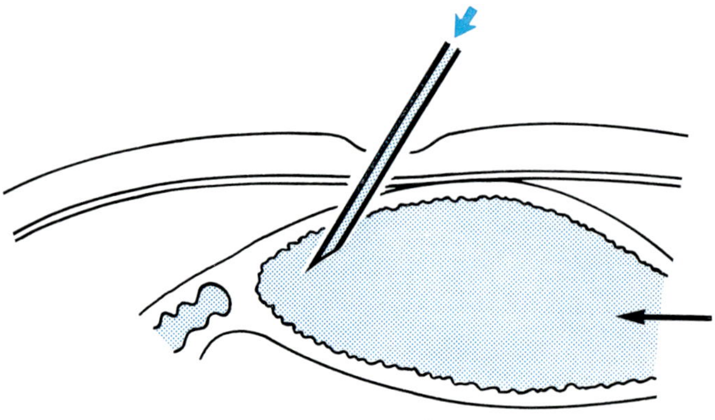

Figure 15

(4) After perforating the peritoneum the needle may be forced into the greater omentum (Fig. 16), which then becomes inflated like a sponge when the gas is insufflated. In this case the abdomen may become filled with several liters of gas, and endoscopic exploration becomes highly difficult or impossible.

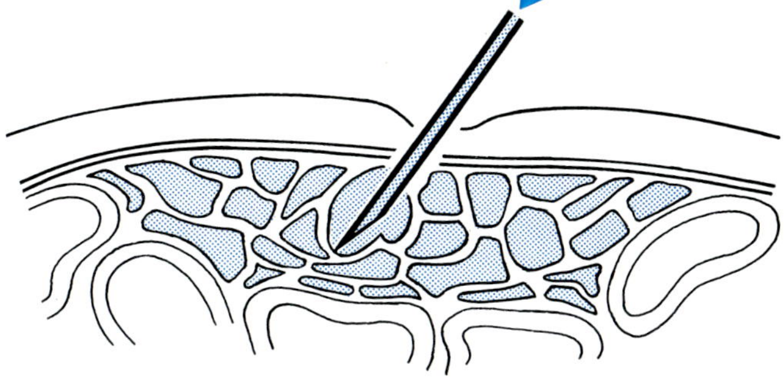

Figure 16

(5) In the case of an abdomen with postoperative adhesions to the abdominal wall, the tip of the needle may enter into or between these (Fig. 17). A situation now arises similar to the inflation of the greater omentum. In general, depending on the size of the inflated adhesion cavity, limited endoscopic exploration still may be possible.

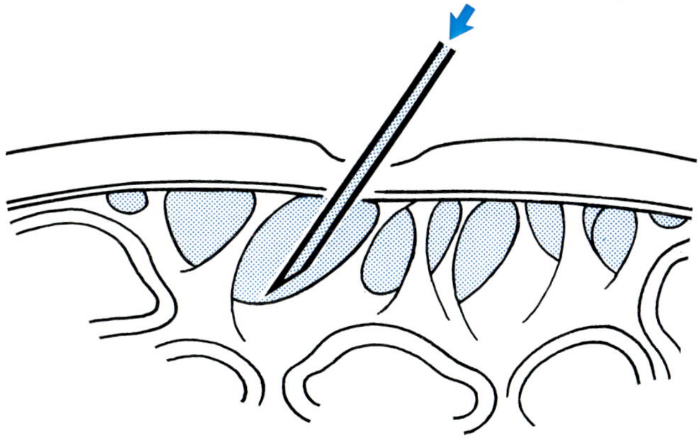

Figure 17

(6) The insufflation needle may be driven too far and may perforate not only all layers of the abdominal wall and parts of the intestine, but also one of the large blood vessels (abdominal aorta or inferior vena cava) (Fig. 18). Alternatively, if the needle is inserted too far caudally in the umbilical area, it may penetrate one of the arteries or veins beyond their bifurcation in the pelvis. In the subsequent insufflation, the gas may be introduced intravascularly into the bloodstream (see also Fig. 26).

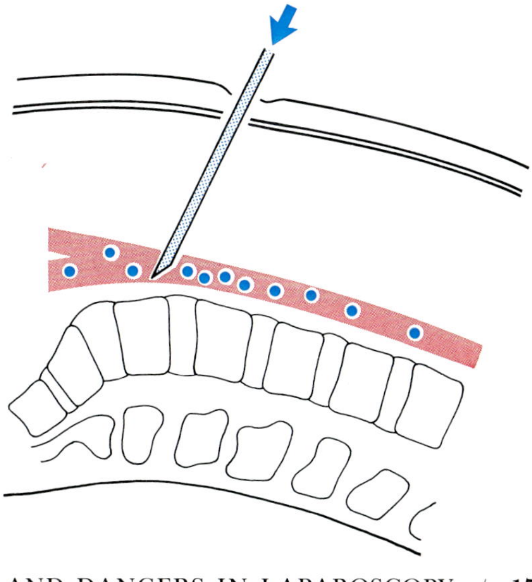

Figure 18

This complication may occur especially if the abdominal wall has not been sufficiently elevated by the insufflation or if, in the case of a very slender patient, the distance from the abdominal wall to the above-mentioned blood vessels was estimated incorrectly.

(7) A mediastinal emphysema (Fig. 19) will result if the needle, inserted too far, impinges not on one of the large blood vessels, but into the retroperitoneal space or the base of the mesentery. Although there is no injury to blood vessels, upon subsequent insufflation of gas the emphysema will extend up into the mediastinum.

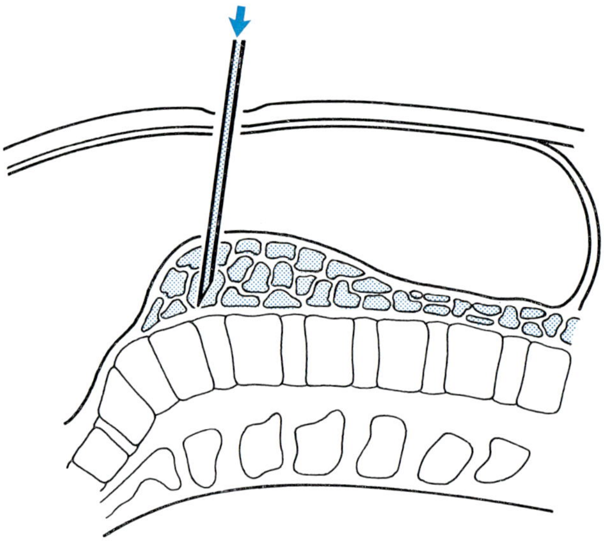

Figure 19

(8) No complication occurs when the properly placed needle reaches the free peritoneal cavity (Fig. 20). Upon subsequent insufflation with gas, the abdominal cavity is in optimum condition for laparoscopy. There is no longer any risk upon subsequent insertion of the trocar bearing the endoscopic lens.

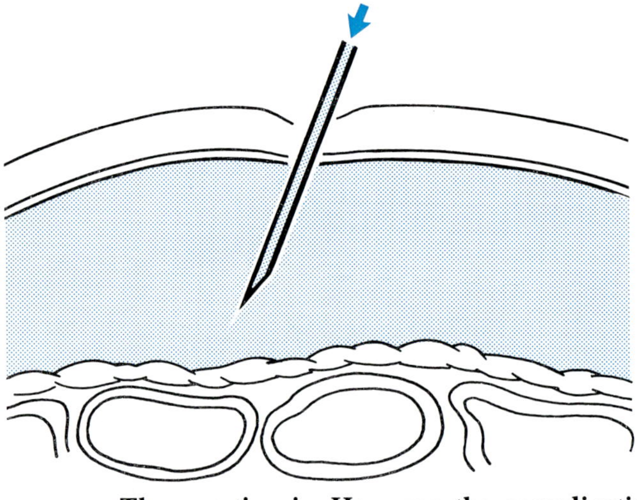

Figure 20

The question is: How can the complications mentioned under (1) through (7) be averted?

Answer: Through the use of proper apparatus and gas insufflation under control as regards volume and pressure (Fig. 21) (the pressure amounting to no more than 5 to 10 mm/Hg and the gas flow to 1 liter per minute), the occurrence of one of the complications described in (1) through (5) above can be recognized quickly and surely.

Complication possibilities (1) to (5) and (7) carry with them no particular risk, however. Only complication (6) requires surgical intervention.

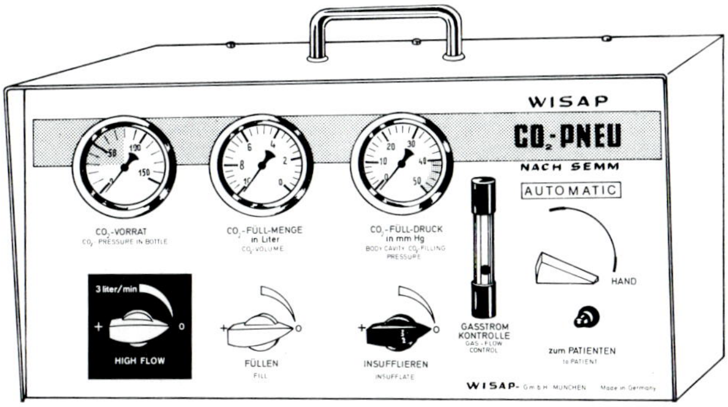

Figure 21

Complications (6) and (7) can be averted through:

(1) knowledge of anatomy (see Fig. 22);
(2) aspiration test (Figs. 145–148); and
(3) laparoscopic scanning (Fig. 28).

A study of Figure 22, showing the pelvic anatomy drawn to scale, makes clear how far removed the aorta and vena cava are from the point of puncture. The distance from navel to aorta, and that from aorta to the skin of the back, are as one-third to two-thirds (see also Fig. 141).

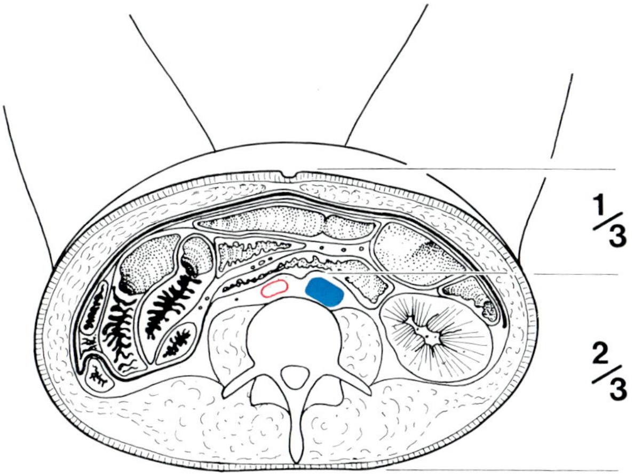

Figure 22

2. THE INFLATION OF THE PNEUMOPERITONEUM

In the inflation of the pneumoperitoneum, the following complications may arise (assuming correct positioning of the needle).

(a) The wrong gas may have been selected, e.g., nitrogen. Since this gas is insoluble in body fluids, any small amounts not entirely removed after termination of the laparoscopy will cause subphrenic discomfort that may endure for from a day to a week.

(b) The gas may be insufflated too rapidly or at too high a pressure, which may lead to circulatory collapse as a result of too much peritoneal stimulation.

(c) Too much gas may be insufflated. The gas pressure compresses the vena cava and also leads to elevation of the diaphragm (Fig. 23). Consequences of this

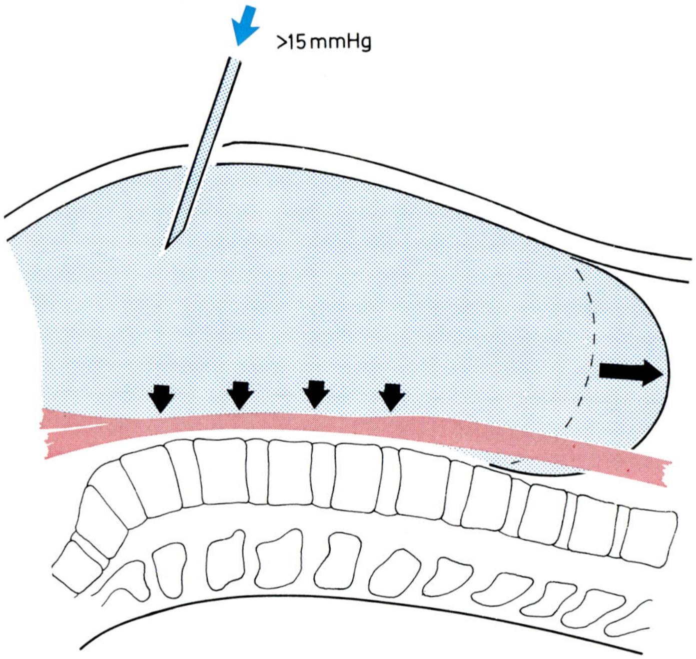

Figure 23

are a marked decrease of return flow of blood from the lower extremities and a reduction of the volume of respiration because of elevation of the diaphragm.

Possible complications (a) to (c) are eliminated through use of the CO_2-Pneu-Automatic insufflator (Semm).

(d) If however, the inadvertent puncture of a large blood vessel has been overlooked through neglect of the aspiration test (Figs. 145–148), then, even with the use of quickly reabsorbable carbon dioxide gas, cardiac arrest may occur after insufflation of about 500 ml of gas. Carbon dioxide can be tolerated intravenously or intra-arterially only up to a total volume of about 150 ml/min. Amounts in excess of this tend to cause dangerous gas emboli; a similar well known example, because of its insolubility, is nitrogen, about 10 to 20 ml (equal to atmospheric air).

These complications do not occur if the insufflation is performed in conformity with the principle:

The volume of insufflation is determined solely by the intra-abdominal pressure.

Formerly, it was general practice to limit the quantity of gas insufflated by an estimate based on the stature of the patient. The danger to the patient, however, lies not in the volume of gas in the pneumoperitoneum but in the pressure at which the abdomen is inflated.

3. THE TROCAR RISK

The organs that are the chief goal of the examination determine the choice of the point of insertion of the laparoscope. The region of the navel is best suited for a general scan of the pelvic organs, and therefore is preferred by gynecologists—not least for cosmetic reasons. As early as 1935, however, Boesch warned against puncturing the linea alba. Because of its single aponeurotic layer and the absence of large blood vessels, this location would seem favorable, but there is danger of a subsequent herniation of the omentum (Fig. 416), the intestine, and so on. Therefore, we have recommended for the past ten years, for cosmetic reasons, the inferior margin of the navel as the proper point for insertion of the trocar (Fig. 164). For the actual paracentesis, however, the part of the muscle 2 to 3 cm lateral to the point of incision in the skin (Z-track insertion, see Fig. 166) is to be recommended.

After the pneumoperitoneum has been regularly and optimally induced, the

Figure 24

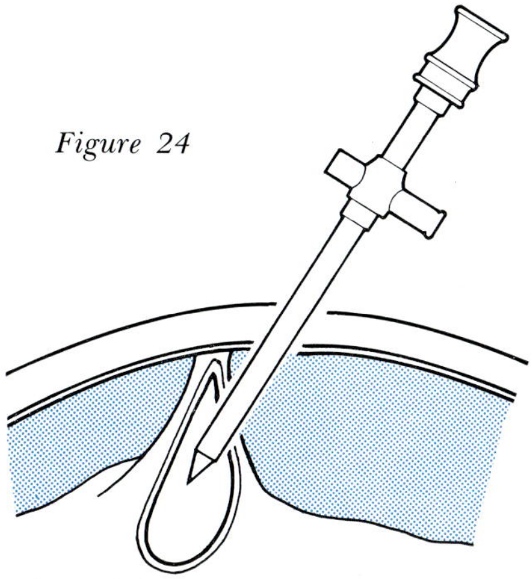

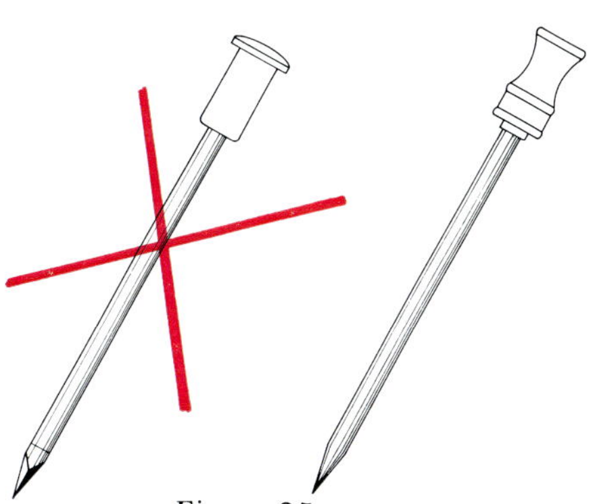

Figure 25

following risks arise from the introduction of the trocar (size determined by the diameter of the laparoscope used):

(a) The trocar, being thicker than the insufflation needle, may strike a loop of intestine adhering to the abdominal wall that proved no obstacle to the insufflation needle. The intestinal loop would not be drawn into the path of the trocar until after the peritoneal cavity was inflated (Fig. 24).

Such a complication can be safely recognized and prevented with the aid of the probing test (Figs. 157, 158) before insertion of the trocar.

(b) The trocar may injure a blood vessel in the abdominal wall in the vicinity of the point of insertion. This complication is more likely if a sharp, pyramidal-tipped trocar (Fig. 25) is used. If only cone-tipped trocars are used, the danger of this complication can almost be eliminated, since blood vessels lying in the way are normally pushed aside by a conical trocar, whereas the sharp edge of the three-sided tip may injure or sever a vessel.

(c) The trocar sometimes is inserted too forcibly after initial, too hesitant attempts fail, and then may jab too far in, perforating one of the blood vessels (Fig. 26) mentioned under Inflation of the Pneumoperitoneum (7) (Fig. 18).

Figure 26

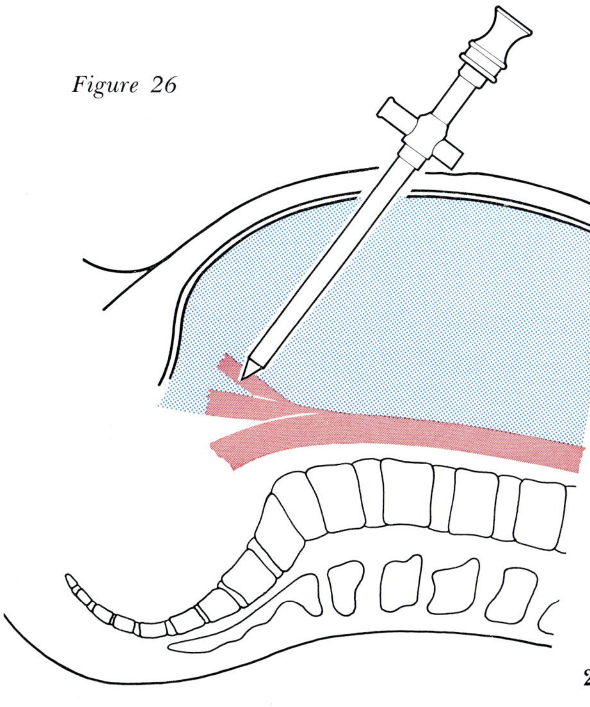

Too deep penetration of the trocar into the abdominal cavity can be avoided as follows:

As described later, **the trocar must never be driven in by the force of the operator's arm muscles.** Instead, it should simply be slipped through the abdominal wall by gentle pressure of the hand and wrist. The little finger also acts as a brake on the momentum of this insertion.

For a full understanding of how far-reaching may be the effect of such a risk, the following is worth noting. It is possible that the tip of the insufflation cannula, as well as that of the trocar, may pass parietally through the peritoneum and injure a blood vessel in the area of the dorsal wall of the pelvis without any blood immediately flowing into the free abdominal cavity. Blood does indeed escape from the blood vessel, but spreads out only retroperitoneally at first (Fig. 27). This retroperitoneal hematoma may spread laterally along the pelvic wall as far as the renal calyx without one drop of blood being visible in the open peritoneal cavity!

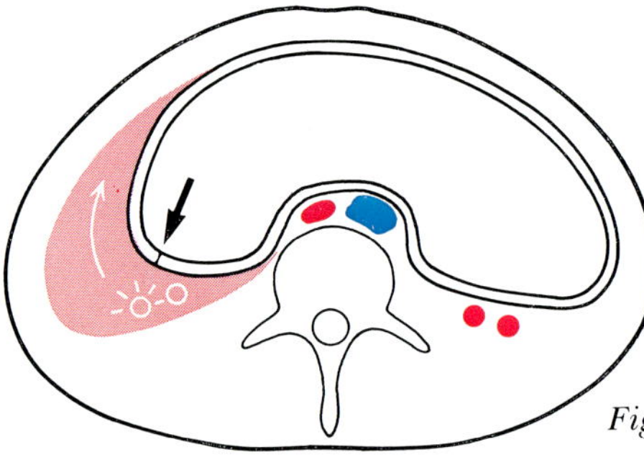

Figure 27

Unfortunately several such cases, interpreted in the past as being incidental to anesthesia, terminated fatally. The irreversible drop in blood pressure was stated to have been caused by the anesthetic, since the diagnosis was: "no bleeding in the peritoneal cavity." However, a conscientious operator should have recognized the retroperitoneal hematoma by virtue of the discoloration of the parietal peritoneum, especially if he had checked both sides for color comparison.

In a case I once observed, the bifurcation of the right iliac vein was slit at the right side by the insertion of an 11 mm trocar, using arm pressure. I had suspected such a lesion immediately after the impingement of the trocar against the pelvic wall. The endoscopy team reported the diagnosis to me as "cause of sterility: bilateral hydrosalpinx"! The lesion at the bifurcation of the internal and external iliac veins had remained undetected. No one on the team had checked the right lateral pelvic wall in the vicinity of the appendix and ascending colon, despite the anesthetist's remark that "the patient is not doing too well" (he had detected a drop in blood-pressure). About ten minutes after the lesion in the blood vessel, the peritoneum was hanging out into the abdominal cavity, black as a thundercloud! An immediate suture of the blood vessel overcame the complication.

In my experience of fatalities resulting from injury to blood vessels, this diagnosis was *not* made because of lack of knowledge of the above-mentioned early symptoms. The following basic rule should become familiar to every physician active in pelvic laparoscopy:

In case of an "anesthetic episode" during laparoscopy, **always suspect injury to a blood vessel** in the region of the aorta, the vena cava, or their branches.

If the anesthetist reports a drop in blood pressure, the operator should immediately scan the entire abdominal cavity with the endoscope, bearing in mind that the blood escaping from an injury to a blood vessel almost never enters the free abdominal cavity at first. This is why the cul-de-sac is free of blood. The massive bleeding spreads retroperitoneally (Fig. 27).

If the anesthetist announces "anesthetic episode" or "cardiac arrest" (Fig. 28):

(1) Stop insufflation of gas immediately.

(2) Lower intra-abdominal pressure to 8 mm Hg.

(3) Do *not* immediately withdraw the endoscope, but ensure by a complete scan that there is no retroperitoneal bleeding. Otherwise, valuable minutes will be lost before opening the abdominal cavity and clamping off the injured vessel, a delay that in my experience can contribute to the death of the patient.

Injury to an intra-abdominal blood vessel, whether during the blind puncture with the insufflation needle or because of overly deep insertion of the trocar, is *the most dangerous complication in laparoscopy.* It can be obviated if the safety tests and manipulations detailed in the following chapters are performed routinely.

Perhaps at this point statistics from another discipline may serve to elucidate. Among *student* air-pilots, accidents, especially fatal ones, are practically unknown. Pilots with 100 or more hours of flight time behind them have the highest fatality rate, for by then they feel they are over the hump, and time-consuming checks of motor and gauges now seem superfluous. "I know what I'm doing now!" Famous last words! The high accident rate in private flying is thus self-explanatory.

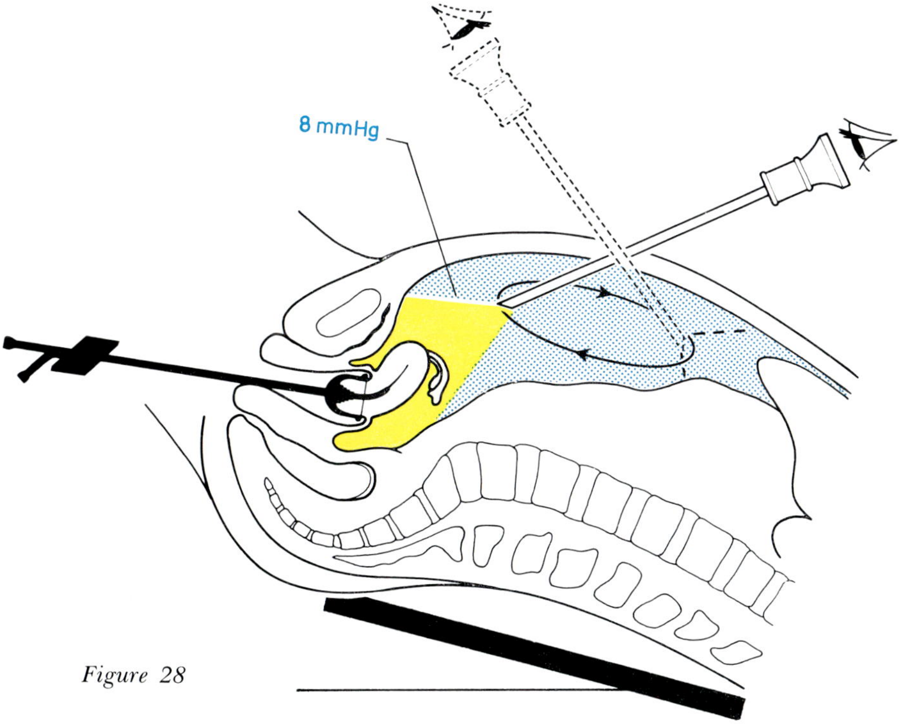

Figure 28

The risk of injury with the trocar is considerably greater in the lower abdomen than in the upper, but it becomes much less as the diameter of the trocar is decreased, and with it the force needed for the initial puncture. The modern slender endoscope for pelvic laparoscopy is especially adapted for this particular technique, and so is called a "pelvic laparoscope."

4. THE OPTICAL RISK

The laparoscope, of course, is monitored visually during insertion into and manipulated within the abdomen (Fig. 29). Skillful management can obviate any contact with the bowel.

However, injuries are possible when employing a laparoscope with an electronic flash device at its distal end. Since this part projects perhaps 2 cm beyond

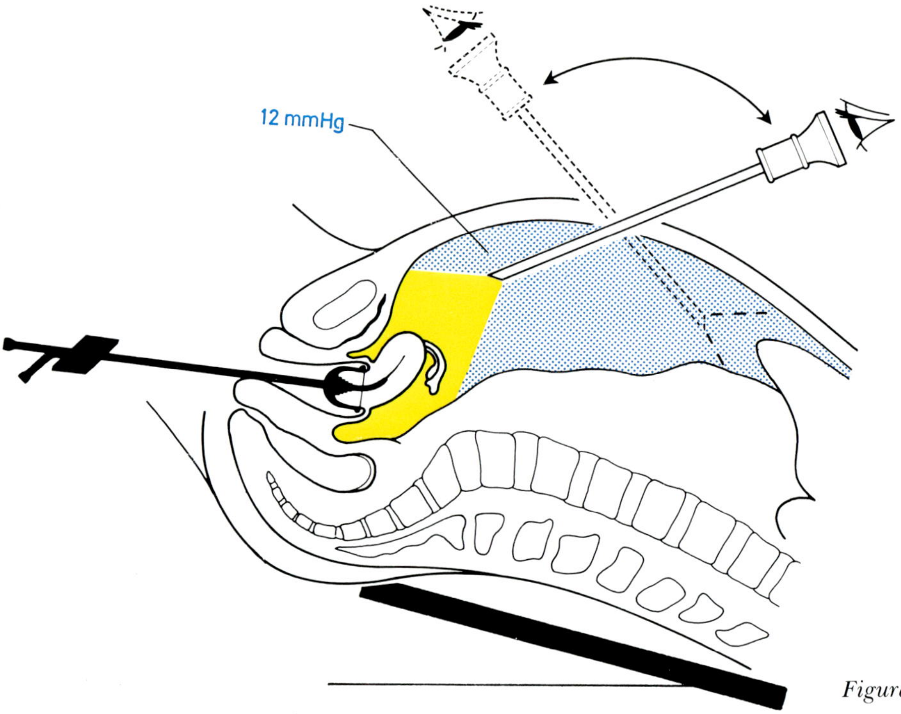

Figure 29

the optic (Fig. 113), injuries, especially in the vicinity of the mesosalpinx, have occurred in the course of attempts to visualize the adnexa. Such complications can be avoided by use of the 180° direct-forward laparoscope (Fig. 39).

Laparoscopes of older types (Fig. 47), in which a distally mounted light source (called "hot light") is itself introduced into the peritoneum, must be regarded today as unacceptable for laparoscopic use.

Diagnostic complications with unfortunate consequences may arise if the monocular nature of the laparoscope leads to misinterpretation of the optical findings. Therefore, the absolute prerequisite to the performance of laparoscopy is thorough training in *surgical* gynecology.

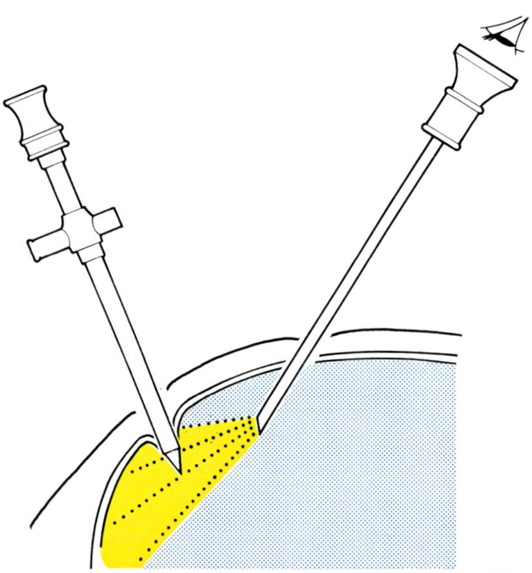

Figure 30

5. THE SECOND PUNCTURE

Complications in connection with the second puncture (necessary 90 per cent of the time, even in purely diagnostic procedures) are confined to possible perforation of one of the larger blood vessels in the abdominal wall. The second puncture, therefore, is performed only after a painstaking translumination of the abdominal wall from within (Fig. 30). By this means, the vascular pattern in the layers of the lower abdominal wall can be clearly visualized. Only in very rare instances is there any risk of injuring a major vessel when making the preliminary incision with the scalpel. Thus, the subsequent insertion of the trocar through the skin and the peritoneum is continuously monitored optically or endoscopically, respectively (Fig. 30), obviating perforation of even subperitoneal vessels. In addition, use of the cone-tipped trocar (Fig. 25) in the second puncture serves to prevent blood vessel damage.

Any vascular damage that still may occur can be repaired by the technique described in Chapter VI, Section 13.

In making the second puncture, we distinguish between two possibilities.

(1) Second Puncture for Further Diagnostic Purposes

The instrument used is the 3-mm suction probe (Fig. 31; see also Figs. 64–67), with which organs that may be blocking the line of vision can be gently displaced. The tubes, appendix, etc., can be atraumatically elevated entirely by suction, and fluids can be extracted from the cul-de-sac for cytologic, chemical, and other purposes. This 3-mm second puncture becomes necessary in almost all diagnostic laparoscopies and involves almost no risk.

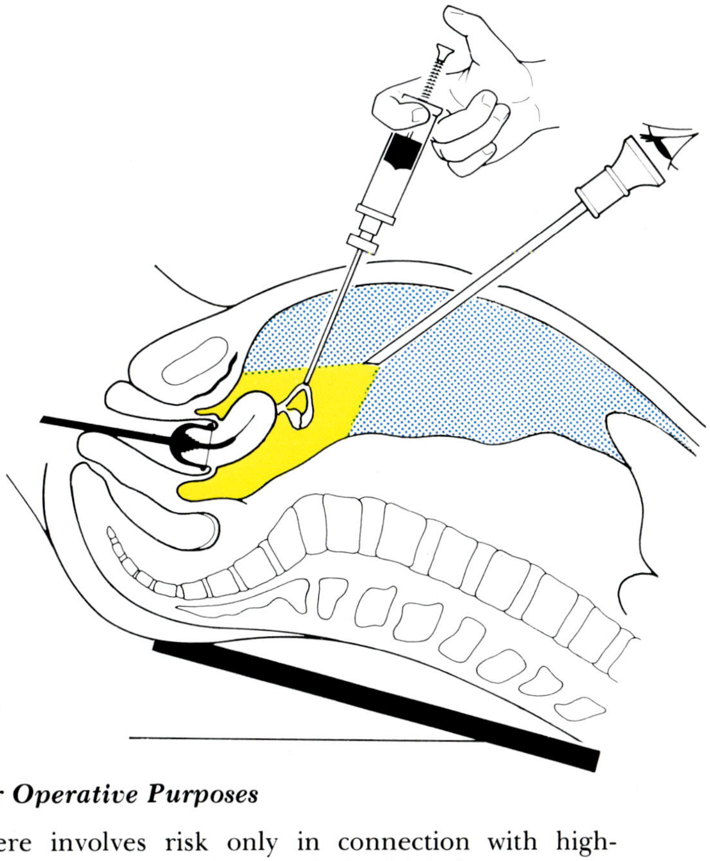

Figure 31

(2) Second Puncture for Operative Purposes

The second puncture here involves risk only in connection with high-frequency current, and then only if the insulation of the high-frequency instrument (scissors, atraumatic forceps, etc.) is defective. In such cases, thumb-sized coagulation effects in the abdominal wall and extensive necroses have been observed that subsequently were repairable only through complicated surgery.

It is assumed, however, that the use of high-frequency current will be banished entirely in the future from the field of gynecologic endoscopy, at which time this source of danger will disappear.

6. PERFORATION BY THE INTRAUTERINE PROBE

The danger of perforating the uterus when inserting the uterine probe into the uterine cavity is no greater than the risk of perforation in any intrauterine procedure. In laparoscopy there is at least the special advantage that such perforation can be detected as soon as the laparoscope is inserted. If the suction intrauterine cannula is not properly placed, this can be seen immediately if: (1) the uterus is not noticeably elevated and steadied; and (2) on monitoring the uterus and bladder with the laparoscope, the tip of the probe can actually be seen (Fig. 32).

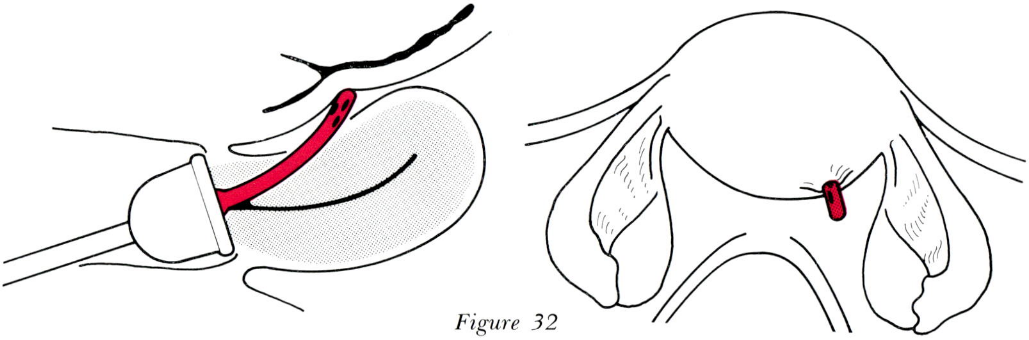

Figure 32

When excessive pressure has been used in tubal dye insufflation, a blue discoloration of the uterus and mesosalpinx may occur through extravasation of the dye into the uterine blood vessels (Fig. 33). Although this complication involves no risk, it may indicate in many cases that the insufflation probe was not placed safely within the cavity but has penetrated the endometrium (Fig. 33).

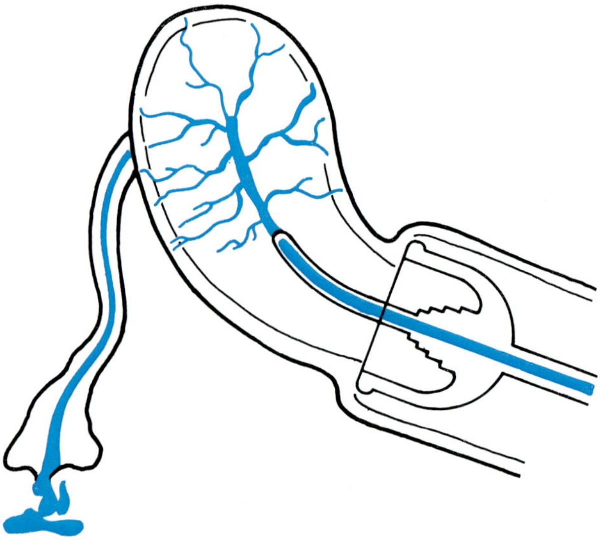

Figure 33

7. DANGER RESULTING FROM EXTENDED PROCEDURES

The risk to the patient during laparoscopy increases exponentially as ancillary operative steps are undertaken in conjunction with the basic diagnostic procedure.

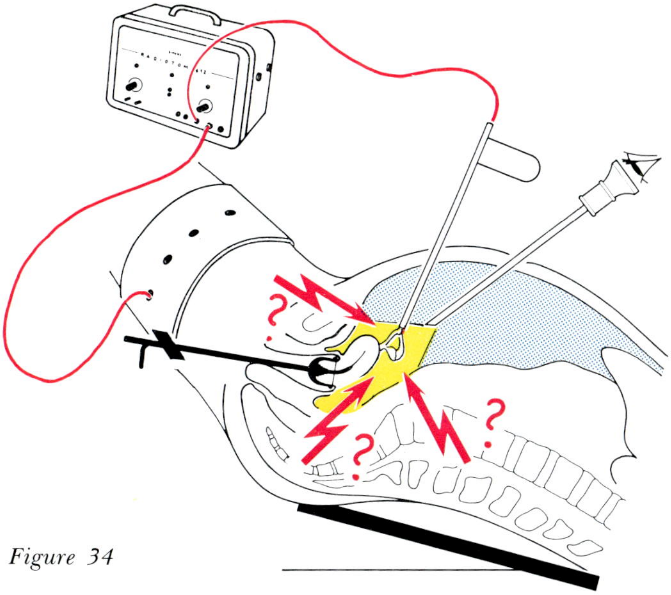

Figure 34

Such steps as a rule require the use of heat for the coagulation of small vessels. If this heat is produced by high-frequency current, the operator has no way of foreseeing what risks lie in store, since high-frequency current may seek unpredictable routes into the abdomen from its point of application to the surface of the skin (Fig. 34; see also Chapter IV, Section 8b).

The increased risk factor involved in the use of high-frequency current is reduced to a minimum if the low-voltage instruments developed by the present author are employed, namely his Sterilization Unit or the Endotherm (Figs. 78 and 81). With these the heat can be localized and precision-controlled as to duration and temperature within 1 degree Centigrade, even in close proximity to the bowel or blood vessels.

When puncture cannulae and scissors are being employed in addition to the use of heat (Fig. 35), a precise means is necessary for determining size, and partic-

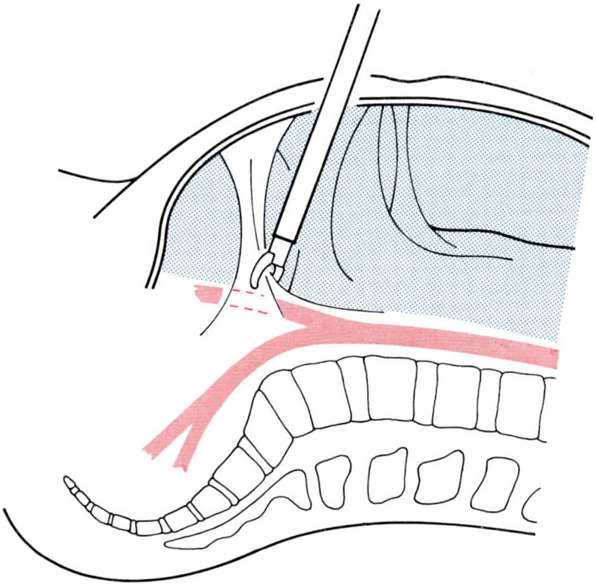

Figure 35

ularly depth, in the visual field. Such surgical procedures often are desirable and of great value in obviating the need for a taxing laparotomy. As a rule, however, they should be undertaken only by an operator with wide experience of several hundred diagnostic laparoscopies. Especially in severing adhesions in appendectomy scars and in the adnexa, the monocular nature of the visualization can result in faulty estimation of depth, leading to possible injury to the major pelvic vessels. Surgical peritoneoscopes (Fig. 36) borrowed from the laparoscopic instrumentarium and intended for use in the upper abdomen are unacceptable in operative pelvic laparoscopy.

8. RELEASE OF THE PNEOMOPERITONEUM

Provided the maximal intra-abdominal pressures indicated in Chapter III, Section 2, have not been exceeded, sudden release of the pneumoperitoneum via the trocar sleeve involves no risk. When the Z-track insertion method is used (Fig. 166), the several layers of the deflating abdominal wall will immediately and automatically slip over one another. With an incision in the midline there is the possibility in rare cases that a small tongue of omentum may herniate or be pinched (Fig. 416). The bowel also may protrude into the residual oval gap in the fascia and become adherent there.

Incomplete expulsion of the carbon dioxide gas presents no problem. The resorption rate from the abdominal cavity amounts to about 100 ml of CO_2 per minute. Larger quantities of gas inadvertently retained (e.g., in the event of a trocar-sleeve slipping out too soon) have no negative postoperative effect, other than occasional shoulder pain secondary to subdiaphragmatic CO_2 collection.

9. ANESTHESIA

The total risk at laparoscopy can be equated to that of general anesthesia. The decision as to whether general anesthesia can be performed at all parallels the consideration as to whether laparoscopy is indicated for a particular patient. (See also Chapter VI, Section 5.)

In principle, laparoscopy is possible even under local anesthesia. Its employment depends mainly on the attitude of the patient. It is recommended that the navel be pretreated with an anesthetizing ointment and that the local anesthetic then be injected liberally around the intended puncture point. After the start of insufflation, the abdominal cavity can be additionally sprayed with a procaine mist or the like. In a centrally anesthetized patient, even the insertion of the suction-intrauterine cannula and elevation of the uterus are painless. Surgical laparoscopy under local anesthesia is limited to sterilization.

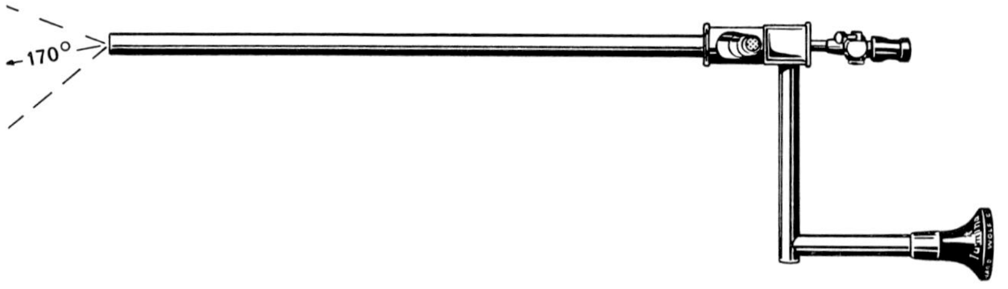

Figure 36

10. CHOICE OF INSTRUMENTS

In view of numerous complications and misadventures in the choice of instruments in past years, this important matter will be considered very carefully in the forensic domain in the future. Particular attention must be paid to the technologic sophistication of the instrumentarium employed.

The thick optics, 11 mm in diameter, customary in upper abdominal laparoscopy should be restricted exclusively to scientific photography and cinematography in pelvic laparoscopy. Such diameters are no longer needed for clinical laparoscopy. In order to visualize the abdominal cavity with the eye alone, the light emitted by thin cold-light fiberoptic cables is sufficient. The low photosensitivity of available still and movie film, however, requires the use of high-intensity illumination for satisfactory photography within the abdominal cavity, so that the diameter of the photoendoscope is a function of the thickness of the fiberoptic cable.

Today there are offset "operative peritoneoscopes" (Figure 36 shows a cold-light model after Palmer-Jacobs) that have long been familiar in laparoscopy for the diagnosis of hepatic disease. The advantage of these is that they enable the operator to visualize the abdomen and at the same time manipulate instruments through a single incision, the instruments being inserted parallel to the visual axis.

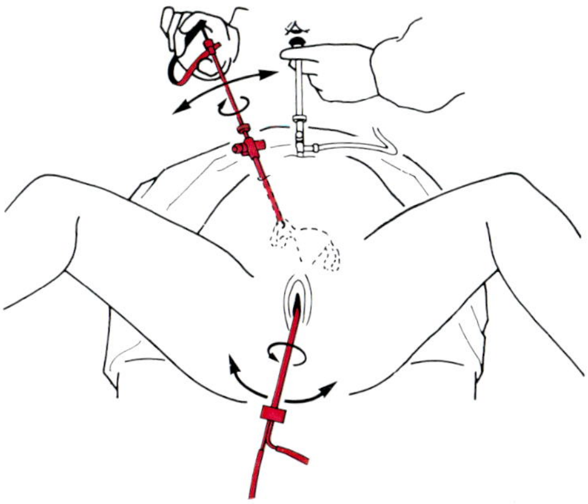

Figure 37

However, handling such endoscopes entails the greatest manual dexterity and faultless topographic knowledge, especially in the presence of adhesions.

Because of the monocular nature of the image afforded through the endoscope, the exact location of instruments inserted along the optical axis is difficult to judge, and a side view of the organ being dealt with can never be obtained. If the liver is being inspected, the side view is not necessary, but in pelvic laparoscopy it is the very cornerstone of visualization of the adnexa.

The offset operative laparoscope is advantageous in requiring only a single puncture, but there are certain disadvantages—particularly an increased surgical risk because of: (1) minimum trocar diameter of 11 mm; (2) insufficient manipulability; and (3) imprecise estimation of distances.

In summary, it may be said that the double puncture technique today is less risky and diagnostically more valuable. The surgical instrument, usually poised at an angle of 50° to 90° to the line of sight, is easy to localize, even with monocular vision. In addition, the second entry offers the possibility of grasping any organ and displacing it independently of the laparoscope (Fig. 37).

IV
The Laparoscopic Instrumentarium

1. THE LAPAROSCOPE

Endoscopes are neither telescopes nor microscopes with regard to their lens systems. They possess their own typical characteristics.

Subject to their specific fields of application, endoscopes were developed on the basis of the ground rules and experience of artisans and masters in select optical workshops. As a result of incomplete understanding between theoreticians and practitioners, optical artisans and physicists, physicians and endoscope-makers, endoscopes left something to be desired until the early 1960s, especially in the field of gynecologic endoscopic photodocumentation. No other endoscopic discipline makes such rigid demands on the field of vision and the aperture as does gynecologic laparoscopy, because of the great relative depth of the pelvic area with which the optical system must deal. Although detailed endoscopic photography from other disciplines such as bronchoscopy and cystoscopy was producing satisfactory color pictures, the color slides and films in gynecology had been poor. The physicist Hopkins between 1960 and 1967 designed a completely new endoscopic instrumentarium with numerous improvements. In place of the glass lenses previously used (Fig. 38, *A*), the light is now transmitted by quartz rods and refracted by "air lenses" (the rod-lens system).

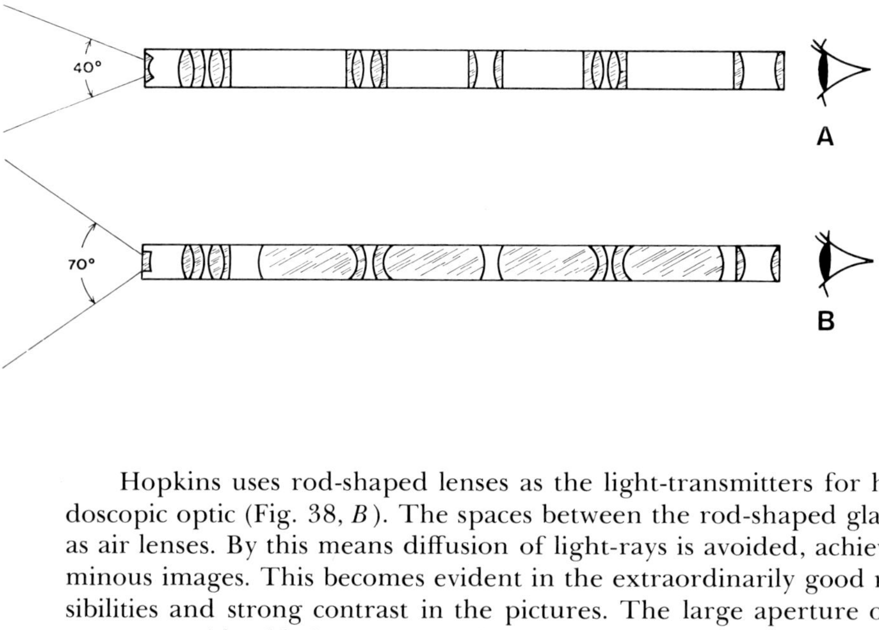

Figure 38

Hopkins uses rod-shaped lenses as the light-transmitters for his modern endoscopic optic (Fig. 38, *B*). The spaces between the rod-shaped glass elements act as air lenses. By this means diffusion of light-rays is avoided, achieving highly luminous images. This becomes evident in the extraordinarily good resolution possibilities and strong contrast in the pictures. The large aperture of the rod-lens system considerably increases brightness, so that the diameter of the laparoscope can be relatively reduced without loss of light-efficiency and brilliance, i.e., it can be slenderer yet still maintain the same excellent optical properties. This has led to the production of extremely slender endoscopes, among them the laparoscope used for pelvic visualization.

As a result of this new impetus, Franke succeeded through the use of com-

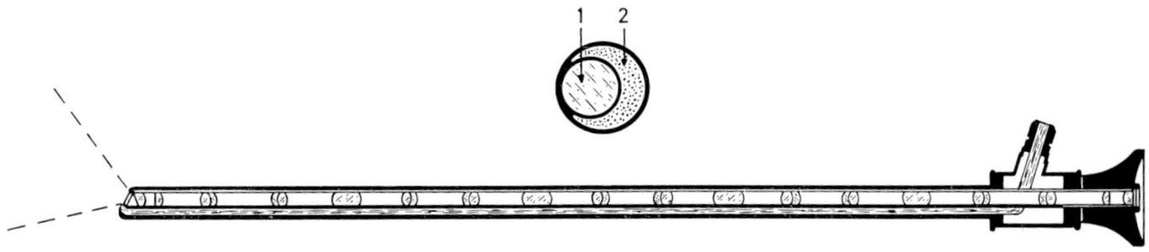

Figure 39

puters in creating new optical systems, even for the earlier conventional scopes, some of which were used to still greater advantage in the production of high-efficiency endoscopes of the narrowest diameters (e.g., Lumina endoscope, Fig. 39: (1) optical system; (2) glass fibers).

Unfortunately the manufacturers at present still use terminology confusing to the layman in describing the angle of vision afforded by each of their laparoscopes, the angle of deflection of the axial line of vision being effected by obliquely angled lenses or by mirrors and prisms. Thus they call: 180° = direct-forward; 172°, 165°, 155.5°, 135° = forward, prograde, or foreoblique; 90° = right-angle or orthograde; 60° or less = retrograde.

Figure 40 provides a graphic chart (from Leising and Rosenbruch, 1971) in which the angles of vision shown one above the other represent the same angles for the observer, but are numbered differently by different manufacturers.

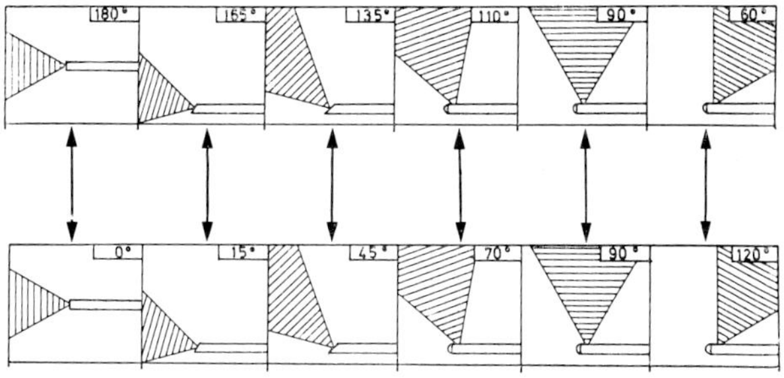

Figure 40

The following laparoscopes are used for diagnostic purposes.

Lumina-Optic

Laparoscope (Semm modification), Figure 41,1: scope with fiberoptic light conduction; 5 mm trocar with sleeve having nipple for attachment of CO_2-gas hose, angle of vision 160° (foreoblique).

The trocar sleeve with automatic gas-tight closure necessary for the above (Fig. 41, 2) has an outside diameter of 6 mm and the scope is 30 cm long.

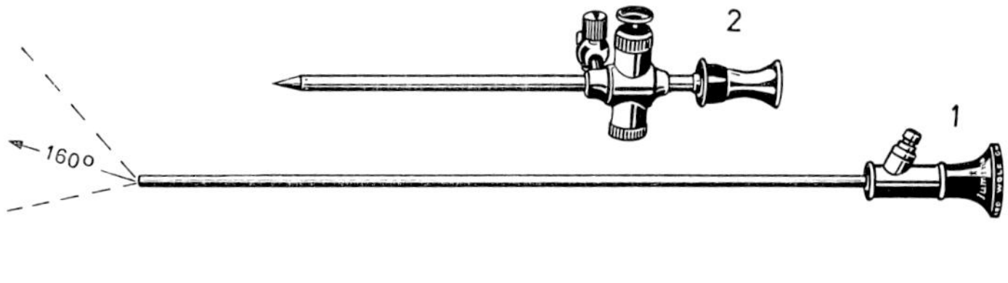

Figure 41

Hopkins Laparoscope

Laparoscope (Semm modification) (Fig. 42,1), 5.8 mm diameter, visual angle 30° (foreoblique with fiberoptic). Here too the trocar sleeve (Fig. 42,2) has a nipple for CO_2 gas insufflation.

The 30° (or 150°; see Fig. 40) deflection of the visual axis affords not only a direct forward visual field but also the possibility of somewhat prograde inspection of the adnexal region.

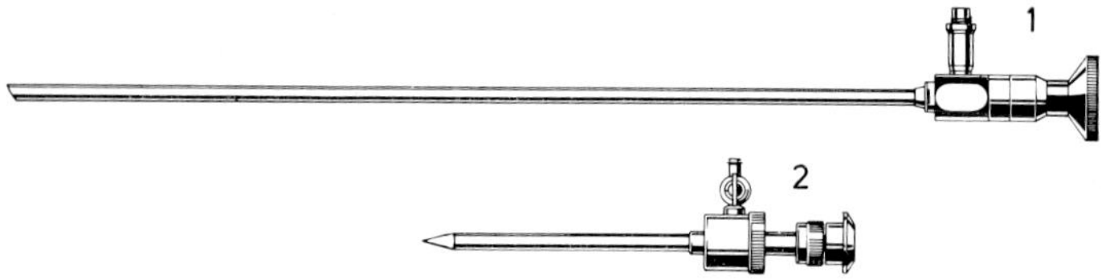

Figure 42

The introduction of flexible fiberoptic endoscopic instruments in gastroendoscopy began in 1957, the idea of conducting light by means of transparent fibers having been patented as early as 1928.

In the field of intestinal endoscopy, the rigid scope today has been abandoned in favor of a flexible one, making inspection of the entire intestinal tract possible from both cranial and caudal aspects. Lens systems can be rendered flexible only to a limited extent (Fig. 43), but the optical image can be transmitted through any required convolutions (Fig. 44) via neatly bundled glass fibers (Chapter IV, Section 2). The difference in the image is evident, however, in the pictures of a pen nib seen in Figures 43 and 44. The resolution of the image in the flexible endoscope is limited by the large number of individual glass fibers

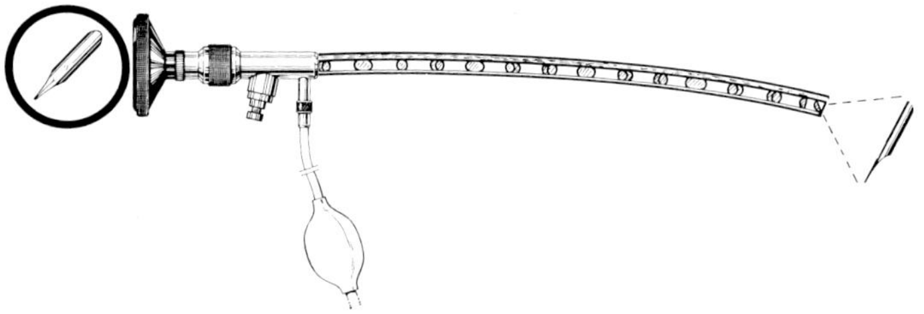

Figure 43

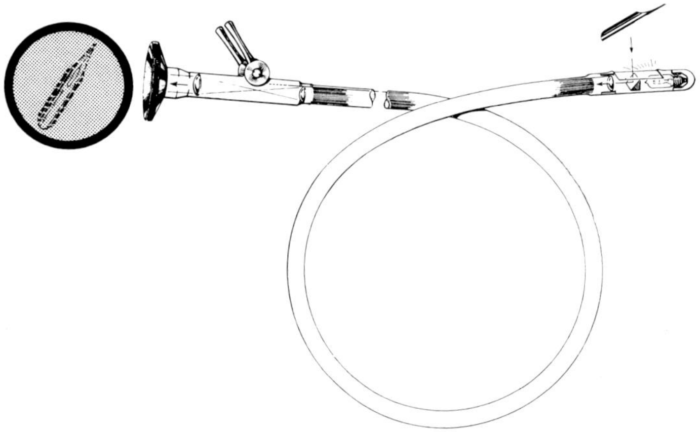

Figure 44

(some 50,000 or more fibers, each 10–15 μ in diameter and in identical arrangement at the two ends of the cable).

The price differential between the rigid and the fully flexible fiberoptic laparoscopic systems is something like 1:10. Flexibility of the endoscope itself is not essential to the techniques of laparoscopy presented in this volume.

Especially in the presence of fat accumulations and adhesions in the abdomen, the existence of blind areas in the visual range emphasizes the necessity of seeing more with the aid of a flexible scope. It is very doubtful, however, whether increased field of vision in abdomens with adhesions, etc., can be equated with expanded diagnostic possibilities in laparoscopy.

In culdoscopy, however, with the patient either in the knee-elbow position (Fig. 45) or in the extreme pelvic elevation (Fig. 46) recommended by Palmer, a fully flexible culdoscope might be of great service in the genital region.

The fully flexible endoscope would be of great significance if in the future gynecologic endoscopy again abandoned the transabdominal route in favor of the transvaginal approach. A fully flexible endoscope would be a real boon in culdoscopy, but the very real problem would remain of positioning the patient satisfactorily. This can be done only on specially constructed operating tables and confronts the anesthetist with real difficulties.

In abdomens with adhesions serious difficulties in orientation would arise for the culdoscopist that could be resolved only by simultaneous recourse to the fluoroscope, as is the case in gastroendoscopy. The direction in which the culdoscope points poses orientation problems when a flexible scope is used, and furthermore, fluoroscopy would have a deleterious effect on the gonads.

Therefore, it is safe to say a culdoscopy no longer can be the method of choice in the present stage of the techniques. A classic example is the impossibility of diagnosing endometrial implants in the vicinity of the uterosacral ligament at culdoscopy, although 80 per cent of all genital endometriosis is localized in the ligaments (Fig. 377).

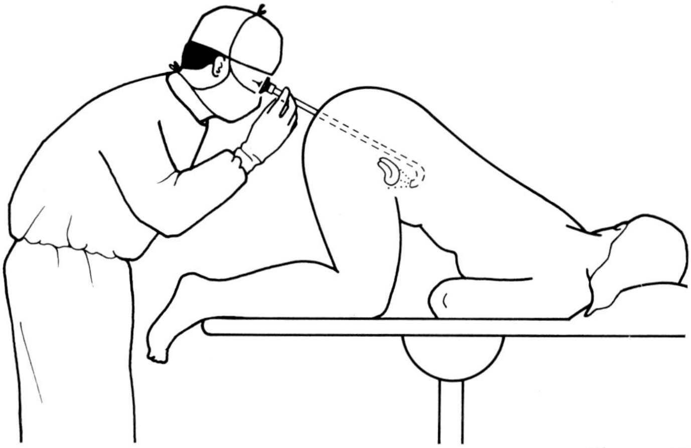

Figure 45

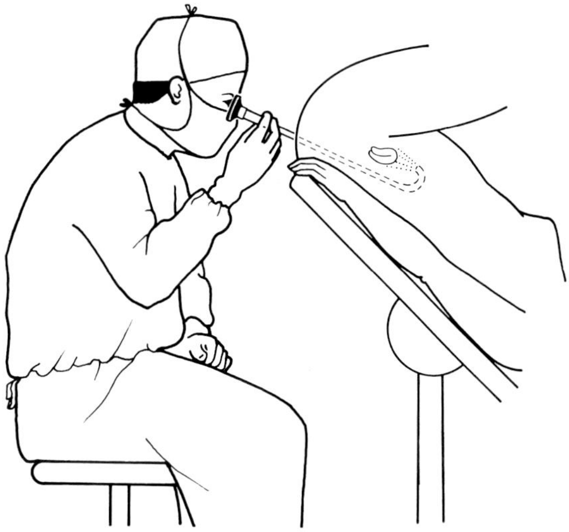

Figure 46

2. THE LIGHT SOURCE IN ENDOSCOPY

Until the middle 1940s, the angle of vision in the endoscope was dependent on the source of light being located at the distal end of the scope in the form of an incandescent bulb or electronic flash device (Fig. 47). The construction of a direct-forward scope was not feasible.

Since an incandescent bulb converts up to 97 per cent of electrical energy

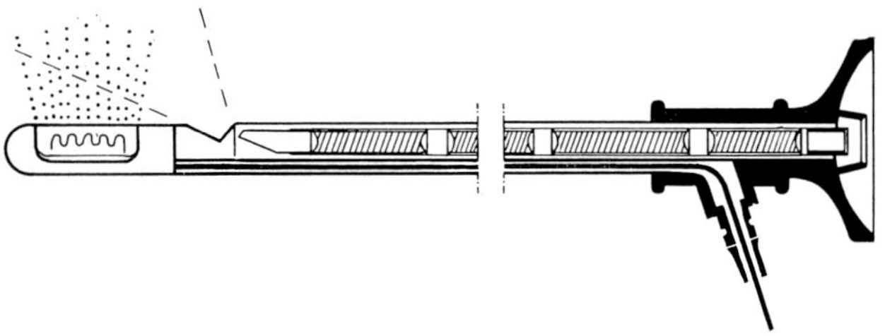

Figure 47

into heat and only about 2 per cent into visible light, endoscopy of the lower abdomen was highly risky. The tip of the scope, whose location in the abdomen could not be monitored visually, became very hot, especially when the current had to be stepped up to provide light for photography. Contact with the bowel, often unavoidable despite the greatest dexterity and care, resulted in burns.

The practically loss-free passage of light through quartz rods, known since the turn of the century, has been available for medical purposes since 1965, and has made possible completely new approaches in the engineering of endoscopes, particularly of laparoscopes with direct-forward optics.

Principle of the Flexible Fiberoptic Cable

If light falls upon the end surface of a smooth quartz rod it enters it, and is repeatedly and totally reflected internally from the lateral surfaces of the rod until it emerges at the far end (Fig. 48). These rods are insulated in order to preclude the lateral escape of the light from fine, sharply-bent fibers, 10 to 70 μ in diameter. Any number of bends then may exist between the light and the ob-

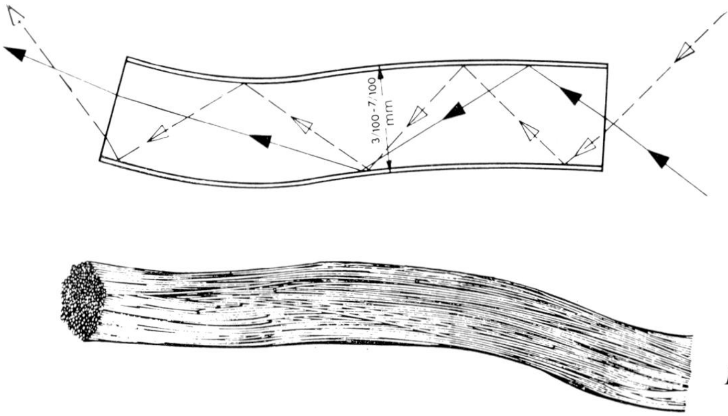

Figure 48

server at the other end. The optical insulation consists of a thin sleeve-layer of a different glass having a lower index of refraction (n), that of the core (n 1) being 1.62, and that of the sleeve-layer (n 2) 1.52, for example.

Bundles of such light-conduction fibers achieve the desired transmission of the image. Because of their flexibility they are ideal for transmitting intense light from an external source into the abdominal cavity, and do so with almost no loss of intensity, yet without any heat. Use of extremely clear glass holds absorption losses at a minimal level. This is especially important in laparoscopy, since faithful color rendition of the image is critical for evaluation of the organs visualized.

Cost differential in such bundles of light-conducting fibers is less dependent on the external sheath of the bundle (plastic, flexible metal, etc.) than on the caliber and light conductivity of the individual fibers. The latter is a function of the quality of the glass, i.e., of the indices of refraction of the core and sleeve glass of each fiber.

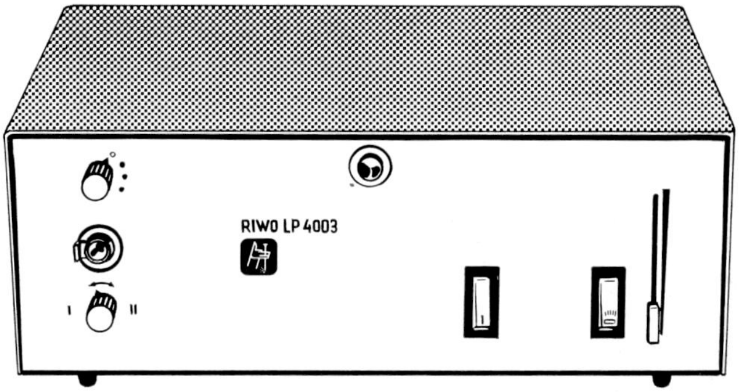

Figure 49

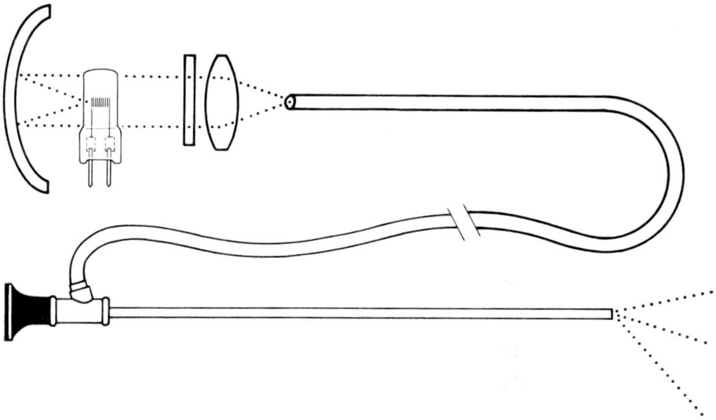

Figure 50

Since 1965 all endoscopes (Fig. 50) have utilized this so-called "cold light" (Fig. 49). The light source is kept outside the operating area (usually 1.5 m away). We use iodine-vapor-tungsten bulbs of from 75 to 250 watts, which provide particularly effective light yield for endoscopic purposes as a result of their punctiform focus. They work as follows:

> The tungsten, which evaporates under high pressure as the coiled filament heats up, mixes with elementary iodine and forms a violet-colored tungsten iodide inside the bulb. When the light is extinguished the tungsten iodide decomposes again into elementary iodine and tungsten, and some of the latter reverts back onto the metal filament. The remainder of the tungsten is deposited on the glass wall of the bulb, but the next time the lamp is used some of this same tungsten may fall back on the filament as the lamp cools. This prevents progressive darkening of the glass bulb from tungsten build-up, and thus the effective life of the bulb is prolonged.

In modern lamps for endoscopy (Fig. 51) these halogen light-bulbs are always installed in pairs, so that if the first one fails the other can be switched on immediately. Since the sudden failure of a light bulb could have serious consequences (e.g., in case of hemorrhage during surgery), *no* lamp containing only one bulb should ever be used as a light source in pelvic laparoscopy.

Brightness controls, as well as color filters for special surface studies, are integral in all such lamps today as a matter of routine.

3. THE PNEUMOPERITONEUM (CO_2 Pneu-AUTOMATIC INSUFFLATOR)

In internal medicine for decades the pneumoperitoneum was induced by using air, which was cautiously pumped in by hand (Fig. 52) with large-caliber squeeze

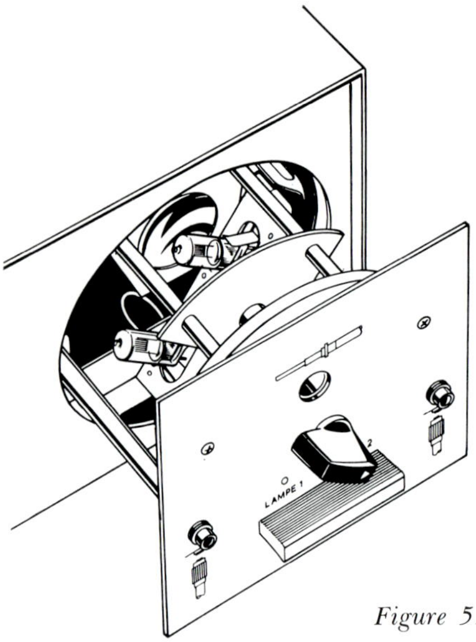

Figure 51

bulbs or rubber balloons. The unanesthetized patient's tolerance to abdominal distention was the guiding factor for the degree of inflation. An anesthetized patient has no such objective control, however, and therefore in laparoscopy an insufflator fully automatic as to volume and pressure (Fig. 53) must be used to admit the gas (see also Fig. 21).

Today the following general considerations govern the choice of gas for insufflation.

Nitrogen is completely insoluble in bodily tissues and fluids; about 10 to 20 ml in the human bloodstream is enough to cause fatal gas emboli. Since gas by the liter is used to induce the pneumoperitoneum, nitrogen is entirely unacceptable.

Air consists of up to 79 per cent nitrogen and 21 per cent oxygen, and thus is just as unsuitable as pure nitrogen. Since nitrogen is not resorbed for days or months, a patient could often suffer subphrenic discomfort for long periods after laparoscopy, as in the days when gynecologists used air to effect tubal patency.

Oxygen is a physiologic nonflammable gas, well endured by the tissues and resorbable, but dangerous. Since high-frequency coagulation is still being used today to stop bleeding, the presence of oxygen involves a risk of combustion, since water in the tissues is decomposed by electrolysis and forms the highly explosive oxyhydrogen gas.

Nitrous oxide is quite soluble in blood and body tissues, as is carbon dioxide. It is nonflammable alone, but in the presence of flammable substances it behaves like pure oxygen in supporting combustion. Since, in the abdominal cavity, we must always be prepared for inadvertent intestinal puncture or injury and the consequent presence of flammable intestinal gas, the same is true of NO_2 as for O_2. Moreover, 3 to 5 liters of nitrous oxide in the abdomen in addition to a general anesthetic make the total anesthetic effect unpredictable, especially if there is also intravascular absorption of the gas.

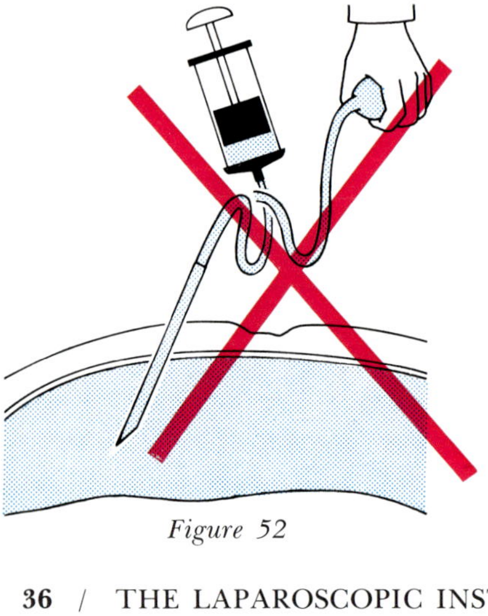

Figure 52

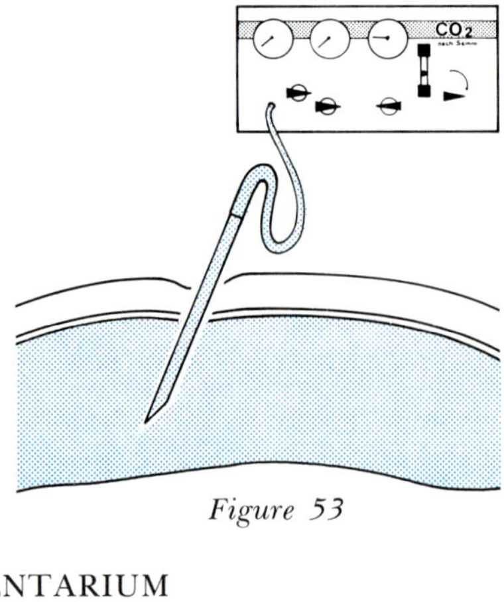

Figure 53

Carbon dioxide gas is ten times as soluble in blood and body tissues as is oxygen. This is true not only of its physical solubility but also of its chemical bonding to an alkali reserve. Carbon dioxide gas can be absorbed into human veins or arteries in amounts up to 100 cc/min without any observable long range adverse effect on the P_{CO_2} metabolism of the individual. Only when the amount thus introduced is increased to 150 to 200 cc/min do tachycardia and circulatory disturbances arise. In the case of an open foramen ovale (about 40 per cent of foramina ovales are functionally open to gas), even CO_2 insufflation presents a danger of emboli.

For safety's sake it has long been customary in gynecology to use CO_2 gas for pertubation of the fallopian tubes, so it is naturally the gas of choice for laparoscopy. Internists offer the objection, to date not statistically proved, that carbon dioxide gas causes slight burns at laparoscopy without anesthesia, perhaps through dissociation of the CO_2 to H_2CO_3 in the abdominal cavity. This is of no consequence in laparoscopy, in which general anesthesia is always the rule.

Other gases, such as argon, helium, etc., have thus far attained only theoretic importance (they are indifferent to water vapor, and do not fog the lens, for example), but they are not yet commercially available for routine use.

Based on the facts that: (1) the pressure in the vena cava amounts to about 15 to 20 mm/Hg and may even assume negative values on elevation of the pelvis; and (2) the unanesthetized patient complains of respiratory difficulties at intra-abdominal pressure above 20 mm Hg, the maximum intra-abdominal pressure for the pneumoperitoneum at first was set empirically at 15 mm Hg. Subsequent first-hand experiments on circulation and respiratory volume in the anesthetized patient have confirmed that, up to this level, neither circulation nor respiratory volume is negatively affected through phrenic elevation. In Chapter III, Section 2, and Chapter VI, Section 9, the risks and dangers attendant upon insufflation of a gas into the abdominal cavity were catalogued and instruction given on how those that may arise can be recognized.

Studies and experiments conducted for several years, starting in 1954, led to development of the CO_2 Pneu-Automatic Insufflator (Fig. 54). This apparatus controls the insufflation of carbon dioxide gas as to time, volume, and pressure. The

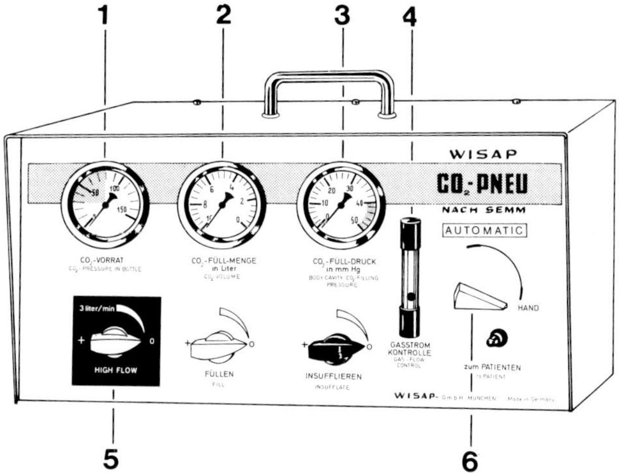

Figure 54

most important component of this machine is Dial 3, "Intra-abdominal Pressure," which gives a constant reading of the exact insufflation pressure as well as the actual intra-abdominal pressure within a range of 0 to 10 mm Hg.

Dial 2, "CO_2 Volume in Body," indicates the volume in liters of the intra-abdominal gas bubble established. This is especially valuable in monitoring the ratio between the pressure and volume of the gas bubble. This ratio provides an early warning if preperitoneal or omental emphysema are induced inadvertently. The "Gas-flow Control," (4), monitors the free passage of gas into the abdomen by the gentle and constant hovering of the little ball. Irregular hovering of the ball immediately indicates that the tip of the insufflation needle is not where it should be.

After filling the pneumoperitoneum to an intra-abdominal pressure of 12 to

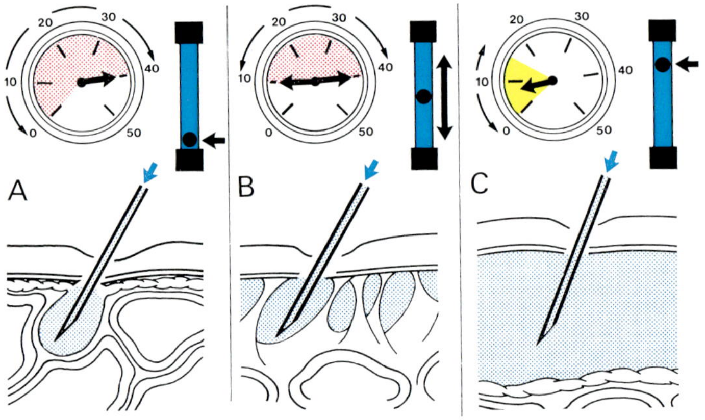

Figure 55

14 mm Hg, the operator switches Dial 6 from "hand" to "automatic." Now an automatic refill device takes over the steady replacement of any gas losses through resorption or leaks in the system. The intra-abdominal gas bubble thus remains constant, and the operator is free to give his undivided attention to his manipulations. Dial 1, "CO_2 Cylinder Contents," shows how much gas is still in reserve in the supply tank.

A, B, and *C* in Figure 55 demonstrate the way in which the insufflation problems listed in Chapter III, Section 2, can be detected instantly on Dial 3.

A. The insufflation needle has entered a closed adhesion-pocket. Dial 3 immediately shows maximum deflection (40 mm Hg) in the red sector. The hovering ball (6) drops back to its starting position.

B. The insufflation needle has reached the free abdominal cavity but has collided with strands of adhesion. Dial 3 fluctuates back and forth between maximum pressure and 10 mm Hg, and the ball rises and falls within the average range.

C. The insufflation needle is in optimal position in the abdominal cavity. After the operator lifts the abdominal wall in the grasp of his hand and shakes the needle to dislodge possible omental shreds, the dial indication drops back to the level of the internal resistance of the insufflation circuit (about 4 to 8 mm Hg before start of insufflation). The ball hovers steadily in the upper part of its tube.

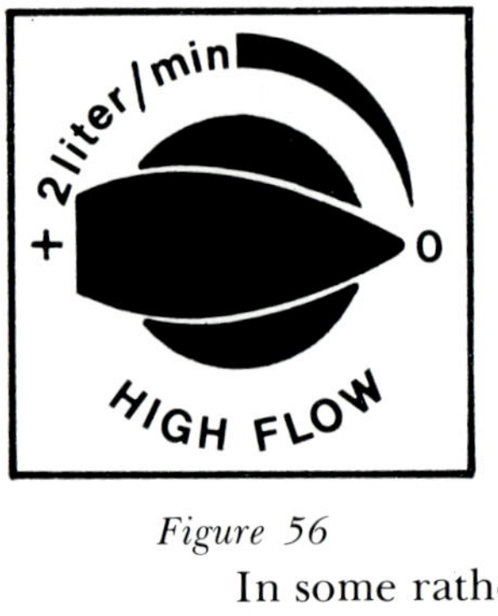

Figure 56

In some rather extensive endoscopic procedures the loss of gas through leaks in the system or exchange of instruments is greater than can be replaced reliably by any automatic device. In such cases the "High Flow" is used (Fig. 56), which replaces the lost gas at a rate of about 1 liter per minute, saving valuable time.

This "High Flow," however, must be used **only after the laparoscope has been inserted into the abdomen** and the operator has assured himself visually of the **completely unrestricted circulation** of this increased gas flow.

The "High Flow" also is needed, especially during photographic and cinematographic work, if the pneumoperitoneum has to be released and replaced because of troublesome vapor formation in the abdomen.

The High-Flow plays no part in the original inflation of the abdomen. For safety's sake *it must under no circumstances be switched on during blind insufflation.* To this end, the knob has a spring device that shuts it off automatically when released to permit its being accidentally left on.

Finally, the use of the concept "blind puncture" is no longer justified. By watching the dials of the automatic insufflator the surgeon "sees" whether or not the inserted needle tip has reached the free abdominal cavity.

The various anatomic situations that may arise in the insertion of the needle, as listed in Chapter III, Section 2, can be read directly from the dials of the insufflator by the indications of gas-flow and volume of the intra-abdominal gas bubble. The prerequisite for absolute safety in these readings is strict observance of the operative procedures laid down in Chapter VI, Section 9.

In monitoring the intra-abdominal pressure during the progress of insufflation, the operator is faced with one serious problem. At first any insufflation machine measures the flow-resistance inherent in the feed-hose and the insufflation needle. If this resistance is greater than the intra-abdominal pressure at a given moment, the pressure may not be measured during insufflation of the gas.

It was not until after it became practicable to reduce the resistance in an insufflation needle, as in the Verres needle (Fig. 57), to below 5 mm Hg with a gas-flow of 1 liter per minute that the way became clear for the development of an automatic carbon dioxide insufflator. If the gas is permitted to escape into the open

Figure 57

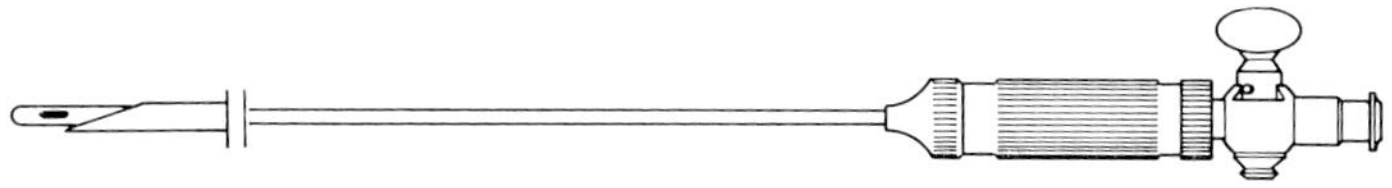

air, the body-pressure dial (3) (Fig. 54) should read only 5 to 6 mm Hg. This test should be made before laparoscopy is begun, so that an imperfectly cleansed needle can be replaced before insertion (see also Chapter VI, Section 9b).

Steptoe has recently suggested attaching a second hose to the Verres cannula, through which the pressure within the gas bubble can be read on a continuous basis. This is necessary when using Verres needles having a flow-resistance greater than 4 to 6 mm/Hg/liter/min. The spring mechanims of the needle becomes less effective, however, as additional caulking is added.

This spring mechanism in the automatic needle (Fig. 58, *A*: (1) insertion through the skin; (2) the peritoneum is reached; (3) after the resistance of the peritoneum is no longer present the blunt insufflation cannula shoots out beyond the sharp point of the needle) was first used by Goetze in 1918 and modified in 1922 by Verres. It propels the blunt cannula out beyond the tip of the needle as soon as the peritoneum has been perforated (Fig. 58, *B*). This averts the danger of puncturing the bowel through too brusque a jab from the insufflation cannula.

For the present there is no need to substitute any other gas for carbon dioxide in gynecologic techniques, but if unforeseen considerations should make this desirable in the future, the Semm insufflator with its automatic safety features can be converted for such substitution at any time. The insufflator, for reasons we will refrain from discussing here in the gynecologic setting, has also been used for many years with NO_2 in laparoscopy of the upper abdomen of unanesthetized patients.

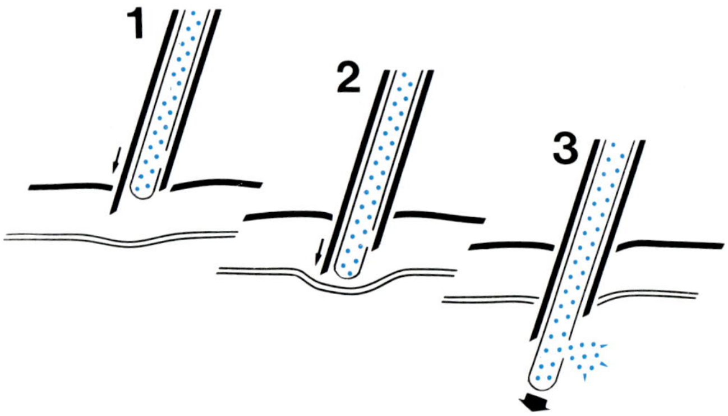

Figure 58A

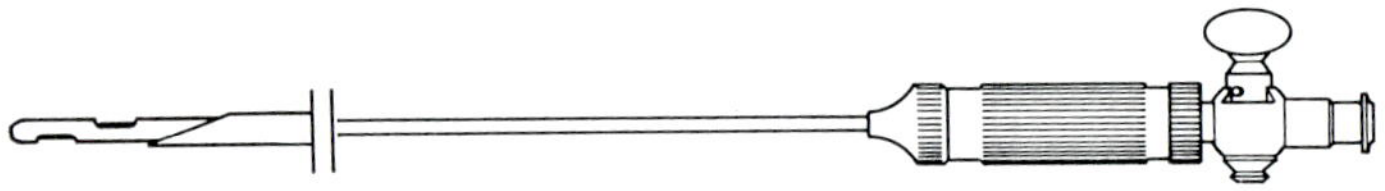

Figure 58B

4. THE SUCTION INTRAUTERINE CANNULA

In order to obtain clear views of the cul-de-sac and the adnexa from the direction of the navel, it is necessary to elevate the uterus out of its normal anatomic position in the pelvis to an extreme anteflexion. Previously this had been accomplished regularly with the instrumentarium developed for salpingography by G. K. F. Schultze, or with one of its many variants (Fig. 59). In this procedure the cannula is more or less loosely poised in the uterine cavity with the aid of a tenaculum, but this loose fixation reduces the effective displacement of the uterus.

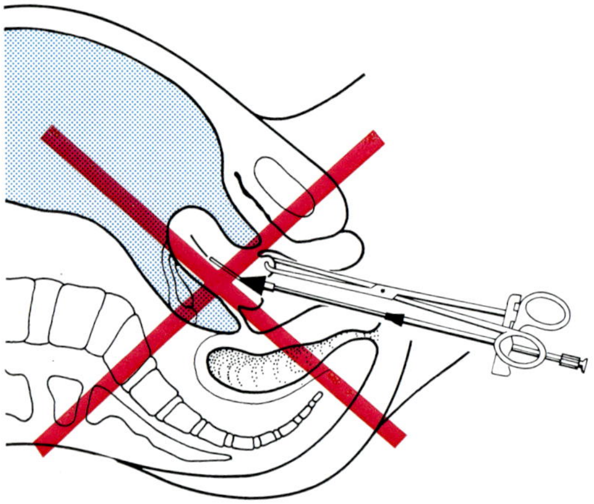

Figure 59

On the other hand, the suction intrauterine cannula (Fig. 60) is placed by suction at the distal 2 or 3 cm of the cervix. The shaft of the cannula and the uterus thus can be moved as one, and the uterus can be readily displaced three-dimensionally within the pelvis. The anterior wall of the uterus can be brought right up against the symphysis pubis in such a way that, even in an abdomen encumbered with fat, a clear view into the cul-de-sac is afforded without needing to put the patient into a position of extreme pelvic elevation. The 15° pelvic elevation generally recommended for laparoscopic purposes is quite sufficient when using the suction intrauterine cannula.

By moving the shaft of the cannula laterally and by rotating it, the uterus can be moved about and the adnexa readily brought into the field of vision. Figure 61 shows the Semm suction intrauterine cannula for insufflation of gas or instillation of dye into the fallopian tubes. In the illustration, (1) identifies the multiperforated tip of the cannula for insufflation of gas or instillation of fluids; (2) is the suction-cup, available in three different sizes; (3) is the orientation disk, indicating which way the curved intrauterine tip is turned; (4) is a nipple for attaching a hose for intrauterine instillation; and (5) is a nipple attaching the suction hose.

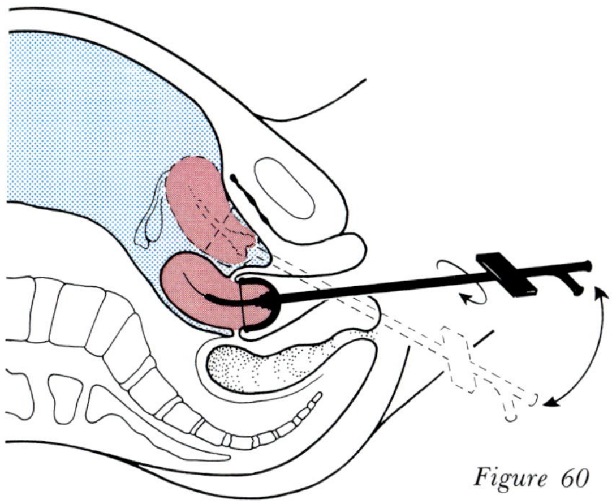

Figure 60

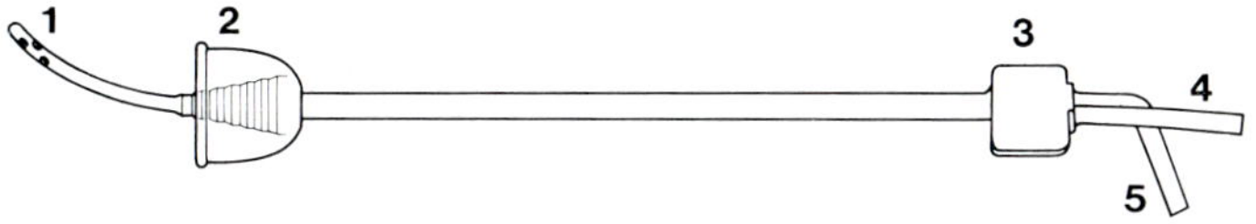

Figure 61

The multiperforated intrauterine cannula affords the additional possibility of insufflation of gas or instillation of blue dye for testing tubal patency. The usual intermediate glass container for the dye is attached to the patient's thigh (Fig. 62). From the innsufflator, the dye is pumped into the uterine cavity under controlled pressure and volume. The suction cannula comes in three sizes (Fig. 63).

Before inserting the suction cannula, the anterior lip of the cervix (see Fig. 132) is grasped and the depth of the cavity is determined by sounding. This is essential, since possible stenosis of the inner cervix might easily be overlooked in cases of sterility. The proper-sized cannula is selected on the basis of the size of the portio vaginalis of the cervix and the sounded depth of the uterus.

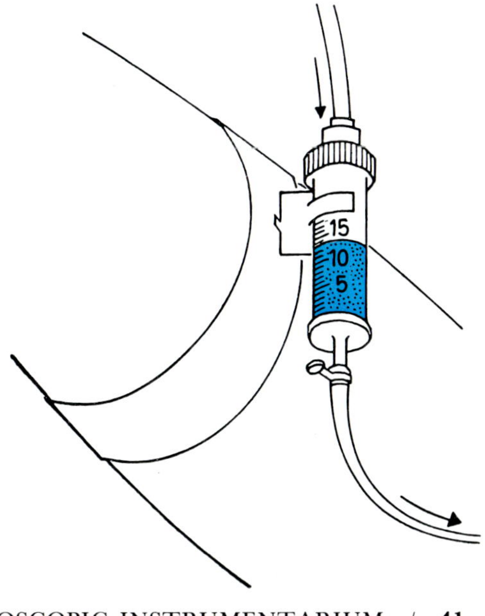

Figure 62

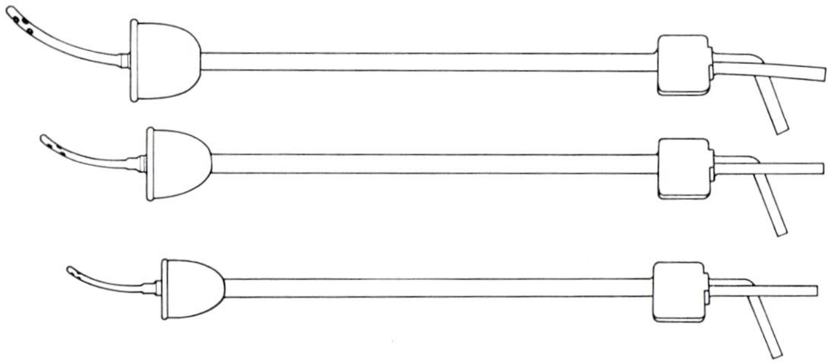

Figure 63

The suction intrauterine cannula can be used only in a nonpregnant uterus. In postpartum sterilization, which is performed most advantageously when the uterine fundus is three to four finger-breadths below the navel, the cannula must *not* be inserted into the puerperal uterus because of the risk of infection. If sterilization is to be carried out immediately following interruption of pregnancy, and the abdomen is free of adhesions, the largest dilator used should suffice for elevation of the uterus. If, however, a dubious topography is revealed at laparoscopy, use of the suction intrauterine cannula is recommended for better mobilization of the uterus.

5. THE SUCTION PROBE

The suction probe performs the following functions: (1) palpation and displacement of organs; (2) attachment to and elevation of organs; and (3) aspiration of free fluids.

Optical visualization of the entire pelvis from the direction of the navel usually is not immediately feasible. The adnexa hang into the cul-de-sac and can be

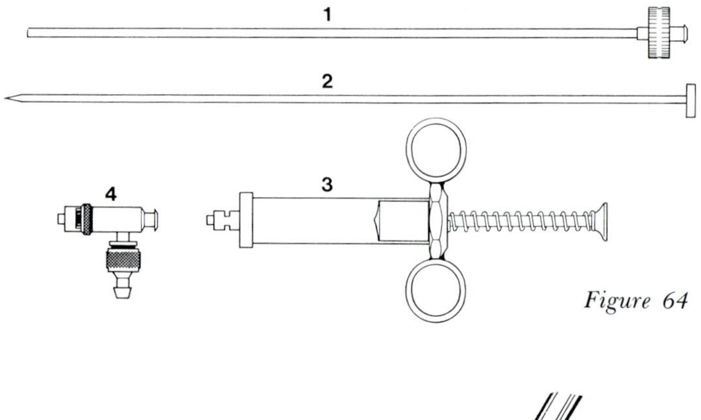

Figure 64

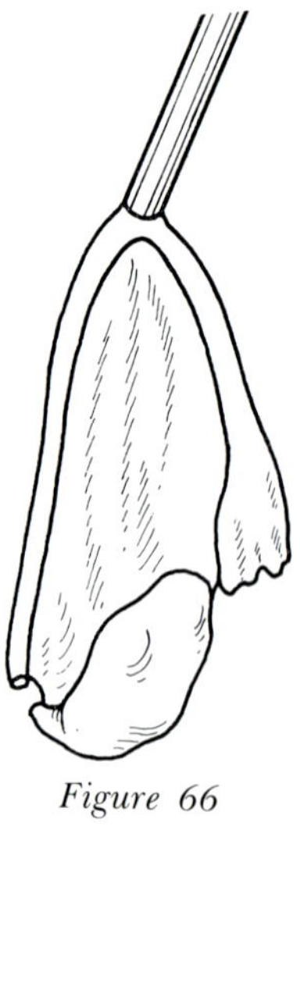

Figure 66

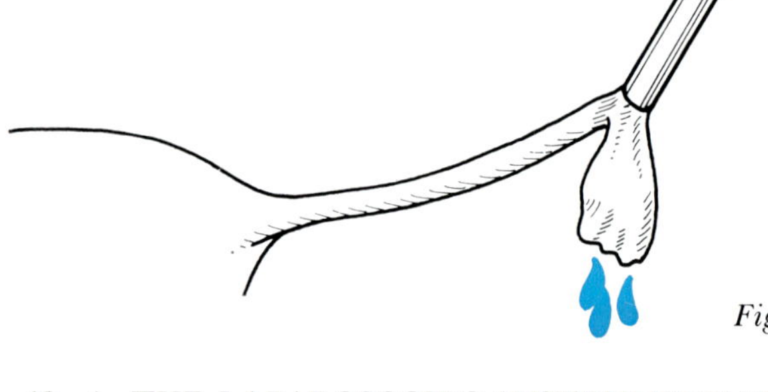

Figure 65

inspected only to an extent of 30 to 40 per cent, and the ovaries often hide the ampullae, so that endometrial implants thus hidden are impossible to diagnose. In most instances a second puncture is necessary to permit elevation of the fallopian tubes. The suction probe with its outside diameter of only about 3 mm can be used for this purpose, the spring action of the attached 10-ml syringe being capable of creating a suction of approximately 50 gm.

The suction probe consists of four parts (Fig. 64): (1) suction probe proper; (2) trocar; (3) 10-ml syringe with automatic refill spring; and (4) T-valve for suction and extraction of fluids. After perforation of the abdominal wall, the trocar is removed and the syringe attached. The operator depresses the spring-plunger of the syringe and applies the suction tube to the organ to be elevated, then releases the plunger (Fig. 65), causing the organ to adhere by suction to the end of the tube. Figure 66 demonstrates the strength of the suction action of the probe, showing an entire normal adnexum (tube and ovary totally extirpated) being elevated by suction power alone.

The aspiration of fluid from the cul-de-sac can be done in either of two ways: (1) by removing the 10-ml syringe and substituting a hose connected to a suction pump (taking care to remove only fluid and not the pneumoperitoneum); and (2) by attaching a T-valve between suction probe and the 10-ml syringe and pumping out the fluid manually (Fig. 67).

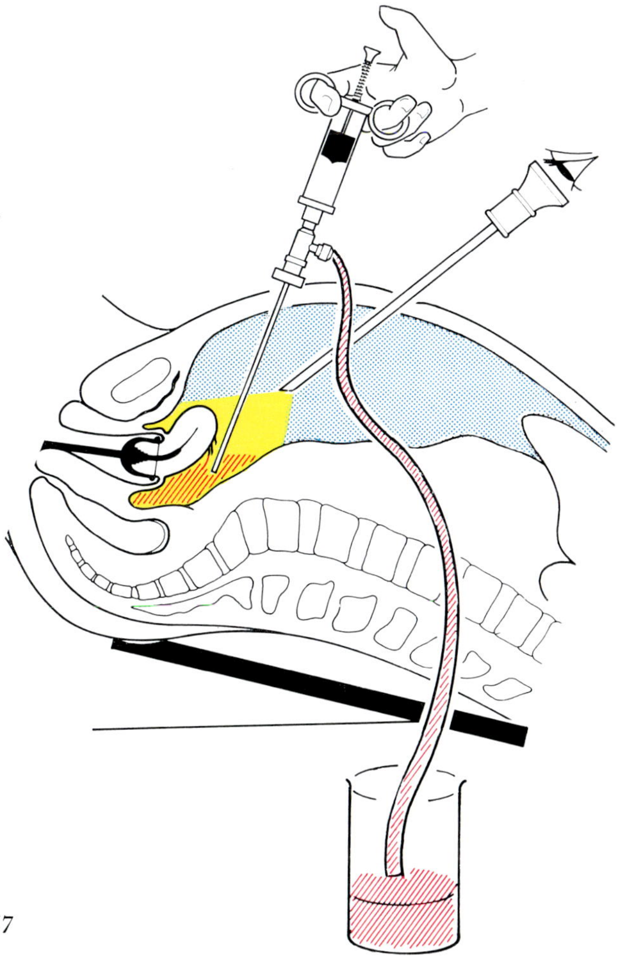

Figure 67

6. THE OPERATIVE INSTRUMENTS

The enormous technologic advances to date with regard to endoscopes and light and the achievement of constant pneumoperitoneum size make possible in ever greater measure minor surgical corrections in the pelvis in the course of laparoscopic procedures. A prerequisite for such undertakings is the double-puncture technique, since the impossibility of three-dimensional vision through the endoscope is a contraindication for surgical measures along the optical axis at laparoscopy. Lacking the perspective afforded by the second puncture (Fig. 37), even the seasoned operator is not immune to misjudgments in displacing individual organs by means of a suction probe, or through grasping forceps in order to identify the true topographic location.

Using a 6 mm trocar, the following instruments can be introduced through the second puncture.

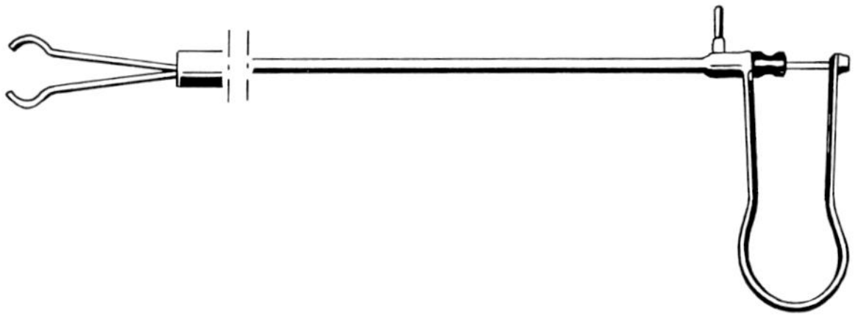

Figure 68

The instruments most used are the suction probe (5 mm model for use with the 6 mm trocar) and the grasping forceps (Fig. 68). The latter may be employed both as a probe and a forceps; in the latter instance, its jaws can be used to grasp the tubes and mesosalpinx, and displace or elevate them.

Since the forceps is insulated as a coagulation forceps for use with high-

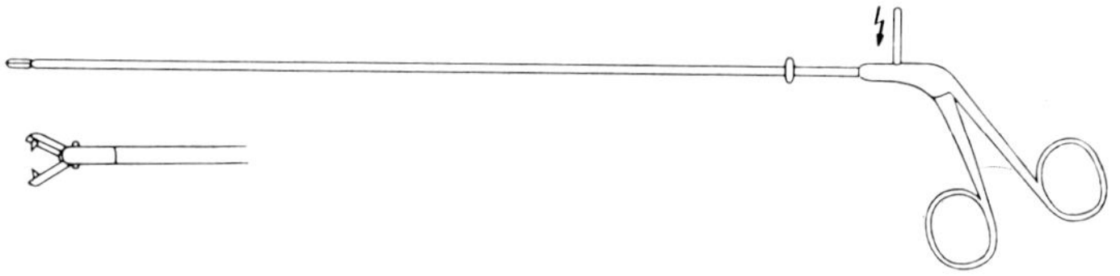

Figure 69

frequency current, it can serve also for coagulation of linear adhesions, endometrial implants, etc., and for tubal sterilization.

Nowadays, however, the grasping forceps is used only for grasping and displacing maneuvers, and low-voltage coagulation forceps are used only for coagulation purposes.

The biopsy forceps (Fig. 69) is used chiefly for removal of pieces of tissue. Two "mouth-teeth" assist in grasping the excised tissue, a step otherwise frequently difficult in the case of a firm, smooth ovary. No excision forceps alone can remove large enough tissue specimens. Therefore, the tissue should be merely grasped and crushed with the forceps. Then the trocar sleeve is advanced, compressing the jaws of the biopsy forceps, and the tissue is gripped between them in order to punch out (Fig. 70) the specimen of tissue. Then, turning the trocar sleeve will excise large pieces of tissue, which is especially important in the resection of a cystic sac after ovarian puncture.

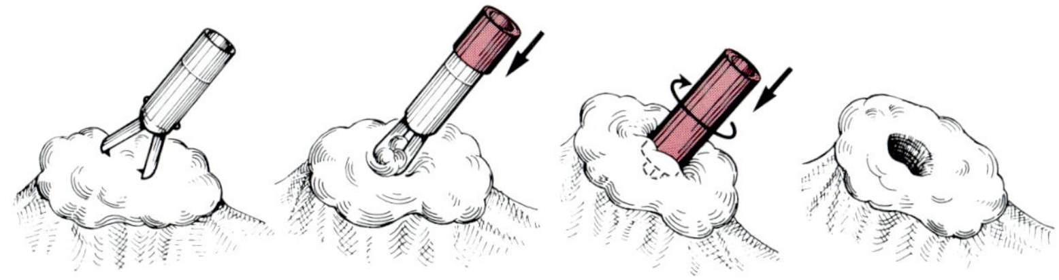

Figure 70

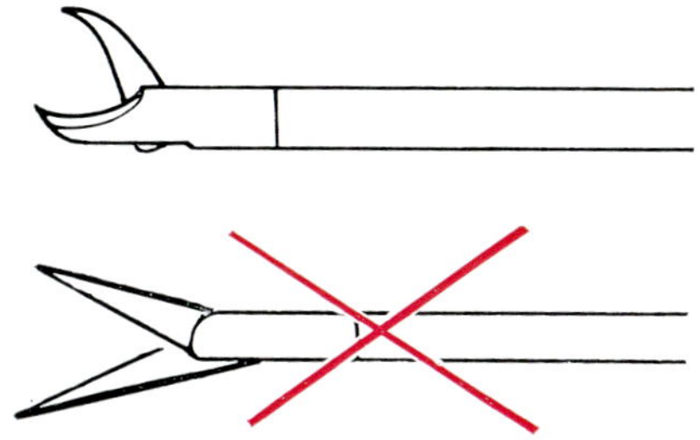

Figure 71

Tissue bridges, linear and velamentous adhesions (for example, at laparoscopy in cases of sterility) are cropped, usually after coagulation, with Frangenheim hook-scissors (Fig. 71). The concavely curved shearing jaws prevent the tissue from sliding out of the bite while being severed. Scissors with straight jaws are

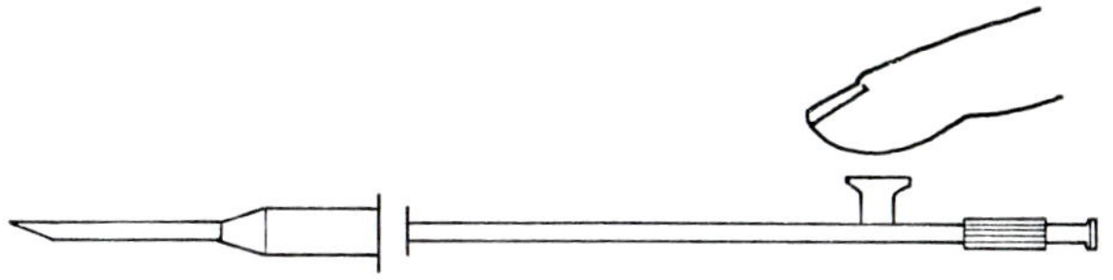

Figure 72

not suitable for endoscopic work, since the pieces of tissue being severed are usually hanging free in space and tend to slide out of the bite of straight jaws.

The puncture cannula (Fig. 72) is used to puncture cyst walls and to extract fluid from the cul-de-sac for cytologic examination.

In the puncture of ovarian cysts it is necessary that the cyst be firmly steadied; otherwise the tip of the needle may slip off and accidentally strike a blood vessel. The best way is to prop the ovarian cyst against the anterior wall of the uterus in order to hold it steady (see Fig. 383).

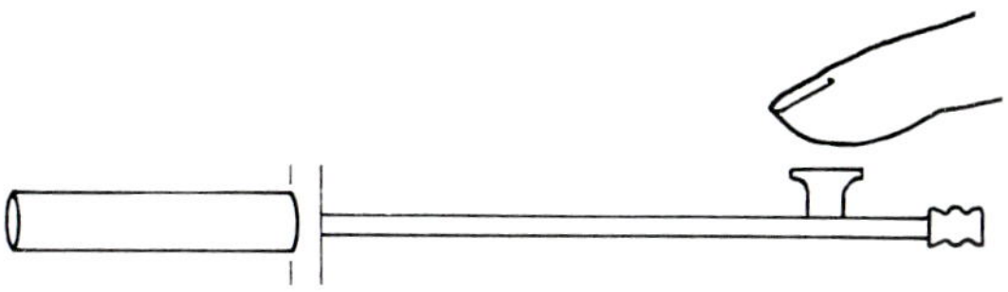

Figure 73

For extraction of larger amounts of fluid—for example, ascites or coagulated blood after surgery on the adnexa—an aspiration cannula with a wide lumen is used (Fig. 73).

In order not to lose the aspirate, it is collected in a special suction flask (Fig. 74), coupled to a suction pump or the suction hose of an anesthesia apparatus. In order that the operator need not be dependent on the continuous suction of the apparatus, at the center of the rubber cork of the flask there is a thick tube with a flared top to which a finger is applied. By lifting the finger, the suction can be interrupted at will if, for example, the tip of the suction cannula inadvertently attaches itself to a portion of tissue. After shaking this occluding bit of tissue loose, the finger closes the flared tube again and suction resumes. When extracting internally located ovarian cysts, it is advisable to lift and replace the finger at rhythmic intervals. This causes any pieces of tissue that are attached to the tip to drop away forcibly from the cannula, and thus the contents of the multichambered cyst can be intermittently but completely extracted.

There is a special suction cannula for extraction of ova (Fig. 75), 300 mm

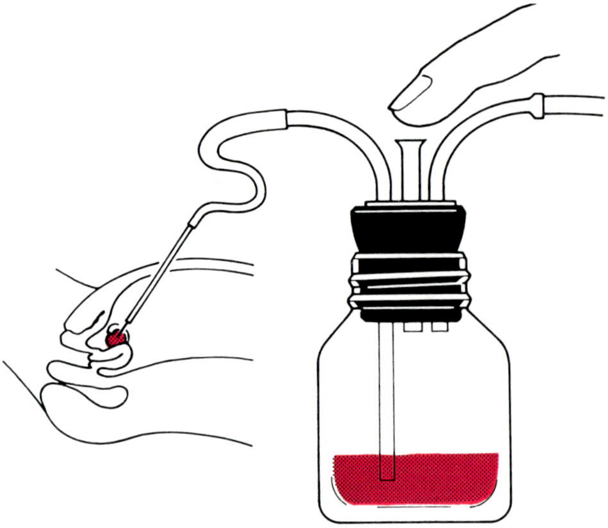

Figure 74

long and 0.8 mm thick. There is a trocar for inserting it into the abdomen, 150 mm long and 1.5 mm thick. This ovum-aspirating cannula can be inserted into the abdomen under visual control at any point in the abdominal wall without leaving a scar. For this purpose, a location for the puncture is selected that lies in a straight line opposite to the ovum. A 90° puncture angle is technically the best approach possible. For suction, a 1 ml or 2 ml sterile spring-syringe is recommended, into which the aspirate can be drawn directly for further disposition (see Figs. 407–409).

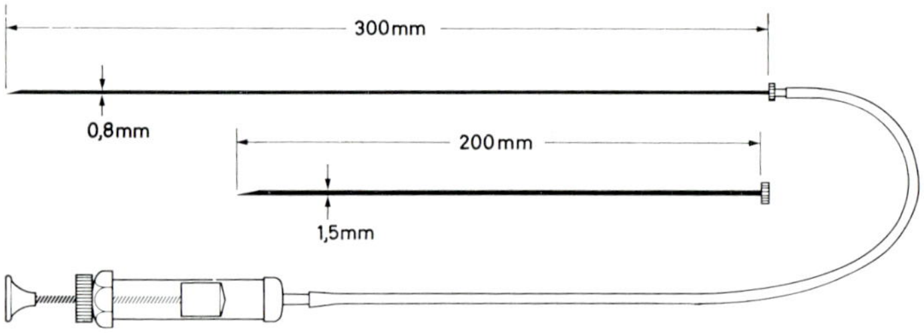

Figure 75

For coagulation of any kind in connection with laparoscopy, only low-voltage current should be employed, i.e., 5 volts AC or DC (Chapter IV, Section 8, a–c). The newly-developed Semm low-voltage coagulation forceps (Fig. 76), in which under electronic control only the small jaws are heated to coagulation temperature, coagulate precisely and without danger to the environment, and linear adhesions close to the bowel or blood vessels can be safely coagulated with accuracy to within 1 mm. At the same time it is possible to coagulate endometrial implants on the dome of the bladder, for instance, without any in-depth injury.

At present forceps of different shapes are available.

(1) Semm crocodile coagulation forceps, chiefly for tubal sterilization (Fig. 76); tubal sterilization by coagulation with low voltage is performed under control of the Tubal Coagulator Unit (Fig. 78). Without endangering the mesosalpinx, 6 mm of tube can be safely coagulated. The crocodile forceps can be used for tubal

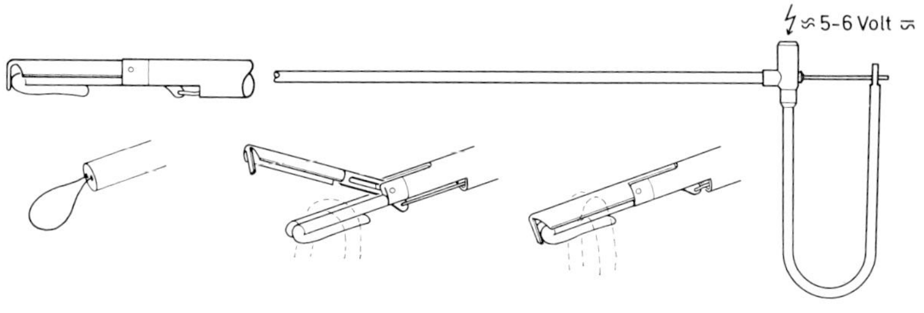

Figure 76

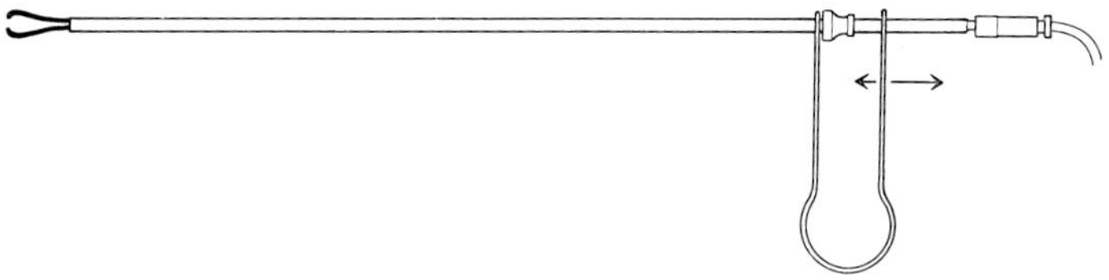

Figure 77

coagulation in connection with various operative techniques: (a) laparoscopy; (b) culdoscopy; (c) posterior colpotomy (culdotomy); and (d) tubal sterilization following cesarean section.

This forceps supplants all earlier surgical sterilization procedures. Since 1964 we have no longer performed bloody tubal ligations (e.g., Pomeroy, Madlener, Labhardt, etc.). For sharp transsection of the tube following coagulation, the tubal scissors were created (Fig. 79), so constructed that only the muscular part of the tube is cut and the underlying vascular bundle is spared.

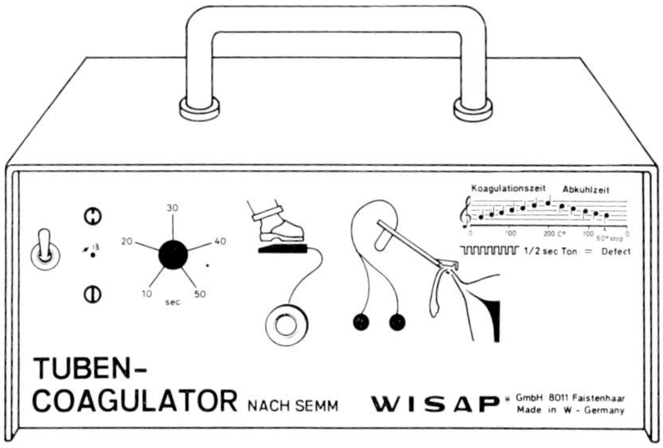

Figure 78

(2) The Semm atraumatic coagulation forceps (Fig. 77) for all laparoscopic coagulation procedures.

For coagulation of cylindric biopsy wounds in the ovaries, or for thermal destruction of ovarian tissues on a large scale (e.g., in the Stein-Leventhal syndrome), the ball-tipped coagulation electrode is used (Fig. 80). This is heated and

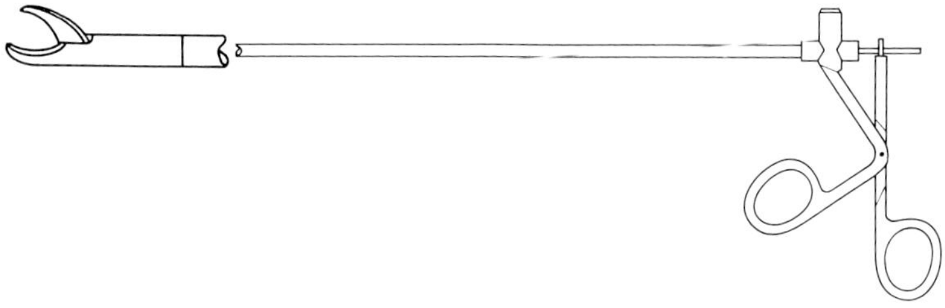

Figure 79

operated electronically, just like the coagulation forceps, at a low voltage from the control unit. The spherical contact surface ensures a uniform distribution of the heat.

The Endotherm (Fig. 81), an electronic control unit, is used as the source of current for the atraumatic coagulation forceps. Here, also, forceps temperature and coagulation time are controlled and monitored electronically. At the same time, acoustic signals alert the operator to the successive steps in the procedure.

Experiments on temporary sterilization with tantalum or plastic clips and Silastic rings are under way at several places (e.g., Gutierrez, Najar, 1973; B. Bleier, 1973; Hulka, 1973).

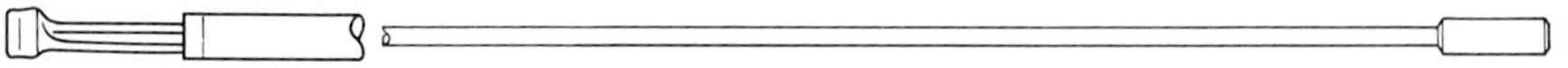

Figure 80

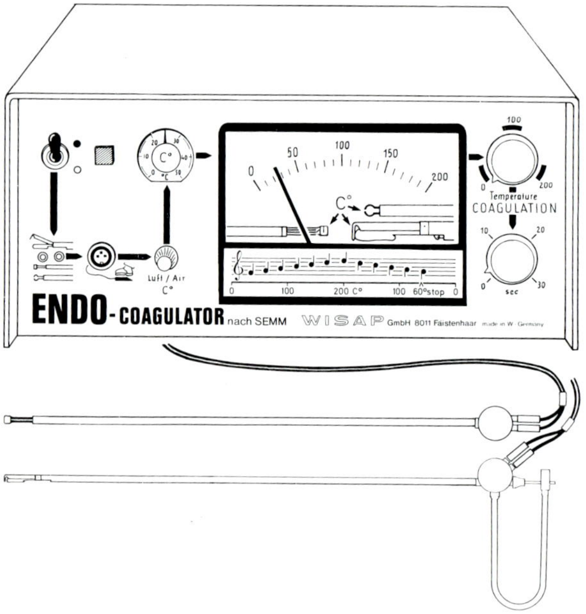

Figure 81

Single or multiple ligation of the tubes (Semm, 1973) is now being tried out. In this operation, a suture is placed around a tube through the mesosalpinx and ligated by means of a silver ring (Fig. 82).

(*a*) By means of the threading forceps, a thick suture is threaded through the mesosalpinx and around the tube.

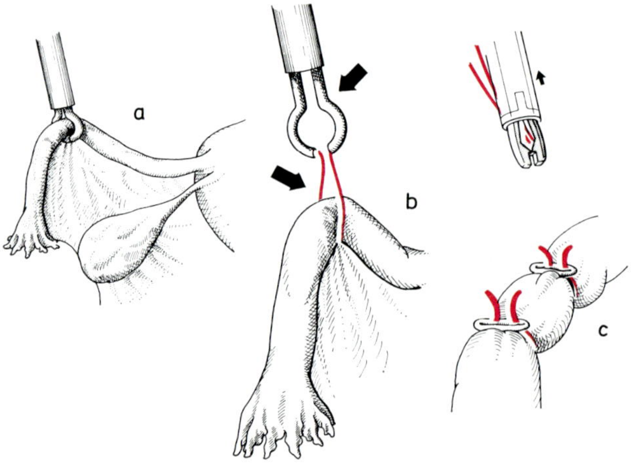

Figure 82

(*b*) The suturing forceps is opened and withdrawn from the trocar sleeve.

(*c*) The suture is ligated firmly around the tube with the ring-pinching forceps.

Figure 83 shows the instrumentarium needed for the temporary ligation technique:

A, Suture thread with spiral guide.

B, Threading forceps (shown with jaws opened).

C, Trocar with trocar sleeve for *A, B,* and *D* (8-mm diameter for second puncture).

D, Ring-pinching forceps with suture cutter.

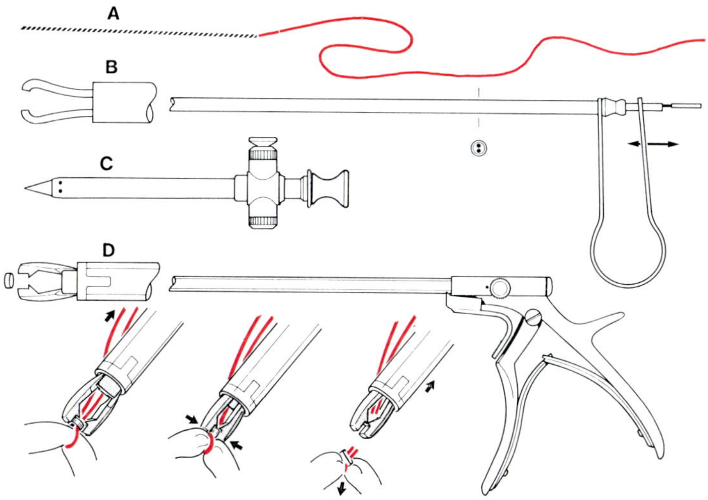

Figure 83

The sketches at the bottom of the illustration show the pinching of the ring and cutting of the suture: (1) placement of the pinching ring against the tube; (2) a pull on the suture to make it snug around the tube, closing off its lumen; (3) firm closure of the forceps jaws, which simultaneously pinches the ring and cuts the suture off.

The tubes may be ligated either once or twice; there is as yet no practical experience as to the relative value of single or multiple ligation.

7. BLOOD VESSEL CLAMPS

As mentioned frequently in the foregoing chapters, injury to blood vessels cannot be avoided with 100 per cent certainty, especially upon insertion of the Verres needle or the trocar, even though all precautionary measures are conscientiously observed. For this reason, it is essential to have an optimal instrumentarium ready at hand for clamping off medium and large vessels in case such an accident occurs. The standard clamps in normal use in gynecologic surgery serve only to crush the vessels. This, however, so injures the intima of the vessel that subsequent vascular plastic surgery of dubious prognosis becomes necessary. The clamp must close off the vessel so elastically that its intima are not damaged. Figure 84 shows a set of vascular clamps with which the femoral vessels—and in an emergency even the abdominal aorta and inferior vena cava—can be closed off temporarily with confidence and without damage to the laminar layers of the inner walls.

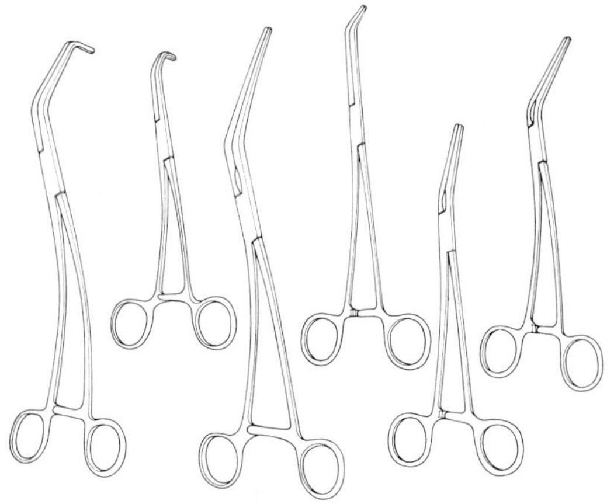

Figure 84

A *sterile* set of vascular clamps *must* be ready at hand *during any laparoscopic procedure.* Even though the need may not arise for years, the precaution must *never* be overlooked (see Chapter III, Section 3).

Once injury to a major vessel has occurred, the damaged vessel is clamped off at sufficient distance proximally and distally from the injury; it can then safely await arrival of the vascular surgeon.

It is a mistake to clamp off large vessels with the clamps customarily used in gynecologic surgery, such as parametrial clamps and the like.

8. ELECTRICITY IN LAPAROSCOPY

Thanks to a technologic breakthrough known as "cold light," the patient in diagnostic laparoscopy is no longer subjected to the dangers of electric injury. But this is not the case with operative laparoscopy, in which high-frequency electricity is being used to an ever greater extent to stem bleeding, to destroy endometrial implants, and more recently for tubal sterilization. The First American Congress of Laparoscopy in 1973 established the fact that routine use of high-frequency electricity is leading to more and more severe burns, sometimes with fatal outcome, as a result of human or technologic failure. In retrospect, it may be noted that high-frequency current was introduced somewhat recklessly into endoscopy, and especially laparoscopy, without prior physical and technologic deliberation.

High-frequency current in its very essence is a surface phenomenon. In electrical conductors, both metals and electrolytes, it deploys on the surface. In penetrating into the interior of the human body, it mainly follows such routes as blood vessels and the intestines, the contents of both being high in salt and other electrolytes. At the point of emergence from these paths into the peritoneum, regardless of the intensity of the current, there is field intensification, which means generation of heat and consequent burns.

In general surgery, in which high-frequency current was introduced in the 1920s, it is used exclusively in surface applications, but in laparoscopy it has to be conducted into the closed abdominal cavity via body tissues. In reaching the operative site it selects its own routes, which vary unpredictably from patient to patient and are in no way subject to the operator's control.

For general comprehension, a short review of the fundamental physics of the high-frequency technique is given later in this chapter.

In the past ten years, we have undertaken experiments (Semm, 1965, 1966a, 1966b, 1966c, 1967) calculated to eliminate high-frequency current from gynecology because of its inherent dangers. In the course of this work we found that temperatures of 500° C, which are common in high-frequency "scarification," are by no means necessary for coagulation of benign lesions of the cervix or for tubal sterilization. From the surface of an electronically heated probe (Fig. 85) the 80 to

90° C temperature, which is all that is needed for coagulation of protein, flows to the surface of the cervix, thermally denaturing the ectopic tissue without causing burns. Biologic studies on thermocoagulation of the cervix and subsequent healing were the basis for the development of the low-voltage coagulation technique for tubal sterilization.

The biologically denatured coagulation surface is shown in Figure 86 (vaginal portion of the cervix five hours before total extirpation, denatured for 15 seconds at 90° C). In the vicinity of the probe, the enzyme reaction of the 1,3,99,1-suc-

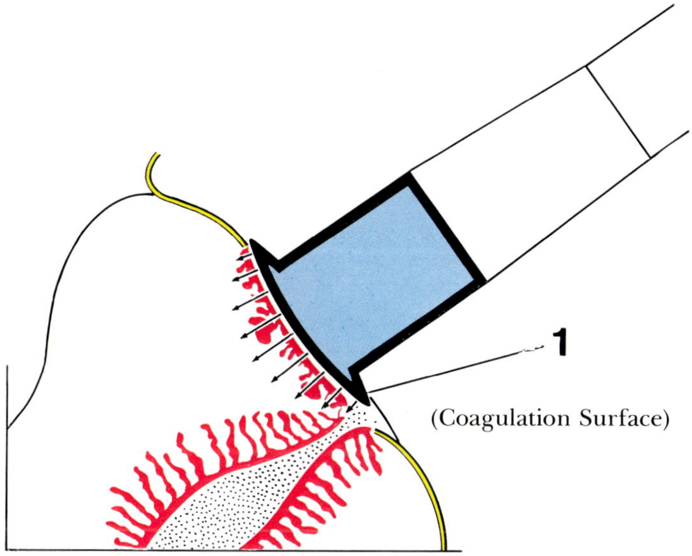

Figure 85

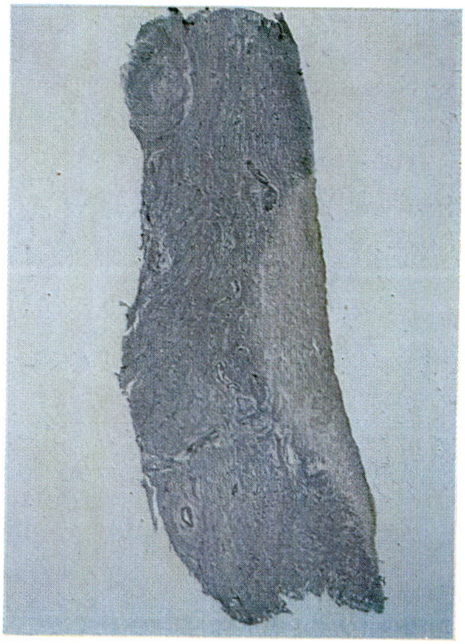

Figure 86

cinodehydrogenase is negative. This area is bloodlessly necrotized and subsequently replaced by regeneration of new tissue from its edges. The tissue sequestration usually seen in high-frequency scarification does not occur.

The coagulation technique on the cervix is painless and can be performed in the physician's office. After four to six weeks the cylindric glossy epithelium and the cervix presents its original nonpathologic appearance. On the other hand, thermocoagulation has the advantage over cryotherapy of benign erythroplasia in that it permits the desired splitting of nabothian cysts. Also, injudicious freezing of the cervix, a nonphysiologic procedure, could lead to delayed damage. Figure 87 shows the control unit for the coagulation probe (Semm's Coagulator).

Temperatures of up to 700° C occur when high-frequency current is employed for tubal sterilization, regardless of whether the instrumentarium is labeled "unipolar" or "bipolar." Figure 88 (from Larbig and Göltner, 1974) (temperature readings in the fallopian tube during electrocoagulation: I at 20 watts, II at 30 watts) documents temperatures arising in the tubes with the use of wattages in the 20 to 30 range when the atraumatic coagulation forceps and high-frequency current are employed.

The temperature of the forceps is given in Figure 89: temperature in the forceps after coagulation is designated "1" and flame- and spark-formation as "2."

> Immediately after the current is shut off, the jaws of the forceps have reached a temperature of 100° C if no sparks were produced during the coagulation (a phenomenon which cannot be ruled out, even at 30 watts). After coagulation, accompanied by flames or sparks, the temperature at the jaws of the forceps was 360° C, and it was still 130° C two minutes after the coagulation.

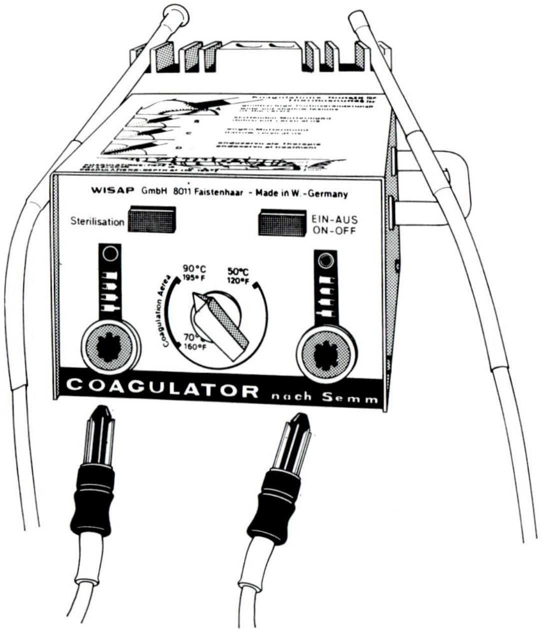

Figure 87

Figure 88

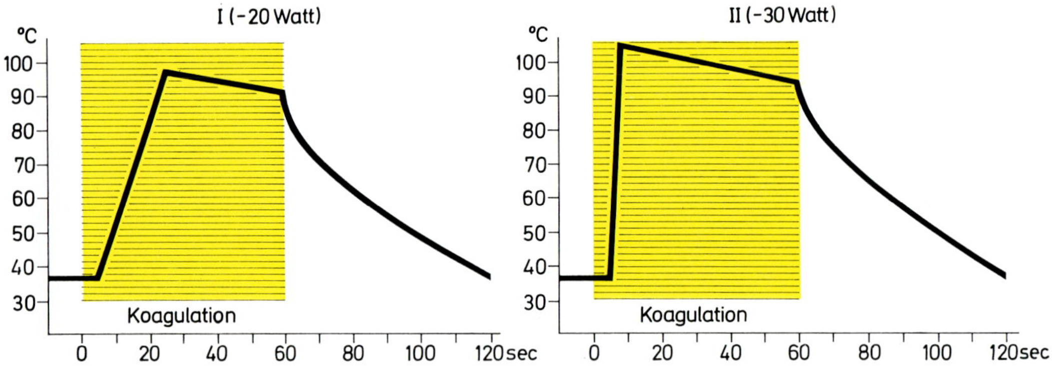

Figure 90 is a graph of temperature readings in the tube when flames and sparks occurred. 1 thru 6 are power settings of the high-frequency generator corresponding to 10 to 100 watts. The graph demonstrates what happens when the wattage exceeds 20 to 30, which might be regarded as commonplace with generators in general use today.

With 50 to 100 watts the fallopian tube tissue is heated to 450 to 600° C, i.e., it is first desiccated and then partially carbonized. To avoid thermal injury to adjacent organs, three to four minutes' cooling time would be necessary.

Low-voltage or "galvanic" current at about 5 volts is quite sufficient to produce the heat energy necessary for endoscopic work. The instruments then require no insulation and have proved their worth in thousands of coagulations of erythroplasias of the cervix (Semm, 1963 ff.). This low-voltage technique was developed for further endoscopic purposes during the period 1970 to 1973. Special control units, such as the Tubal Coagulator and the Endotherm, greatly increase the range of possibilities in laparoscopic therapy and surgery. Figure 91 shows the temperature range during low-voltage coagulation in tubal sterilization. Area 1: heating time; Area 2: coagulation period; while there is still water in the tissue,

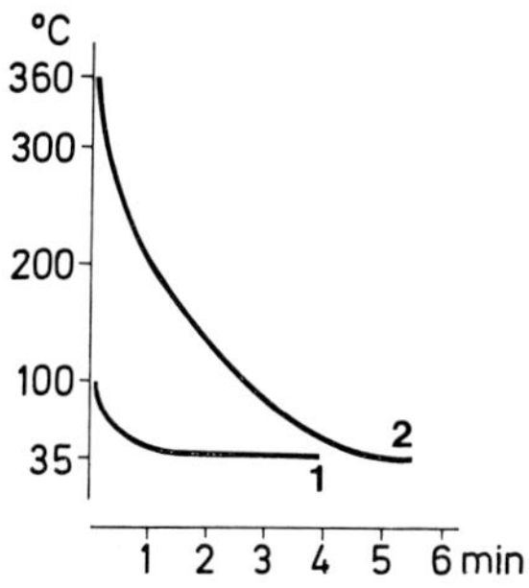

Figure 89

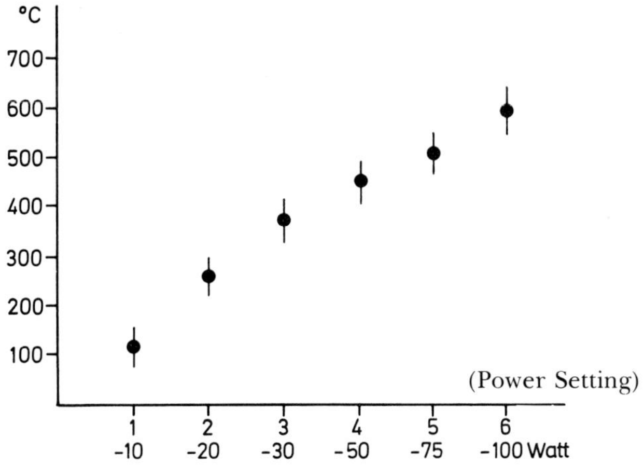

Figure 90

the temperature cannot exceed the boiling point; Area 3: the water is vaporized in the area within the grasp of the crocodile forceps, and with that the tissue temperature reaches the electronically controllable maximum range. Experiments have shown the biologic effectiveness of high-frequency and low-voltage currents to be the same, since the tissues, once denatured, are killed as completely as they can ever be. (See Fig. 468.)

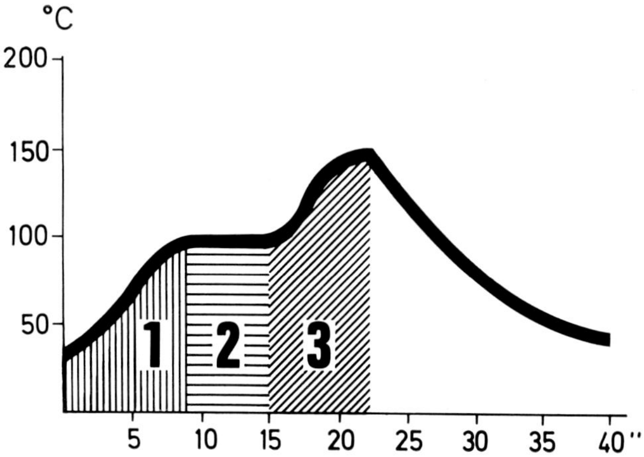

Figure 91

Since the high-frequency procedure today is still the more usual one, the two techniques are described here side-by-side.

High-Frequency Current

Medically applied high-frequency current means AC at about 400,000 to 3 million oscillations a second, or 0.4 to 3.0 MHz.

Such currents are produced conventionally with the aid of tubes or, more recently, with transistor circuits. Because of their high rate of oscillation they have no influence on nervous or muscular control potentials. In surgery these currents can be used at wattages from 30 to 300 and voltages from 100 to 400 for coagulation and severance of tissue as required. As already mentioned above, this high-frequency current deploys chiefly on the surface of metals or electrolytes. Within the range of general surgery this is quite harmless, since all such surgical use is limited to the surface of the body. An open incision into the interior of the body merely creates additional surface (Fig. 92).

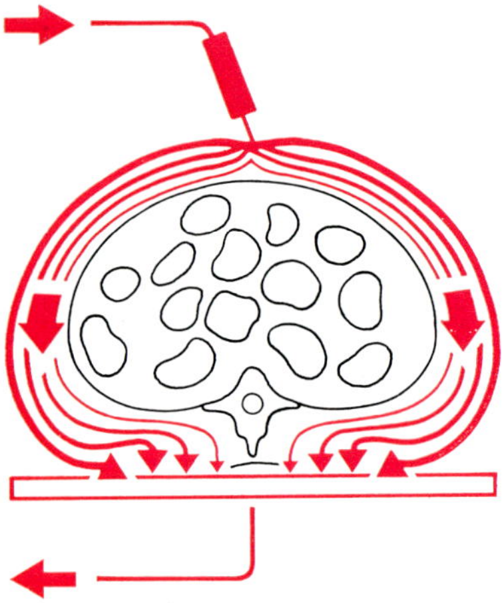

Figure 92

However, many endoscopists are using the therapeutic properties of high-frequency current for cutting and coagulating *inside* the closed cavities of the body without stopping to consider the paths taken by the current (Fig. 93).

It is important to understand the biophysical basis of therapeutic use of high-frequency current in achieving cutting and coagulation effects.

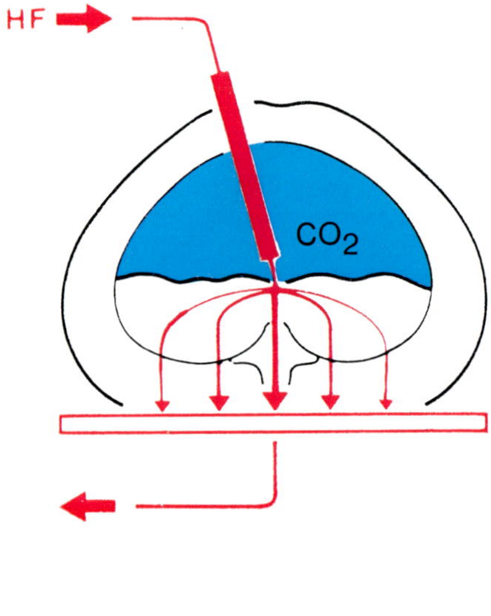

Figure 93

There are three possibilities that illustrate the local effect of destructive heat generated by high-frequency current (Fig. 94).

Fulguration

In this case there is a spark discharge between the tip of the electrode and organ surface without direct contact between them. The development of heat is limited to the tissue surface visible within the spark range.

Coagulation

This is heating of the tissue to the boiling point under the influence of high-frequency current.

Electrocautery

This requires separation of the tissues with an electric knife or biopsy forceps. The cut surface may be either smooth and even or rough and uneven, depending on the quality of the current produced by the high-frequency generator.

Tissue separation with smooth margins can be effected by electrocautery by means of an uninterrupted parallel undampened high-frequency current, which can be produced with tube or transistor generators. If one superimposes on this current a dampened oscillation, as is used exclusively in fulguration, one achieves, in addition to heating of tissues to the boiling point, explosion of the cells and subsequent formation of an uneven cut surface.

On a large surface, the so-called "indifferent plane," high-frequency electricity moves in a broad base over human skin and is conducted by it, thanks to its electrolyte content, to the punctiform active electrode, a scalpel or ball coagulator. As long as the conductivity (resistance) of the skin remains unchanged, the resistance to conduction increases as a result of field intensification in the neighborhood of the active electrode. In step with the power of the high-frequency generator, electrical energy thereby is converted to heat. Under the influence of this heat, water vapor in the tissue causes it to explode, or to melt or burn up. Small blood vessels shrivel immediately by the coagulation effect, so that tissues severed by cautery bleed little or not at all.

However, if the active electrode is located *inside* the abdomen, the current must flow from the active to the inactive one via the abdominal cavity. In accordance with the law that a current always follows the path of least resistance, it follows a blood vessel or the intestinal contents, especially when (after ingestion of spinach, for example) the intestinal contents are especially rich in electrolytes. At some point along the way, behaving according to its nature as a surface current, it diverges from the vascular or intestinal path in order to reach the active electrode located on the peritoneum, the second available bodily surface. At each point

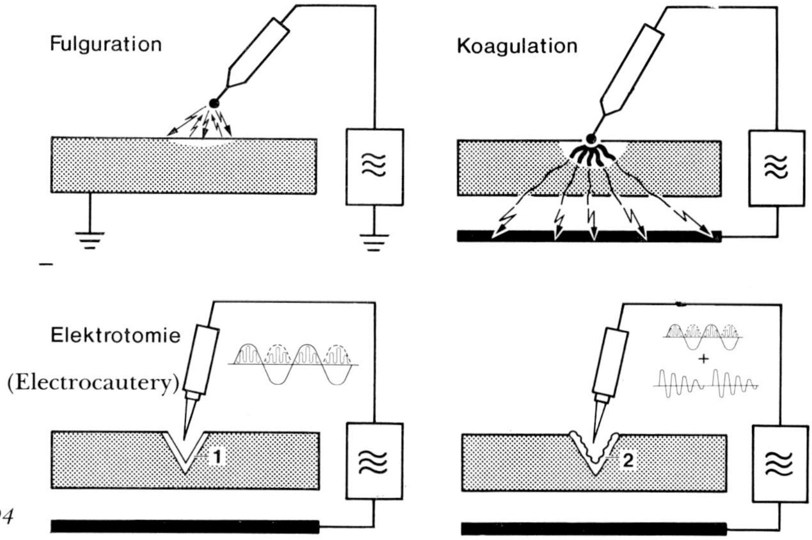

Figure 94

where the current diverges from a blood vessel or intestinal contents to the peritoneum, a field intensification can arise just as is intended at the active electrode. Since no one can predict at what point it will leave the tissue for the peritoneum, high-frequency current for intra-abdominal use is inherently unpredictable from the physical standpoint. The numerous recorded accidents involving intestinal burns afford evidence of these theoretic and physical principles. The sketch in Figure 95 shows the locally unpredictable path of the high-frequency current to the fallopian tube (see also Fig. 239).

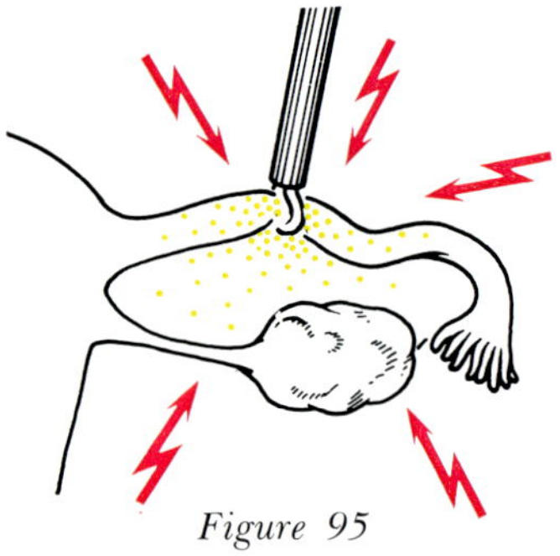

Figure 95

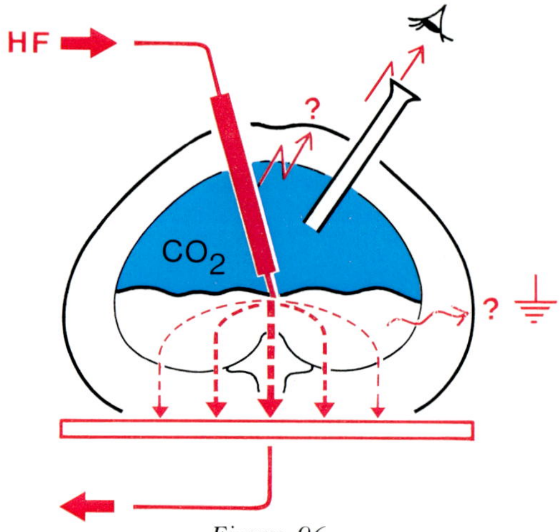

Figure 96

High-frequency current follows the rule and seeks the path of least resistance, so it is not surprising that on occasion it passes via the instruments to the operator, himself an excellent conductor (Fig. 96). At the point of transfer, since this usually is a minute point of contact, the operator sustains burns of, for example, the eye, nose, hand, etc.

In view of the unexpected frequency of burns in the course of sterilizations, the Complications Committee of the American Association of Gynecologic Laparoscopists was formed to investigate such accidents. On the basis of its deliberations (published by Corson, Patrick, Hamilton, and Bolognese in 1973) the following basic recommendation on electrosurgical high-frequency units for laparoscopic purposes was promulgated.

*General Recommendations for Electro-Surgical Units for Laparoscopic Procedures**

1. Maximum output should be approximately 150 watts cutting, and 50 watts coagulating into 500 ohms.

2. Power output should be independent of load impedance variations between 100 and 1000 ohms, so control setting changes are necessary.

3. Power output should not vary with normal line voltage fluctuation.

4. Open circuit voltage should be high enough for fulguration but should not be so high that breakdown of insulation of instruments or surgical gloves is likely.

5. The output should contain adequate filtering to block low frequency currents that may stimulate muscular contraction in the patient, even under general anesthesia.

---

*From J. Reprod. Med., *11*:, No. 4:163, 1973.

6. Ideally, isolated output circuitry is preferred over grounded designs. Such a unit would not operate if the cable from the return electrode were inoperative.

7. A warning tone and light indicator should signal when the unit is energized to minimize accidental activation.

8. The return electrode (plate) must adequately disperse current returning to the unit. At least 10 square inches of area per 100 watts of power is recommended. Return cables should be inspected and routinely replaced depending on frequency of use.

9. Radio frequency interference generated by the unit that might interfere with pacemakers and monitors should be reduced to a minimum through design and shielding.

10. A circuit breaker, or at least a fuse, should be incorporated to protect the electrosurgical source.

11. A thermal cut-off protection should be provided to protect the unit from high operating temperatures. Fans to dissipate internal heat are undesirable because of the risk of cross contamination between cases. If a fan is present, a replaceable filter should be provided.

12. Footswitches should be easily cleaned and waterproofed against accidental spillage of operating room fluids. They should have proper mechanical design allowing a surgeon to reposition the footswitch without accidentally depressing a control pedal.

13. Electric cables should be sturdy and long enough to provide for adequate positioning between the patient and the outlet.

14. Service is a major consideration. Qualified personnel should be available for rapid on-site repair and to instruct operating room attendants in proper usage.

The following recommendations were made for the use of endoscopic instruments in connection with high-frequency generators.

*Specific Recommendations for Laparoscopic Apparatus to be Used with Electrosurgical Units**

1. The telescopic eyepiece should be electrically insulated from the shaft to protect the operator from shocks and burns.

2. A fiberglass sheath should be employed to protect against patient skin burns at the incision site.

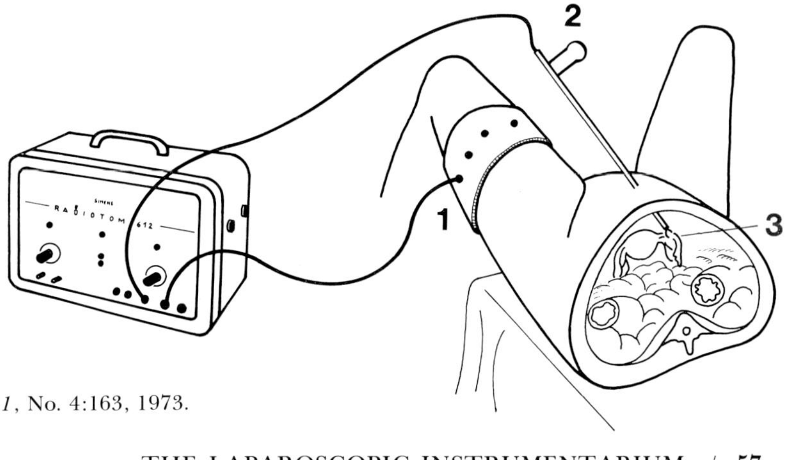

Figure 97

*From J. Reprod. Med., *11*, No. 4:163, 1973.

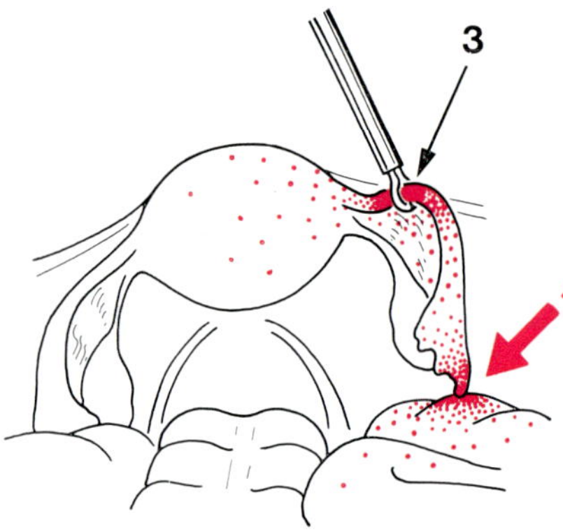

Figure 98

3. Forcep handles should be totally insulated to protect the operator and abdominal wall skin of the patient.

4. Future laparoscopic design should include a bipolar coagulation instrument to eliminate the return electrode plate. A hand-operated circuit control to replace foot activation would reduce inadverent open circuit activations.

The logical conclusions from these two American safety warnings are that **high-frequency current is definitely contraindicated for endoscopy,** but neither a manufacturer nor a surgical team can observe all these precautions fully at all times.

As an illustration of high-frequency current, the risks are depicted again in Figures 97 and 98:

Schematic depiction of the thermally endangered tissues in high-frequency cautery. The electrical energy is led to the body via the large leg electrode (1 in Fig. 97); it is led away from it at a punctiform spot and bundled in the direction of the tip of the coagulation instrument (2, Fig. 97), in this instance an atraumatic grasping forceps (3, Fig. 98). As the current intensity builds up, the tissue in the vicinity of this bundling, usually conical in shape, heats up in the direction toward the instrument, that is, the tip of the cone. We normally observe the maximum development of heat in the immediate vicinity of the tip of the instrument. But since the electric current always follows the path of least resistance, it often does not take what might seem the shortest path, that in the present instance appears to be from the uterus to the oviduct or mesosalpinx. So it is possible for an unnoticed short-circuiting shred or bridge of tissue to conduct the current: for example, the bridge depicted in the drawing (4, Fig. 98), formed by the tubal ampulla in contact with a loop of the small intestine. The high-frequency current

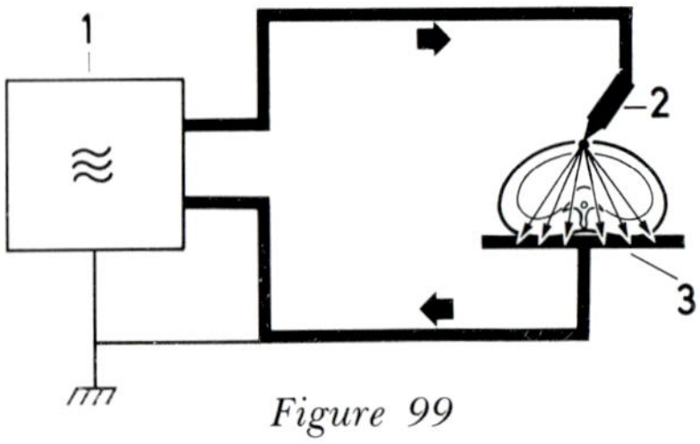

Figure 99

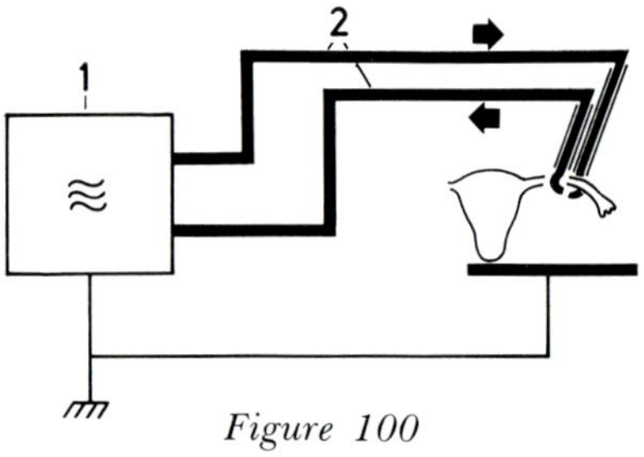

Figure 100

now diverges from the electrolyte-containing intestine to the oviduct at an almost punctiform spot; because of the field intensification the intestinal wall is heated, and the critical temperature of 55° C is exceeded. The consequence is a necrosis of tissue and a puncture, sometimes visible immediately and sometimes not until 24 to 48 hours later. The same situation occurs when adhesions are being coagulated. Here too, the bases of linear adhesions on the intestine are also heated.

In gynecologic endoscopy the use of current *from high-frequency generators* developed originally for *major surgery* is *no longer acceptable.* The recommendations of our American colleagues of high-frequency generators with an output of 150 watts for cutting and 50 watts for coagulation become questionable when it is realized that the fallopian tubes can be optimally coagulated with low voltage at an output of 5 to a maximum of 10 watts. The coagulation of the tubal ostia at hysteroscopy, which we also once performed with high frequency at 30 to 40 watts, we now do with low voltage at about 5 watts.

The resistance of human tissue is not constant, making the coagulation effect incalculable. One is forced to work with an overdose of electric current to avoid an unsatisfactory coagulation effect.

Since, in America especially, tubal sterilization is the main indication for laparoscopy, the "bipolar sterilization forceps" was developed recently (Fig. 102). This instrument markedly reduces the risk of high-frequency current applications. The differences between unipolar and bipolar electrical systems are seen in Figure 99 (1. = high-frequency generator, 2. = active electrode, and 3. = neutral electrode) and Figure 100 (1. = high-frequency generator, 2. = nongrounded high-frequency electric current).

Summary

Use of human tissues as electric resistance in order to produce heat no longer is the method of choice for coagulating tissues during endoscopic procedures.

The same also is true of the recently recommended bipolar technique (see Sec. 8c), when it is limited not only to tubal coagulation but also to lysis of adhesions.

Coagulation with Low Voltage

From 1970 to 1973, before the development of low-voltage coagulation forceps, I performed experiments for coagulation of the oviducts by the bipolar forceps technique customary in neurosurgery (Fig. 101). Histochem-

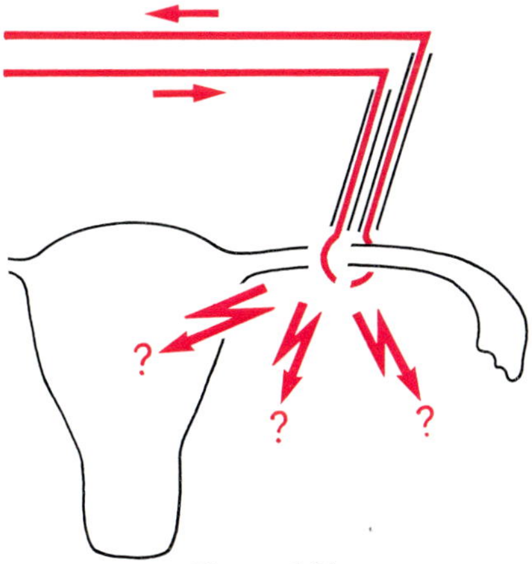

Figure 101

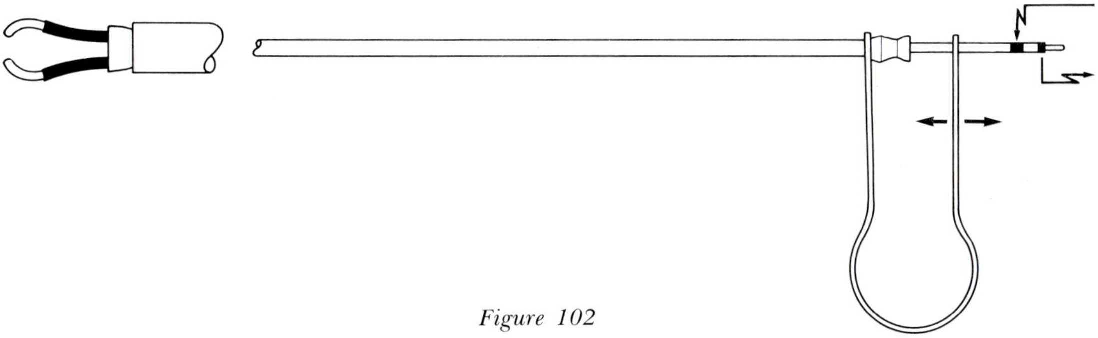

Figure 102

ical experiments had shown that the oviducts can be optimally coagulated in this way. However, clean electrodes were a prerequisite. Two successive coagulations with the same forceps are *not* feasible, since necrotic remnants of tissue insulate the metal jaws. With polished jaws, a high-frequency of 20 to 30 watts is required to achieve the coagulating temperature against the resistance of the tissue electrolytes. A great disadvantage of the bipolar technique is the sparking frequently observed as a result of the close mutual proximity of the electrodes. This gives rise to temperatures of over 500° C, and thus to charring of the tissues (Figs. 89 and 90). The danger inherent in the bipolar forceps, therefore, is not reduced perceptibly. The danger to the patient from high-frequency is merely lessened. The coagulation process in tubal sterilization, for instance, is not controllable, so that a clean and clear-cut surgical procedure is not possible. For this reason, the high-frequency generator has been banned from our own gynecologic endoscopy room since the end of 1972.

The modern low-voltage coagulation technique depends in principle on the

Figure 103

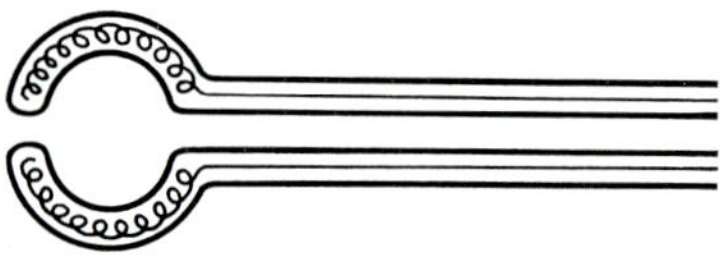

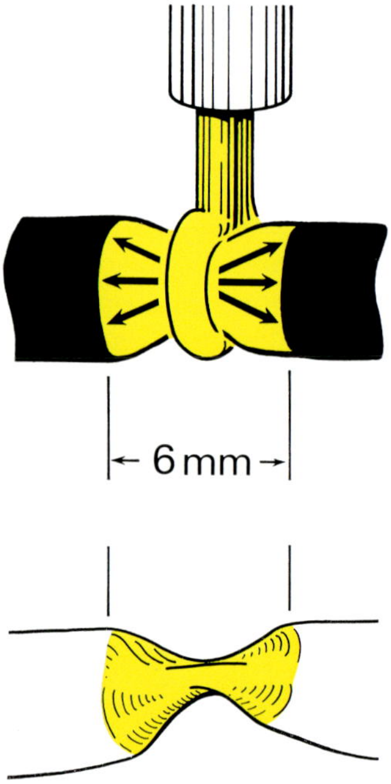

Figure 104

regulated heating of a resistance wire at the jaws of, for example, the atraumatic forceps (Fig. 103).

For heating purposes, either AC or DC at a maximum of 5 to 6 volts is required. The temperature of the jaws is regulated electronically. They emit a constant heat attuned to the coagulation requirements, i.e., to the mass of the tissue being coagulated. The sketch in Fig. 104 shows that the heat flows only to the tissue in actual contact with the forceps. No tissues are coagulated except those that can be monitored directly by the eye. The constancy of the "physiologic" coagulation temperature in the oviduct in the course of low-voltage sterilization is shown by the temperature curve in Figure 91. Charring of tissue and similar dangers are therefore impossible (cf. the temperature curve for high frequency in Figures 88–90).

The new coagulation technique with weak current became possible through the construction of my new switching and regulating apparatus. Its working principle is represented in Figure 105. There is a current and volt regulator that is not

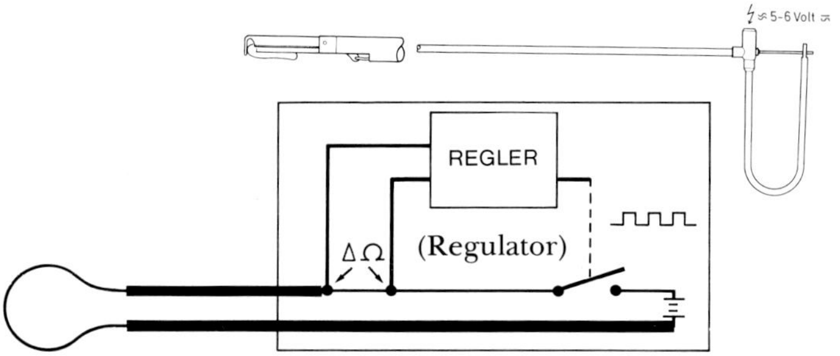

Figure 105

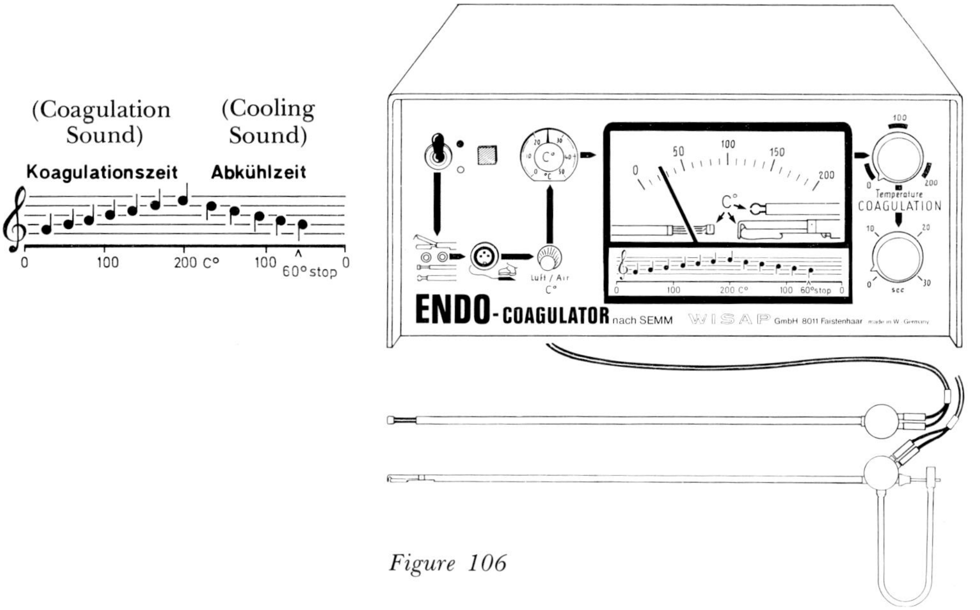

Figure 106

influenced by the temperature within the loop of the forceps, and which supplies the electrical energy according to the preselected dial setting. The tissue in touch with the heating wire (i.e., forceps jaws, point coagulator, wire loop) is heated to a selected constant temperature without contacting the electric current. The tissue is then coagulated by shear thermal conduction.

The practical use of this regulation system is being realized in the Semm Endocoagulator (Fig. 106). This apparatus for the first time permits the combined use of three instruments: (1) punch coagulator; (2) crocodile forceps; and (3) atraumatic coagulation forceps. Thus, coagulation of the tube, adhesions, endometriosis, and so on, can be accomplished without any electric hazard for the patient, although 5 volts of current are not injurious in this system, which precludes contact with the patient's body.

The Endocoagulator shows optically and acoustically the progress of the coagulation effect. An increasing sound frequency is produced as the local tissue temperature rises. This whistle indicates the boiling point and stays at the same frequency until the last water has been evaporated. Only after complete evaporation of the tissue water within the grasp of the forceps has occurred can the temperature reach the chosen maximum temperature value. Depending on the thickness of the mass of tissue to coagulate (fine adhesion, tube, fat, etc.), the end-temperature is set at 120 to 190 degrees. After discontinuing this heating current, the decreasing sound frequency remains in a linear relationship to the decreasing temperature. The operator then knows when the coagulated tissue has cooled so that the forceps can be removed without danger. The cooled tissues may then be allowed to fall back safely into the abdominal cavity.

On a large dial the same process can be followed visually. A built-in synchronizer that beats in five-second intervals limits the coagulation time to proved values. The coagulation effects, whether monitored acoustically or optically, are controlled by depressing a foot pedal while viewing through the endoscope. All instruments used in this system are made of stainless steel and may be readily autoclaved.

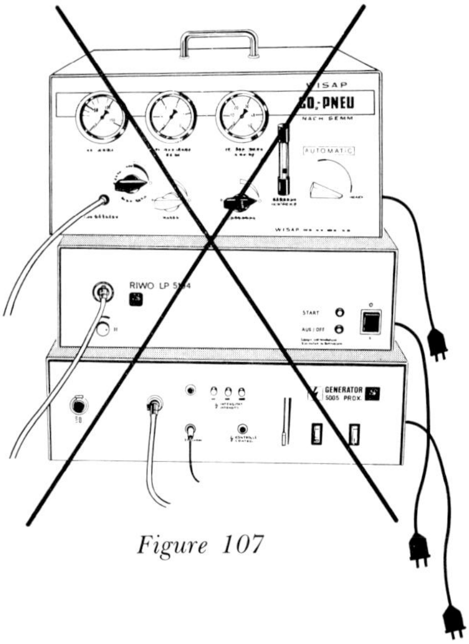

Figure 107

Instead of a blind and uncontrolled burning with high-frequency current, we have regulated protein coagulation at preselected levels of electric current today. Figure 104 demonstrates the very limited site of action possible with low current coagulation instruments. The coagulation effect is controlled to the millimeter (see also Figs. 345–347).

Thus modern optics, gas control, cold light, and electronics have transformed,

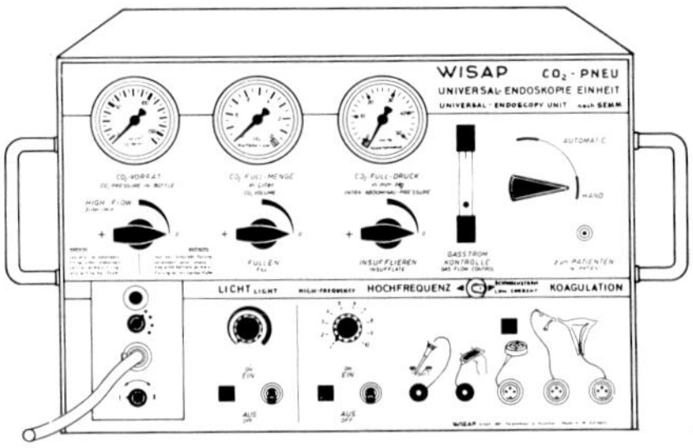

Figure 108

simplified, and improved—in short, revolutionized—our procedures in pelvic laparoscopy.

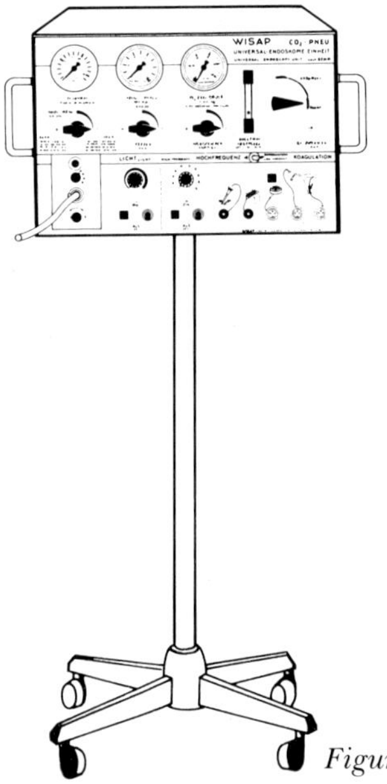

Figure 109

9. COMBINATION APPARATUS FOR CARBON DIOXIDE, LIGHT AND ELECTRICITY FOR LAPAROSCOPIC USE

As one technologic advance follows on the heels of another these days, it is not unusual to find varied pieces of apparatus stacked up in our endoscopy rooms

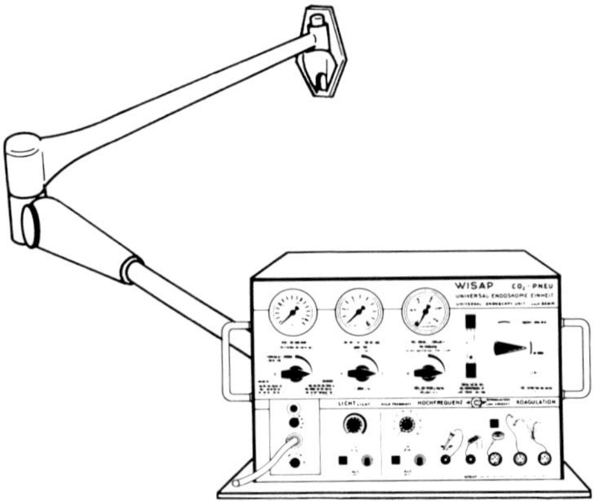

Figure 110

(Fig. 107). Lately, however, manufacturers have been producing units that combine all the energy sources and controls in a single housing: gas, light, and electricity for endoscopic needs, with both high-frequency and low-voltage current to meet all the requirements of this transition period. All the knobs, dials, and indicators are on a front panel where they can be read easily. Such combinations, known as Universal Endoscopy Units (Fig. 108), allow the operator to monitor all the dials at a glance, and thus the risks inherent in the complexities of the laparoscopic procedure are reduced. The equipment is mounted on a space-saving cart or wall-mount (Figs. 109, 110).

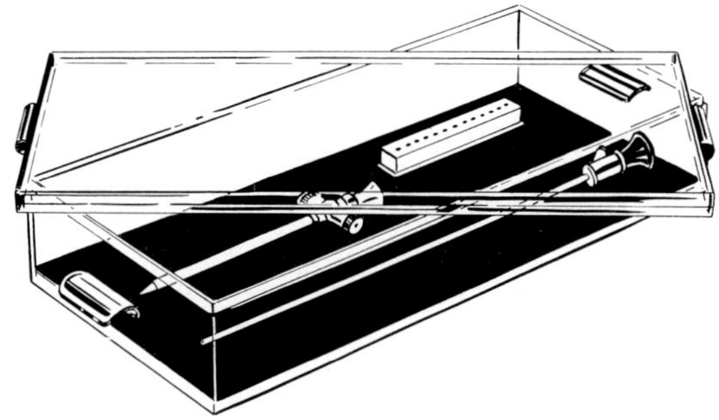

Figure 111

10. CARE AND STERILIZATION OF LAPAROSCOPIC INSTRUMENTS

Special directions for care and sterilization of the various endoscopic instruments are supplied by the individual manufacturers. The following basic rules apply to the lenses. The least harmful method of sterilization is doubtless by means of formalin tablets in either a metal or see-through container (Fig. 111). A disadvantage of this method is that efficient sterilization takes about 24 hours.

Next, there is gas sterilization. It should be ascertained in advance from the manufacturer whether his instruments will stand the pressure variations involved in gas sterilization, from vacuum to a pressure of 2 to 4 atmospheres.

Some manufacturers recommend autoclaving the laparoscope. The rapid heating (up to 120° C) of the nonhomogeneous structural elements of the optical system (glass, metal, and plastic) undoubtedly has an effect on the life of the instrument.

All metal parts, including the insulated instruments such as atraumatic forceps, biopsy forceps, etc., can be autoclaved without fear of damage, and can be put into the instant sterilizer without harm.

In the case of the latest fiberglass trocars, etc., in common use in America as a means of lessening danger from the ubiquitous high-frequency current, the manufacturers' directions should be followed to the letter. No doubt in the future these fiberglass instruments will give way to sturdy, long-lived metal instruments intended for low-voltage use with the sterilization unit and the Endotherm.

The endoscopic instruments must be not only sterilized but also thoroughly cleansed. After each endoscopic procedure the trocar, forceps, etc., must be disassembled (Fig. 112), painstakingly cleaned, rinsed in silicon oil, and only then subjected to sterilization. If this rule is neglected before sterilization, tissue fluids and blood may become encrusted in the 30 cm-long hollow instruments. On subsequent use, particles of foreign substance may become dislodged from the improperly cleaned instruments and find their way into the next patient's abdomen.

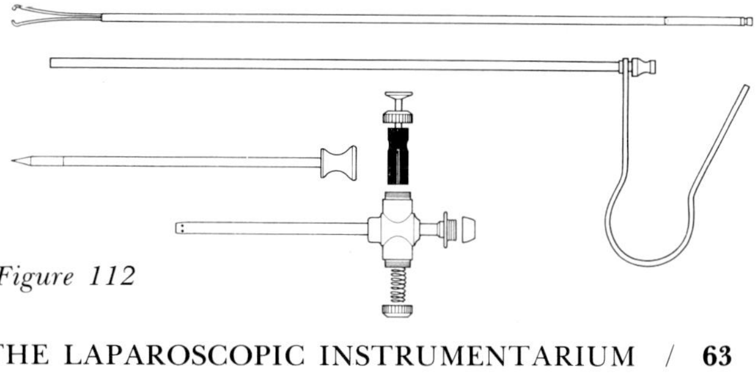

Figure 112

V

Laparoscopic Documentation

1. THE LAPAROSCOPIC PHOTO

The desire to capture the endoscopic image photographically and thus achieve documentation goes back to the beginnings of photography. Photographic exposures were achieved even with the endoscopes of Desormeaux and Stein (Fig. 7). In the years that followed, experiments were made with incandescent tungsten bulbs introduced inside the body, using brief overload illumination to produce the light needed. However, for many years the long exposure times (1/5 to 1/30 second) and the small, indistinct pictures were far from satisfactory.

It was not until it became technologically possible to mount an electronic flash-bulb at the tip of the endoscope (Fig. 113)* that well-lighted photographs at fairly short range inside the abdomen could be obtained. A gynecologist, Thomsen, in 1953 was the first to take color photographs of the cul-de-sac by the use of an intracorporeal flash. Camé in Switzerland carried this technique over into laparoscopy in 1954, and Fourès in France produced such an apparatus in 1955. The German Society of Electrotechnicians permits no more than 24 volts for use in connection with the human body. The firm of Richard Wolf, in cooperation with Lent, in 1961 developed an electronic flash capable of functioning under this limitation.

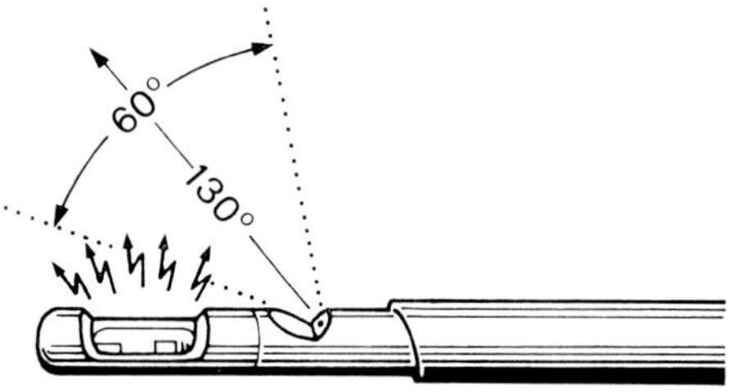

Figure 113

This epoch-making advance in upper abdominal laparoscopy led to the appearance of the first worthwhile laparoscopic color atlases (e.g., Beck, 1968). However, this technologic advance was not yet sufficiently developed for application to gynecologic laparoscopy, because of the distally located flash-bulb and the consequent impossibility of a direct-forward 180° line of vision. The latter is especially important in laparoscopy in order to facilitate topographic scanning of the pelvis.

In addition, the discharge of the electronic flash for 1/800 second in the abdominal cavity at 380 volts and 50 to 100 watts per second was dangerous for the

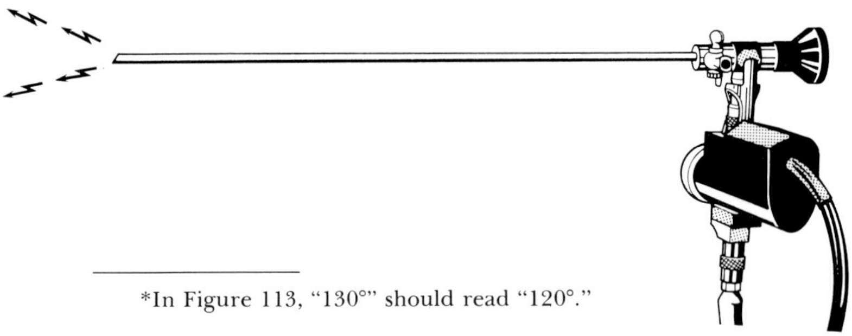
Figure 114

*In Figure 113, "130°" should read "120°."

patient, as evidenced by a sudden twitching sometimes observed at the moment the picture was snapped (Cohen, et al., 1970, p. 65).

Storz tried to lessen the risk by shifting the vacuum flash-bulb into an insulated housing directly beside the eye-piece (Fig. 114), but even with this technique I could not always avoid an electric shock to the patient. In addition, the flash, attached so close to the eye-piece, heated up very quickly in the course of a sequence of photography, resulting in extreme discomfort for the operator.

In 1966 I laid down a rule that *all* electric current for the discharge of electronic flash-bulbs must be eliminated from the immediate sphere of laparoscopic activity. As the fiberglass light cable attained ever greater technologic perfection, this requirement was met by the firm of Richard Wolf (Fig. 115: (1) electronic

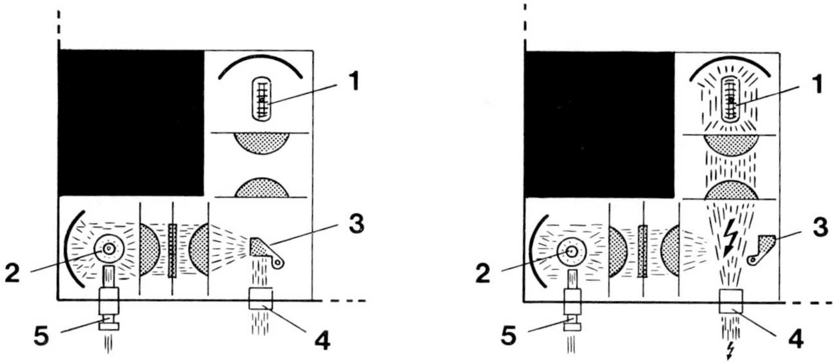

Figure 115

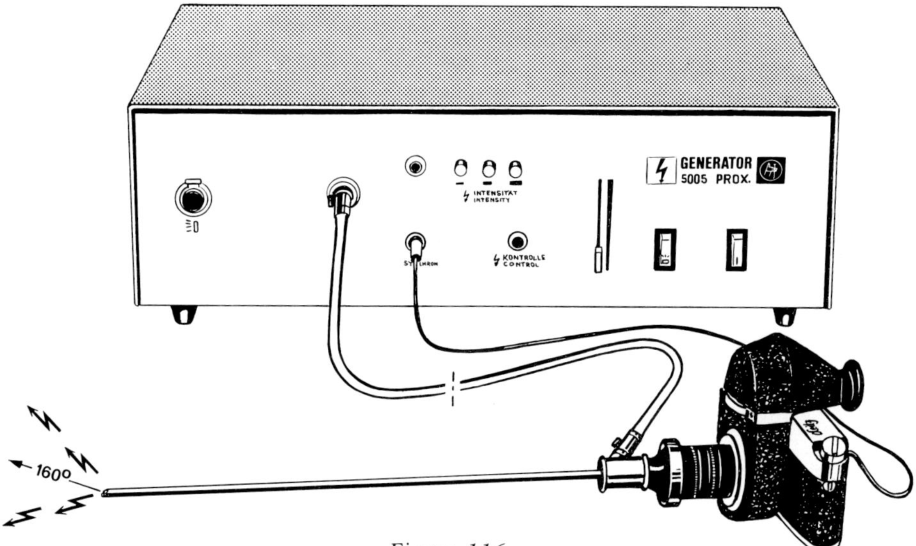

Figure 116

flash-tube; (2) halogen projection lamp; (3) deflection prism; (4) aperture for light and flash; and (5) light aperture). Today the high-efficiency electronic flash occurs far away from the patient, and its light is reflected into the abdomen harmlessly via a fiberoptic cable (Fig. 116).

With this extracorporeal flash, together with the routine diagnostic lens (from

Wolf with 6 mm trocar, or from Storz with 7.2 mm trocar), well-lighted 10 mm color slides or color prints from negative film can be made that are satisfactory for the documentation of routine findings.

For scientific purposes, however, an 11 mm diameter laparoscope, which gives pictures with a diameter of about 30 mm, is necessary. With a 24 × 36 mm format, the upper and lower margins of the round picture made by the circular lens are cropped (see Laparoscopic Atlas section). This set-up affords pictures seen from the vantage point of the navel, with full illumination of the pelvis. The color reproductions in this atlas almost without exception were taken with extracorporeal flash, transmitted to the lens via a fiberoptic cable.

Basic requirements for modern endoscopic photography are as follows.

(1) The electronic flash must be placed far away from the surgical site, i.e., at the other end of a fiberoptic cable.

(2) The fiberoptic cable must be continuous from the light source to the distal end of the endoscope. Even a single break of continuity cuts down the amount of light transmitted by about 50 per cent.

(3) The electronic flash condenser must recharge very rapidly, so that slide sequences covering the course of an operation can be made at intervals of no more than five seconds.

(4) The rectangular endoscopic slide in 24 × 36 mm format is the size of choice and has been achieved since 1969, using 16 mm film.

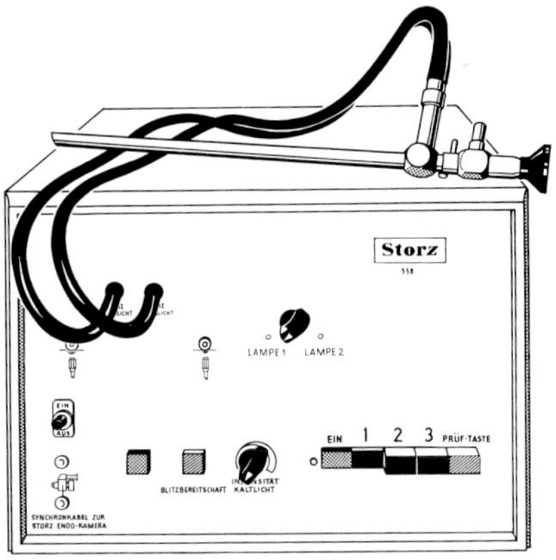

Figure 117

Since great technologic progress is still being made in this field, no further detailed suggestions will be made here about the camera housing, etc. In any case, the mirror-reflex camera with automatic film advance dominates the scene. Mechanical winding of the camera by hand is a great hindrance in laparoscopic photography. The physician who is about to acquire new photographic equipment for use in laparoscopy should first study the latest developments in this field. Recently, the Storz firm introduced a photolight source that eliminates to a large degree all previous lighting problems without requiring acquisition of new optical equipment (Figs. 117 and 118). All that is required is to slide their 11 mm diameter fiberoptic cable over the routine Hopkins optical instrument in order to transmit the intense, bright light over two more fiberoptic cables.

In the present discussion a sharp distinction must be made between simple documentation of findings in routine laparoscopy and scientific photography for teaching and publication. Since no essential changes have come about recently in the light sensitivity of color film, it is not to be expected that the gap between rou-

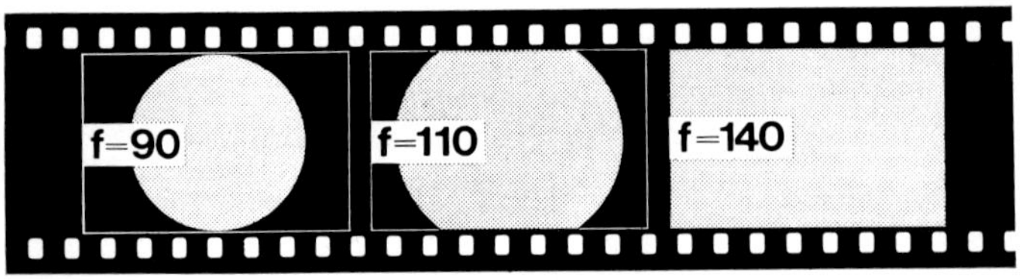

Figure 118

tine and scientific documentation will be reduced in the immediate future. The rapid developments of the last ten years, indicated in Fig. 119, will probably slow to a temporary halt.

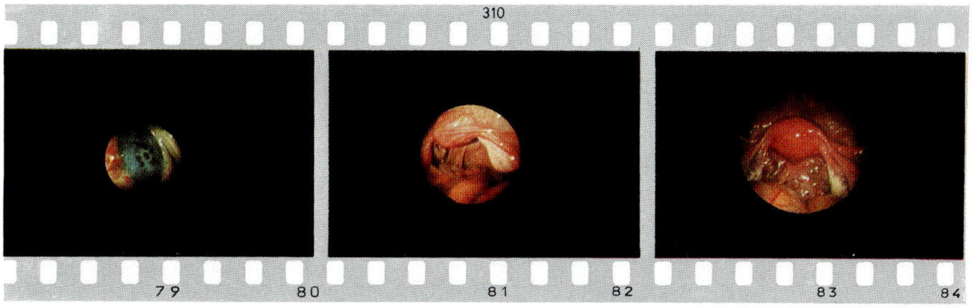

prior to 1965 1965 1966

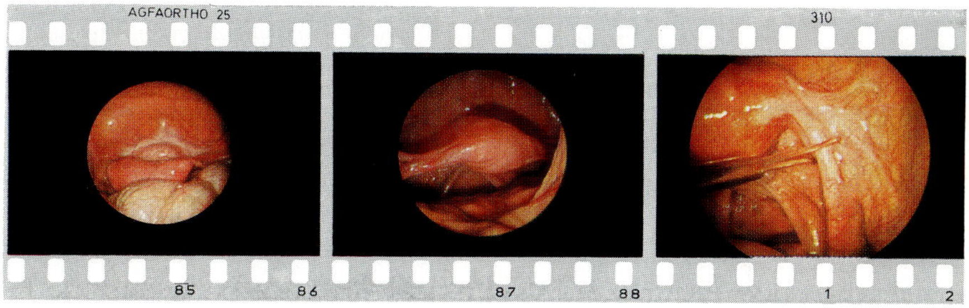

Figure 119 1968 1969 1970

2. LAPAROSCOPIC CINEMATOGRAPHY

Attempts at cinematographic documentation in endoscopy are as old as the development of the motion picture camera itself. Up until 1966, however, all such attempts were unsatisfactory; seven-tenths of the screen remained dark, and only at its center did a small, circular moving picture appear. Not until 1967 to 1968 was it possible (using light from xenon-vapor lamps and a further development of the Hopkins optic and 16 mm color film of 22 DIN speed) to obtain well-lighted motion pictures of the entire pelvis via fiberoptic cable. The combination of light sources used for this cinematography, two xenon-vapor lamps of 450 W (Fig. 120 shows Storz 6000 "Film Fountain": (1) integral light cable; (2) fiberoptic cable to the cold-light source for examination), permits routine laparoscopic cinematography. Today, thanks to finer focusing mechanisms, a single light source is sufficient.

In 1969 there came the final breakthrough to full-screen color movies with the aid of the Lumina optic. Shortly after this the light source was reduced in size to take up no more room than a portable typewriter (Fig. 121, light source for full-screen 16 mm movies from Wolf, with Beaulieu camera).

Since the goal seems to be in sight in the development of quality motion pictures, the following data perhaps may be relevant.

(*a*) *Endoscope.* The 11 mm diameter laparoscope serves as the optical source with its 30° or 180° view (Storz or Wolf). The light is transmitted via one (Wolf) or two (Storz) thick fiberoptic cables all the way to the distal end of the laparoscope (Fig. 122. Storz. (1) 11 mm diameter laparoscope for documentation with Hopkins magnifying lens; (2) 11 mm diameter laparoscope with focusing lens giving exceptionally sharp enlargement; (3) trocar for 11 mm diameter laparoscope).

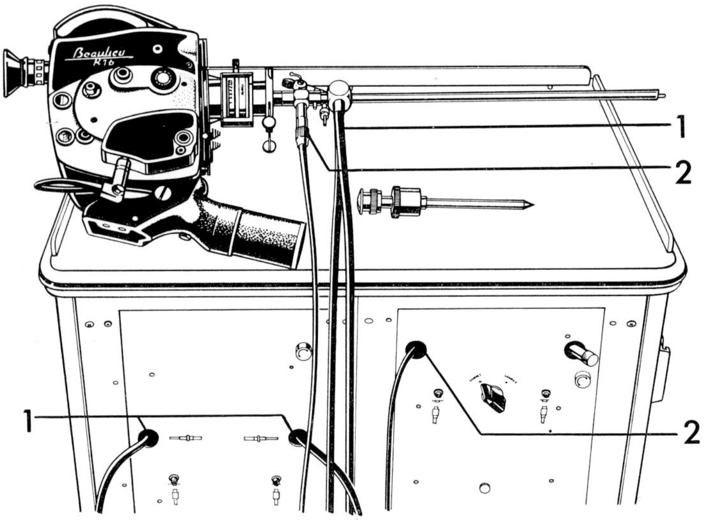

Figure 120

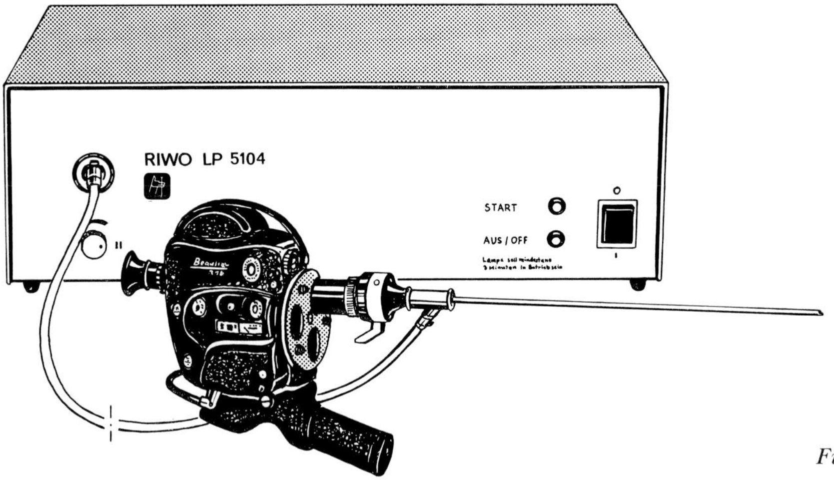

Figure 121

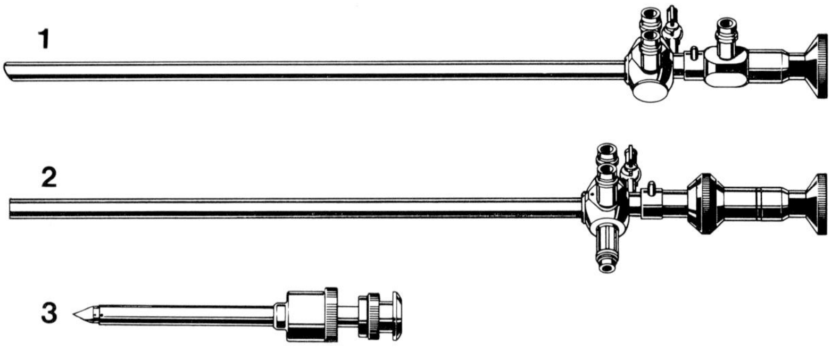

Figure 122

(*b*) The *telephoto lens* must match the eye-piece of the endoscope, the threaded connection to the camera being of international standard. The length of the telephoto lens is limited by the amount of light. The above laparoscopes, using a 90 to 110 mm telephoto lens and 16 mm film, make possible full-screen, well-lighted, panoramic views of the pelvis.

250 to 400 W xenon-vapor lamps serve as light sources. The ignition system requires that the high-pressure lamps be turned on five minutes before filming in order to obtain authentic color rendition.

Until a 16 mm camera becomes available with automatic sector-wheel setting, light-metering through the lens, and an automatic regulator for the intensity of the light source, the optimal illumination for laparoscopic cinematography must continue to be by "feel."

When making movies one should bear in mind that the predominance of red in the pelvis swallows up considerable light (open the diaphragm one or two stops), whereas the ovary, for instance, which is white, reflects light threefold.

Movie Film

Black-and-white 16 mm film is out of the question for laparoscopic cinematography.

Kodak offers 16 mm Ektachrome EF 23° DIN. Recently it has been possible to get well-lit detail shots even with regular film, thanks to the high efficiency lamps available. Color rendition and quality copies are excellent in both instances.

Camera

The Bolex and Beaulieu 16 mm movie cameras are both worthy of discussion. The latter is handier. Its optical light-metering through the lens gives good basis for optical judgments. No automatic aperture is yet available, however. The picture in the Beaulieu finder flickers because of the revolution of the sector-wheel. As a result, correction of focal sharpness while filming, for example to achieve good panning, can be made only with difficulty.

The Bolex gives the better view in the finder, but no light-metering is available; however, experience indicates that this is less than vital, and I prefer the Bolex.

Light sources available to date permit camera speeds of 16 to 64 frames per second, the latter, of course, only for close-ups.

Endoscopic cinematography with 8 mm or Super-8 film no longer presents any difficulties from the point of view of lighting. The wide range of fully-automatic cameras here also permits problem-free filming. The scientific value of these films from the standpoint of reproducibility, however, is very poor. Blowing up 8 mm film to 16 mm leads to undesirable loss of sharpness for endoscopic work. A problem-free presentation of the future perspectives in endoscopy will be attempted in the following section.

3. LAPAROSCOPIC TV AND TAPE RECORDING

Developments in closed-circuit television in recent decades have been on a phenomenal scale. At Expo-1970 in Osaka, Japan, a black-and-white television camera the size of a Super-8 camera was exhibited for the first time. The portable tape-recorder for use with this camera was no larger than the ordinary portable model. In the course of our teaching we are still using one of these to demonstrate laparoscopic findings (Fig. 123).

Since in the endoscopic image the colors all appear as varying gradations of red, the contrast in black-and-white TV appears only in shades of grey, which is unsatisfactory. But, for courses in laparoscopy or demonstrations while teaching, this process (Fig. 123) has been very worthwhile in recent years, making it possible for a number of spectators simultaneously to follow the demonstration and recognize the decisive manipulations.

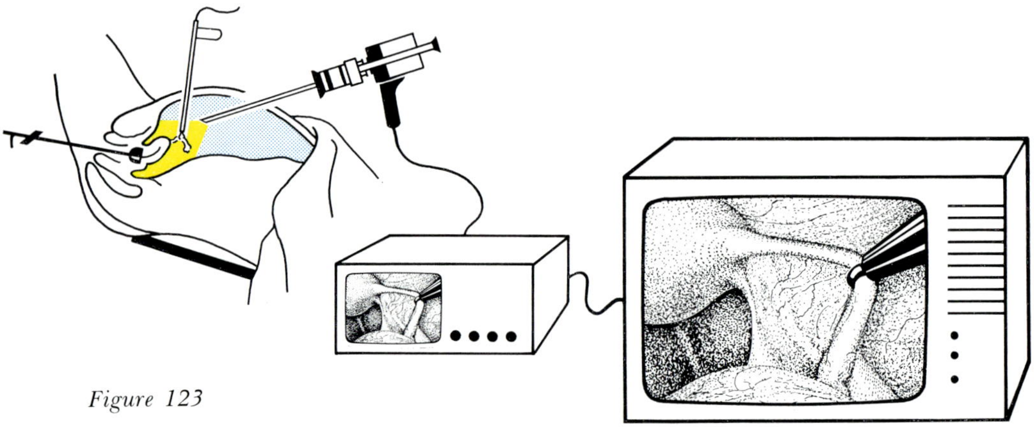

Figure 123

Problem-free endoscopic demonstrations in full color for large audiences were finally achieved through the use of Philips color TV (Fig. 124), a technologically sophisticated portable television camera that gave excellent pictures. Participants in the First European Congress of Endoscopy, Munich, 1970, were

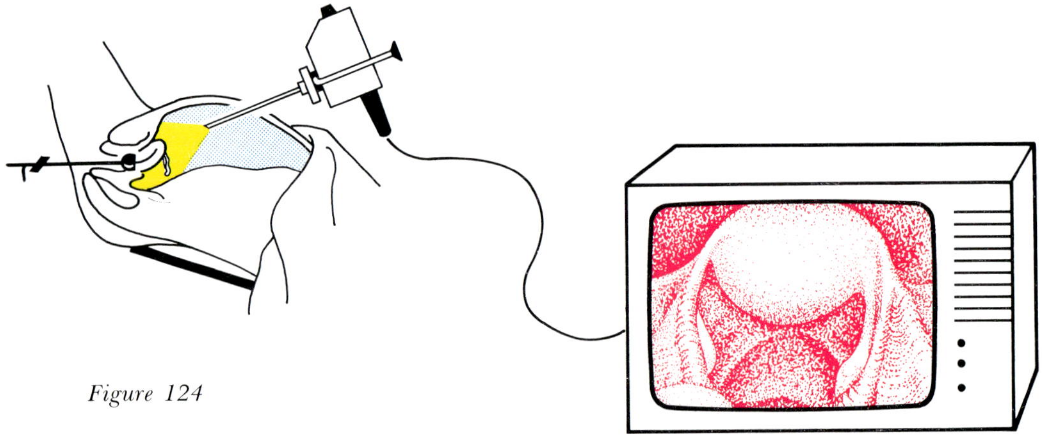

Figure 124

the first to see a giant 60 × 80 foot color demonstration of peristalsis of the ureter in genital aplasia (in conjunction with Eidophor-CIBA).

Now, five years later, the firms of Akai and Sony are manufacturing a small, light, battery-operated color television camera with a tape-recorder attachment (Fig. 125). A situation regarded as utopian four years ago has thus been realized, both in camera weight and price.

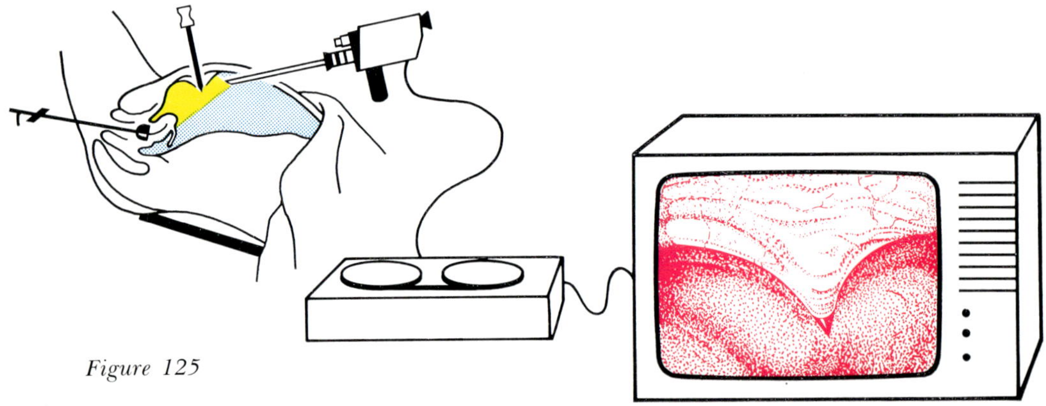

Figure 125

VI
The Technique of Gynecologic Laparoscopy

1. INDICATION FOR AND CONTRAINDICATION AGAINST LAPAROSCOPY

As a result of technologic progress with laparoscopic ends in optics, light, gas-insufflation equipment, ancillary instruments, and electricity, the range of available operational techniques has been expanded tremendously. Technologic advances in photography, cinematography, and television also have made significant contributions. Not only operative techniques, but also diagnostic and therapeutic possibilities can be demonstrated optimally to a sizable group of observers.

Of course, the danger remains that laparoscopy might come to be regarded as too simple a procedure and too conclusive a diagnostic means—one that could be learned by casual observation. It must be stressed, therefore, that laparoscopy represents an operative technique in gynecology that must be taught only as the climax in the course of professional education, one that even then demands intensive training: (1) *because of the necessary insertion of the trocar through the abdominal wall,* and (2) *because of the difficulties involved in monocular vision.*

Indications

Without discounting the importance of the above preamble, it must be realized that the catalogue of indications for laparoscopy in gynecology and obstetrics has been expanded radically. The effective application of laparoscopy leads toward new horizons in diagnostic and therapeutic gynecology.

The list of indications falls under three headings.

NONSURGICAL DIAGNOSTIC LAPAROSCOPY.

1. Differential diagnosis of normal vs. pathologic female genitals.
2. Primary sterility.
3. Secondary sterility or infertility.
4. Prediagnosed (e.g., by insufflation, hysterosalpingogram, etc.) tubal factor in sterility.
5. Postoperative follow-up in sterility cases.
6. Acute lower abdominal distress in early pregnancy.
7. Suspicion of endometriosis.
8. "Second-look" laparoscopy after hormonal treatment for endometriosis.
9. Therapy-resistant bladder irritation (e.g., endometriosis of the dome of the bladder).
10. Chronic distress in the lower abdomen.
11. Congestion of pelvic veins.
12. Chronic salpingitis.
13. Acute or subacute disease of the lower abdomen.
14. Differential diagnosis of intra- vs. extrauterine pregnancy.
15. Chronic pelvic pain.
16. Bleeding of corpus luteum.
17. Differential diagnosis of ovarian vs. adnexal conglomerate tumors and leiomyomata.

18. Differential diagnosis of uterus duplex vs. ovarian tumor.
19. Metrorrhagia in the postmenopausal patient (e.g., granulosa cell tumor).
20. Pathologic amenorrhea.
21. Differential diagnosis of salpingitis vs. parametritis or appendicitis, especially in the puerperium.
22. Substitute for exploratory laparotomy as so-called "second-look" operation in ovarian carcinoma.
23. Genital malformation.
24. Vaginal atresia, with or without internal malformation.
25. Uterine hypoplasia.
26. Search for perforated IUD.
27. Therapy-resistant abdominal distress.
28. Suspicion of uterine perforation.
29. Laparoscopic monitoring of hysteroscopic intrauterine manipulations.
30. Endoscopic monitoring of conventional or suction curettage after perforation.
31. Diagnosis of acute internal bleeding after trauma.

Surgical Diagnostic Laparoscopy.

1. Ovarian sterility; primary or secondary ovarian hypoplasia.
2. Tubal factor: tubal dye insufflation in sterility.
3. Puncture of follicular cyst (e.g., mature) and aspiration of fluids (e.g., for cul-de-sac cytology).
4. Gonadal biopsy in uterine aplasia for sex determination.
5. Suspicion of ovarian carcinoma.
6. Substitution of laparoscopy for exploratory laparotomy in ovarian carcinoma.
7. Suspicion of tuberculosis in the adnexa, genitalia, or abdomen.
8. Suspicion of hormone-active tumors (e.g., granulosa cell tumor).

Surgical Therapeutic Laparoscopy.

1. Tubal sterilization by coagulation in the nonpuerperal patient.
2. Tubal sterilization by coagulation in the puerperal and postabortal patient.
3. Tubal sterilization by ligation.
4. Tubal sterilization with clips (e.g., tantalum clips) or Silastic rings.
5. Local monitoring after abdominal operations for sterility (e.g., Pomeroy, Madlener, etc.).
6. Salpingolysis in connection with tubal dye insufflation.
7. Adnexal correction after sterility operations or conservative operations in connection with tubal dye insufflation.
8. Coagulation of endometrial implants.
9. Ovulation disturbances in the Stein-Leventhal syndrome (partial ovarian resection).
10. Puncture of juvenile ovarian cysts with cyst wall resection.
11. Puncture and resection of "chocolate" cysts.
12. Correction of chronic (nongynecologic) scar tissue in the abdomen.
13. Postoperative lysis of adhesions in the chronically (gynecologically) scarred abdomen.
14. Puncture and resection of hydatids (e.g., on the ampullae).
15. Instillation of medications into the abdominal cavity (e.g., cortisone for prophylaxis of adhesions).
16. Cyst-puncture and aspiration of ascites in overstimulation following HCG/HMG treatment.

17. Correction of herniated omentum after laparoscopy.

Some of these indications require special commentary, for example, *metrorrhagia in postmenopausal women.* Laparoscopy should be employed for elderly women, even with negative findings on palpation and proliferation of endometriosis. In two dubious cases we were able to diagnose pea-sized granulosa cell tumors visually at laparoscopy and verify these histologically by biopsy.

After *difficult and extended operations on the fallopian tubes,* it sometimes is advisable to perform laparoscopy on the fourth to the sixth day in connection with hydropertubation. In this way the start of adhesions can be prevented by aspiration of coagulated blood, etc., through the 4 mm tube, and regrowth can be hindered by instillation of 500 ml of physiologic saline solution plus 500 mg of cortisone.

Biopsy for Sex-Determination of Gonads. Biopsy nowadays replaces the once customary exploratory laparotomy in vaginal or uterine aplasia, and enables the sex of the gonads to be diagnosed beyond the shadow of a doubt (see also Fig. 332).

Chronic Lower Abdominal Pain. A careful choice of laparoscopy in chronic pain of the lower abdomen creates a completely new field of diagnosis and therapy. Patients with lower abdominal pain can often be reassured after laparoscopy that they possess "normal" internal genitalia, and most are relieved of years of psychosomatic abdominal distress and become perfectly healthy. In others, a single linear adhesion is found linking an ovary and the posterior wall of the uterus or the intestine, etc., which has led to complete personality changes in the patient, especially when dyspareunia results. In such patients, usually classified as "hysterical," the decision for laparotomy would not be justifiable, and laparoscopy is clearly the method of choice. In fact, the distress can be cured by a snip of the scissors after coagulation—both at laparoscopy.

Other cases show varying amounts of surface endometriosis that have escaped diagnosis because of completely contrary clinical symptoms.

Contraindications

In laparoscopy we distinguish between absolute and relative contraindications.

ABSOLUTE CONTRAINDICATIONS. If a patient is declared a bad risk by the anesthesiologist, the sum of individual findings leading to his decision amounts also to a contraindication against laparoscopy. In borderline cases the decision should be made in favor of classic exploratory laparotomy, since in these any necessary surgical therapy can be instituted without loss of time.

Special contraindications are acute peritonitis in the upper abdomen, abdominal distention, etc. Laparoscopy is also out of the question in cases of hemorrhagic diathesis.

RELATIVE CONTRAINDICATIONS. *Tumors larger than the fist* do not constitute a primary indication for laparoscopy. Only in borderline cases, when surgery is inappropriate for other reasons, can laparoscopy determine whether postponement of the operation for vital or personal reasons is justifiable or more life-threatening than the immediate operative risk.

This does not apply to *ovarian carcinoma* once it has become larger than the head or has reached the arch of the ribs. Here, primary exploratory laparotomy, which would be very taxing to the patient, can be replaced by laparoscopy, through which sufficient material can be obtained for histology. After appropriate chemotherapy, a repeat laparoscopy may indicate the need for a "second-look" operation.

The first exploratory laparotomy, hitherto customary, can thus be avoided, and the second-look operation becomes the first taxing undertaking for the patient.

Known diaphragmatic hernia. With the patient in a 15° Trendelenburg position, limiting intra-abdominal pressure, and simultaneous intubation anesthesia, diaphragmatic hernia constitutes only a relative contraindication. It is recommended in such cases that the abdomen be inflated to only 8 to 10 mm Hg.

Acute pelvic peritonitis. In such cases, inflation of the abdomen could destroy the physiologic barrier between the lower and upper abdomen caused by exudation of fibrin, thus provoking a dangerous abdominal peritonitis.

It is worth noting here that ailments considered as presenting high risk for upper abdominal laparoscopy, such as respiratory insufficiency, cardiac insufficiency, coronary disease, threatened hepatic decompensation, massive portocavernous collapse, external hernia, and thyroid disease (as described by Rettenmaier, 1969), are of lesser significance in pelvic laparoscopy. This regard to the risk factors is one more reason to distinguish sharply between pelvic and upper abdominal laparoscopy.

When considering the indications and contraindications in laparoscopy, it should always be borne in mind that laparoscopy is a kind of middle ground between bimanual examination in the course of an examination under anesthesia, on the one hand, and exploratory laparotomy on the other. Thus, the one may call for greater, and the other for more limited, intervention. However, it is no service to the cause of laparoscopy to overdo its application and use it in place of exploratory or surgical laparotomy. Laparoscopy serves for the extension of gynecologic diagnostic techniques, and at most for minor surgical undertakings. Its overuse gives it a bad name.

EMERGENCY LAPAROSCOPY. Under this heading there are the following indications:

(1) Acute lower abdominal distress in early pregnancy.

(2) Differential diagnosis of salpingitis vs. parametritis and appendicitis, even in the puerperium.

(3) Suspicion of uterine perforation.

(4) Conventional or suction curettage after perforation with endoscopic monitoring.

(5) Correction of herniated omentum after laparoscopy.

(6) Cyst-puncture and aspiration of ascites in overstimulation after HCG/HMG treatment.

(7) Suspicion of intra-abdominal bleeding after trauma.

The immediate clarification at laparoscopy of gynecologic illnesses, which in classic gynecology would have required a waiting period of days or weeks, sometimes with hospitalization of the patient, is advantageous for both patient and physician, and the time spent in bed by the patient is shortened considerably.

Further discussion of indications can be found in the individual descriptions of the endoscopic color pictures in the Atlas section.

2. PREPARATION OF THE PATIENT FOR LAPAROSCOPY

Psychologic Preparation

The psychologic guidance and explanation offered to the patient with regard to laparoscopy is basically different from that for gynecologic laparotomy. The latter is a matter of surgical intervention in the face of a life-threatening pathologic prognosis, such as extrauterine pregnancy, removal of a large growth such as a uterine leiomyoma, or the restoration of fertility.

Laparoscopy, on the other hand, is primarily a diagnostic procedure that may:

(1) Entail minor surgical measures during the procedure.

(2) Lead a priori to, e.g., tubal sterilization carried out by coagulation.

(3) Require immediate laparotomy in conjunction with laparoscopy if the diagnostic findings warrant it, or if a complication occurs during laparoscopy that can be controlled only at laparotomy.

The physician must bring the patient to a psychologic understanding of the intended laparoscopy from these three aspects, advising her of the minor and low-risk nature of the procedure and its great personal advantage for her in perhaps avoiding a laparotomy. The operator however, must ask the patient beforehand whether:

(1) He has her consent to perform any operation medically necessary during the same session of anesthesia; or

(2) She prefers to have operation postponed.

Even though such measures become necessary in fewer than 1 per cent of cases, the operator must always explain to the patient in advance the ordinary anesthetic risks and the possibility that the laparoscopic technique may make it necessary to expand the procedure beyond mere diagnostic measures.

He also must explain that a second 5 mm puncture in the right or left lower abdomen may be undertaken if required in order to obviate the possibility of more extensive surgery. The patient must understand that at least 36 to 48 hours' hospitalization may be necessary. Especially in the case of treatment for sterility, the patient must be prepared to spend four to six additional days in the hospital in order that the tubal patency achieved at laparoscopy can be maintained through a series of hydropertubations.

The psychologically correct education of the patient is important because laparoscopy is a diagnostic procedure which must leave a favorable attitude in the mind of the patient, inasmuch as the same procedure may at some future time again be necessary for her.

Physical Preparation of the Patient for Laparoscopy

The full diagnostic and therapeutic potential of laparoscopy can be realized only if this procedure is as respected clinically as laparotomy and as appropriately prepared for. A few years ago anesthesia finally became established as a modern field of medical specialization. In the same way, laparoscopy must integrate its requirements into its techniques.

3. HOSPITALIZATION

For General Diagnostic and Surgical Laparoscopy

Laparoscopy can be performed at any time from infancy to old age, depending only on the indications, contraindications, and medical state. The day before the laparoscopy the patient is hospitalized in accordance with local custom, subjected to laboratory studies, and given an enema.

For Special Laparoscopy Such as Tubal Diagnosis, Diagnosis of Endometrial Implants, etc.

In such cases the patient is scheduled on the basis of her menstrual cycle. For diagnosis of the fallopian tubes the same preparations are made as for pertubation or hysterosalpingography, i.e., the eighth to the 12th day is optimal with a normal 28-day cycle. For diagnosis of endometrial implants laparoscopy should be undertaken between the 18th and 25th days, since small implants occasionally are overlooked in the first third of the cycle.

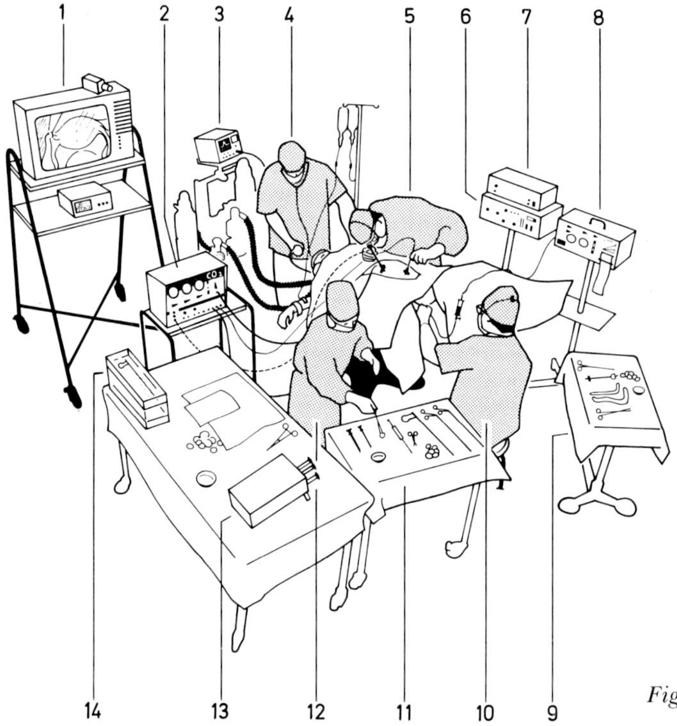

Figure 126

4. THE LAPAROSCOPIC OPERATING ROOM

The operating room for gynecologic laparoscopy must conform to all modern requirements of anesthesia and recovery (Fig. 126). If laparoscopy is performed casually (as is common practice) in a small anteroom of the operating suite (for the sake of better facilities for darkening the room), it is imperative that an adjacent large operating room be vacant and waiting throughout the procedure. In this connection it is important to repeat here the remarks of the father of gynecologic endoscopy, Palmer, which were later echoed by Thoyer-Rozat and other endoscopists:

> Celioscopy is a surgical procedure which must not be performed by a gynecological surgeon who is not himself capable of performing a laparotomy should occasion arise.

It is self-evident that only a fully accredited and experienced gynecologic surgeon must be allowed to perform laparoscopy or even be present in the immediate vicinity of the surgical table.

A normal operating table that permits the patient to be placed in the typical gynecologic positions and the head to be lowered by 15° (Trendelenburg) is satisfactory for laparoscopy (see Fig. 126).

5. ANESTHESIA

The patient is subjected, under supervision of the anesthesiologist, to the standard preoperative tests including blood studies, and is premedicated as for laparotomy.

There are three basic possibilities in anesthesia for laparoscopy.

Local Anesthesia

Palmer tried out the possibilities of performing laparoscopy under local anesthesia from 1948 to 1954. The inflation of the abdomen with the pneumoperitoneum, the insertion of the trocar, and the absolute necessity of rendering the uterus mobile with a vaginally inserted probe, all make laparoscopy a very unpleasant experience for the patient, even if the local anesthetic is expertly placed.

Since the patient very well may require repeated laparoscopies in her lifetime, it is desirable to avoid giving her a phobia about the procedure. Only in highly motivated patients should laparoscopic sterilization, for example, ever be dealt with under local anesthesia.

Epidural Anesthesia

The possibility of performing laparoscopy under epidural anesthesia has been investigated, chiefly by Frangenheim. Essentially the same qualifications apply here as for local anesthesia.

General Anesthesia

Following the general view held by other specialists, we have performed laparoscopy exclusively under general anesthesia for the past ten years. The patient is intubated and a stomach tube is put in place so that the stomach may not become distended as a result of hyperventilation preceding the intubation.

Because of the frequent use of electric current for coagulation purposes, *the use of inflammable* or *explosive gases in anesthesia is totally unacceptable.*

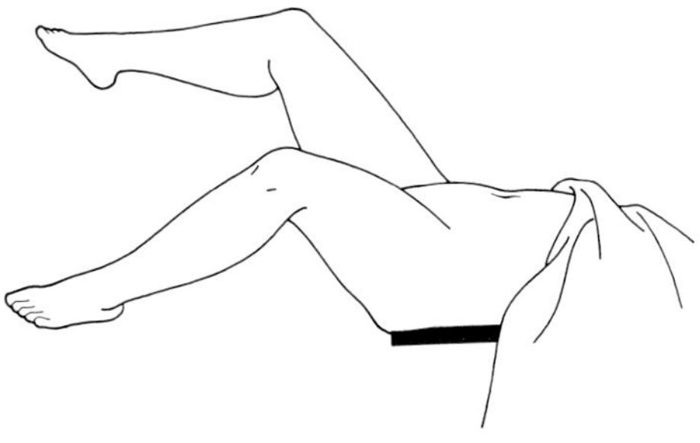

Figure 127

6. POSITIONING THE PATIENT

For laparoscopic purposes the patient should optimally be placed in typical gynecologic position (Fig. 127), e.g., dorsal lithotomy. The essential requirement is that the buttocks should extend a little beyond the table edge, so that the suc-

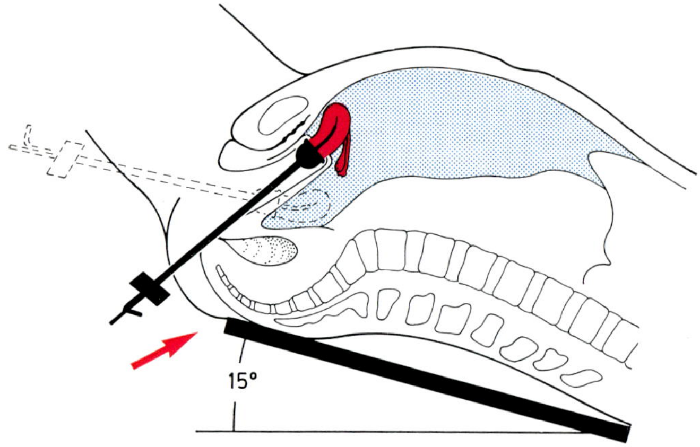

Figure 128

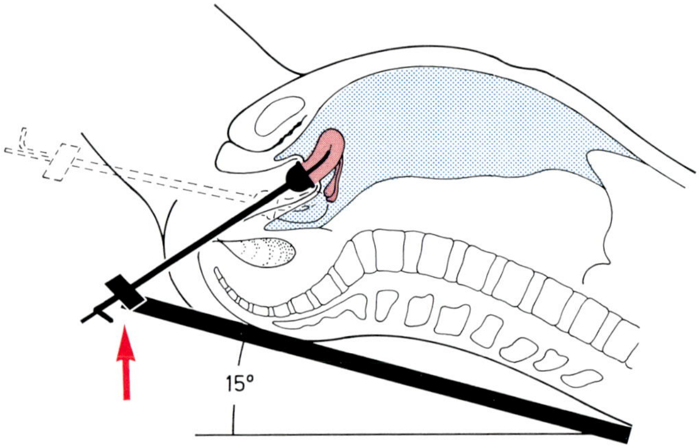

Figure 129

tion intrauterine cannula can be freely moved in a dorsal direction during the procedure (Fig. 128). If the table extends beyond the buttocks, the freedom of mobility of the probe is severely limited. The uterus cannot be maximally moved up against the posterior wall of the symphysis and the cul-de-sac can be only partially inspected (Fig. 129).

Laparoscopy to all intents and purposes is an intra-abdominal procedure. The legs must be draped and the abdomen disinfected according to the general rules of asepsis, just as at laparotomy.

During the preparatory measures the patient remains horizontal. As soon as the insufflation of gas begins, however, she is lowered to a Trendelenburg position with her head lowered about 15 degrees. This is necessary in order that the bowel will fall naturally toward the upper abdomen from the inception of insufflation (Fig. 130).

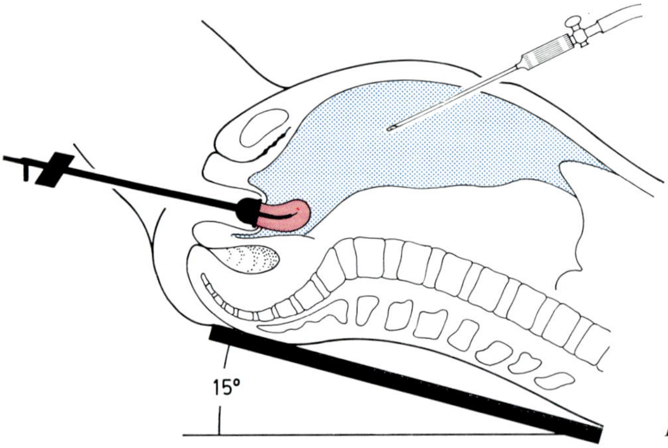

Figure 130

7. PREPARATION OF THE GENITALS

When the patient is fully asleep and covered with sterile sheets, the operator first inspects the internal female genitals bimanually. This prelaparoscopic bimanual inspection (Fig. 131) is extremely important and must *never* be omitted. In this way the operator orients himself to the size, mobility, and position of the uterus, as well as to the relationship to the adjacent organs that may be palpated. These palpation findings are of the greatest importance for the subsequent optical correlation of size of the various organs to be seen in the pelvis.

Since the uterine cavity must be probed prior to any laparoscopy (except when early pregnancy is suspected), the bimanual inspection serves also for diagnosing ante- or retroflexion, which is important for the insertion of the uterine sound. By this means the operator also satisfies himself that the bladder is empty, and he can perform a catheterization if necessary. A full bladder limits the overview of the pelvis to a great extent (Fig. 197). Finally, the proper positioning of the patient is again checked (Figs. 128 and 129).

After inspection and cleansing of the cervix, its outer lip is grasped and the

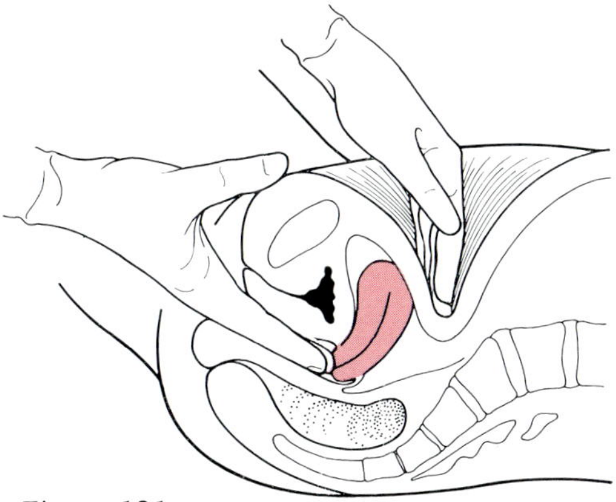

Figure 131

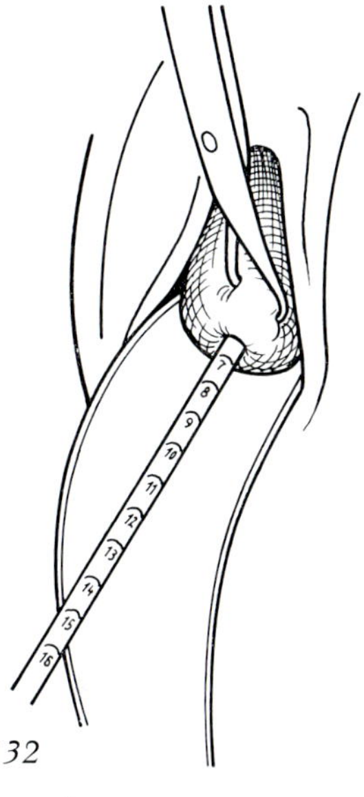

Figure 132

depth of the uterus is determined (Fig. 132). This is of great importance, especially in cases of sterility, since possible stricture of the internal os can thus be diagnosed.

Next, the suction intrauterine cannula is introduced into the cervical canal in a direction conforming to the ante- or retroflexion of the uterus. With a re-

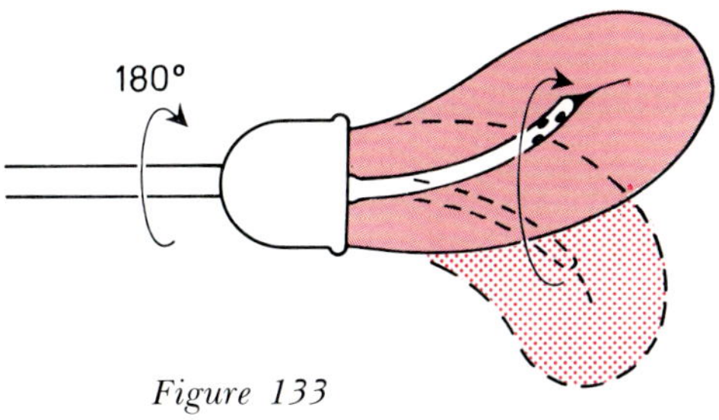

Figure 133

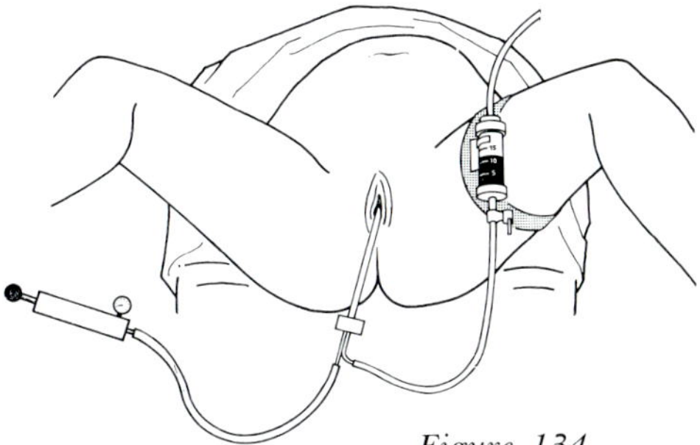

Figure 134

troflexed uterus, the curvature of the cannula is rotated cautiously anteriorly after insertion (Fig. 133) before placing the bell of the cannula over the cervix by suction. With the diagnosis of sterility, the insufflation tube of the cannula also is coupled by a hose to the intermediate dye-container (Fig. 134). When the suction cup is placed firmly over the cervix by about 2 to 3 cm, the body of the uterus and the shaft of the cannula projecting out of the vagina form a rigid unit, allowing the uterus to be moved about at will three-dimensionally.

Other intrauterine probes dating back to the insufflation instruments for x-ray contrast media in hysterosalpingography (G. K. F. Schultze) have one great disadvantage: they are fixed only loosely to the cervix by means of tenacula (Figs. 59 and 60), and the effective radius of motion of an intrauterine probe fixed thus loosely in the cavity is sharply limited. This means a reduced field of vision at laparoscopy.

If sterilization is to be performed following abortion, it is recommended that after curettage the uterus be elevated with the thickest dilator used for dilation of the cervical canal to obviate the danger of perforation.

8. CONTRAINDICATION AGAINST THE SUCTION INTRAUTERINE CANNULA

Pregnancy

When early intrauterine pregnancy is suspected, e.g., in a differential diagnosis between extra- or intrauterine pregnancy, the intrauterine cannula obviously must not be inserted. In this case the operator makes use of a ring forceps equipped with a medium-sized swab for mobilizing the uterus. Usually it is quite sufficient to insert two fingers into the vagina in order to move the uterus adequately. In many cases digital insertion into the rectum is useful.

Anatomic Idiosyncracies

In case of vaginal aplasia, well-known for instance in the Rokitansky-Küster-Hauser syndrome (Fig. 278), the insertion of the vacuum adapter naturally must be omitted. The internal genital sinus in such cases can easily be demonstrated digitally by depression of the external vulvar region and through the rectal ampulla.

Since laparoscopy is becoming more and more important, even in childhood, the approach may require lysis or dilatation of the hymenal membrane. Since irreparable defloration is unavoidable, permission of the parents or guardians must be obtained in advance.

The suction probe (Figs. 31 and 64–67) may be used where the intrauterine vacuum cannula is of limited value.

9. ESTABLISHMENT OF THE PNEUMOPERITONEUM

In gynecology it is preferable to induce the pneumoperitoneum with carbon dioxide gas, since the historical development of laparoscopy shows that endoscopy of the lower abdomen is particularly fraught with the possibility of complications, and carbon dioxide is a product of biologic metabolism and therefore open to the lowest possible rate of complications. Carbon dioxide: (1) is ten times more readily soluble in the blood and tissues, both physically and chemically, than pure oxygen; (2) involves no danger of explosion, especially important in the presence of electricity so common in laparoscopy; and (3) is available commercially, and therefore accessible to any hospital.

The use of nitrous oxide, as suggested by Siede (1962) for upper abdominal laparoscopy, is accompanied by two risks in the lower abdomen.

(1) The gynecologic patient is under general anesthesia. A theoretically more than lethal dose of about 5 liters of NO_2 in the free abdominal cavity, which may either be resorbed or flow uncontrolled into a blood vessel, represents a real risk in anesthesia.

(2) NO_2 is a nonflammable gas that nonetheless behaves like pure oxygen in the presence of flammable substances.

The inflation of the abdominal cavity with 3 to 6 liters of carbon dioxide gas must be accomplished in stages, alternating with safety tests. These tests (see below), amounting to no more than a few simple wrist motions plus visual monitoring, in no way complicate the procedure, but obviate the risks of this method.

The step-by-step procedure for inducing the pneumoperitoneum runs as follows.

Disinfection of the Navel

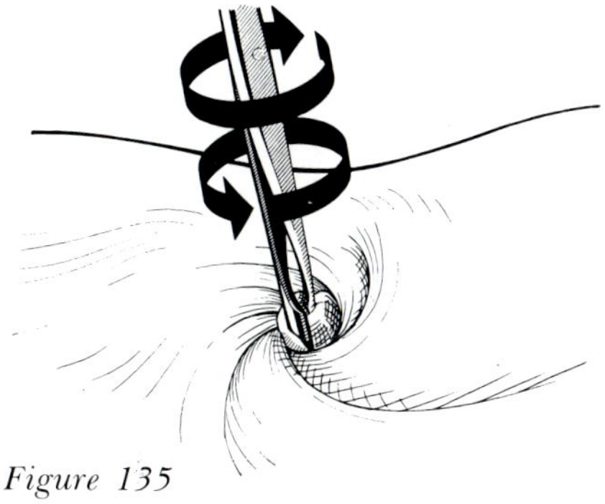

Figure 135

For cosmetic reasons laparoscopy today is always performed through the skin of the caudal aspect of the navel indentation. The disinfection of the navel calls for special care, since it is a traditional view in surgery that the navel is the dirtiest area of the human abdomen.

A cotton swab held in tweezers and dipped in strong skin disinfectant is rotated about ten times to the right in the navel with moderate pressure. This is then repeated with a fresh swab, rotating this time to the left (Fig. 135). The entire abdomen is then disinfected, especially the region of the navel. This technique serves to remove the surface layer of hardened squamous epithelium and cleanse the navel itself thoroughly. In rare cases in which the navel is unusually dirty, an additional pass with tweezers is necessary. Using this technique, we have not seen a single instance of navel infection in ten years.

The Needle Test

In order to be able to monitor by the dials any obstacles to insufflation in the abdomen, the insufflation resistance of the gas tube and of the injection needle must be less than 5mm Hg at a flow speed of 1 liter of gas per minute. If the

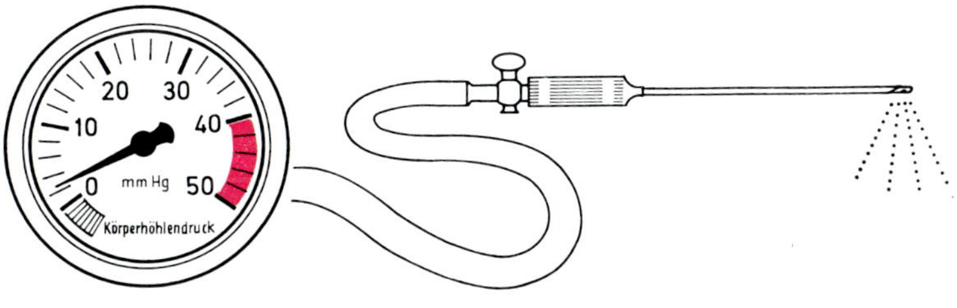

Figure 136

needle is placed incorrectly, i.e., if there are hindrances to the flow of gas such as the peritoneum (preperitoneal emphysema), omentum (omental emphysema), etc., the fact can be detected only within the range of 0 to 10 mm Hg. Higher pressures simply inflate the resistant membrane with no change of its registering on the dials. The result would be one of the complications mentioned in Chapter III, Sec. 2. We have modified the Verres needle to the extent that the flow resistance is less than 5 mm Hg when 1 liter of gas is flowing freely out into the atmosphere.

For the needle test the knob marked "INSUFFLATE" on the CO_2-Pneu-insufflator (see Fig. 54) is turned on. On turning the right-hand knob to "HAND" the "BODY CAVITY FILLING" dial must register no higher than 5 mm Hg (Fig. 136). If the pressure reads higher, it means either that the needle was not properly cleansed or that it is defective and must be exchanged.

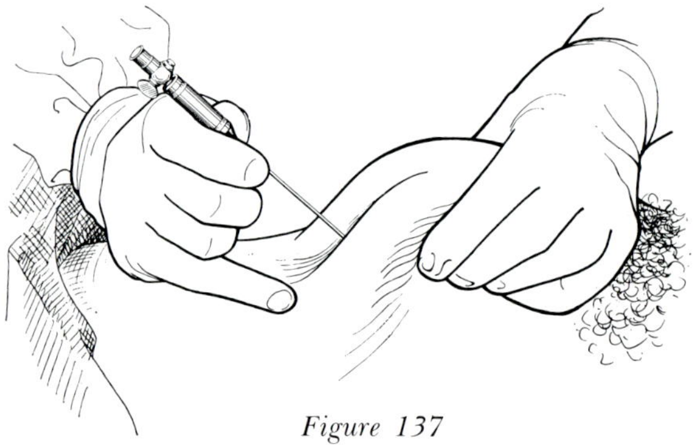

Figure 137

Insertion of the Verres Needle

The tip of the Verres needle is aimed with the right hand at the caudal slope of the navel indentation. Then with the left hand (a left-handed operator of course must reverse these directions) lift the abdominal skin as much as possible. The actual insertion of the needle through skin and umbilical fascia is done using only a wrist motion. The little finger serves as a guiding support for the hand (Fig. 137) so that the latter will not topple forward upon overcoming resistance to perforation.

During the course of this slow wrist motion insertion of the needle, the operator, with the aid of the spring mechanism of the needle, must keep track of each

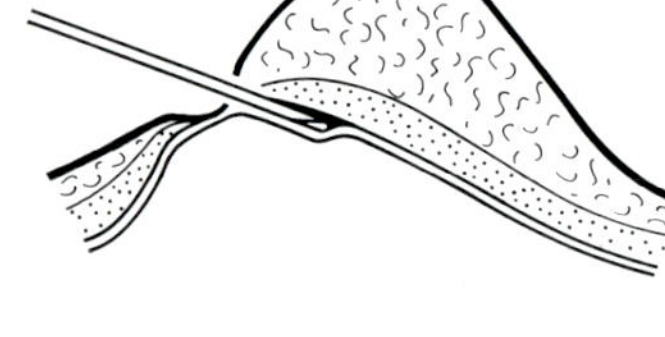

Figure 138

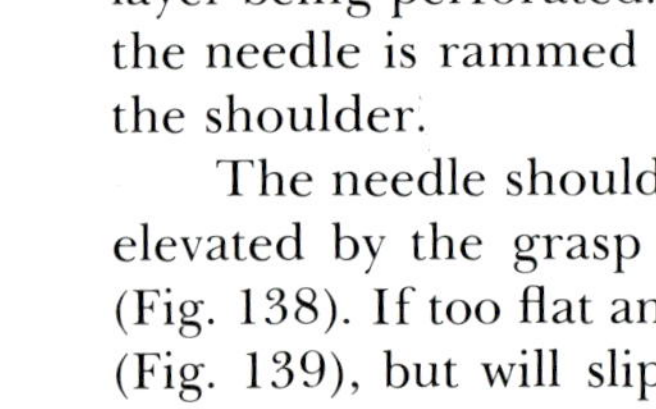

Figure 139

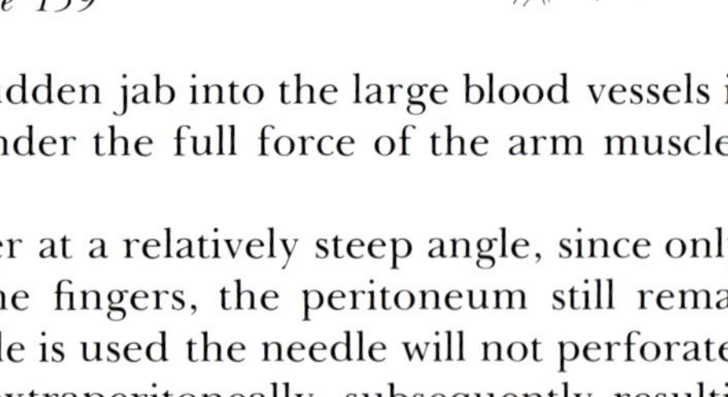

Figure 140

layer being perforated. A sudden jab into the large blood vessels is possible only if the needle is rammed in under the full force of the arm muscles swinging from the shoulder.

The needle should enter at a relatively steep angle, since only the skin can be elevated by the grasp of the fingers, the peritoneum still remaining horizontal (Fig. 138). If too flat an angle is used the needle will not perforate the peritoneum (Fig. 139), but will slip in extraperitoneally, subsequently resulting in a preperitoneal emphysema (Fig. 140).

In making a blind puncture always bear in mind the anatomic position of the aorta and the inferior vena cava. Both vessels lie only a few centimeters below the parietal peritoneum (Fig. 141), especially in slender patients. The relationship of the distance from naval to aorta and that from needle to skin of the back, as shown in Figure 142, is as 1/3 to 2/3, a ratio of which the operator is not automatically conscious.

Figure 141 shows five possible placements of the tip of the needle.

(1) Preperitoneal insufflation causes preperitoneal emphysema.

(2) Subperitoneal induces the desired pneumoperitoneum.

(3) In omentum, causes omental emphysema.

(4) In the bowel, causes inflation of intestines or stomach.

(5) Retroperitoneal location causes gas emboli (Fig. 18) or mediastinal emphysema (Fig. 19).

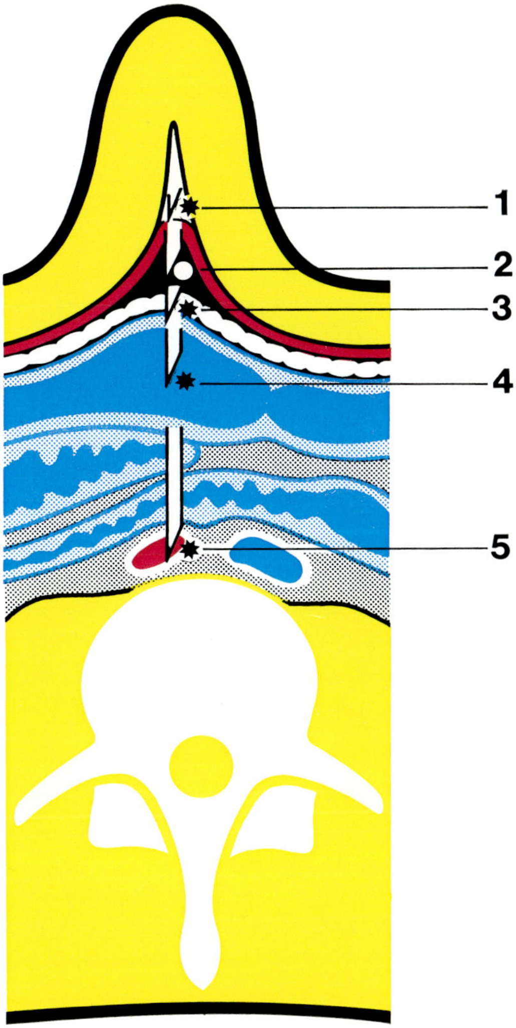

Figure 141

Perforation of the large blood vessels with the Verres needle can be avoided if the operator bears clearly in mind the topography of these vessels in making the puncture.

Perforation at the navel has the advantage that only a few millimeters of tissue must be penetrated in slim patients, and a maximum of only 1 to 2 cm in stout patients (Fig. 142).

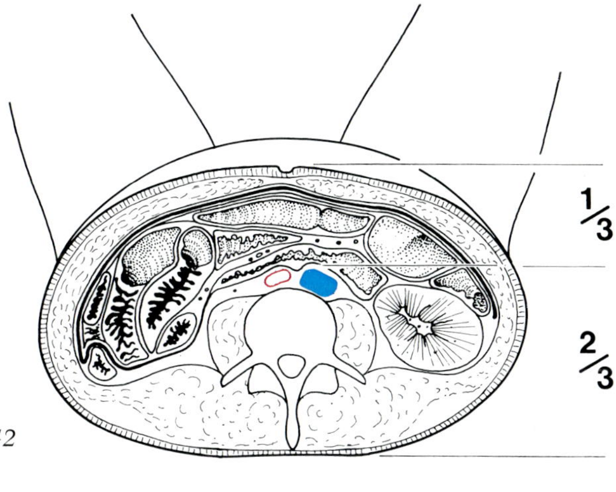

Figure 142

The Verres needle permits fully automatic penetration of the skin with maximum protection for the bowel (Fig. 143).

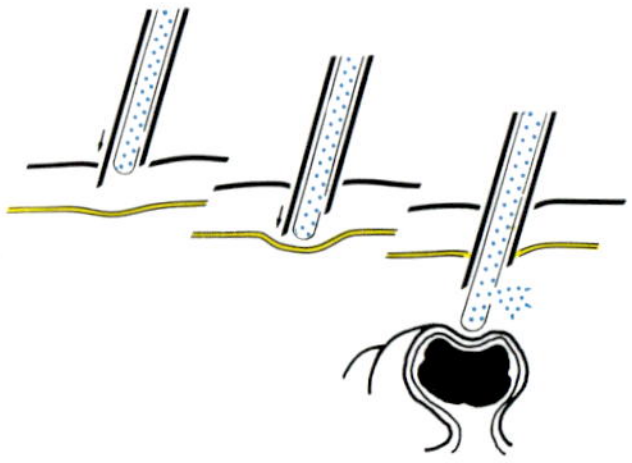

A spring matched to the resistance of the peritoneum allows the dull mandrin to shoot out from the hollow needle past its sharp tip so that the sharp part of the needle can cause no further perforation.

Figure 143

The frequently heard suggestion that, in order to determine whether the tip of the needle is indeed in the open abdominal cavity, the operator should turn it with a circular motion after the puncture is highly dangerous. The moving fingers of the operator at the upper end of the cannula can barely perceive the slight resistance of the omentum or small intestine. Moving the needle in this area can serve only to enlarge the puncture or exacerbate any lesion already caused.

Always remember that penetration of the abdominal cavity is impossible without at least gently touching the intestine (or, still more, the omentum). This lies in direct contact with the peritoneum and is pushed aside by the tip of the needle, no matter how dull the latter may be. A turning motion in this area is never wise. Even with a dull needle, the omentum may be lacerated. A basic warning against this "touch test" is therefore in order. It can lead to unfortunate bleeding.

The optimal sign for a successful puncture of the abdominal skin is a soft hissing sound as the needle enters. This is because, after the perforation of the peritoneum and the shooting forward of the dull mandrin, a negative pressure is produced through the maximal elevation of the abdominal skin by the left hand of the operator, and this immediately causes air to be sucked in. Always wait for this phenomenon, or else attach an open syringe needle to the Verres needle. If the tip of the needle has reached the free abdominal cavity, the sterile salt solution is immediately aspirated (Fig. 144).

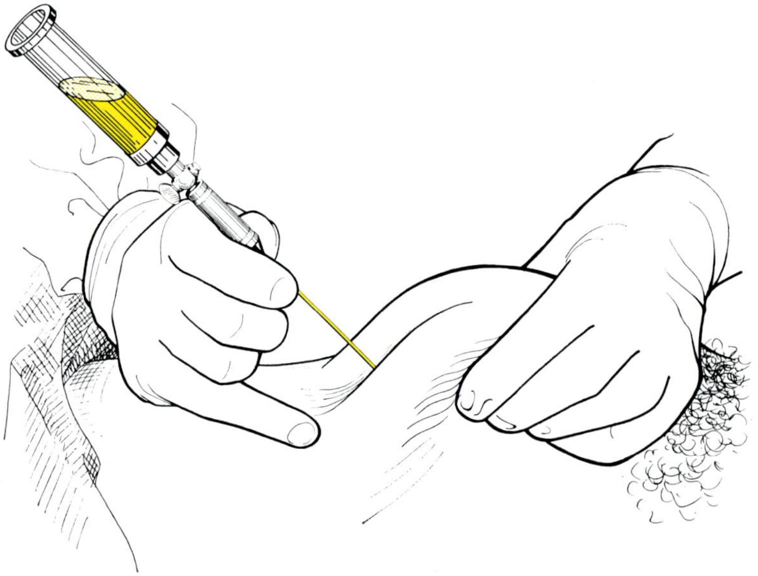

Figure 144

It has sometimes been suggested that, in order to make it easier to insert the Verres needle, a slight split should be made in the caudal slope of the navel indentation with a scalpel. Experiments have shown that this merely provokes unnecessary bleeding. It sometimes happens in very asthenic or postpartum patients that this cut goes too deep through the fascia, and the needle then no longer forms a sufficiently air-tight seal when insufflation starts.

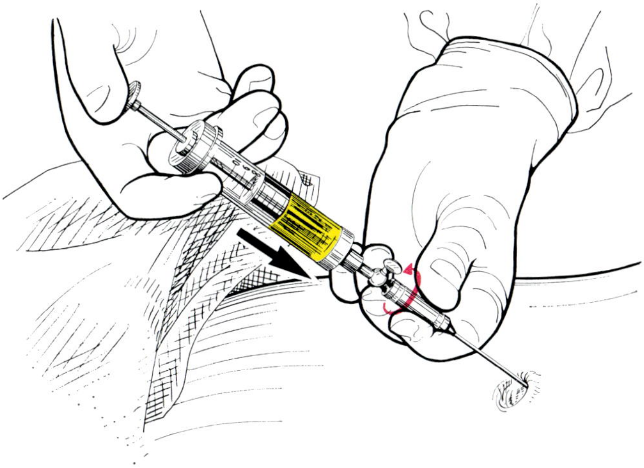

Figure 145

Aspiration Test

If the operator is convinced that he has placed the tip of the needle correctly, about 5 to 6 ml of a physiologic saline solution should be instilled with a 10 ml syringe (Fig. 145). In order that the lumen of the Verres needle can be exposed in all directions, rotate the needle slowly meanwhile.

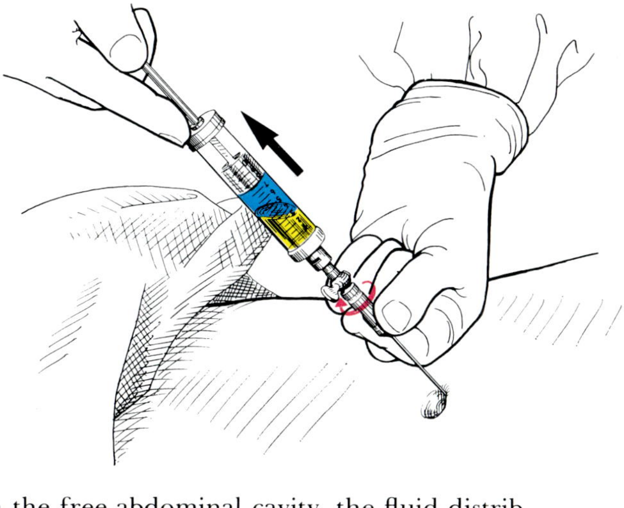

Figure 146

If the Verres needle is indeed in the free abdominal cavity, the fluid distributes itself between the loops of the intestines. The attempt to reaspirate while rotating the needle (Fig. 146) is then unsuccessful. The next step for inducing the pneumoperitoneum, namely the attachment of the gas insufflation hose, can now proceed.

If the Verres needle is not in the free abdominal cavity, the instilled NaCl solution has flowed into tissue or intestinal lumen. The attempt at reaspiration

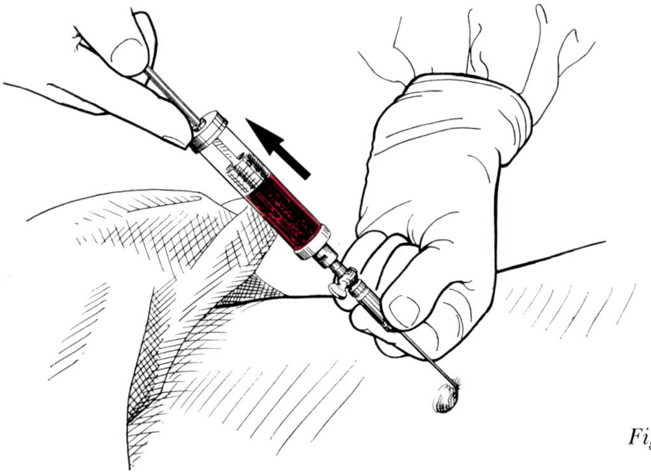

Figure 147

results in a brownish tinge to the reaspirated fluid (Fig. 147). If blood comes back, a blood vessel has been punctured. With such test results as these, the next step (insufflation of the gas) must *not* be taken. The experienced laparoscopist then

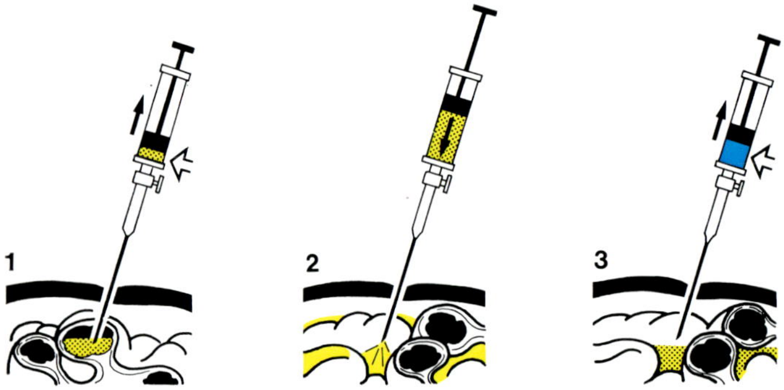

Figure 148

decides on the basis of the indication and the quality of the anesthesia of the patient whether a second puncture can or cannot be ventured.

The sketches in Figure 148 again show whether the fluid flows out into the abdominal cavity and there diffuses (2 and 3: aspiration test negative) or whether it gets into the bowel, where it can be reaspirated (2 and 1: aspiration test positive).

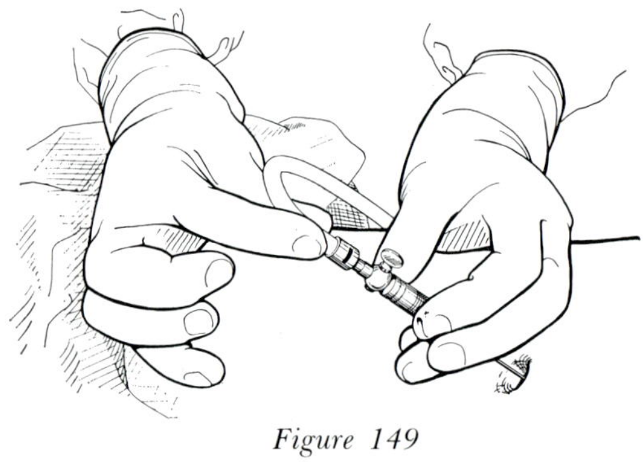

Figure 149

Start of Insufflation

After a successful negative aspiration test the insufflation supply hose from the CO_2-Pneu apparatus is coupled to the Verres needle (Fig. 149). After vigorous elevation of the abdominal skin (Fig. 150), the needle of the Body Cavity Filling dial (see Fig. 54) should be swinging in the negative range, a sure sign that the needle has reached the free abdominal cavity. If this is not the case, however, open the Insufflate valve and at the same time shake the abdominal skin and cautiously move the needle. If the needle has penetrated slightly into the omentum, this maneuver and the gas pressure will shake it loose. A brief increase in the reading of the Body Cavity Filling dial should be followed after two or three seconds by a swinging of the pointer in the 0 range (see Fig. 154).

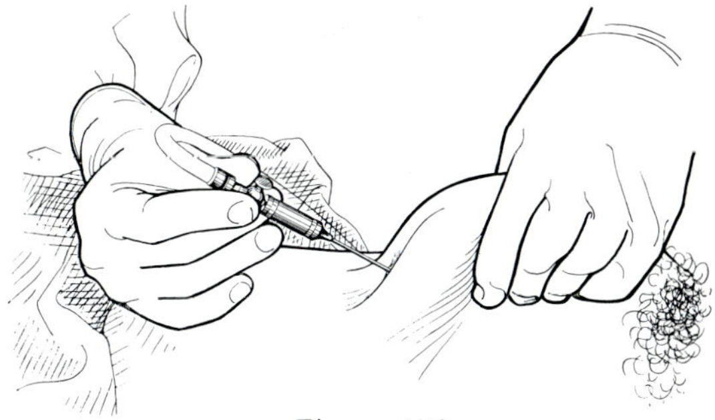

Figure 150

The ball in the flow-through indicator now hovers uniformly in its upper range. The operator can now slowly try to let go of the abdominal skin (Fig. 151), but while he is doing so the dial must not indicate values above 5 to 8 mm Hg. Only in obese patients, where the weight of the fatty abdominal skin plays a part, does the dial show about 10 to 12 mm Hg, a purely mechanical consequence of the weight of the skin.

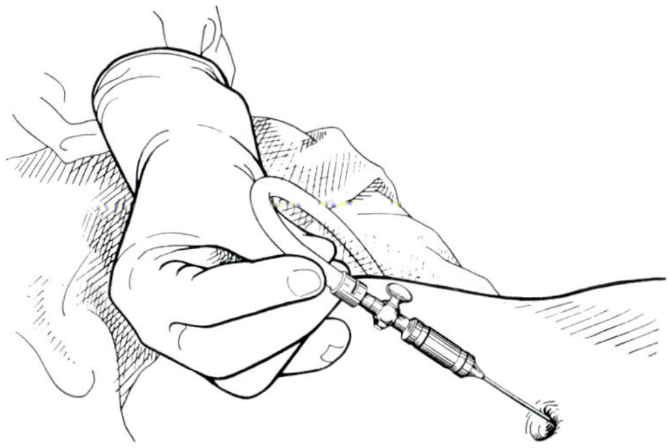

Figure 151

Before insufflation starts the patient is brought to a 15° Trendelenburg position (Fig. 152) in order to let the intestines gravitate from the lower to the upper abdomen in the course of further manipulations. It is not necessary to lower the head any farther than this for the performance of a laparoscopy.

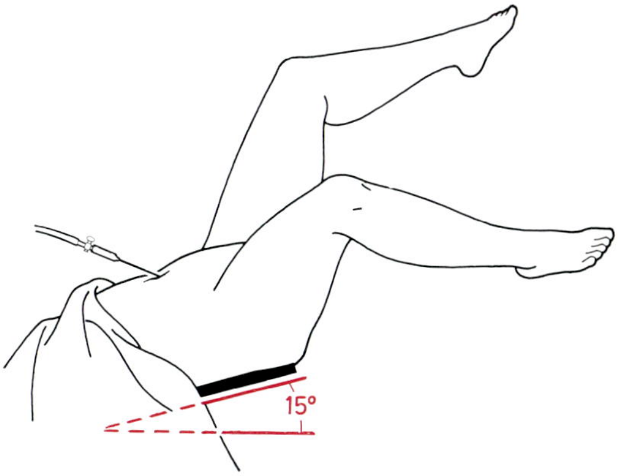

Figure 152

Until about 1 liter of carbon dioxide gas has been insufflated, the Verres needle is held in such a way that the insufflation pressure does not exceed 5 to 10 mm Hg (Fig. 153).

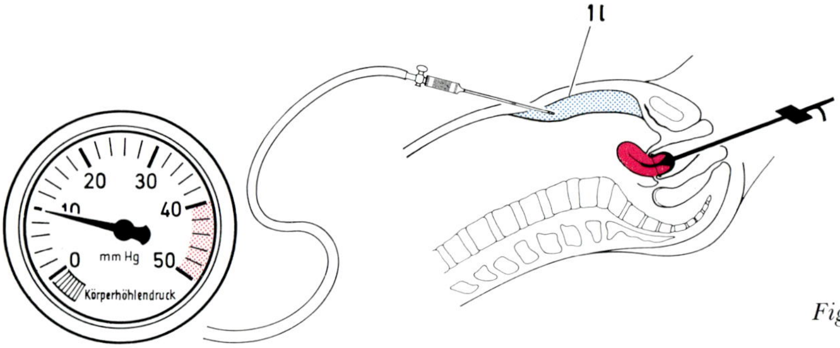

Figure 153

Manometric Test

When about 1 liter of gas has entered under the above conditions, the manometer test is made.

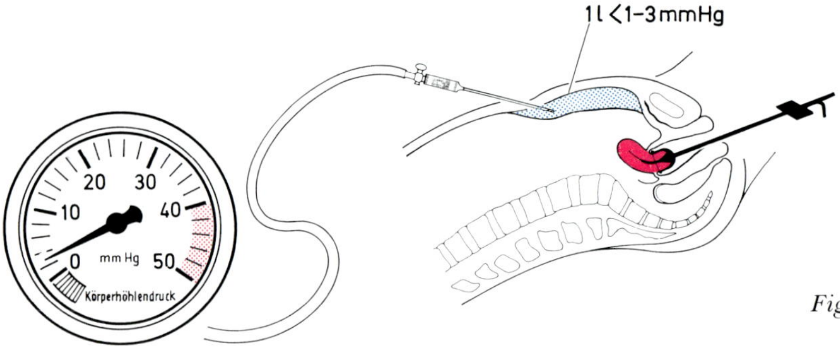

Figure 154

The gas flow is turned off at the Insufflate knob, and the dial must now drop back to about the 1 to 3 mm Hg range. This signals that the 1-liter gas bubble is located safely in the free abdominal cavity (Fig. 154). However, if the dial still shows 8 to 10 mm Hg, some hollow space, such as a preperitoneal emphysema, an omental emphysema, or the bowel, has been inflated. In such cases one is well advised not to consider the time but to try again to release as much gas as possible through the Verres needle. By means of a new insertion of the needle with aspiration test, etc., and depending on the indication and the level of anesthesia of the patient, the operator can try once more to reach the free abdominal cavity.

Very obese patients present problems, and only the experienced operator can decide whether the high dial readings result solely from the thickness of the abdominal wall, i.e., from its weight, or from some complication.

If, after monitoring the dial, the intra-abdominal pressure is determined to be 1 to 3 mm Hg, the insufflation of gas can proceed without further ado until an intra-abdominal pressure of about 10 to 12 mm Hg is achieved (Fig. 155). Since,

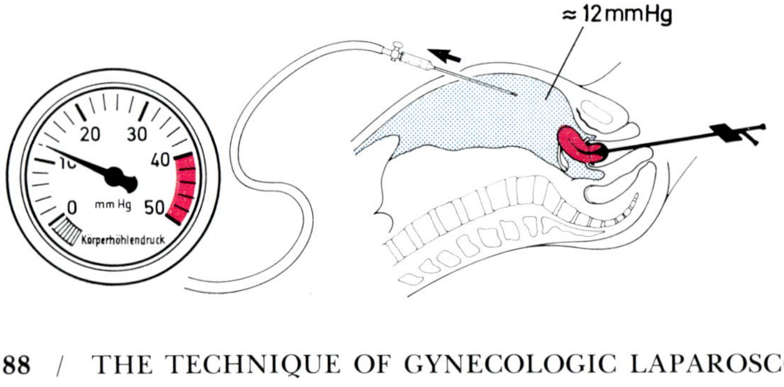

Figure 155

as a matter of principle, the resistance to gas flow is measured via the monofile lead plus the intra-abdominal pressure, the operator stops the insufflation briefly after each liter and measures the intra-abdominal pressure at that stage. When this has reached values of about 10 mm Hg, the next safety measure is undertaken, namely, the probing test.

10. PROBING TEST

Whether by skillful manipulation or by chance, free access to the abdominal cavity is sometimes achieved despite the presence of massive adhesions in the abdomen. The subsequent insertion of the trocar may collide (e.g., after a cesarean section) with a thin ventrally-adhering loop of the small intestine (see Figs. 14 and 24). In order completely to obviate such complications, we routinely perform the probing test.

In preparation we again disinfect the abdominal skin (Fig. 156) 2 to 3 cm below the navel while the insufflation of the pneumoperitoneum is slowly reaching its completion. Then, a 12 mm-long, 0.8 mm-thick cannula mounted on a 10-ml syringe filled with about 2 to 3 ml of physiologic saline solution (left over from the aspiration test) is pushed into the depths of the abdominal gas bubble (Fig. 157). With a light release of the plunger of the syringe (Fig. 158), some gas is aspirated in such a way that a continuous bubbling is observable in the liquid. If

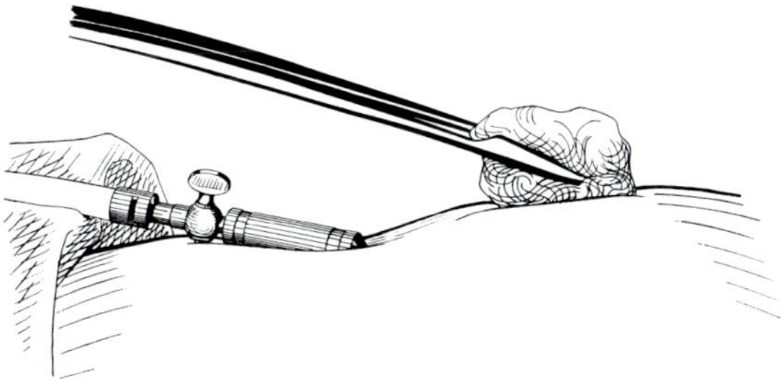

Figure 156

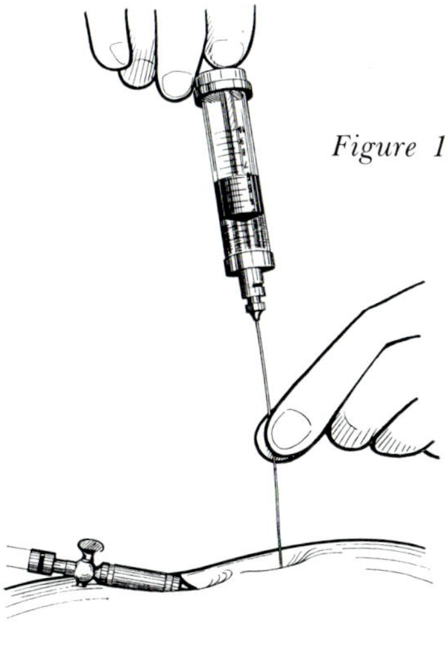

Figure 157

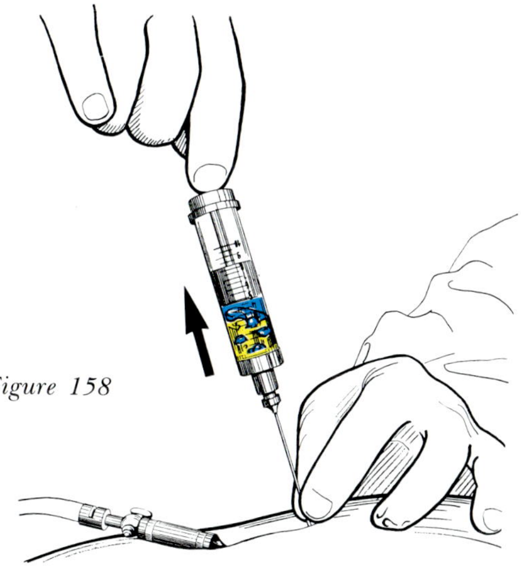

Figure 158

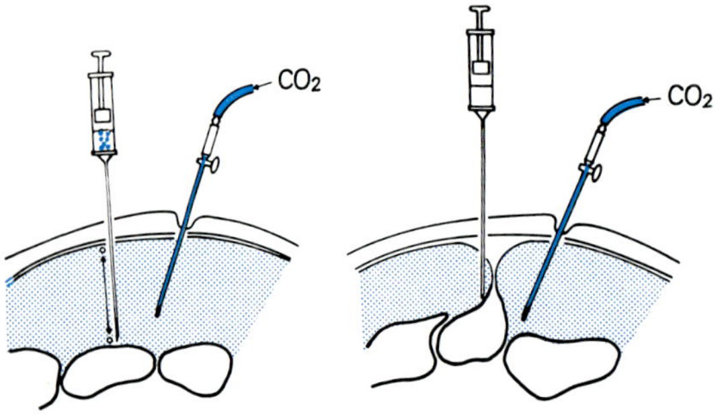

Figure 159

this chain of bubbles is suddenly interrupted, either an adhesion or the bowel is in contact with the tip of the needle (Fig. 159): either can be diagnosed from the direction and depth of insertion of the needle.

If the pneumoperitoneal cavity is probed vertically, the needle is withdrawn until it is in the fatty tissue, and once more is pushed first to right and then to left at an angle of about 45° to detect a possible adhesion (Fig. 160). Velamentous adhesions can be recognized by sudden stoppage of the gas bubbles upon perforation of the tissue. The sketch in Figure 161 illustrates the principle of this.

This probing test is extremely valuable and helps the operator guard against greater complications when the trocar is inserted later. In almost every case an adhesion-free direction for the insertion of the trocar can be found by means of this test.

Figure 160

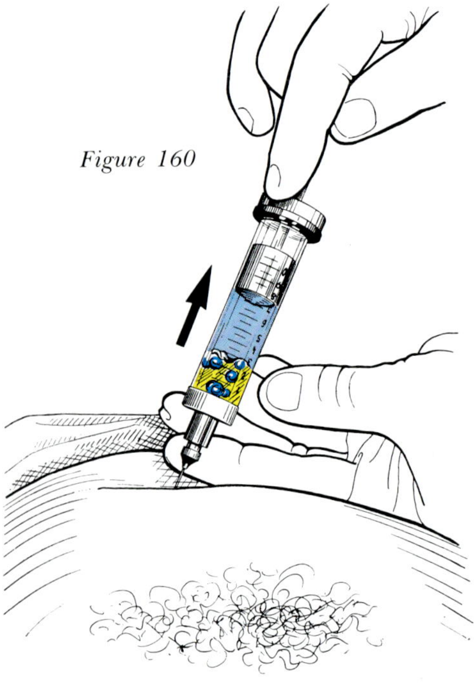

Figure 161

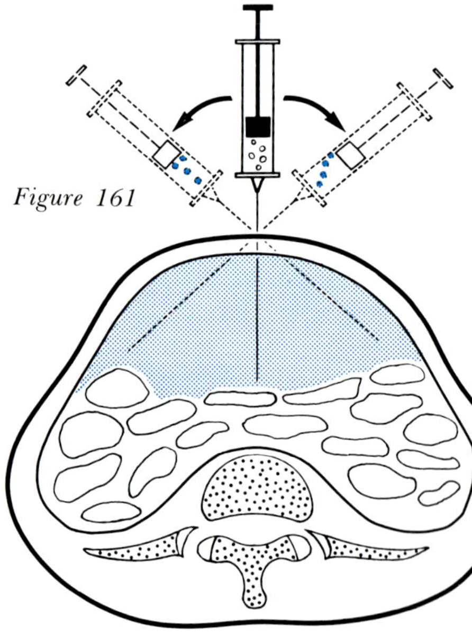

The test also can be performed after the insufflation of the gas has been fully completed, but it is recommended that the test be started at an intra-abdominal pressure of 8–10 mm/Hg, in order to save time.

INSUFFLATION PROBE. When the intra-abdominal pressure (measured after closing the Insufflate valve) has reached 10 to 12 mm Hg (Fig. 162), a sufficiently large gas bubble has been induced for visual monitoring of the abdominal cavity.

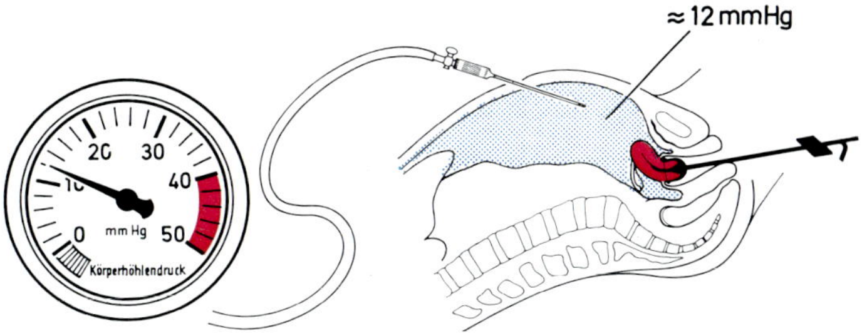

Figure 162

The insufflation is now interrupted and the Verres needle withdrawn. The insufflation hose is then uncoupled from the needle and attached to the trocar.

11. INSERTION OF THE TROCAR

For cosmetic reasons the navel technique generally is preferred today. Moreover, the view from the vantage point of the navel affords the best chance of surveying the pelvic organs and simultaneously concluding the laparoscopy with a general scan of the entire abdomen (see Fig. 29). Sometimes chronic conditions of the lower abdomen turn out to be of gynecologic importance for differential diagnosis through pathologic findings in the upper abdomen, e.g., in the liver.

When the trocar is inserted there is always a danger of puncturing large blood vessels, especially the common iliac artery and vein (see Figs. 18, 26, and 27), if the penetration of the trocar does not slide smoothly through the soft rectus musculature but rather through the tough fascial region. This takes considerable force.

In this connection, we should repeat that the conical tip of the trocar may injure these vessels *without* any blood immediately pouring out into the free abdominal cavity through the peritoneum, which undoubtedly has also been perforated. A blood-free abdominal cavity is *no guarantee* that a large blood vessel has not been perforated. Always watch out for the retroperitoneal hematoma working its way up laterally to the renal calyx.

For reasons mentioned above, the choice of trocar and laparoscope should be subject to the following considerations: (*a*) trocar for routine diagnosis and therapy; or (*b*) trocar for photography, cinematography, or television.

The slimmer the trocar, the less risk in the puncture.

Trocar for Routine Diagnosis and Therapy

For routine diagnostic and therapeutic purposes, the thin (Wolf 6 mm, Storz 7.2 mm) laparoscope is used. It is advisable to keep it in the warmer for an hour or two beforehand (Fig. 174) to preclude undesirable misting of the lens upon entry into the abdominal cavity.

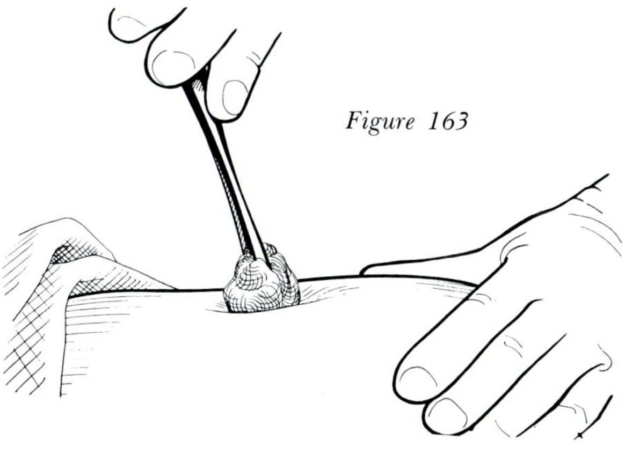

Figure 163

Before inserting the appropriate trocar for the above, the navel is disinfected once more (Fig. 163). Then, the puncture wound from the Verres needle is enlarged in the direction of the caudal slope of the navel indentation, using a slender 6 mm scalpel (Fig. 164) with a horizontal puncture (Fig. 165). Care should be taken to cut through the fascia, making especially sure of this postpartum.

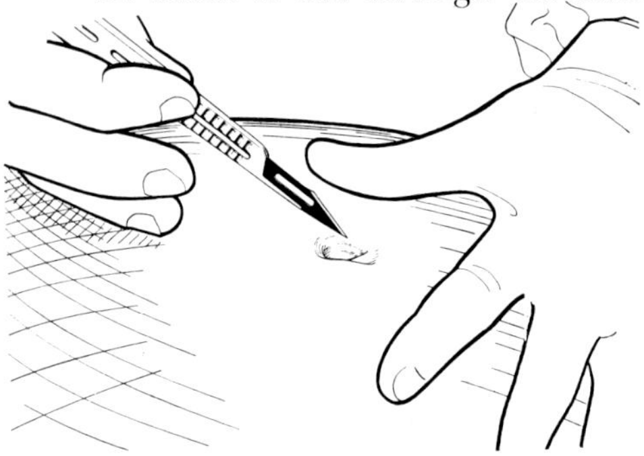

Figure 164

Next follows the insertion of the trocar through the abdominal wall. I purposely do not use the words "pierce" or "thrust." Since the perforation of the linea alba requires considerable force and can give rise postlaparoscopically to incomplete closure of the wound in the abdominal wall and other complications (see Fig. 416), we have been using the Z-insertion technique (Fig. 166) for the past ten years without any complications.

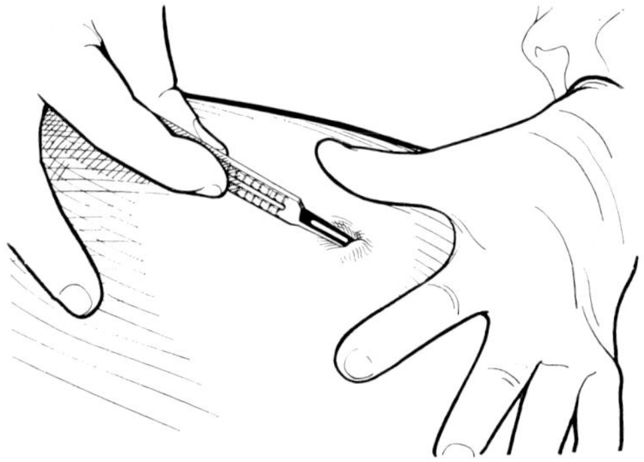

Figure 165

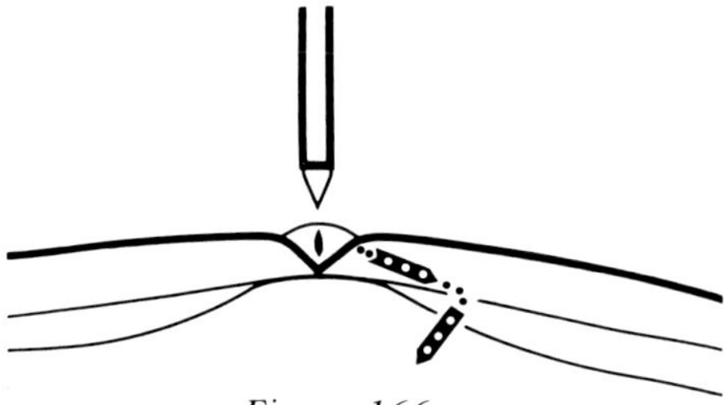

Figure 166

The procedure is as follows. The conical-tipped trocar with attached insufflation-hose is held so that its proximal end comes to lie in the hollow of the hand. The conical tip is first inserted sagittally about 1 cm into the navel incision (Fig. 167). Then turn the trocar 90° to the right (or left, as indicated by the probing finds) and advance it about 2 to 4 cm in the subcutaneous fatty tissue. Now, elevate the abdominal wall maximally with the free hand as for insertion of the Verres needle, so that the tip of the trocar clearly presents subcutaneously 2 to 3 cm laterally from the navel (Fig. 168).

Now, by elevating the trocar, prick the rectus muscle slightly 2 to 3 cm laterally from the navel before aiming the conical tip of the trocar in the direction of the uterine fundus and slowly advancing it through the abdominal wall. The indentation then formed at the right beside the trocar (Fig. 169) gives a clear indication that the rectus muscle has been pierced correctly. If this insertion technique is neglected, the tip of the trocar may slide off the rectus muscle again as far as the linea alba, which can cause an unfortunate hematoma, and the desired effortless Z-insertion effect is lost.

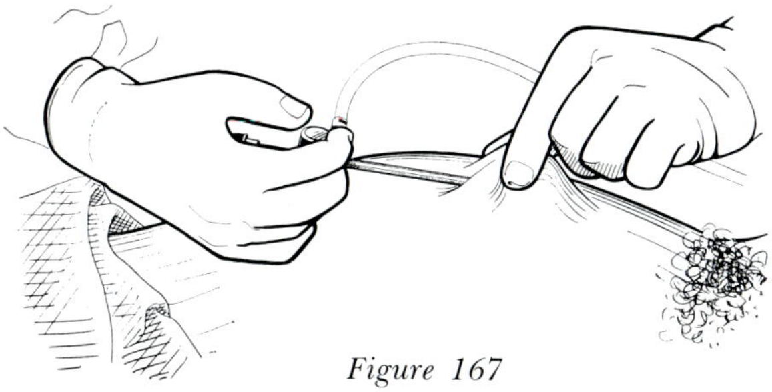

Figure 167

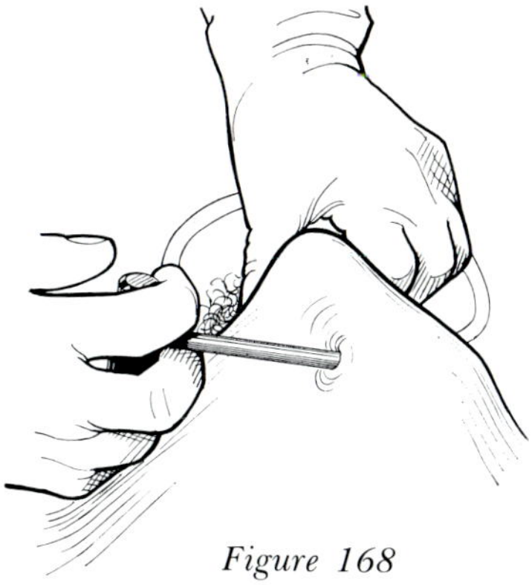

Figure 168

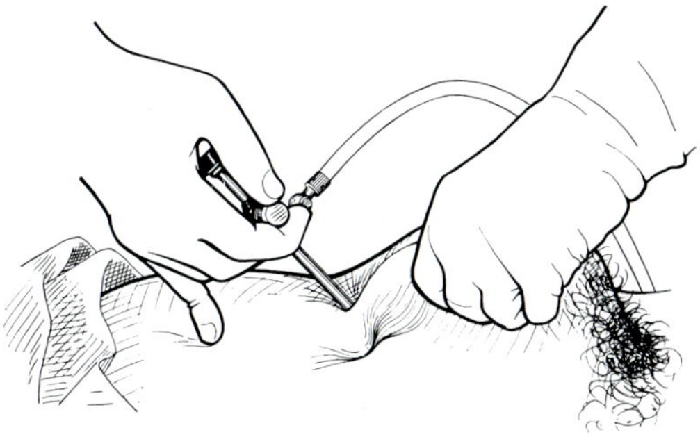

Figure 169

The basic rule when inserting the trocar through the abdominal wall is to make the insertion with a wrist motion, as in the insertion of the Verres needle (see Fig. 137).

The projecting little finger acting as a guide (Fig. 169) guarantees again that the insertion motion does not end in a sudden plunge into the interior of the body as soon as the perforation resistance is overcome.

After the trocar is in place in the abdominal wall, it is withdrawn from its sleeve (Fig. 170). An automatic valve action closes the lumen gas-tight.

After opening the gas cock at the trocar, the Body Cavity Filling Pressure dial *immediately shows the intra-abdominal pressure.*

For further insufflation of CO_2 through the trocar, turn the right-hand knob of the CO_2-Pneu from Hand to Automatic (Fig. 171).

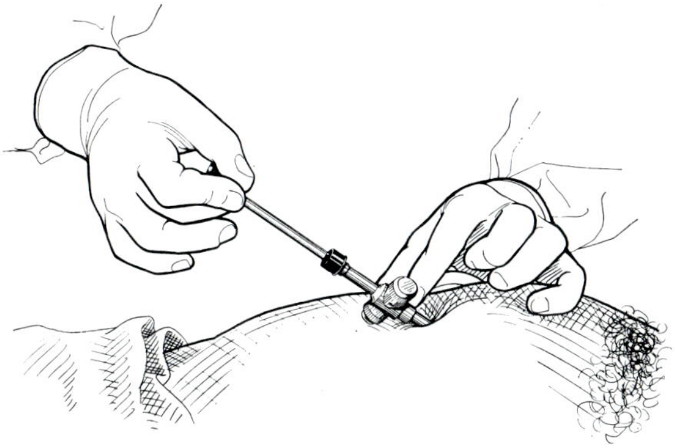

Figure 170

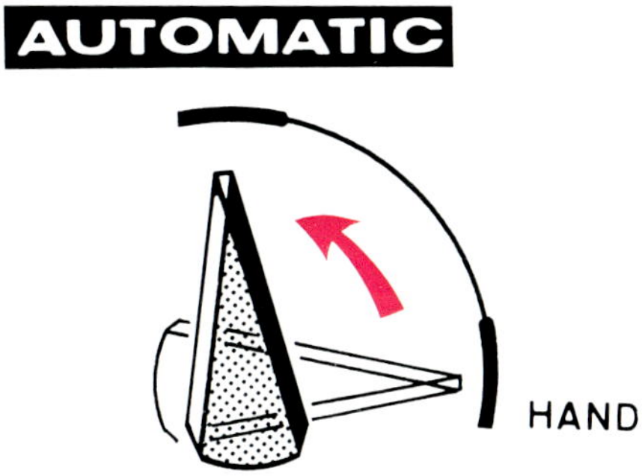

Figure 171

Trocar for Photography, Cinematography and Television

For teaching and research purposes, it is necessary to use the 11 mm trocar in order to make possible the use of lenses with suitable light-conduction cross-section. This trocar is introduced in the same way as described above, but now special precaution and care must be observed. In the first place, the navel incision must be made 1.5 cm larger; otherwise the frictional resistance in the skin will require an unnecessary amount of force for penetration.

When a particularly valuable finding of scientific interest has been made in the course of a routine laparoscopy that cannot be documented to the necessary standard of quality, we use the dilatation instruments (Semm, 1972). This obviates

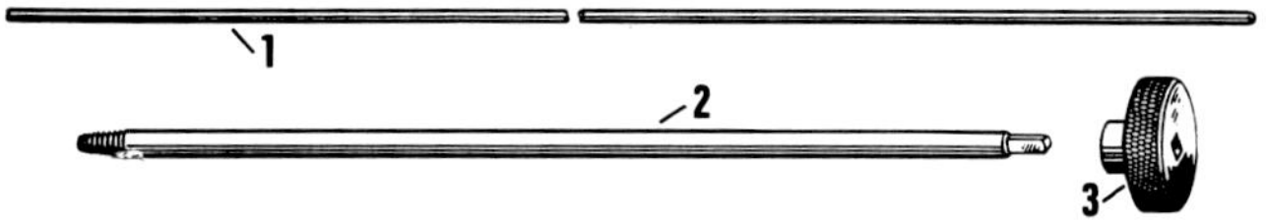

Figure 172

a second puncture with the 11 mm trocar, which might lead to unfortunate bleeding and hematomas in the abdominal wall.

Atraumatic dilatation of the umbilical wound is achieved with the Semm triple dilatation set (Fig. 172: (1) guide rod; (2) threaded dilatator; (3) knurled

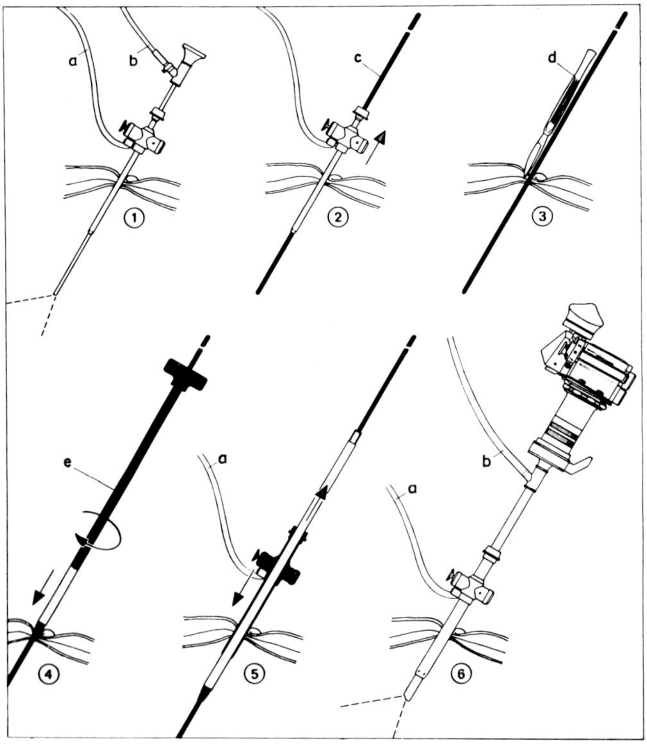

Figure 173

knob) for the small caliber trocar cannula or for the 11 mm photographic/cinematographic trocar, as follows (Fig. 173):

(1) First remove the 5-mm routine laparoscope from its cannula: (*a*) CO_2 gas; (*b*) light cable.

(2) Replace it with a long guide rod (*c*) over which the trocar cannula is withdrawn.

(3) Now enlarge the incision in the skin at the navel caudally with a scalpel (*d*) by a length of about 10 mm.

(4) Push the bluntly conical threaded dilator (*e*) over the guide rod (*c*). Turning this to the right enlarges the opening in the abdomen with minimal damage.

(5) The knurled knob is removed and the trocar sleeve for the photographic or

cinematographic lens is introduced over the threaded dilator with the guide rod through the abdominal wall.

(6) The threaded dilator then can be readily exchanged for the photographic laparoscope.

12. INTRODUCING THE LAPAROSCOPE

The laparoscope that fits the trocar cannula is removed from the warmer (Fig. 174) and introduced instead of the trocar. The insertion should be monitored visually so that any injury will be detected instantly. The direct-forward laparoscope or the one with angled visual field at 30° or 150° (see Fig. 40) permits a quick survey for orientation, the operator having already established the topography by the direction in which the laparoscope is aimed. Before insertion of the routine instrument, the endoscopy room should be darkened. There should be only enough subdued light in the room for all maneuvers to proceed efficiently.

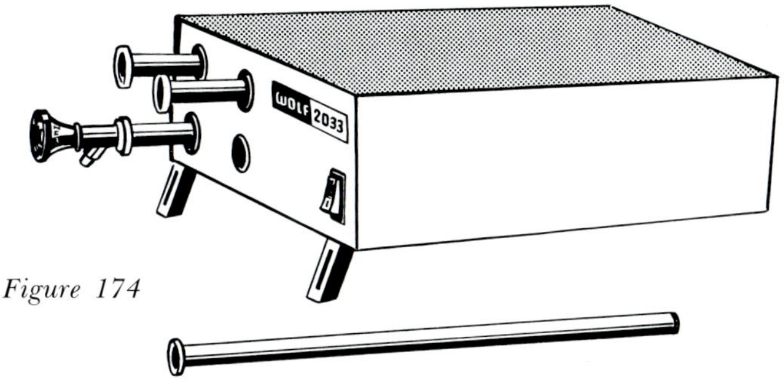

Figure 174

This half-light is not recommended when using the cinematographic lens, since the sharp contrast between light reflected into the abdominal cavity from the xenon-vapor lamps and the darkness of the room is bad for the operator's eyes.

The operator first checks the point of entry precisely and orients himself by means of an all-round survey of the entire abdomen, including the liver, making especially sure that no retroperitoneal hematoma (Fig. 27) is present. Only then does he proceed to inspection of the pelvis. After an orienting survey the uterus is elevated carefully out of the pelvis, and the systematic inspection of the genital organs commences. Upward, downward, and lateral inclination of the uterus by means of corresponding movements of the shaft of the suction intrauter-

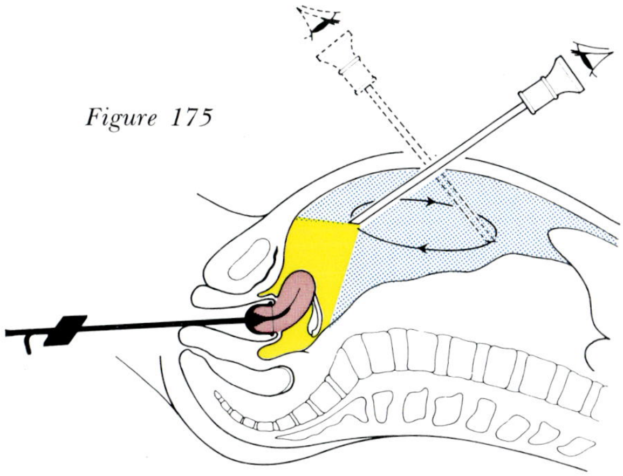

Figure 175

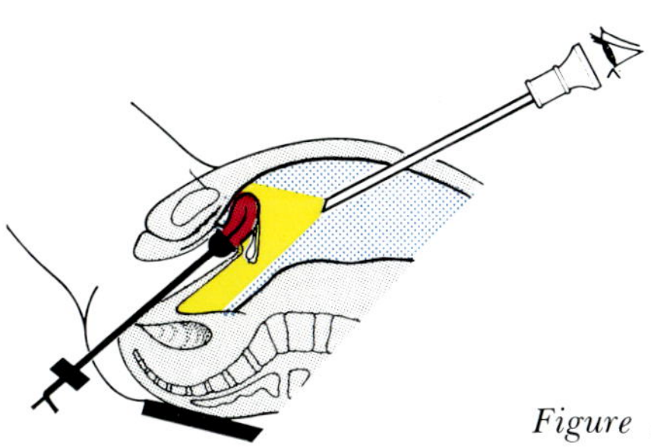

Figure 176

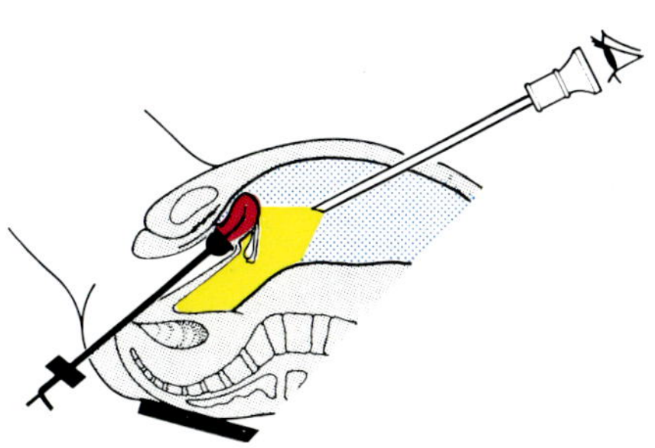

Figure 177

ine cannula facilitates the inspection, as does rotation of the 30° (or 150°) fore-oblique optic (Figs. 176, 177).

If the lens becomes misted or soiled with blood, it can be cleared by brushing it lightly against the wall of the intestine. This suffices for visual scanning, but for photography or cinematography the laparoscope should be withdrawn after each soiling and the lens thoroughly cleansed with sterile physiologic saline solution.

13. THE SECOND PUNCTURE

Until now the only instrument available to us for the second puncture, aside from the simple probe, was the 6 mm trocar for the ancillary surgical instruments (Part A, Chapter 4, Section 6). The probe has served its purpose admirably in hepatic diagnosis, but leaves something to be desired in laparoscopy. However, the newly developed suction-probe (Figs. 31, 64–67) can be used in practically every diagnostic laparoscopy. The trauma to the patient resulting from the 3 mm puncture (preparatory 1.5 mm incision with a slender scalpel) is minimal compared to the tremendous diagnostic value inherent in its use.

All the organs can be manipulated by the suction effect of the probe (e.g., oviducts, tubal ampulla, mesosalpinx, ovary, omentum, and appendix) without the slightest danger of injury. Therefore, the second puncture is recommended in all laparoscopies in which the first scan determines that further surgical measures

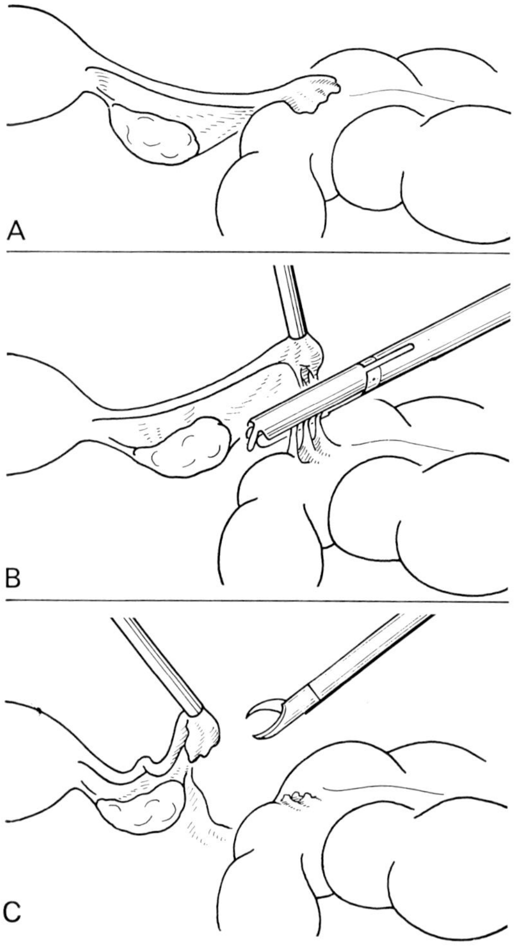

Figure 178

are not necessary but that a second puncture with a larger trocar would be justified.

A further application of the suction probe is in order if therapeutic surgical intervention is required and some additional organ fixation becomes desirable. Figure 178 demonstrates a situation that frequently occurs. The tubal ampulla has become adherent to the colon after an appendectomy (*A*). By elevating the ampulla, the adhesion is stretched so that it can be coagulated (*B*) with the low-voltage crocodile forceps, and then detached (*C*).

The location for the second puncture in operative laparoscopy depends on which organ is to be manipulated. That is to say, if the manipulation is to occur in the left lower abdomen, the second puncture should be made on the right side, and vice versa. If there is already an abdominal scar in the abdominal wall, e.g., an appendectomy scar, the 5 mm incision needed for the second puncture is made within the existing scar. Since the second puncture is monitored both internally and externally, the danger of injury to a blood vessel is practically negligible. The second puncture obviously should not be made too close to the navel, in order to avoid any collision with the laparoscope.

First, bring the lens close to the inside of the abdominal wall and determine the exact pattern of its vascular system by means of transillumination. After

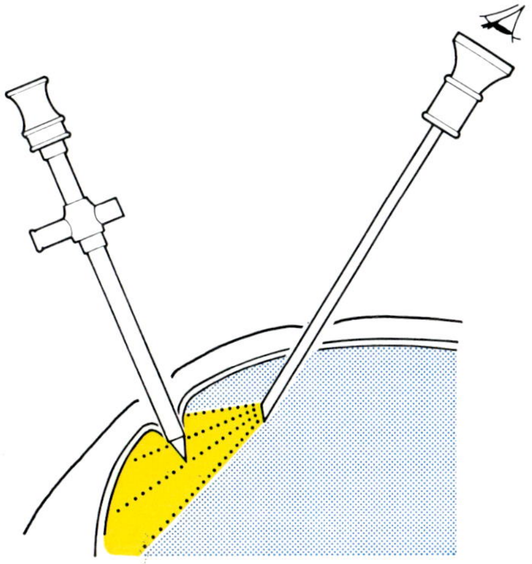

Figure 179

selecting an area free of blood vessels, or clear from any old appendectomy scar, the skin incision is made with a slender 6 mm scalpel. Then, insert the 6 mm trocar for the second puncture with its relatively blunt conical tip into the incision, again using the Z-track insertion method (see Fig. 166), and monitor through the lens the further penetration of the trocar through the peritoneum (Fig. 179).

Through this second puncture, all the instruments listed in Chapter IV, Section 6, can be inserted alternately and exchanged without noticeable gas loss.

The trocars for the second puncture have the same diameter as those for the laparoscope (except for the trocar for ligation of the tubes). Thus, at any time the optic can be inserted into the second puncture when it is necessary to make an inspection in the vicinity of the navel, or to lyse adhesions more accessible through this second aperture (Fig. 180).

The second puncture, however, can also be used to monitor visually any complication or unclear situation in the vicinity of the umbilical puncture. For this purpose a second laparoscope may be used or, if one is not available, the laparoscope already in the navel puncture. From the second puncture (Fig. 180) the navel puncture itself can be inspected closely with the original laparoscope still in

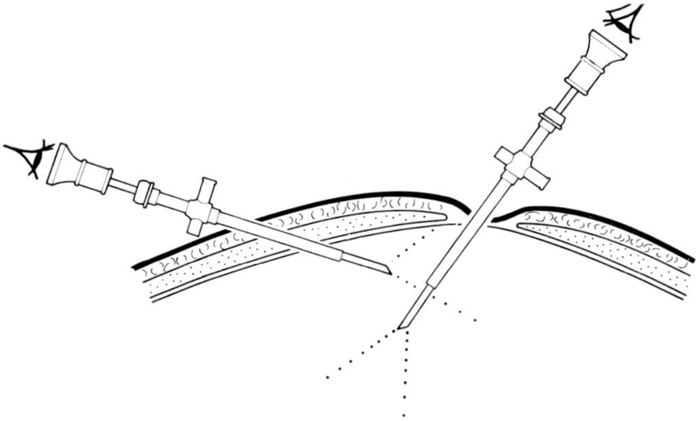

Figure 180

place. This becomes necessary, for instance, when in the immediate vicinity of the navel a loop of small intestine is adherent to the abdominal wall, and it is not possible to be sure from the umbilical vantage point whether it was injured in the first puncture.

In cases of adhesions or vascular anomalies, troublesome bleeding may arise in the umbilical region in rare instances. If this occurs, the location of the bleeding can be spotted through the second puncture and stemmed by a simple surgical procedure (Fig. 181). With a very large surgical needle, the abdominal wall can be pierced from outside under endoscopic supervision as seen from the second puncture, and the bleeding vessel can be sutured with this one large stitch.

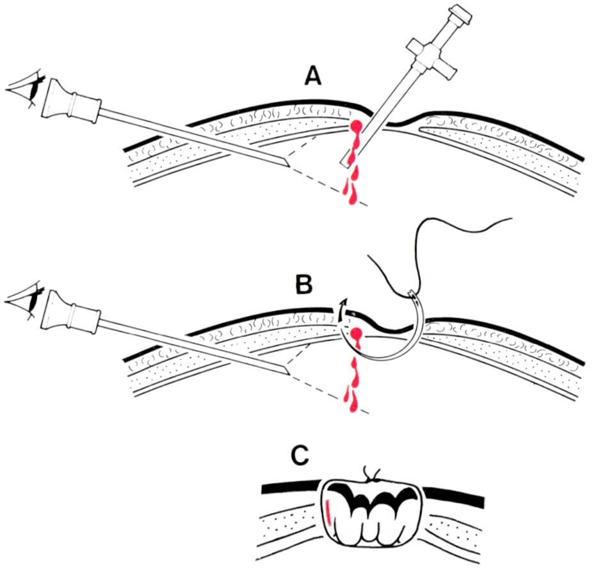

Figure 181

We achieved complete success twice within ten years with this technique. This simple means of staunching the flow of blood should always be borne in mind in cases of bleeding from the abdominal wall, and laparotomy becomes unnecessary. The technique also was effective in dealing with the complication of a herniated omentum shown in Figure 416.

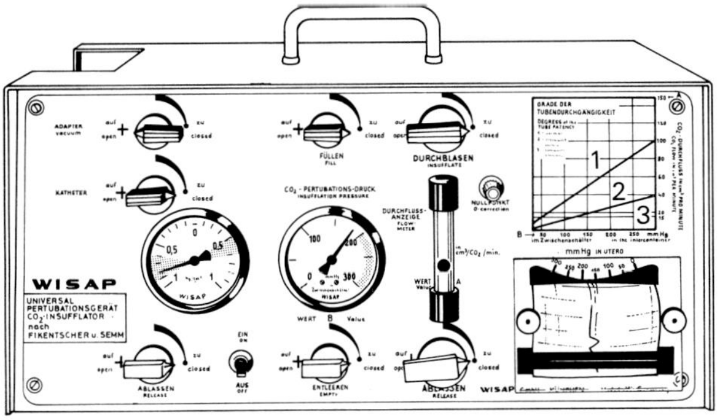

14. TUBAL INSUFFLATION OF DYE DURING LAPAROSCOPY

In the diagnosis of sterility patients, both hysterosalpingography and tubal insufflation of dye are routine procedures today. It has become almost obligatory in these patients to perform a laparoscopy and evaluate the tubal patency by this technique. The blue dye (Chapter VII, Section 2) can be plainly seen in the reservoir attached to the intrauterine vacuum sound in Figure 182. For this purpose, a pressure of 100 to 300 mg Hg must be supplied in order adequately to evaluate the tubal status (see Fig. 423). Using either the suction or atraumatic probe, the entire tube and ampulla can be visualized.

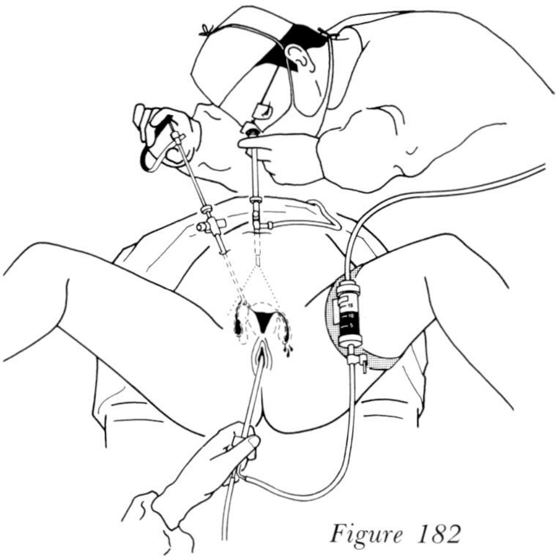

Figure 182

15. CONCLUDING THE LAPAROSCOPY

After completing the required procedures the entire abdominal cavity should be scanned once more (see Fig. 28). Then, under continued optical surveillance, the laparoscope is withdrawn from the trocar sleeve. After the valve is opened, the gas flows out of the abdominal cavity. Since the intra-abdominal pressure never exceeds 10 to 15 mm Hg, no circulatory shock results from the quick release of the gas, even through the 11 mm cannula. The complete discharge of the gas is accelerated and aided by gentle massage of the abdominal wall and by elevating it while slowly drawing out the trocar sleeve. At the same time the patient is restored to the horizontal position.

The suction intrauterine cannula is removed after release of the vacuum in the adapter cup.

16. POSTOPERATIVE CARE OF THE WOUND

After the trocar sleeve is removed the patient's navel, the site of the second

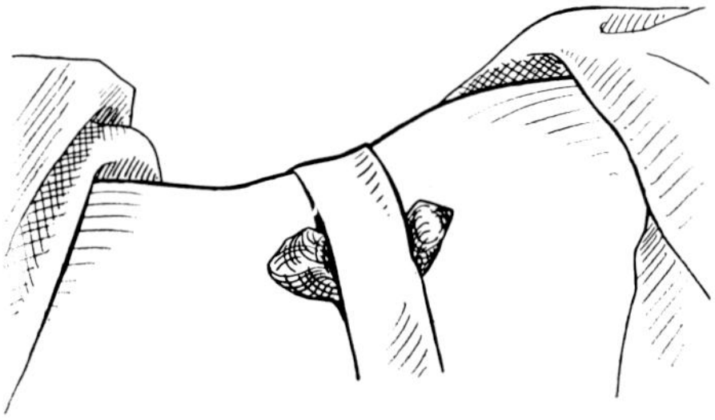

Figure 183

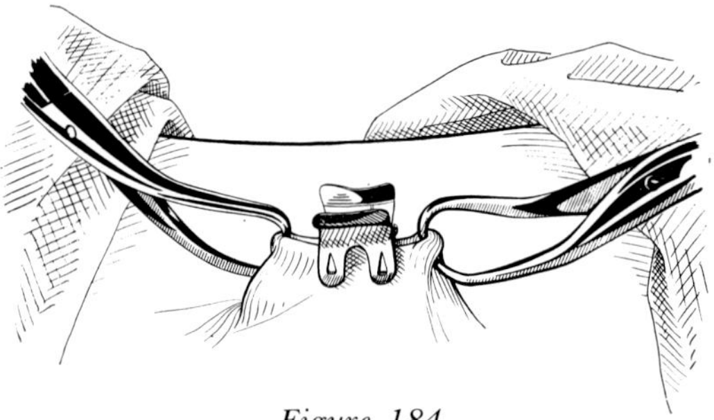

Figure 184

puncture, if any, is disinfected again and the wound is covered with an antibiotic ointment. After using a 6 or 7 mm trocar it usually is quite sufficient to fit a small gauze pad to the edges of the wound in the navel and fasten it with an adhesive bandage (Fig. 183). After using the 11 mm trocar it normally is necessary to use metal clips such as those shown in Fig. 184. These clips are removed on the second postoperative day and replaced with an adhesive bandage. (*Editor's note:* If the edges of the incision are actively bleeding, one or two sutures of 3–0 plain catgut may be quickly and easily placed. These (Figs. 183, 184) sutures need not be removed since they will rapidly dissolve and cause no patient discomfort and minimal tissue reaction.)

17. POSTOPERATIVE CARE OF THE LAPAROSCOPY PATIENT

The primary postoperative care of the laparoscoped patient involves the anesthesia, provided no special surgical intervention is otherwise necessary. For subsequent postoperative care the patients can be subdivided into three groups: (*a*) those who had merely diagnostic laparoscopy without supplementary surgical manipulation; (*b*) those who had tubal dye insufflation or sterility diagnosis; and (*c*) those who had (*a*) and/or (*b*) plus surgical intervention.

With regard to (*a*), if the patient has undergone only endoscopic monitoring of the internal genitalia and the results indicated that no treatment involving hospitalization was needed, the patient (depending on her state of well-being) can be released and sent home with instructions after 24 hours.

With regard to (*b*), the same remarks apply as well for sterility patients who, after their tubes have been studied, have also undergone dye insufflation. Frequently a repetition of the hydropertubation is advisable after two to four days if the indications so suggest.

With regard to (*c*), if surgical measures followed the laparoscopic diagnosis (e.g., cutting of adhesions, massive manipulation of the ampullae, coagulation of endometrial implants, or biopsy of the ovaries) it is safer to prolong the post-laparoscopic hospitalization to three to five days. This is especially true if high-frequency current has been used. Intestinal damage that sometimes occurs in connection with the use of high-frequency current (intestinal burns) does not, as a rule, become symptomatically evident until the third or fourth postoperative day.

If such injuries have not been surgically repaired, the patient frequently is seriously ill by the fifth or sixth day. Indeed, once intestinal contents have escaped into the free abdominal cavity through necroses of the intestinal wall caused by electric field intensification, immediate laparotomy is required. This complication should no longer occur once high-frequency current has been generally eliminated from the laparoscopic scene.

Postlaparoscopic hospitalization also is necessary, especially with operatively treated sterility cases, if an intra-abdominal cortisone treatment with high dosages was inaugurated during laparoscopy to avoid additional adhesions.

Out-patient laparoscopy, now much discussed, in which the patient is merely observed for a few hours in the hospital after the laparoscopic procedures, is subject to a serious complication rate, according to a statistical study by Epple and Funk (1973). That study of 159 patients undergoing ambulatory laparoscopy reported that 48 (11 per cent) were bedridden for up to six days, and 31 (8 per cent) for more than six days. After a standardized two-day hospitalization there has been no need for further bedrest in our own experience of 2000 laparoscopies.

As noted earlier, the psychologic aspect, as well as the diagnostic and therapeutic, should be taken into account in laparoscopy. The patient must retain a favorable memory of the procedure in order that, in an emergency she may in later life harbor no anxiety about the experience and will be able to undergo it again with confidence.

The question of ambulatory laparoscopy is very much in the news at present in connection with tubal sterilization. If it is to be performed with the use of high-frequency electricity, I consider ambulatory laparoscopy to be ill-advised. In this connection it should again be stressed that the laparoscopic method should be judged, not by the hundreds of successful cases, but by the very low rate of subsequent fatality; all such deaths may be ascribed solely to inadequate techniques and methods.

VII
Atlas of (Pelvic) Laparoscopy

With the aid of 224 endoscopic color photographs we can now demonstrate what can be diagnosed at endoscopy and what can be done about it therapeutically and surgically. Each picture is accompanied by a brief comment and line drawing. The pictorial atlas represents a continuation of Chapters I through VI; the possibilities and limitations of laparoscopy are discussed further, together with illustrative color photographs.

In order to give the atlas a certain continuity, the illustrations have been arranged according to the indication groups described in Chapter VI, Section 1,a: (1) nonsurgical diagnostic laparoscopy (Figs. 185–293); (2) surgical diagnostic laparoscopy (Figs. 294–331); and (3) surgical therapeutic laparoscopy (Figs. 332–417). Within these three major groups it has been possible to interpret almost all ranges of indication from the color slides. Since endoscopic color pictures usually are not very intelligible in themselves, owing to the fullness of detail, each is accompanied by an explanatory line drawing. Numerals designate the anatomic and pathologic organs. **The key to the numerals is given at the end of the pictorial section on a fold-out page, which should enable the reader to study both the photographs and the line-drawings with ease. Text and drawings included in the pictorial section clarify the specific procedures.**

1

Nonsurgical Diagnostic Laparsocopy

(a) Differential Diagnosis: Normal Topography vs. Pathologic Genitalia

Fig. 185. As the patient lies on her back, the uterus seen from the navel is retroflexed in the cul-de-sac, even though normally anteflexed. The fallopian tubes and ovaries usually are not visible; they can be seen only if the uterus is elevated as shown on a later slide.

Fig. 186. Because of the variable motility of the utero-ovarian ligament, the ovaries, especially when enlarged, may also appear in front of the uterus. This explains why the location of ovarian cysts is sometimes determined as being in front of and sometimes behind the uterus. In this connection, it must be borne in mind that when a woman stands erect the ovaries hang almost vertically by the infundibulopelvic ligaments.

Fig. 187. When the uterus is elevated with the aid of the suction intrauterine cannula, a view is afforded into the cul-de-sac. Both adnexa can be seen at the same time, which is of importance for judging the sizes of various organs. The left ovary has a corpus luteum in bloom.

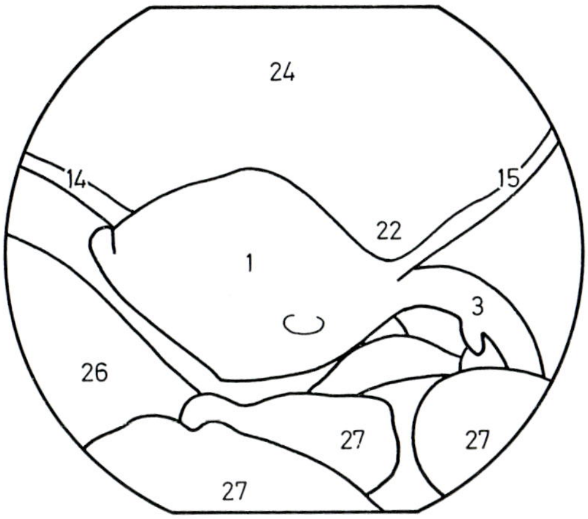
24
14
15
22
1
3
26
27
27
27

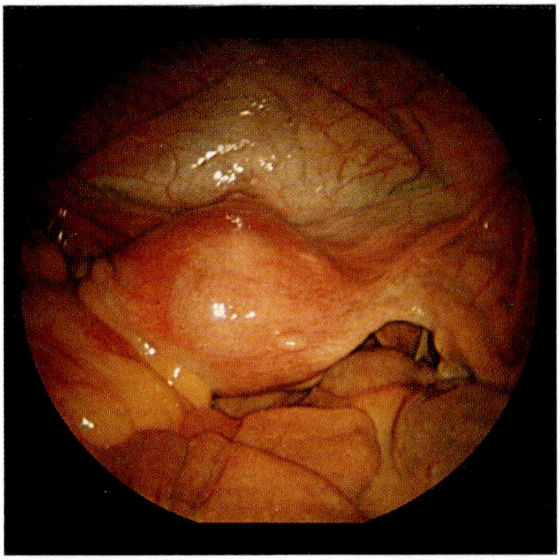

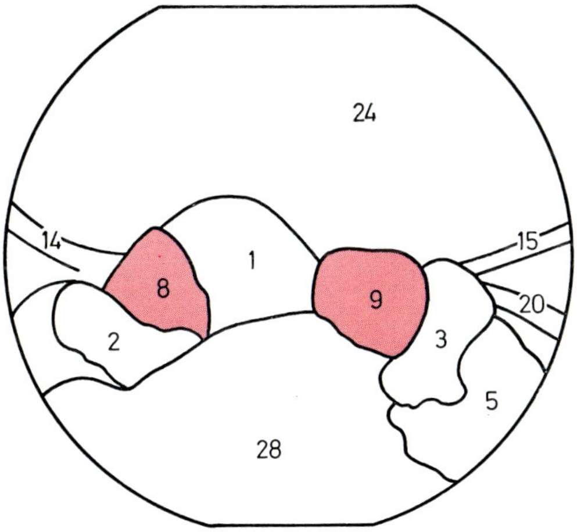
24
14
15
8
1
9
20
2
3
5
28

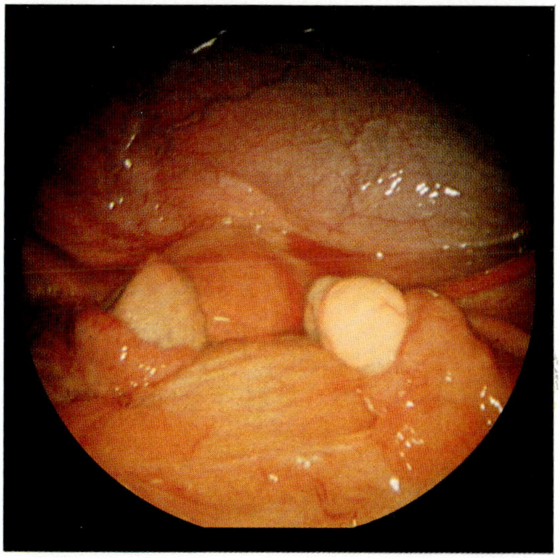

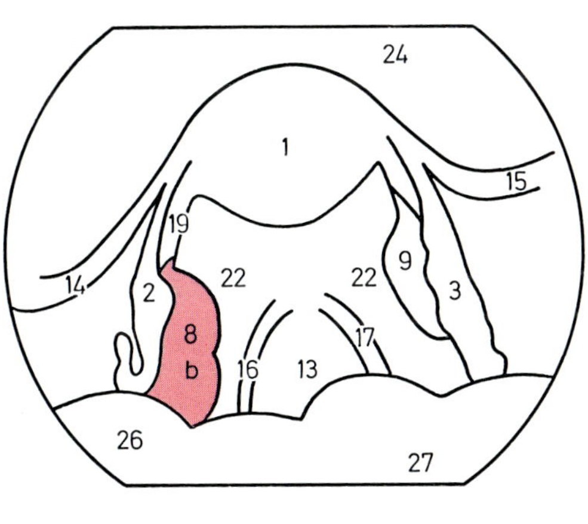
24
1
15
19
22
22
9
14
2
3
8
b
17
16
13
26
27

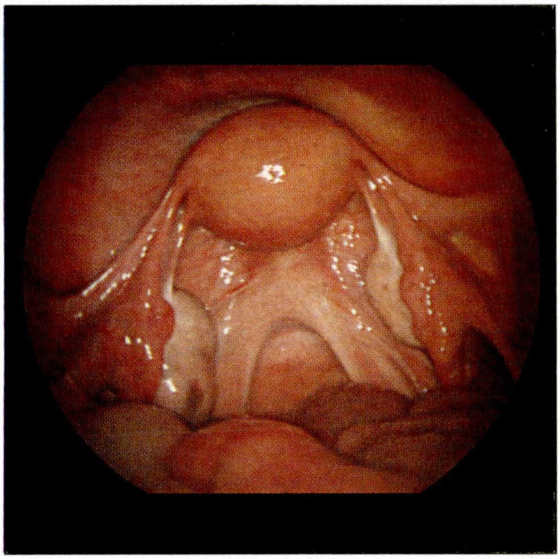

Fig. 188. By inclining the uterus laterally with the suction intrauterine cannula, a clear view is afforded into the cul-de-sac and of the right broad ligament dorsally and the left ventrally.

Fig. 189. By advancing the laparoscope, whose lens system gives a clear focus at most distances, the fine structure of the adnexa can be appreciated. Here the right uterosacral ligament is quite sharply defined.

Fig. 190. With the shaft of the suction intrauterine cannula fully depressed, the uterus is elevated maximally up against the symphysis and the ligamental apparatus of the uterus is tensed. This affords a clear appraisal of a possible asymmetric pattern of the ligamental structure. The left uterosacral ligament here is strikingly thicker than the right one. The arrow (→) indicates a maturing follicle.

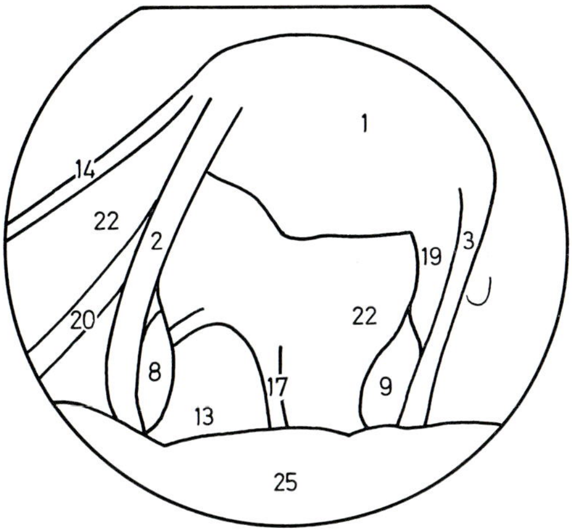
14
22
2
1
19
3
20
22
8
17
9
13
25

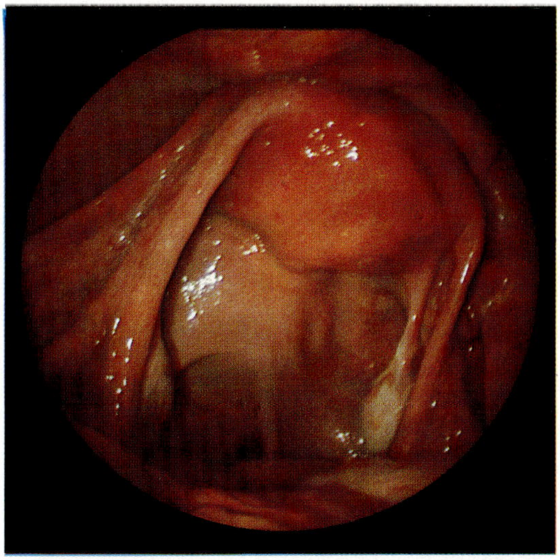

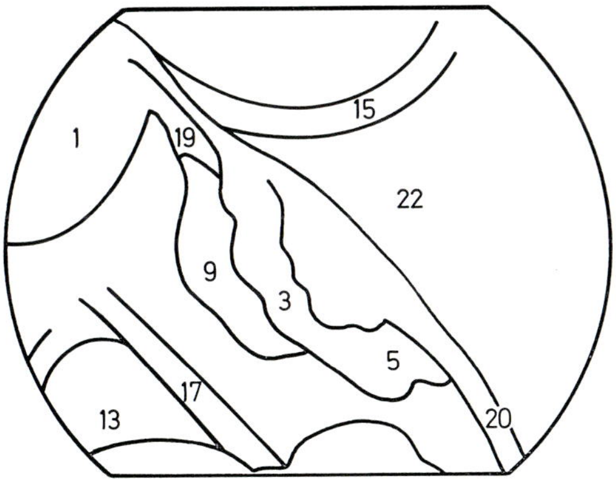
15
1
19
22
9
3
5
13
17
20

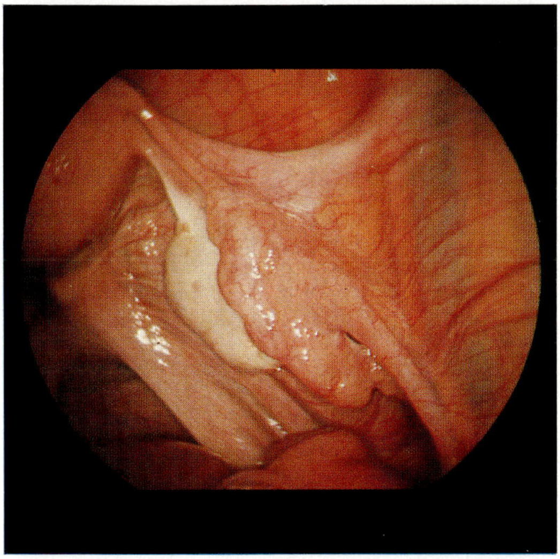

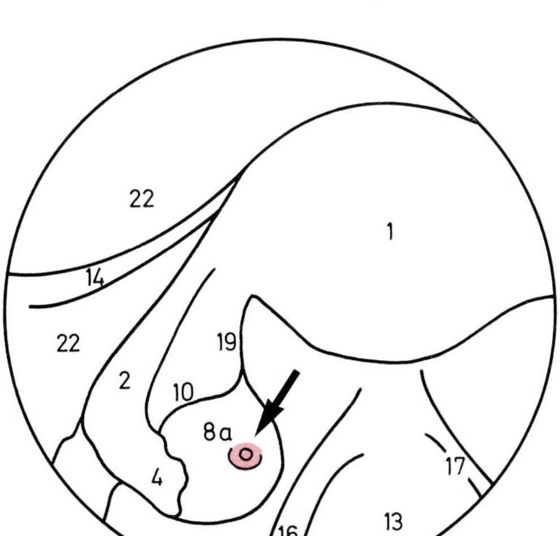
22
1
14
22
19
2
10
8a
4
17
16
13

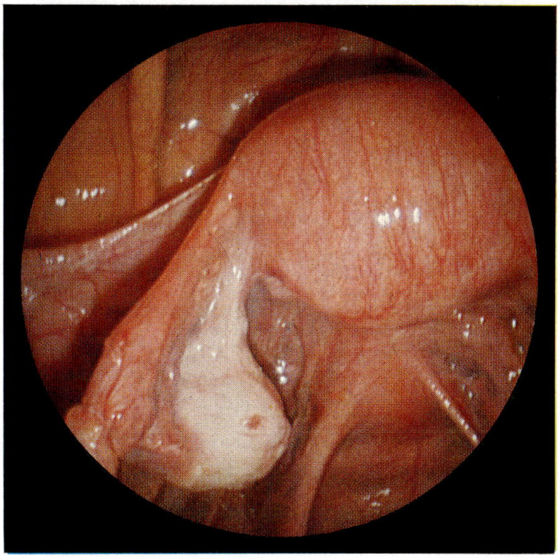

Fig. 191. Outside the pelvis, the object most subject to inspection is the appendix. Here we see a noninflamed, very long, but normally shaped appendix hanging into the pelvis. Any inflammation of such an appendix usually is very difficult to differentiate from salpingitis on the right side, since the typical symptoms of both inflammatory pictures overlap.

Fig. 192. After appendectomy the scar ideally should lie free of adhesions at the caudal end of the tenia of the ascending colon.

Fig. 193. Here the Verres needle has penetrated into the omentum at the start of the carbon dioxide gas insufflation, and the omentum has not been shaken free soon enough by elevation of the abdominal wall (see Fig. 16). The carbon dioxide gas has produced an omental emphysema. At this extent it does not yet obscure the view, nor does it represent any risk to the patient, either during laparoscopy or postoperatively.

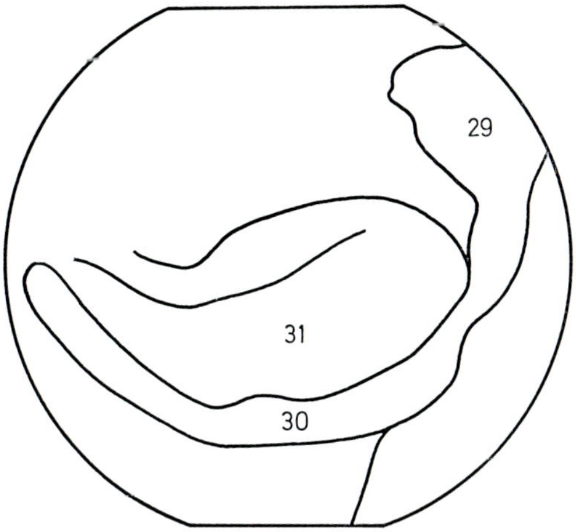
29
31
30

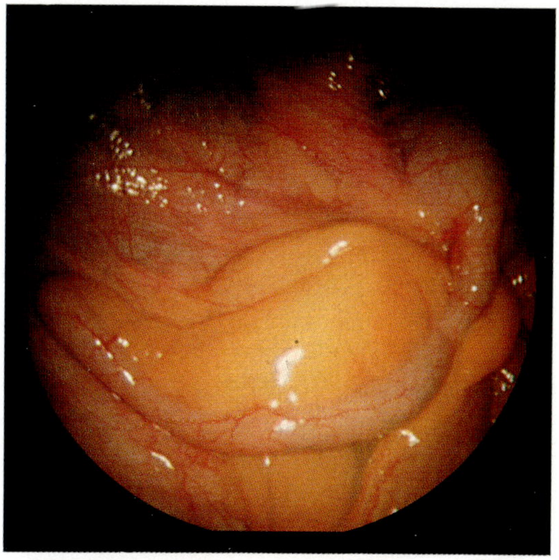

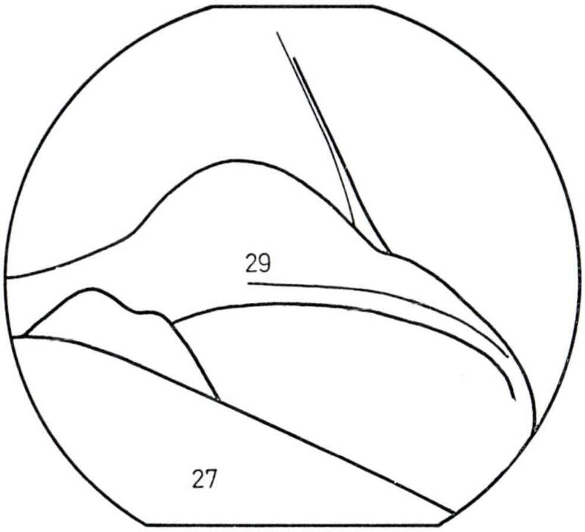
29
27

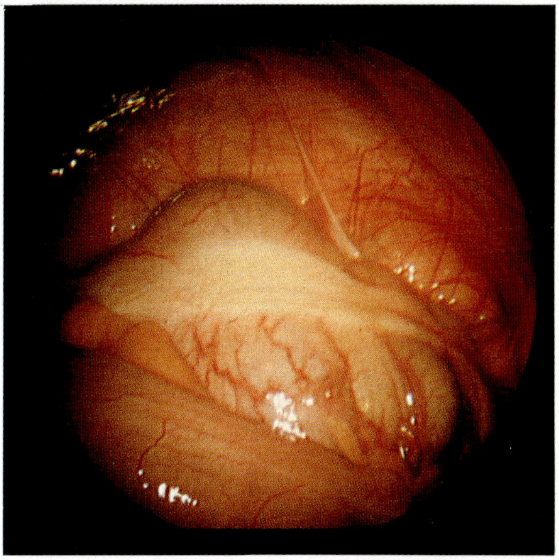

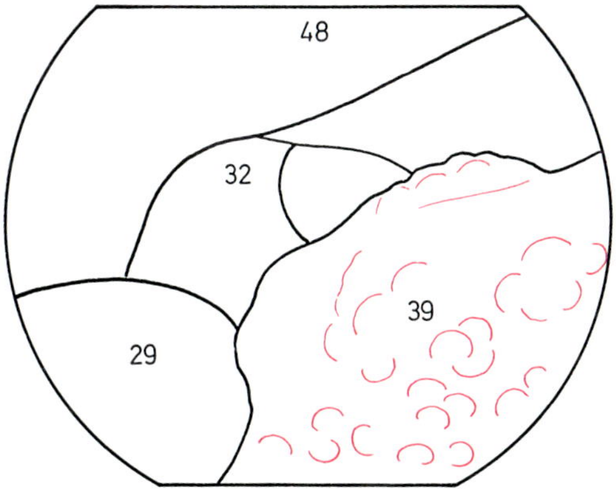
48
32
39
29

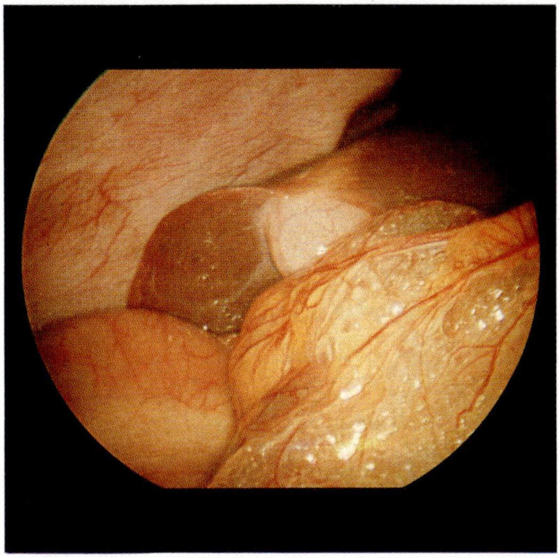

Figures 194–196 demonstrate how difficult it is, especially in obese patients, to penetrate the parietal peritoneum. If the peritoneum lies tightly against the abdominal fascia, it is perforated simultaneously with the latter by the Verres needle or trocar tip. If, however, there is a layer of fat between them, the peritoneum may be pushed forward several centimeters into the abdominal cavity along with the tip of needle or trocar.

Fig. 194 shows the loosening of the peritoneum from the fascia (see also Fig. 138) caused by the tip of the trocar. Since this event cannot be monitored optically in the case of the Verres needle, the possibility of forming a preperitoneal emphysema is great, even when the greatest care is exercised (see also Fig. 13). This event, however, can be promptly detected when using the Semm insufflator by continuous monitoring of the intra-abdominal pressure and the resistance to inflow, second by second. A preperitoneal emphysema cannot be detected by percussion.

Fig. 195. Here, in an obese patient, the tip of the trocar has not yet perforated the parietal peritoneum until it has advanced far into the abdominal cavity. By optical monitoring of the second puncture, injury to a blood vessel such as the inferior epigastric artery in the abdominal region can be prevented completely.

Fig. 196. This trocar perforated the peritoneum in the close vicinity of the inferior epigastric artery. Because a *conical* tip was used, the vessel escaped injury and was merely pushed aside. If a three-sided pyramidal trocar had been used in this case (see Fig. 25), this vessel probably would have been severed by the sharp edge of the trocar, or at least would have suffered a tangential cut. This picture demonstrates the importance of my insistence on a conical-tipped trocar. If such a complication does arise, laparotomy is not required; the vessel can be ligated at laparoscopy in the manner shown in Figure 181.

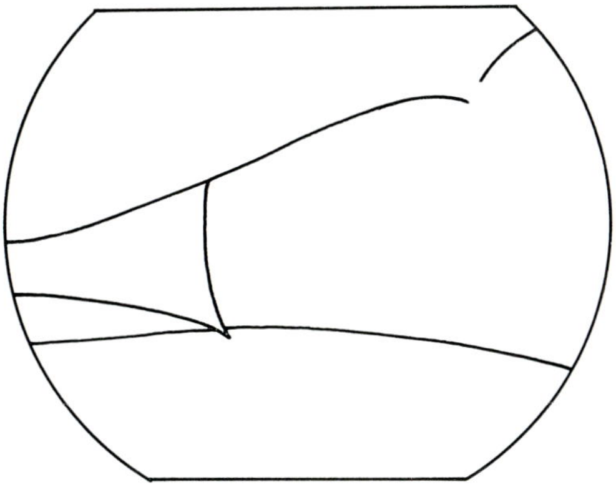
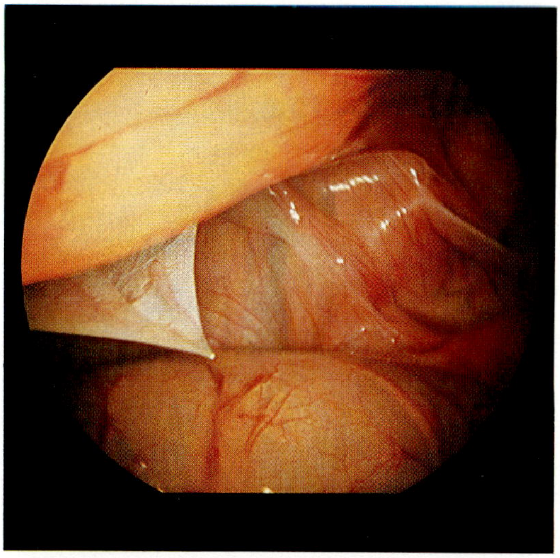
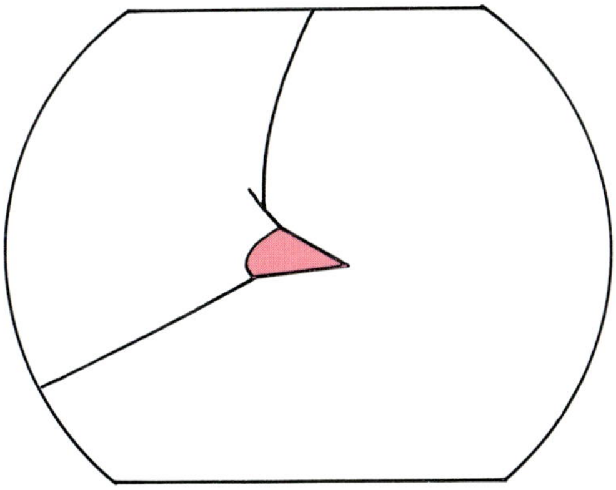
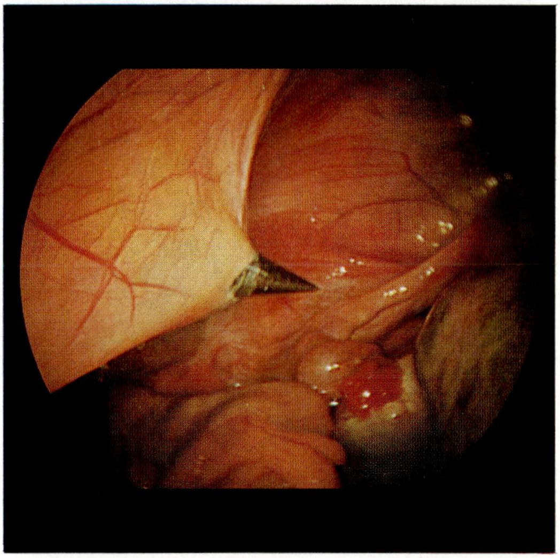
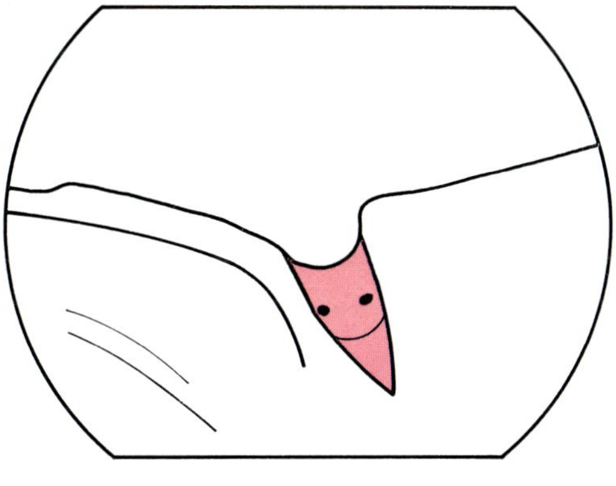
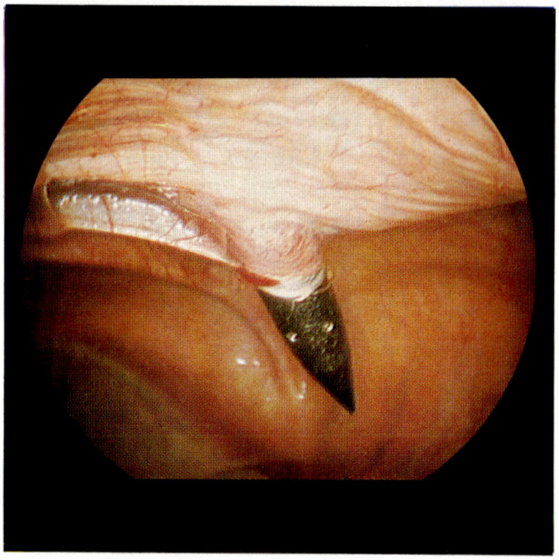

Fig. 197. An essential prerequisite for laparoscopy is a completely empty bladder. If this requirement is not observed, the view into the pelvis is partially obscured; the inspection of the cul-de-sac in particular is impossible. The arrow (→) demonstrates endometriosis.

Fig. 198. The value of routine catheterization of the bladder is shown by the picture. A catheter inserted even slightly into the bladder causes the dome of the latter to bulge out sharply. The metallic color of the catheter actually is clearly detectable through the ischemic bladder wall.

Fig. 199. The view into the pelvis is severely limited in very stout patients, since even the inside of the abdominal cavity is lined with fat. Even with careful catheterization the fat-lined dome of the bladder hangs down on the uterine fundus. The view into the cul-de-sac is rendered difficult by the masses of fat on the omentum and by the epiploic appendices.

The over-all yellow-red color, so clearly seen in this photograph, is typical in the obese patient.

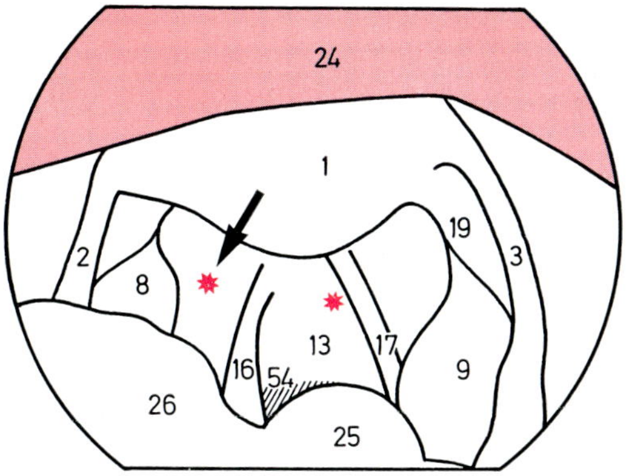
24
1
2
19
3
8
13
17
16
54
9
26
25

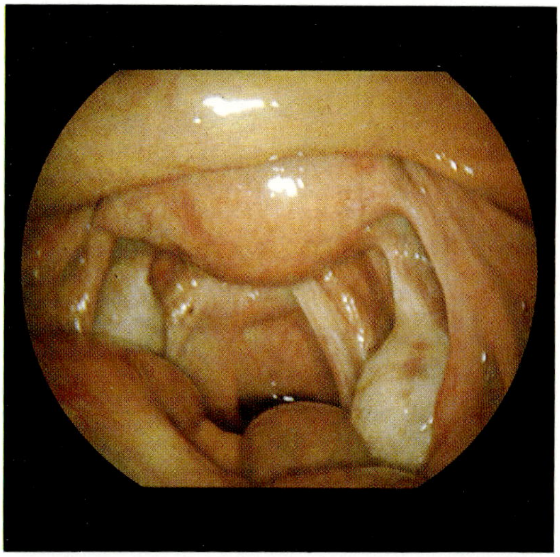

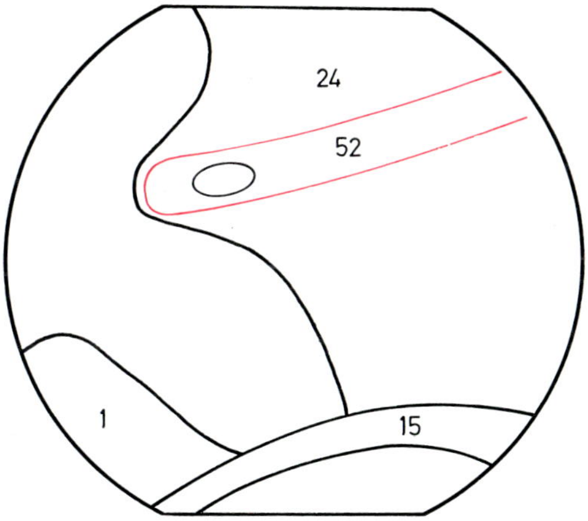
24
52
1
15

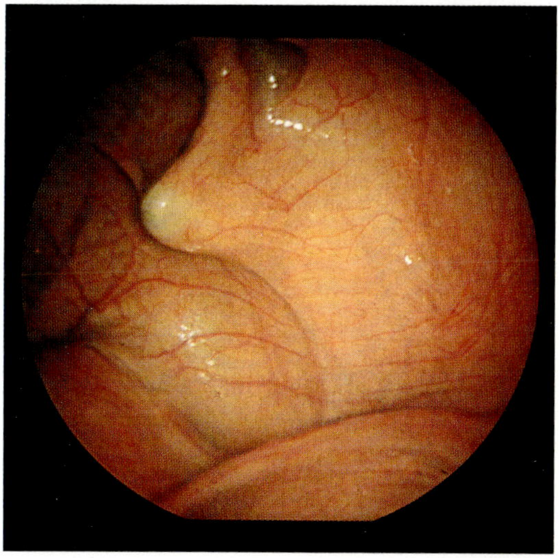

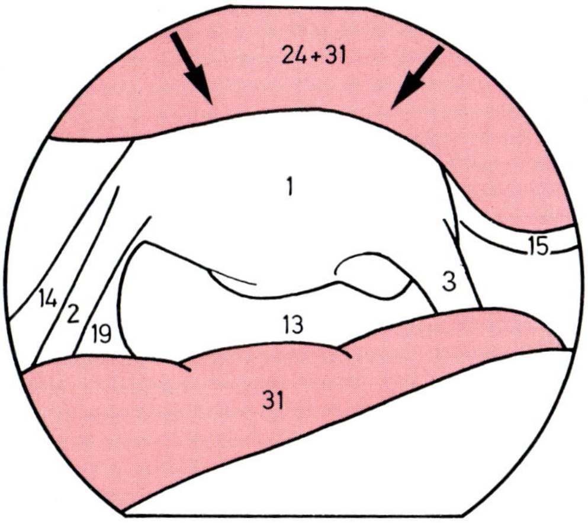
24+31
1
15
14
2
19
3
13
31

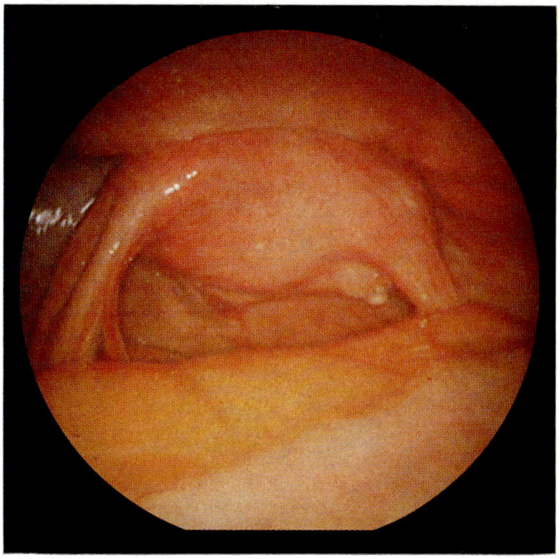

Fig. 200. It is fundamental in gynecologic laparoscopy to routinely view the upper abdomen. Lower abdominal pain occasionally has its origin in the upper abdomen, and for this reason inspection of the liver should not be omitted. Here is seen a liver of normal size with its sharp edge. The gallbladder is tense, but the surface vascularity does not suggest that a chronic inflammatory process is present.

Fig. 201. The surface of the liver seen is uneven and shows trabecular markings, and the gallbladder appears ready to rupture. Further medical evaluation and liver function tests would be advisable with these findings.

Fig. 202. Under the sharp edge of the liver lies a tensely filled gallbladder with very prominent vascularity. Chronic cholecystitis was found to be the source of this patient's referred lower abdominal pain.

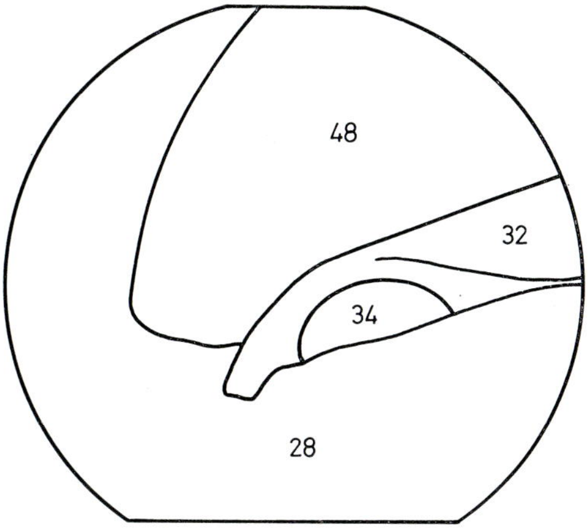
48
32
34
28

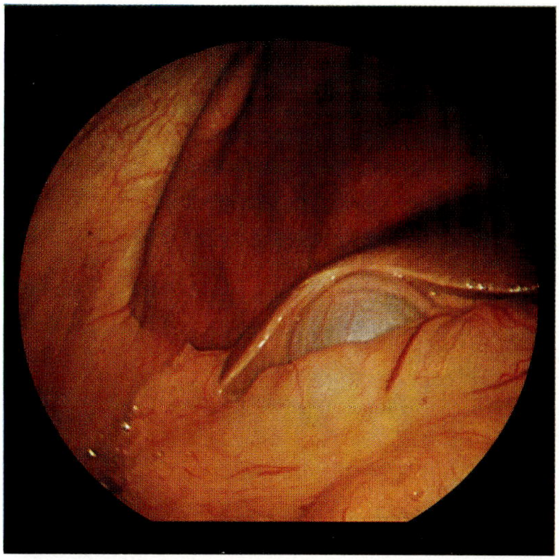

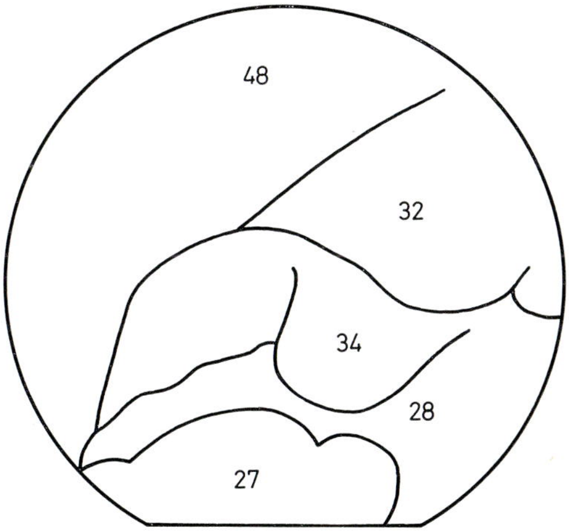
48
32
34
28
27

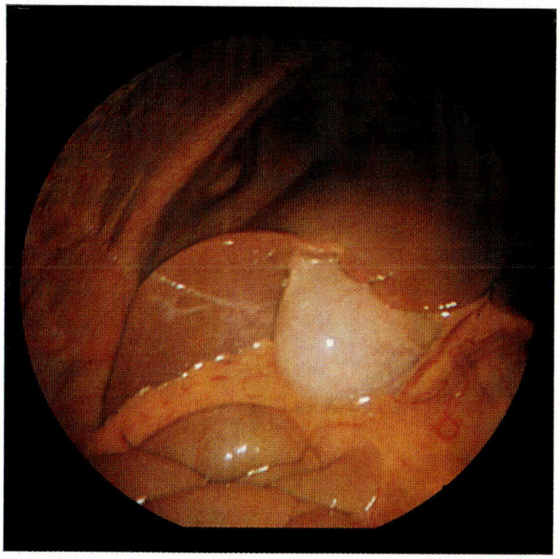

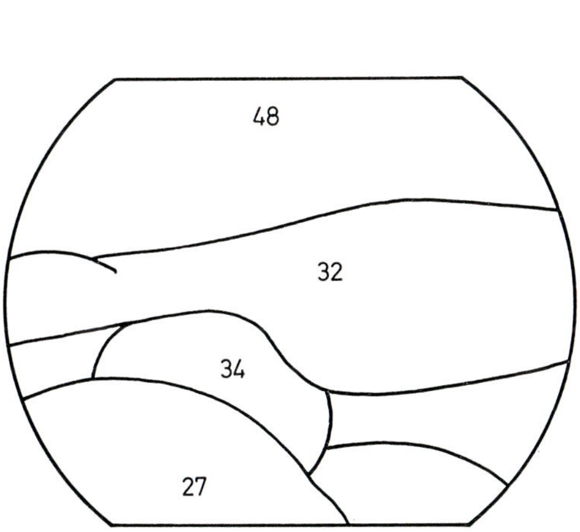
48
32
34
27

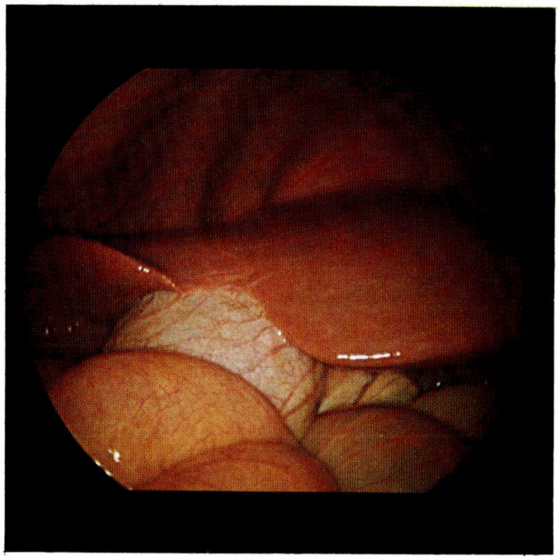

(b) Primary and Secondary Sterility

Fig. 203. Primary or secondary sterility constitutes one of the major indications for diagnostic laparoscopy. Visualization alone of the internal female genitalia, however, usually is not diagnostically revealing; it must be augmented by tubal dye insufflation and/or biopsy of the ovaries. Only rarely can occlusion of the tubes, as seen in this picture, be recognized through nodular formations in the vicinity of the cornual region of the tubes. These may be caused by intramural myomas. However, it is usually a matter of mucosal excrescences of the uterus by encapsulated nodules, which we designate as adenomyosis. In the present case the latter diagnosis is very probable, especially in view of the fact that there also is endometriosis in the cul-de-sac.

Fig. 204. Occlusion of the oviduct can be recognized here macroscopically by the knobby deformity of the right tube. It is a matter of endometriosis in the form of a tubal adenomyosis, now called salpingitis isthmica nodosa, resulting from extrauterine endometrial mucosa. In addition, an extensive endometriosis is recognizable in the cul-de-sac. The bleeding implants lead to brownish discoloration of the 10 to 15 ml of exudate in the cul-de-sac.

Fig. 205. As a result of endometrial implants in the left uterosacral ligament, the latter is finger-thick. The cul-de-sac is filled with about 20 ml of dark brown serous fluid from the bleeding implants.

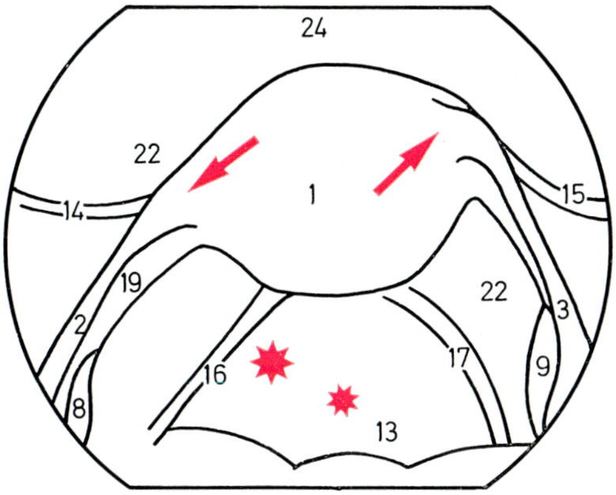
24
22
14
1
15
19
22
2
3
16
17
9
8
13

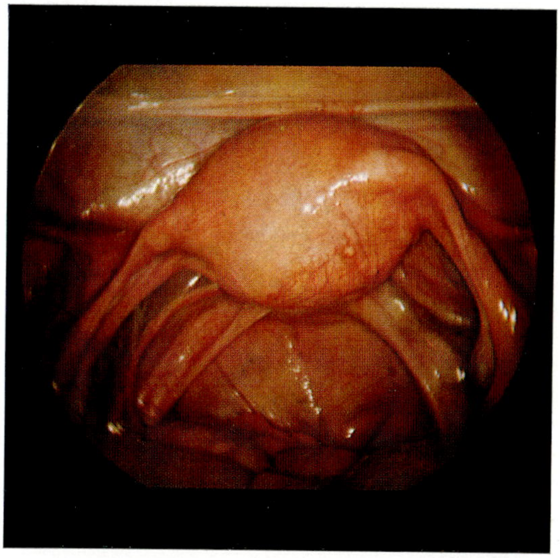

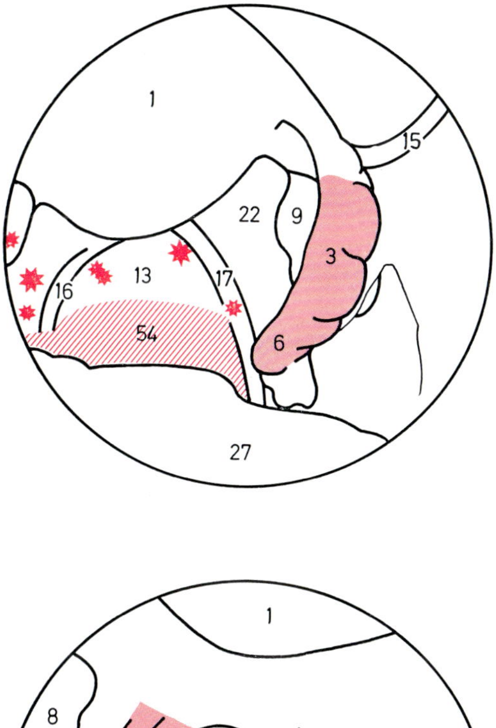
1
15
22
9
3
13
16
17
54
6
27

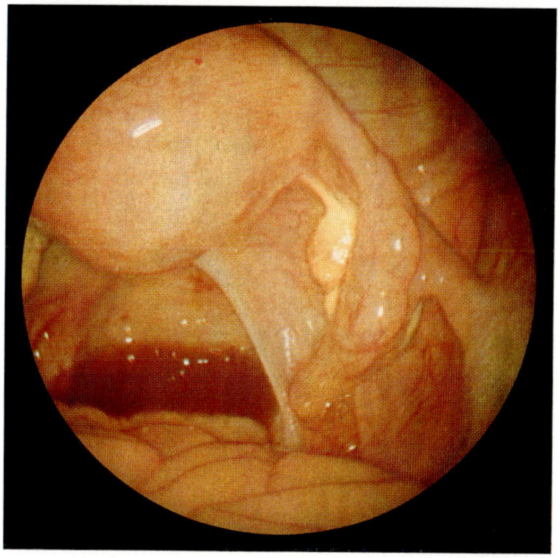

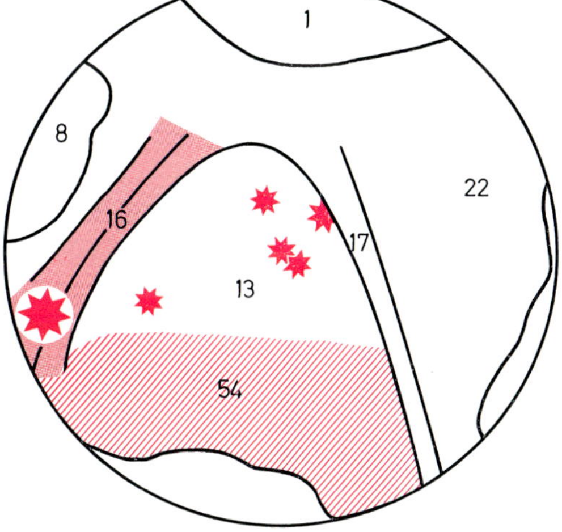
1
8
22
16
17
13
54

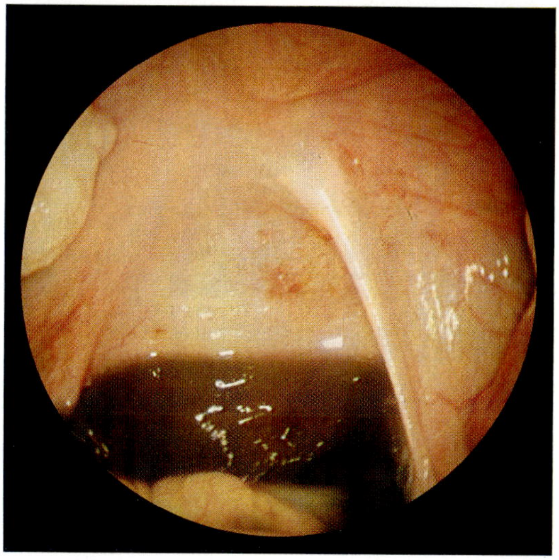

(c) Laparoscopic Monitoring of the Postoperative Site After a Sterility Operation

Fig. 206. This laparoscopic view six months after a sterility operation shows that the neotubostomy performed on the right tube was not successful. The "newly-created" tubal ampulla is hanging almost sequestered on the mesosalpinx of the tube, which is again occluded. The mesosalpinx is being elevated with atraumatic forceps. In the cul-de-sac the insufflated dye that has oozed from the left tube can be seen.

Fig. 207. Six months after a fimbriolysis in the region of the left ampulla, this laparoscopic picture shows that the tubal ampulla is closely adherent with the ovary in numerous S-bends and is occluded. The ampulla cannot come into contact with the matured follicle. The tube appears engorged because of the insufflated dye, which is under a pressure of 200 mm Hg.

Fig. 208. If a sterility operation is performed without adequate measures against postoperative adhesions (e.g., without the use of hydrocortisone flushing, etc.) a very disappointing picture is sometimes seen postoperatively. Here we see the situation after resection of the right tube with implantation. The cul-de-sac is broadly obscured by adhesions, and the uterus can scarcely be elevated.

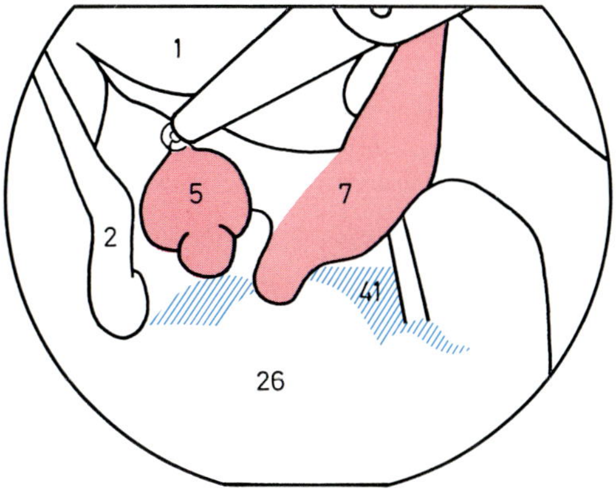
1
2
5
7
41
26

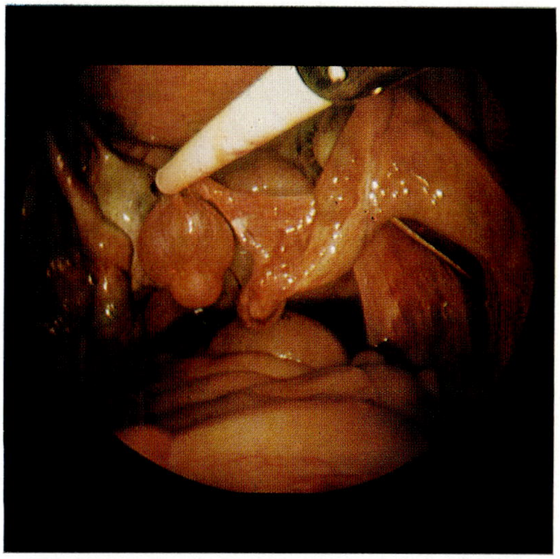

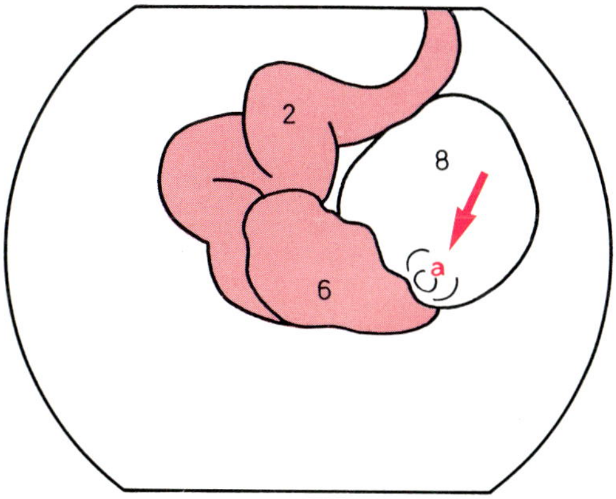
2
8
a
6

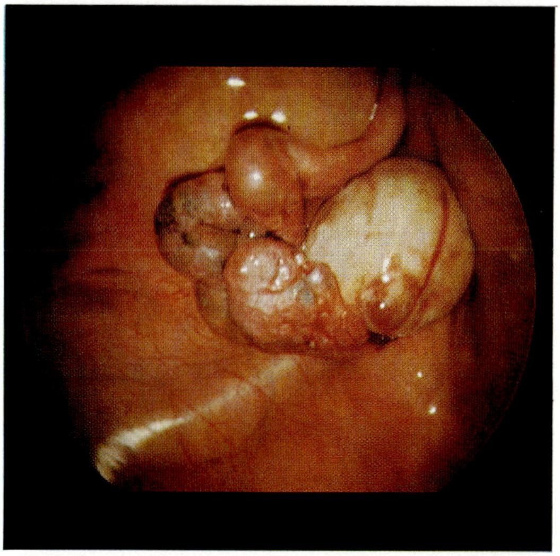

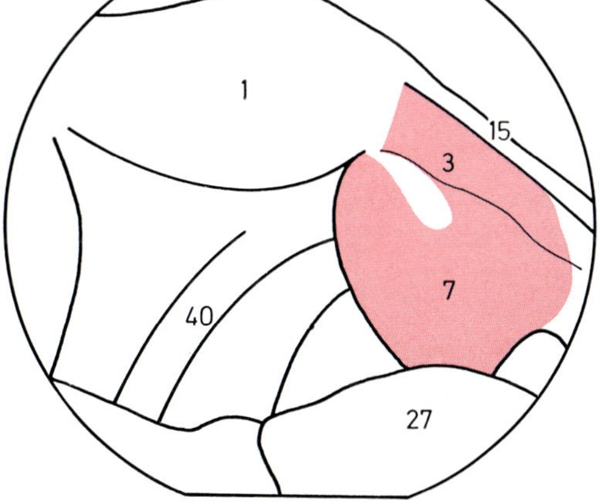
1
15
3
7
40
27

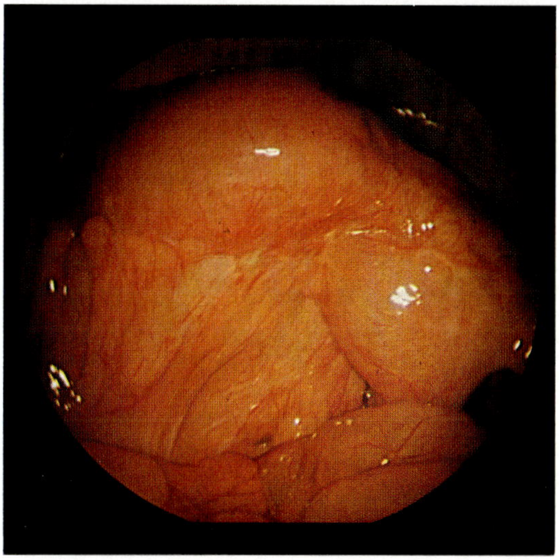

(d) Acute Lower Abdominal Distress in Early Pregnancy

Fig. 209. In early pregnancy a differential diagnosis between extrauterine and intrauterine pregnancy presents difficulties. On the basis of this laparoscopy a pigeon-egg sized dermoid was diagnosed in a patient with an eight-week sized intrauterine pregnancy.

Fig. 210. This hydropic graafian follicle was found in a patient two months pregnant with colicky lower abdominal distress. Such thin-walled follicular cysts can readily be removed by suction during early pregnancy. The wall of the cyst is resected at several places with the biopsy forceps and coagulated (see Figs. 383–400).

Fig. 211. Colicky lower abdominal distress in early pregnancy often has no genital causation, and is interpreted as acute appendicitis, which often results in an unnecessary appendectomy. In the present case, however, a fully normal appendix was revealed in a patient three months pregnant. There was no surgical intervention.

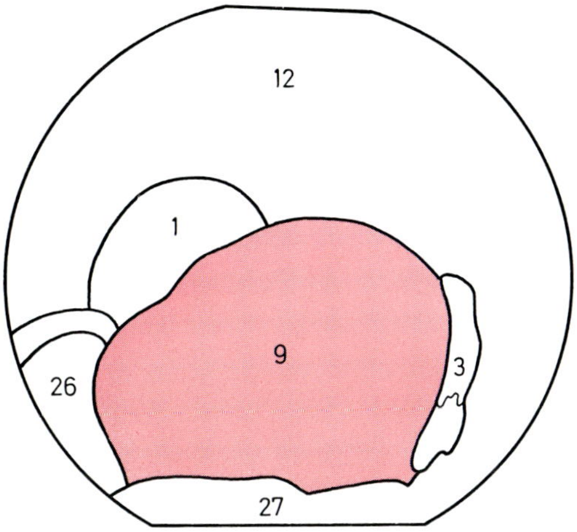
12
1
9
3
26
27

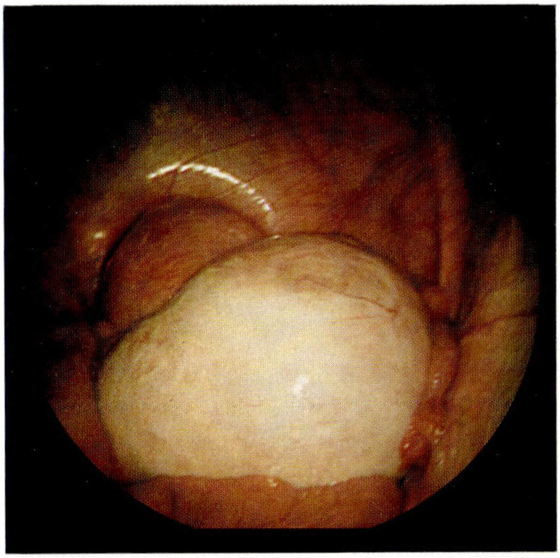

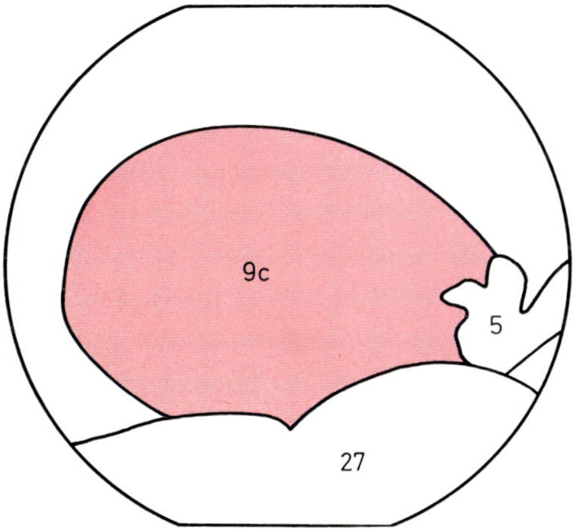
9c
5
27

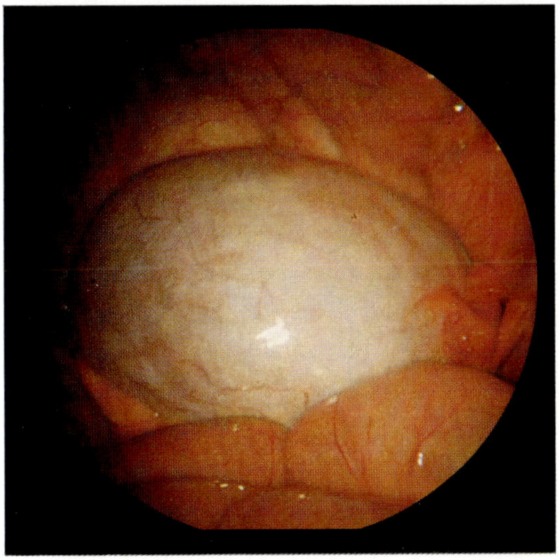

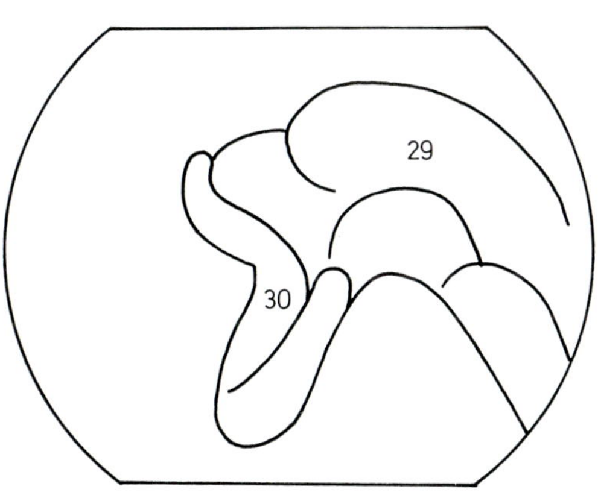
29
30

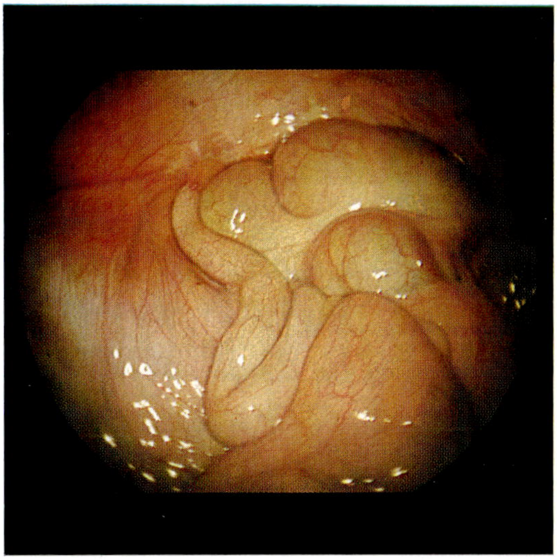

(e) Suspicion of Endometriosis and "Second-Look" Laparoscopy After Hormonal Treatment of Endometriosis—Therapy-Resistant Inflammation of the Bladder (e.g., Resulting from Endometriosis on the Dome of the Bladder)

Fig. 212. With endometriosis, the "menstrual blood" produced from the endometrial implants often is found in the cul-de-sac before elevation of the uterus.

Fig. 213. Bladder distress of long years' standing often is caused by endometriosis. These implants of endometriosis on the dome of the bladder led to crusty thickening and adherences in the vicinity of the anterior wall of the uterus.

Fig. 214. After the elevation of the uterus, numerous endometrial implants no larger than the head of a pin were visible in the vicinity of the left broad ligament. Such implants usually cannot be felt by palpation, and thus escape routine detection.

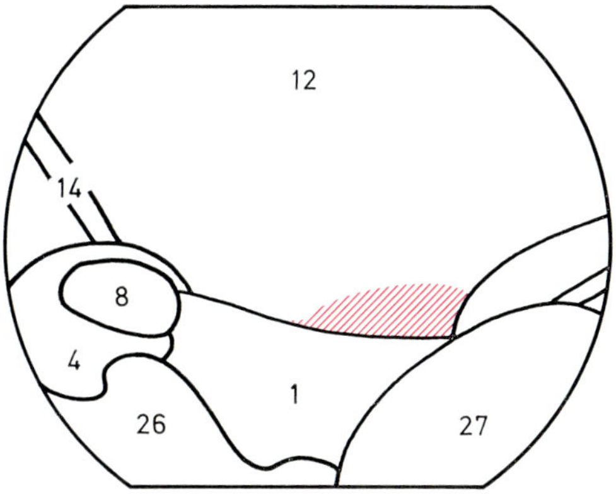
12
14
8
4
1
26
27

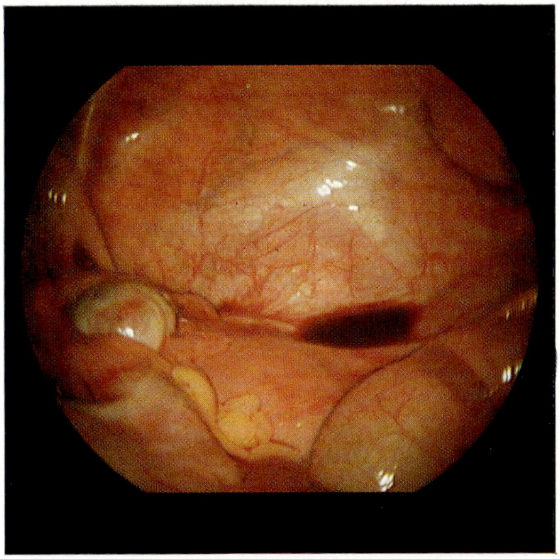

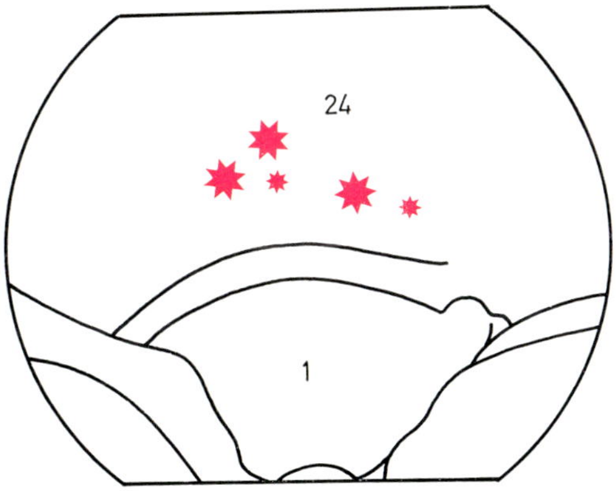
24
1

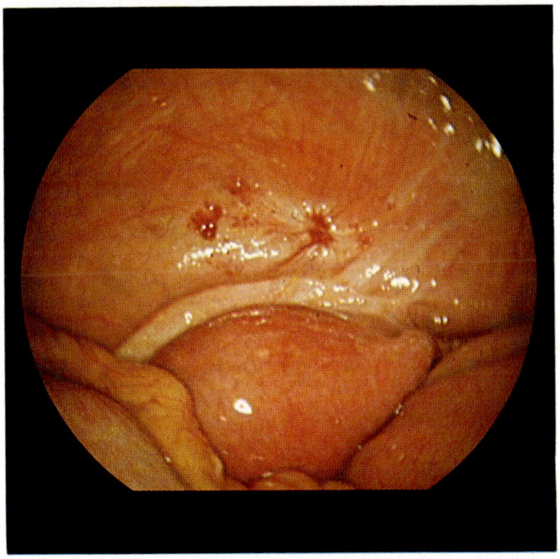

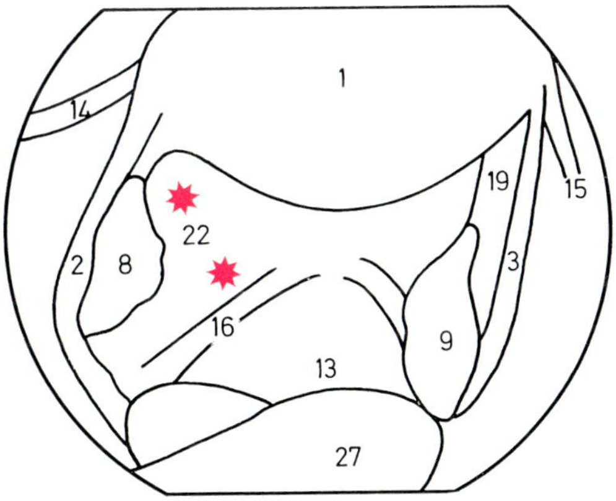
1
14
19
15
22
2
8
3
16
9
13
27

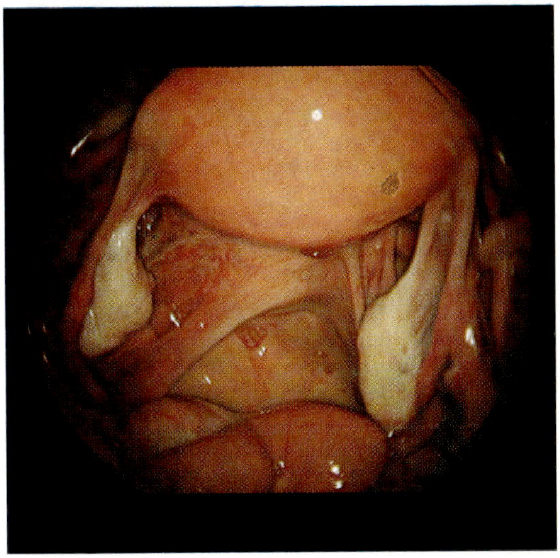

Fig. 215. These endometrial implants lie in the left broad ligament and in the vicinity of the left ureter. After years of kidney ailments on the left side they have now led to an occluded ureter. These implants were successfully eliminated by the aid of Endotherm coagulation without damage to the ureter (see Chapter IV, Section 8c).

Fig. 216. The ovary is a favorite location for endometriosis. Here the white colored ovary appears as large as a human fist, and in several places shows the escaping of the tarry cyst contents (the common terms "tarry" or "chocolate" cyst stem from this condition). On the anterior wall of the uterus, bulging myomatous nodules are clearly visible.

Fig. 217. The left endometriotic ovary, engorged with old blood, is suspended very loosely on its utero-ovarian ligament. The numerous endometrial implants in the cul-de-sac have led to dense adhesions in this region, some of which were broken by elevation of the uterus.

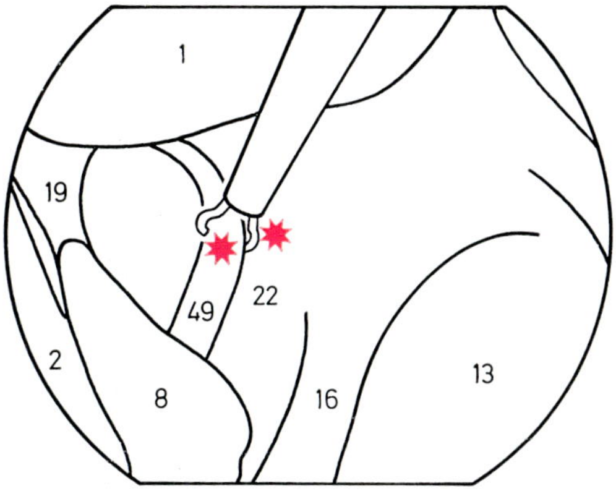
1
19
49
22
2
8
16
13

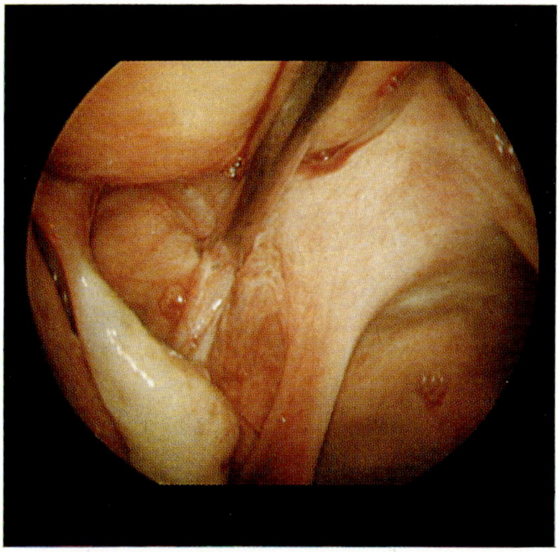

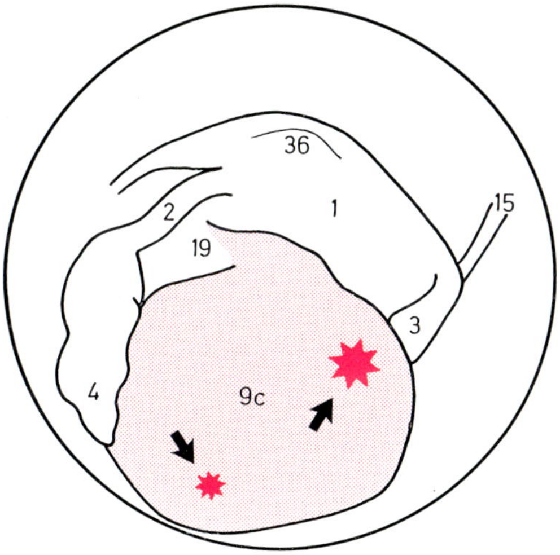
36
15
1
2
19
3
4
9c

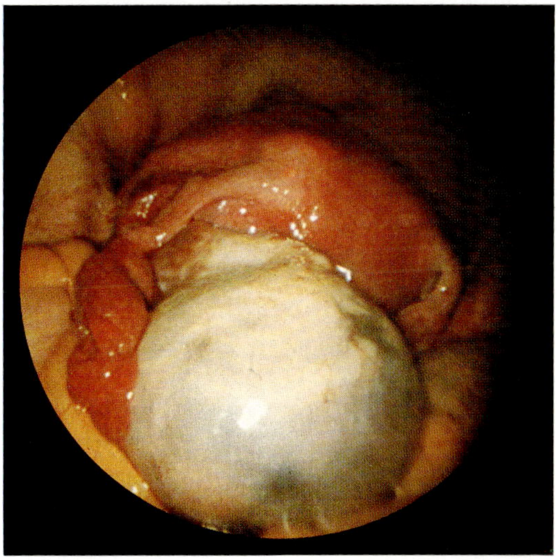

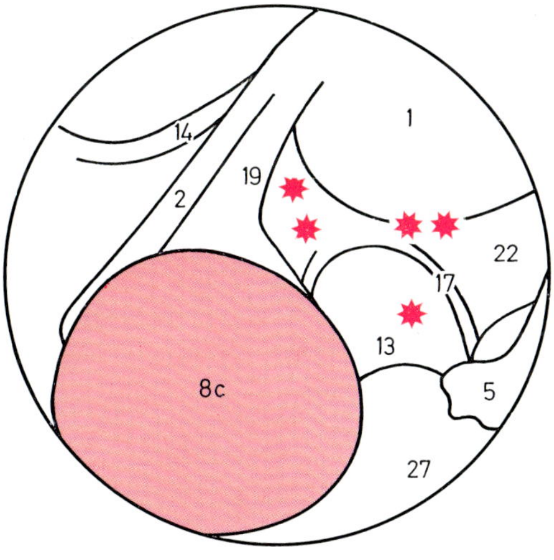
14
1
19
2
22
17
13
5
8c
27

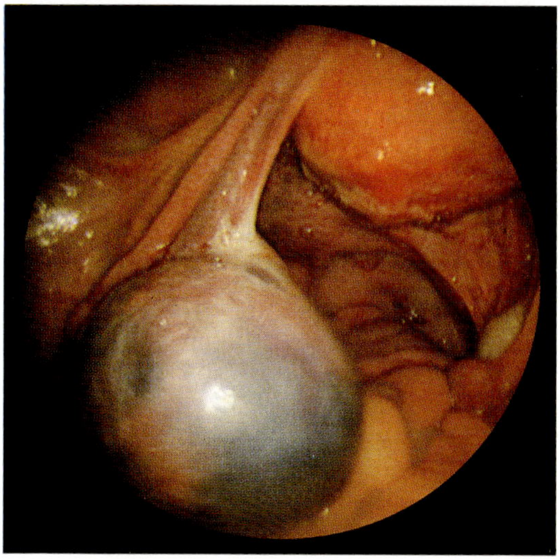

Fig. 218. Upon elevation of the "chocolate cyst" at the left, some of the hematoma is running out of the cyst through a fresh rupture. The right ovary also has become a "chocolate cyst." In the cul-de-sac we find still more pinhead-sized endometrial implants.

Fig. 219. The left ovary, enlarged to the size of a pigeon's egg, has been partially changed into a "chocolate cyst" as a result of endometriosis. In this instance it is confined exclusively to the left ovary.

Fig. 220. Endometriosis often is not immediately evident at the first inspection of the internal genitalia; only on closer examination of the peritoneum can the numerous implants be seen. This is especially true when the laparoscopy is not being performed at an optimal time for diagnosis of endometriosis, i.e., in the last third of the menstrual cycle.

In the case of this same laparoscopy performed during the first third of the cycle, the implants can be recognized only upon closest inspection. The enlargement of the left ovary here is likewise caused by a hematoma resulting from endometriosis, as was revealed upon subsequent puncture of the ovary. The white color of the tunica albuginea is deceptive as a result of a wrongly chosen time for differentiating between ovarian endometriosis and a follicular cyst.

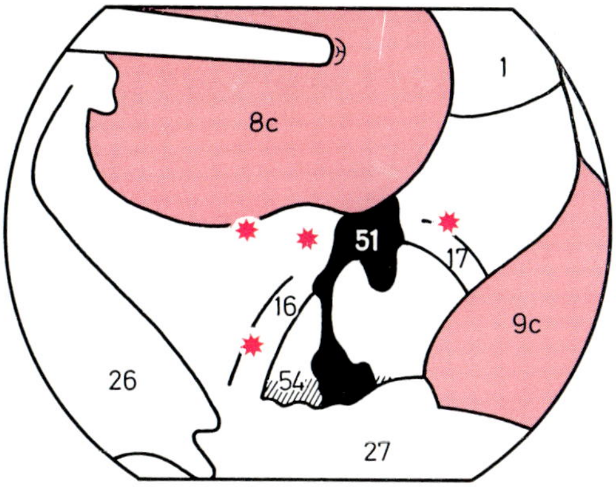
1
8c
51
17
16
9c
26
54
27

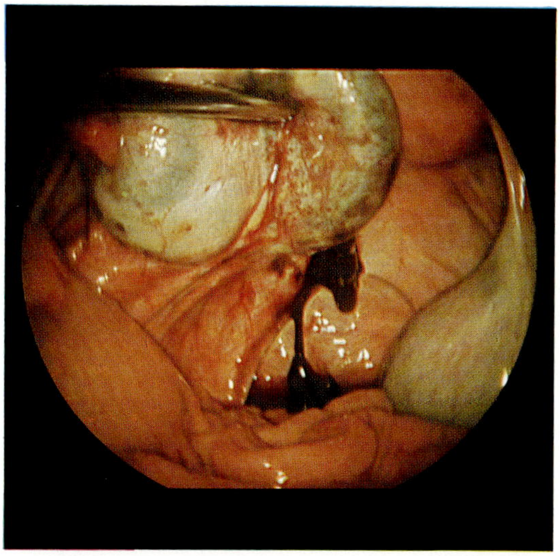

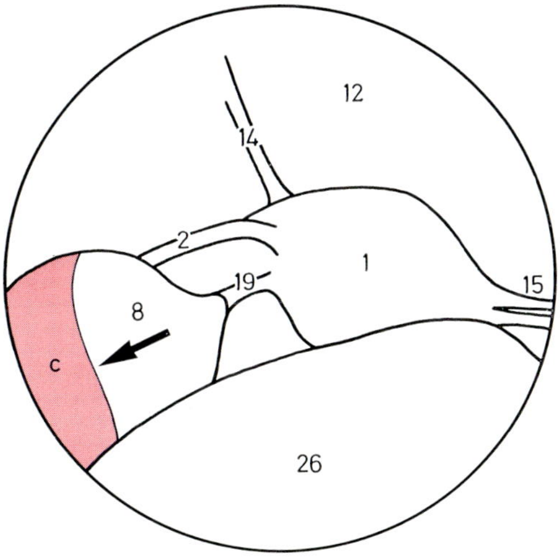
12
14
2
1
19
15
8
c
26

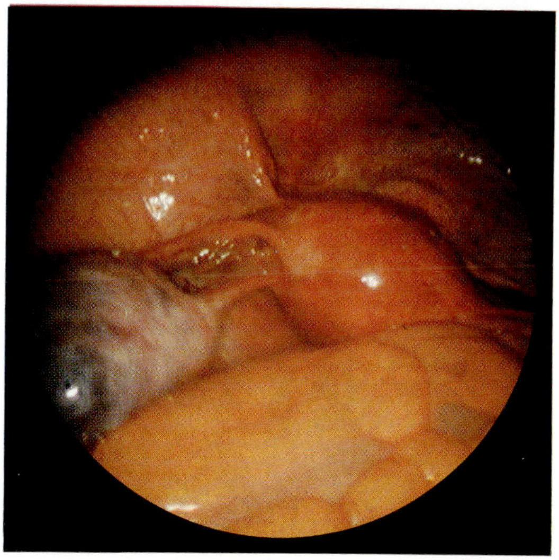

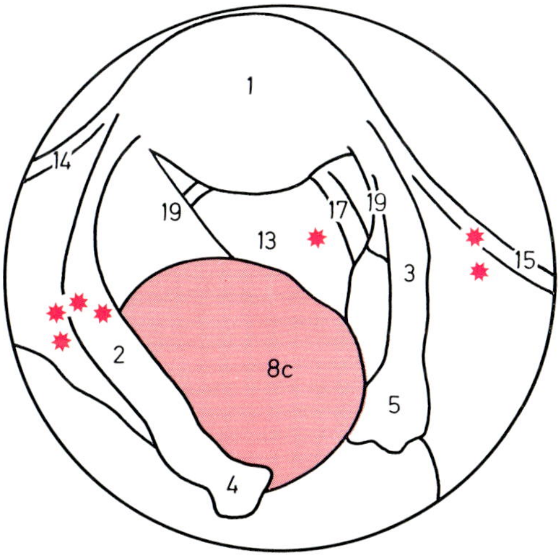
1
14
19
17
19
13
15
3
2
8c
5
4

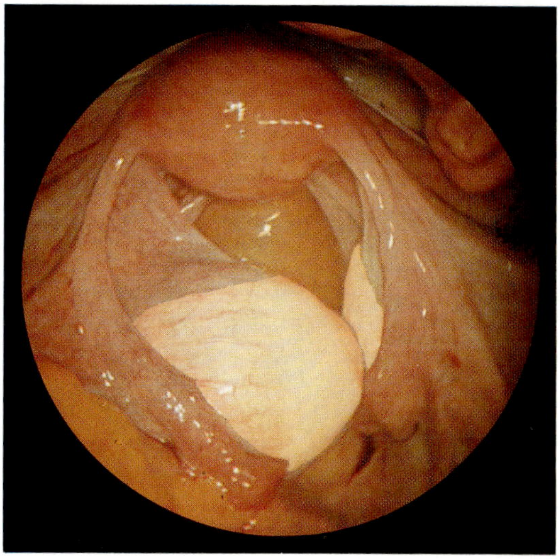

Fig. 221. Endometriosis is an especially fruitful field for laparoscopy, because the implants not only are diagnosed but can be treated during the same session. This picture shows the coagulation of implants in both uterosacral ligaments during laparoscopy. Note particularly the additional hypertrophy of the left uterosacral ligament. At the same time, pronounced bilateral varicosities in the form of pelvic congestion can be observed in this patient.

Fig. 222. With the uterus elevated, an old, scarred, cherry-sized implant of endometriosis is revealed in the left uterosacral ligament. In the cul-de-sac there are about 10 ml of clear serous fluid. The left ovary bears the corpus luteum showing evidence of recent extrusion of an ovum. In the vicinity of the right broad ligament, the veins are as thick as a pencil.

Fig. 223. The endometriosis on the dome of the bladder, in combination with a "chocolate cyst," has here led to broad deposits of fibrin, with secondary adherence of the dome of the bladder and the anterior wall of the uterus. Even such massive findings, possible with optical scanning, escape notice in the bimanual examination technique, and for years have gone under the diagnostic name of "chronic inflammation of the bladder."

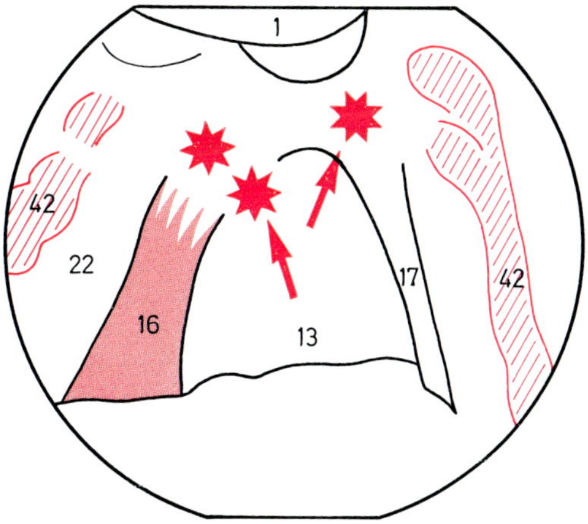
1
42
22
16
13
17
42

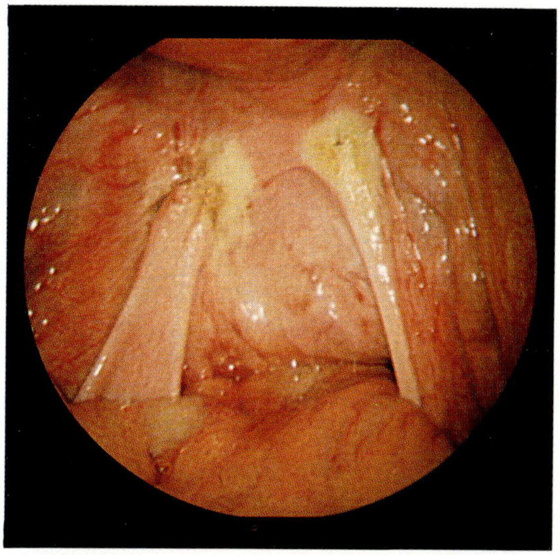

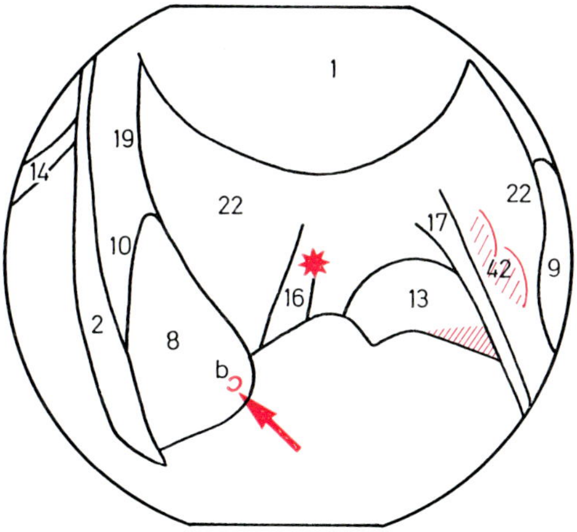
1
19
14
22
10
2
8
b
c
16
13
17
42
22
9

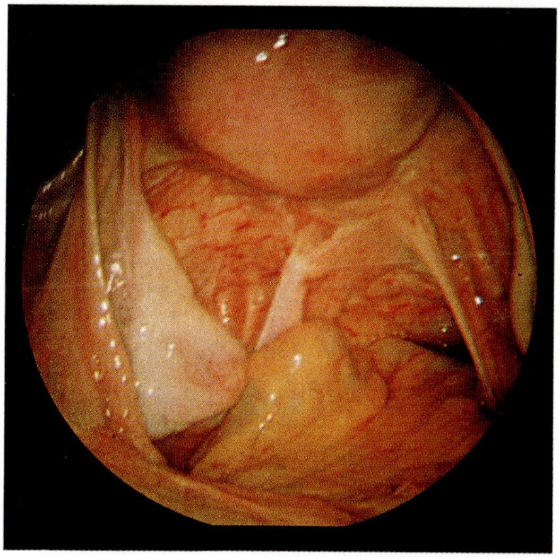

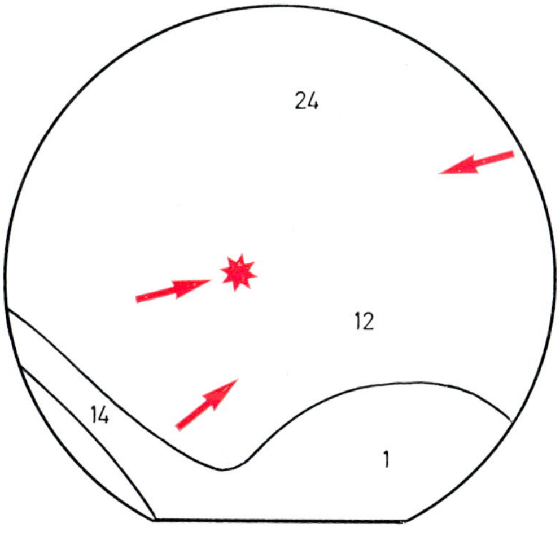
24
12
14
1

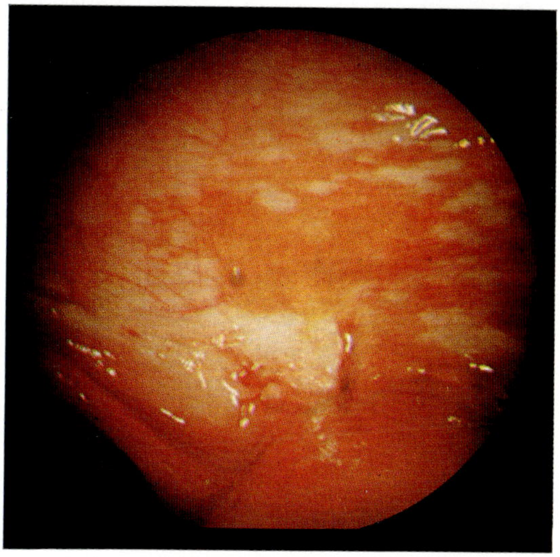

(f) *Chronic Lower Abdominal Distress and Its Laparoscopic Explanation*

Fig. 224. A primary indication for gynecologic laparoscopy is "chronic distress of the lower abdomen." By visual inspection of the pelvis, morphologic causes are diagnosed for which no characteristic pathology can be found in reviewing the case. The patients usually have been undergoing conservative therapy for years.

In these patients, chronic distress in coitus is caused by minor velamentous adhesions that have arisen on the sites of old implants of endometriosis. Moreover, we recognize some split-scars in the peritoneum, a syndrome that has arisen intrapartum (Allen and Masters). Both ovaries carry some retention cysts with the surface of the ovaries becoming irregularly lumpy as a result. The outer configuration of the uterus conforms to an arcuate uterus.

Fig. 225. Here, after a case of pelvic peritonitis, the omentum has become attached to the uterine corpus and fundus, a condition that makes it impossible to view the cul-de-sac even after elevation of the uterus. In cases of fullness of the intestines, phantom tumors often can be palpated in the presence of such adhesions in the lower abdomen.

Fig. 226. Postoperatively after an oophorectomy an adhesion of the omentum to the right round ligament has arisen. Such adhesions in the lower abdomen can be safely and neatly severed nowadays by the Endotherm coagulation technique at laparoscopy (see Chapter IV, Section 8). Such lysis of adhesions no longer involves a repeat laparotomy.

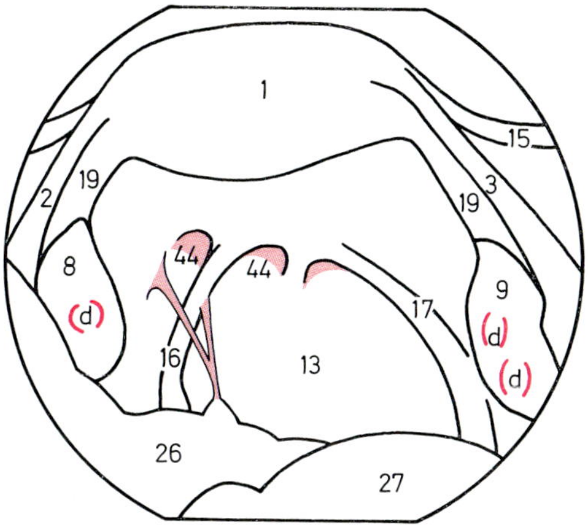
1
15
2
19
3
19
8
44
44
9
(d)
17
(d)
(d)
16
13
26
27

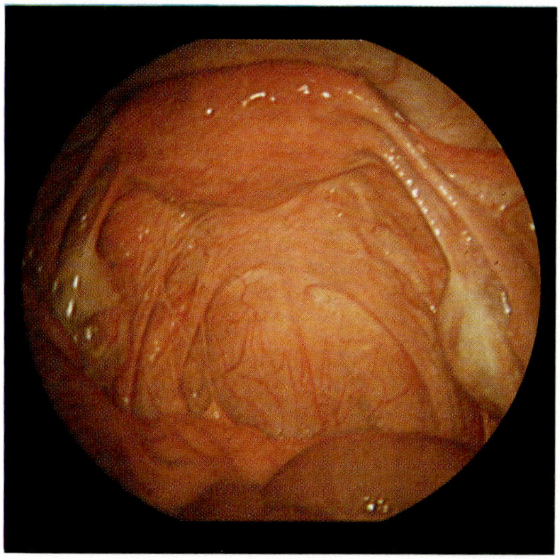

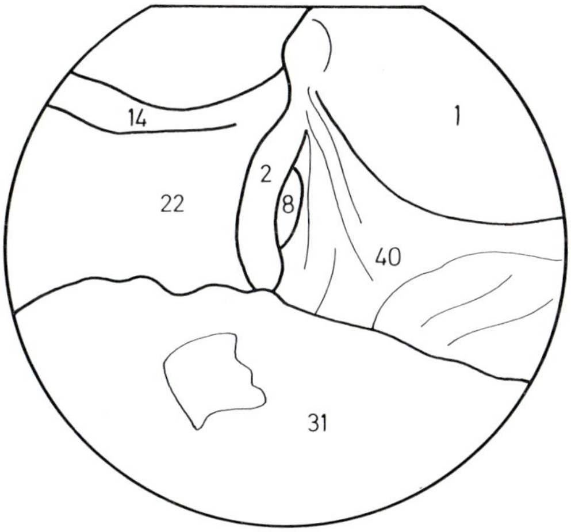
14
1
2
22
8
40
31

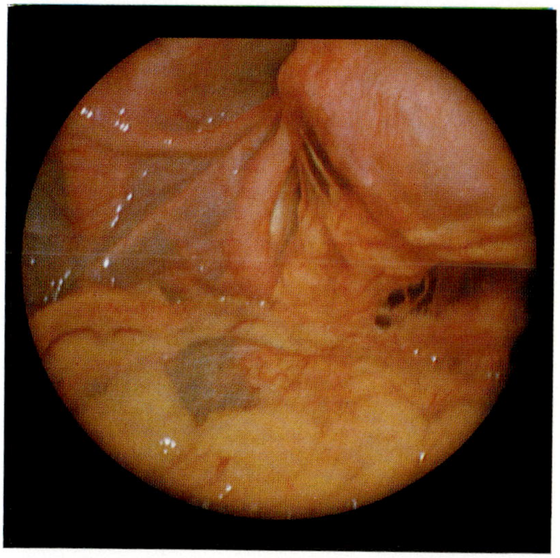

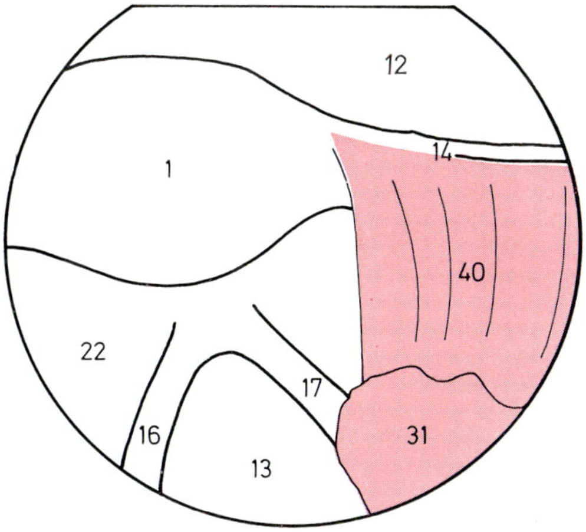
12
14
1
40
22
17
16
31
13

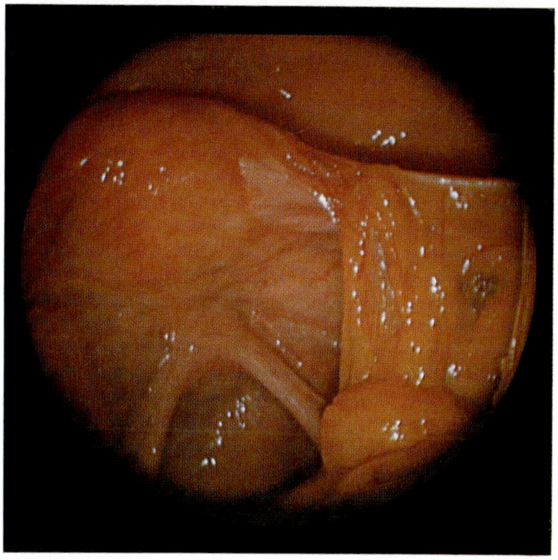

Fig. 227. In this patient, who had not undergone laparotomy previously, broad-based adhesions were found between the omentum and the posterior wall of the uterus, obviously the result of a continuing low-grade pelvic peritonitis. The chronic pains in the lower abdomen also may be caused partially by the pelvic congestion in the region of the right mesovarium and broad ligament.

Fig. 228. After operative suspension of a retroflexed uterus, chronic lower abdominal distress often is noted. Here we see the situation eight years after the procedure as described by Halban and H. Martius. The round ligaments had been attached to the anterior wall of the uterus, and the bladder peritoneum was sutured to the uterine fundus (*arrow*), a method derived from vesicofixation according to Halban-Werth. The nonphysiologic location of the suspensory apparatus explains the chronic distress. Chronic congestion also may have had something to do with the occurrence of the pelvic congestion clearly visible on both sides.

Fig. 229. In the retroflexed uterus the anteflexion technique of Doléris-Gillan also has been used. This picture shows the situation eight years after the operation, which was successful because of its location. The sharp angling of the oviduct (*arrow*) that almost always results often leads to induced tubal sterility.

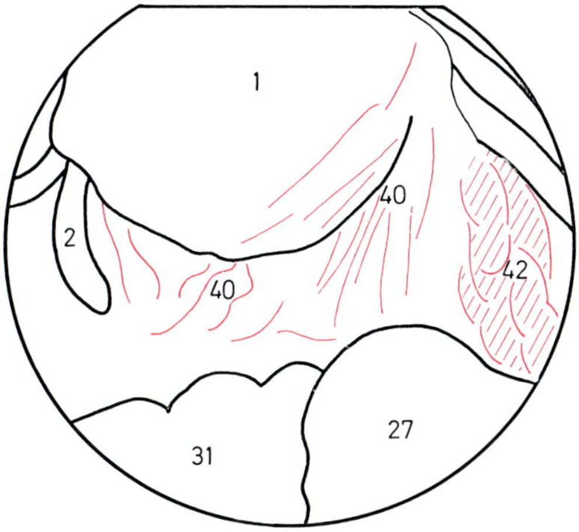
1
2
40
40
42
31
27

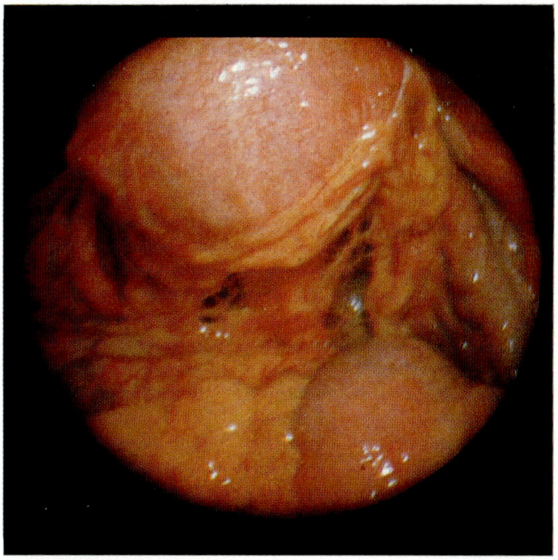

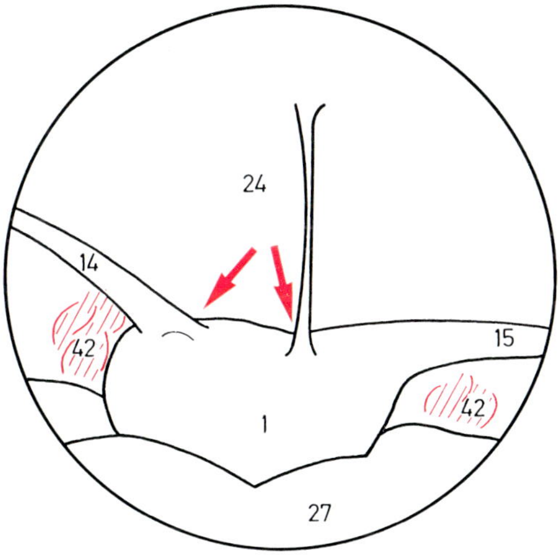
24
14
42
15
1
42
27

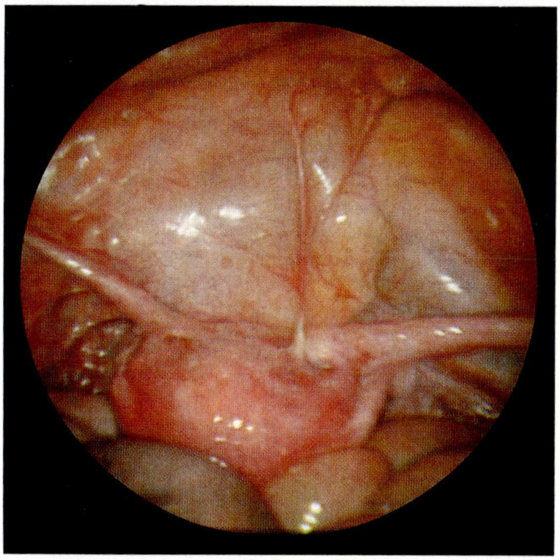

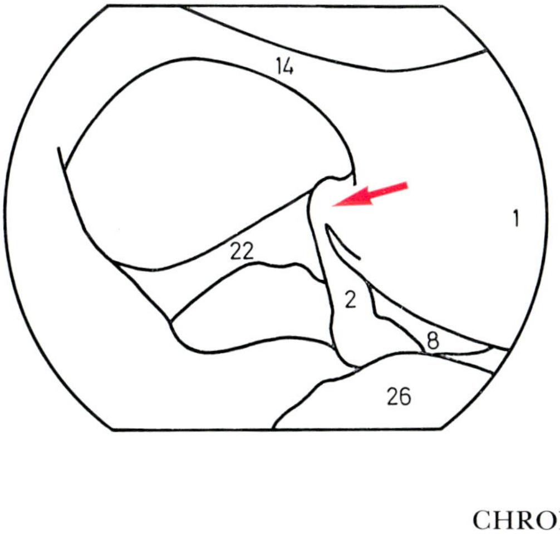
14
1
22
2
8
26

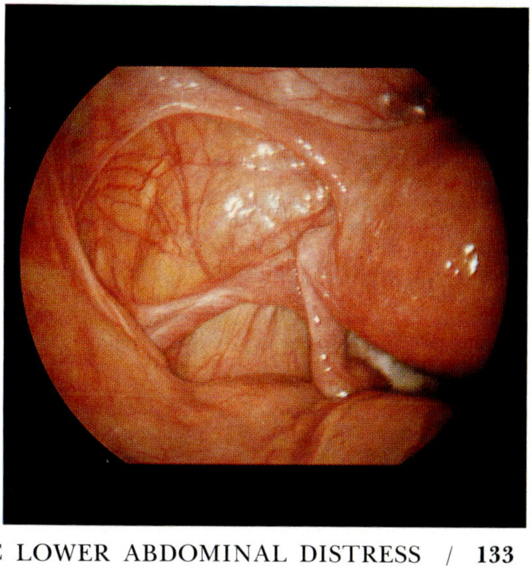

Fig. 230. This retroflexed uterus had been suspended anteriorly ten years earlier (Doléris). Since that time the patient had complained of severe lower abdominal distress. At laparoscopy a fine adhesion (*arrow*) was seen between the dome of the bladder and the fundus, which ran to the rectal ampulla. After coagulation with the crocodile forceps and the Endo-coagulator (Fig. 178), this adhesion, which had been the cause of the patient's complaint, was eliminated with scissors.

Fig. 231. The soft, doughy tumor seen here on the right beside the uterus is diagnosed at laparoscopy as a parovarian cyst. The right tube, much elongated, passes over it in a long curve.

Fig. 232. After a right salpingectomy because of tubal pregnancy, the omentum has become adherent to the fundus, blocking the view into the cul-de-sac. The omentum was successfully separated from the uterus at laparoscopy.

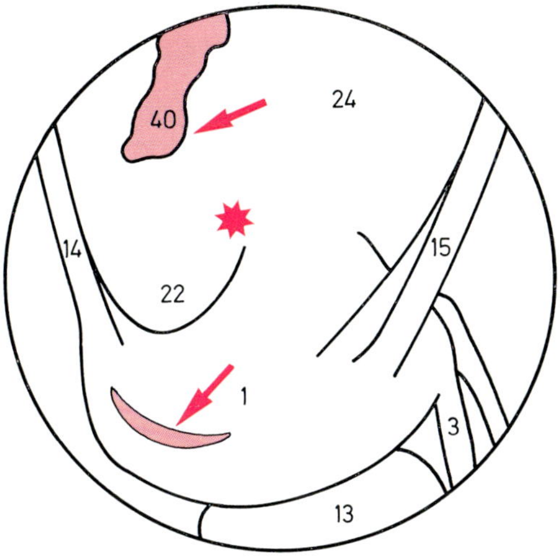
40
24
14
15
22
1
3
13

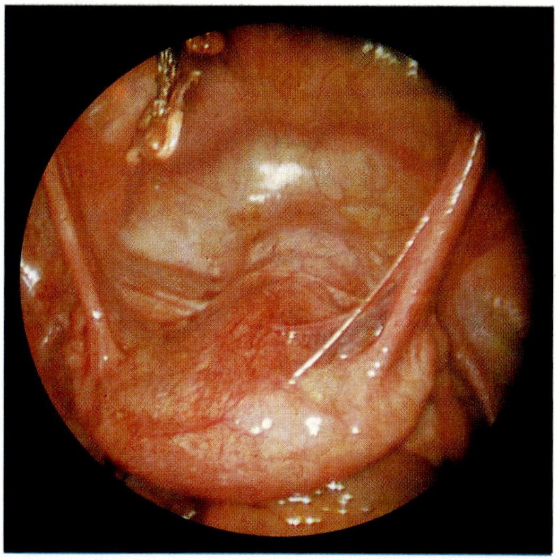

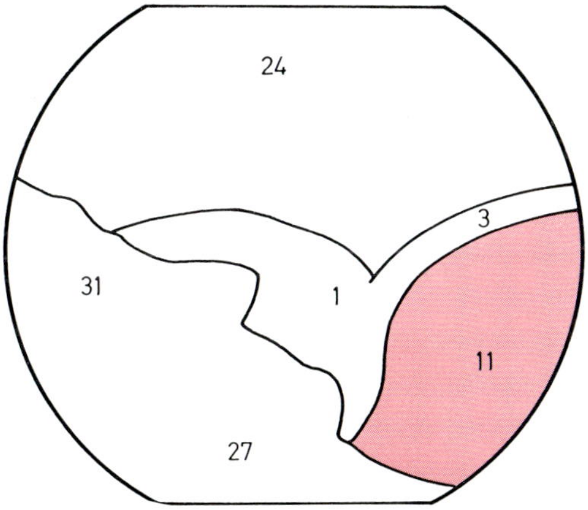
24
3
31
1
11
27

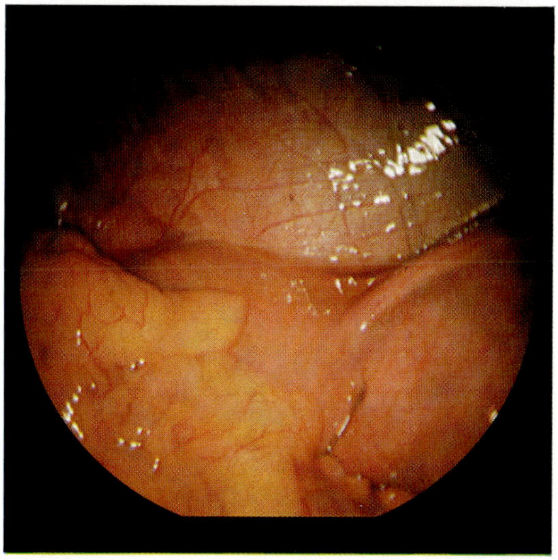

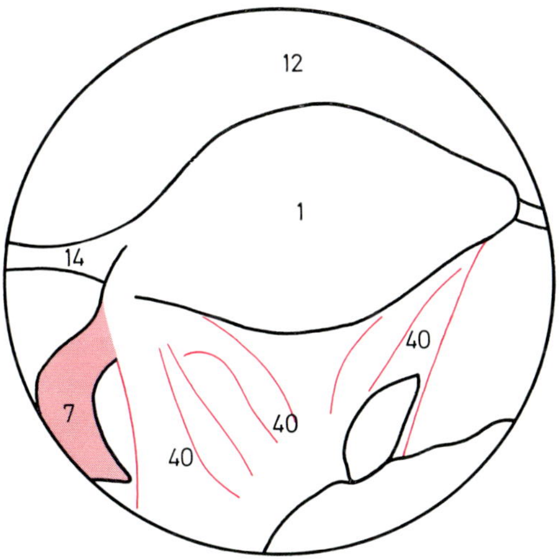
12
1
14
40
7
40
40

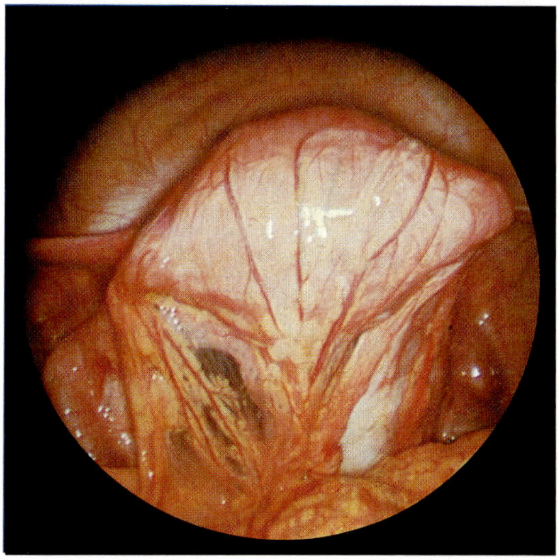

Fig. 233. Obscure lower abdominal distress, especially during coitus, is here explained by the dense linear adhesion running between the posterior wall of the fundus and the rectal ampulla. It apparently arose on the site of previous endometriosis. The severing of this adhesion at laparoscopy led to elimination of this chronic distress.

Fig. 234. In 80 per cent of all appendectomies, laparoscopy reveals an adhesion between the intestinal and the parietal peritoneum. Usually these adhesions cause no discomfort, but in many cases they are the cause of chronic lower abdominal complaints.

Fig. 235. Loops of small intestine are involved in these adhesions, and are drawn ventrally and limited in mobility. In such cases the state of fullness of the intestine determines whether the complaint is one of chronic drawing or rather of colicky pains in the adnexal and abdominal areas.

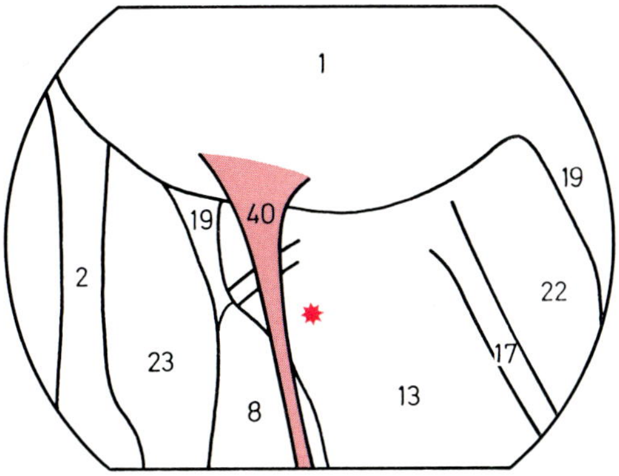
1
19
19
40
2
22
17
23
13
8
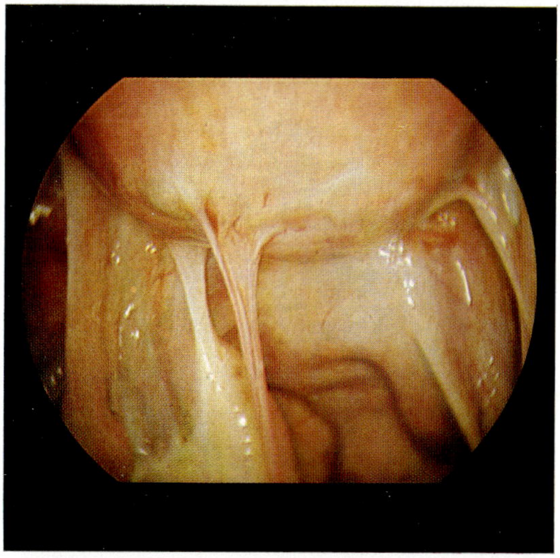

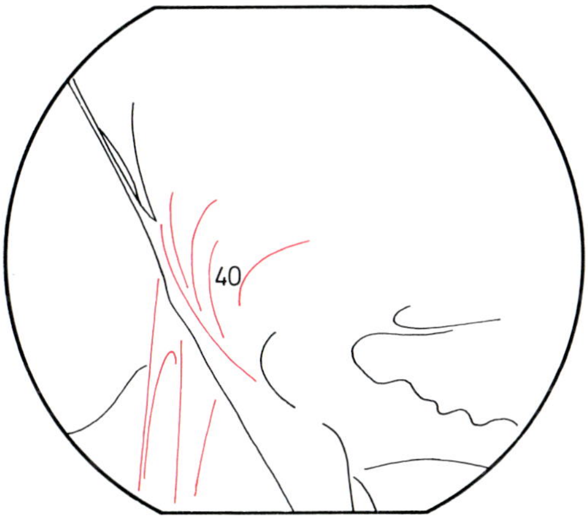
40
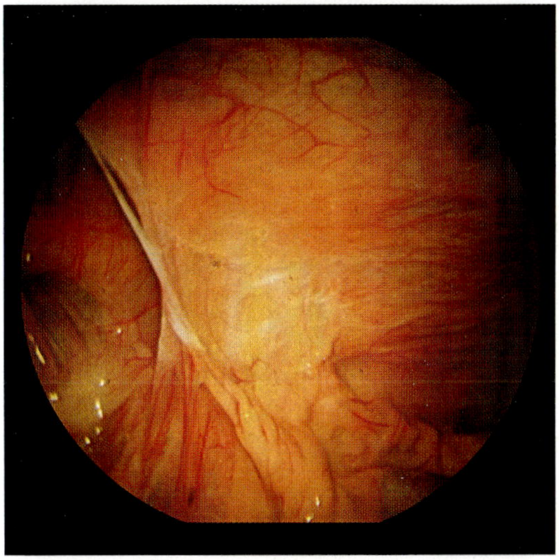

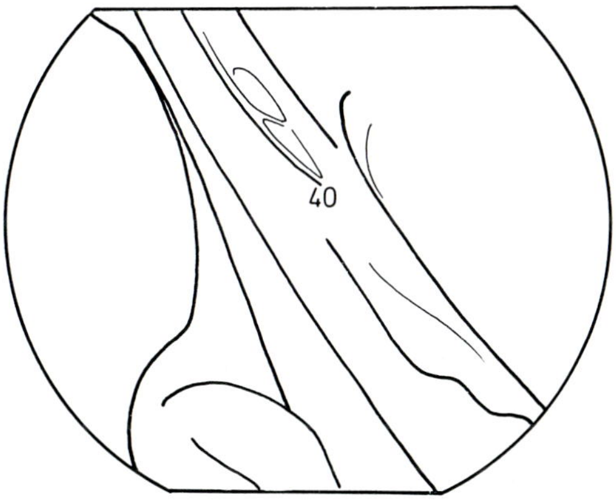
40
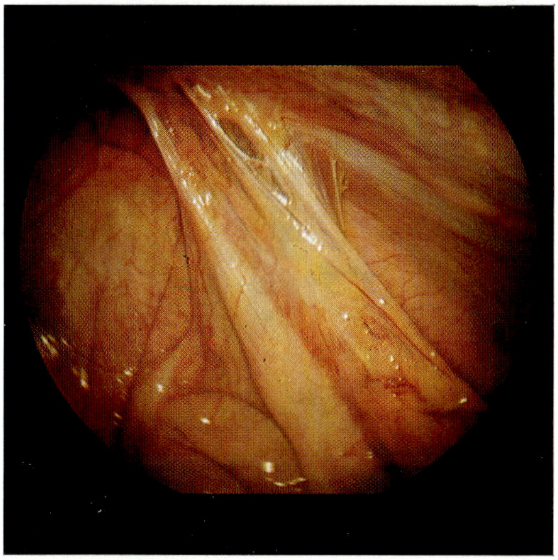

(g) Congestion of Pelvic Veins

Fig. 236. Varicosities in the region of the parametria, particularly of the mesovarium, play a significant role in chronic lower abdominal distress. They apparently occur with greater severity as a result of increased hormonal medication.

In the case shown here, lower abdominal complaints that had persisted for years were caused by varicosities, some of them finger-thick, in the paracervical region. Although the hydrostatic pressure of about 1 m with a 15° elevation of the abdomen is lacking, the engorged varicose vein complexes are clearly recognizable.

Fig. 237. After elevation of the left fallopian tube, the varicosities in the left parametrial region above the uterosacral ligament become clearly visible. The mesovarium is engorged with varicose veins.

Fig. 238. While reclining normally on her back and with the uterus not elevated, this postmenopausal patient also has quite distinct varicosities in the atrophic ligaments of the tube and of the ovary.

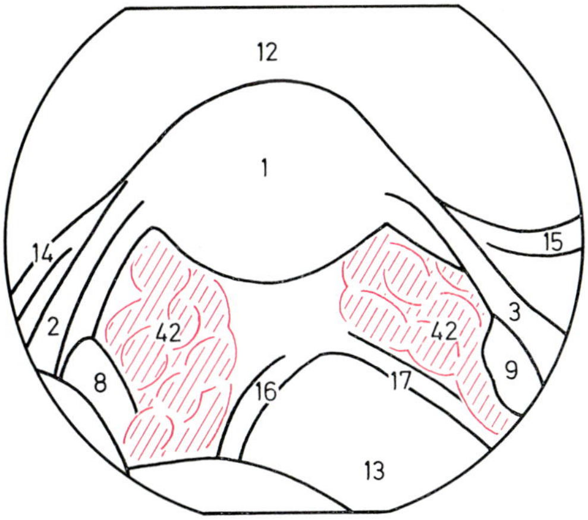
12
1
14
15
2
42
42
3
8
16
17
9
13

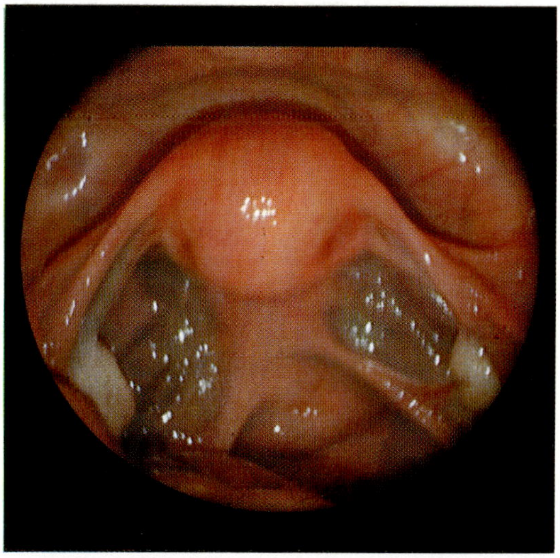

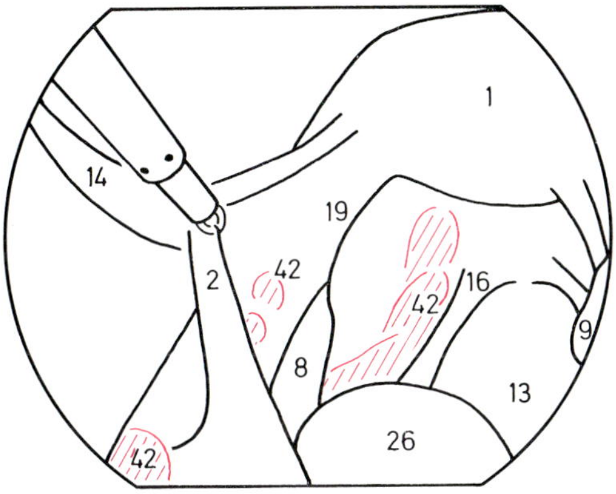
1
14
19
2
42
42
16
9
8
13
26
42

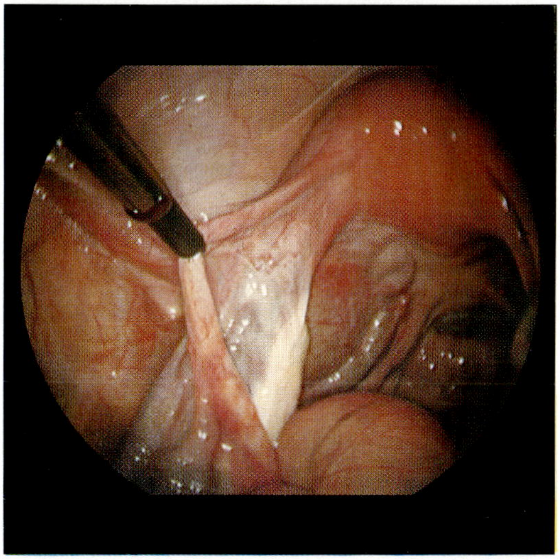

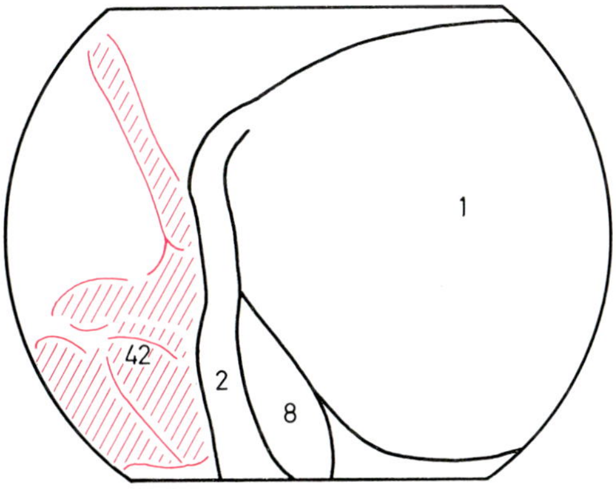
1
42
2
8

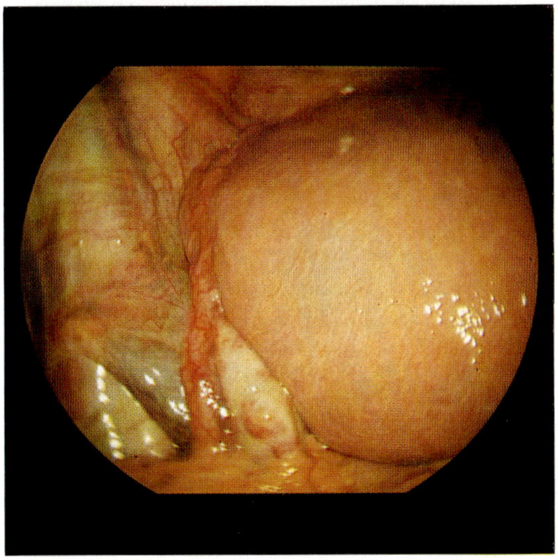

Fig. 239. This gravida nine was sterilized by coagulation of both tubes with high-frequency current. In the region of the left broad ligament the pelvic congestion is clearly visible. The arrows indicate the points where the atraumatic high-frequency coagulation forceps took hold. Note the irregular course taken by the high-frequency current. In the sterilization of the right tube it apparently flowed chiefly from the fundus, but in the left tube it flowed more from the region of the ligament, no doubt because of the high conductivity of the blood in the peritubal varicose vein complex.

Fig. 240. Despite the 15° Trendelenburg position, the varicosities in the broad ligament and in the mesovarium are seen to be still engorged. The picture makes clear the possibility and danger of massive formation of thrombi in the adnexal region in the event of a gynecologic operation or even spontaneously, e.g., postpartum. Upon elevation of this uterus, a few small peritoneal adhesions were torn. A peritoneum with several scars is seen in the right broad ligament, which can be thought of in connection with the Allen-Masters syndrome.

Fig. 241. In addition to a chronic perisalpingitis with peritubal adhesions, some of which were torn upon elevation of the uterus, there are marked varicosities, especially in the region of the left broad ligament and the right infundibulopelvic ligament.

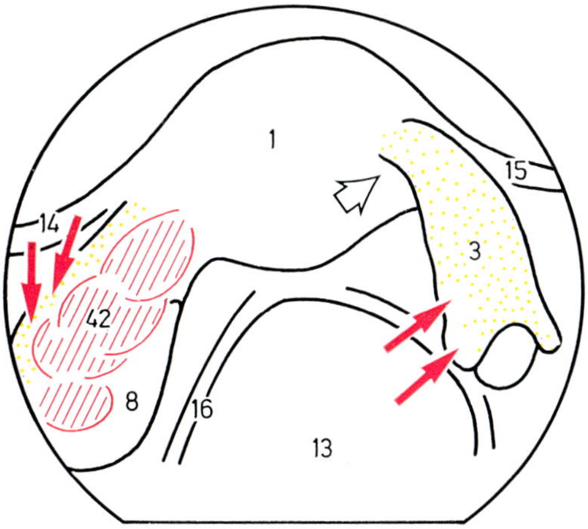
1
15
14
3
42
8
16
13

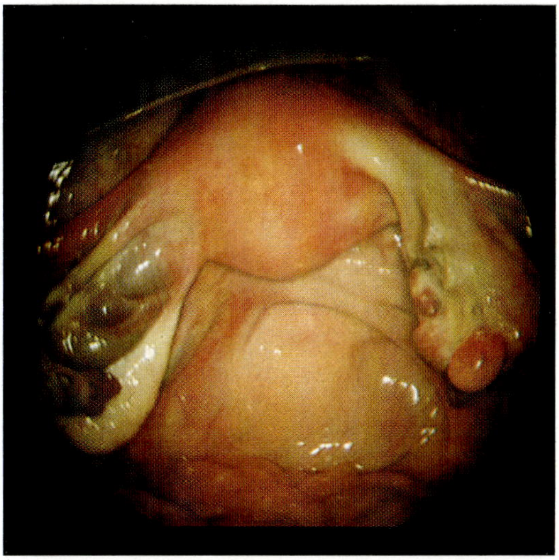

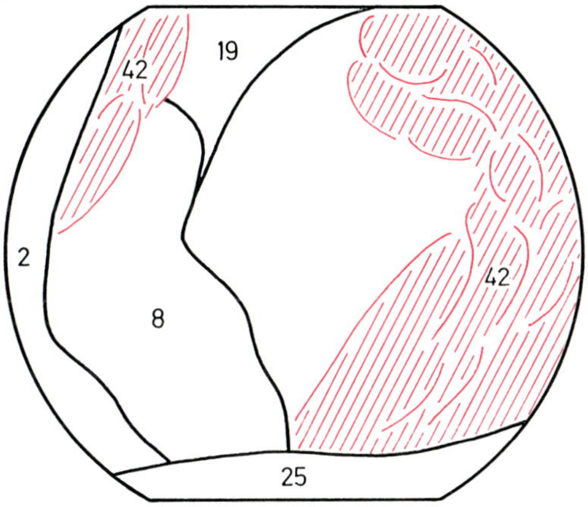
42
19
2
8
42
25

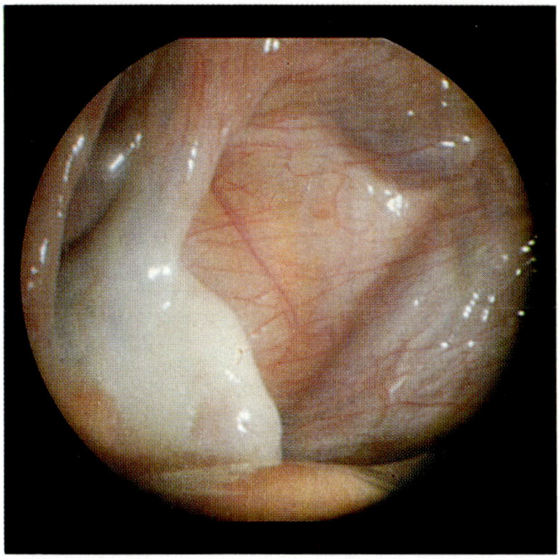

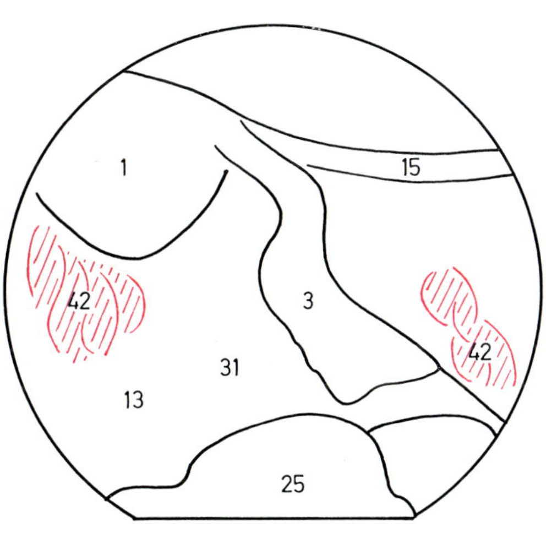
1
15
42
3
31
42
13
25

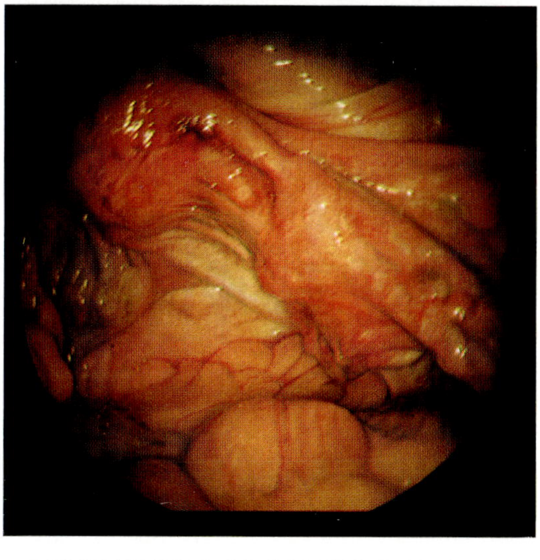

(h) Chronic Adnexitis

Fig. 242. Chronic adnexitis usually is associated with an abdomen full of adhesions. Here the tube, occluded in the form of a sac, can be seen adherent to the right pelvic wall. The old tubal ampulla can be seen in only rudimentary form.

Fig. 243. The left tube is seen here injected in chronic inflammation as a clubbed tube.

Fig. 244. This clubbed tube can be shown only by elevation of the tube in its central part with the aid of atraumatic forceps. The peritubal tissue is inflamed and engorged; the right ovary is distorted by numerous small retention cysts.

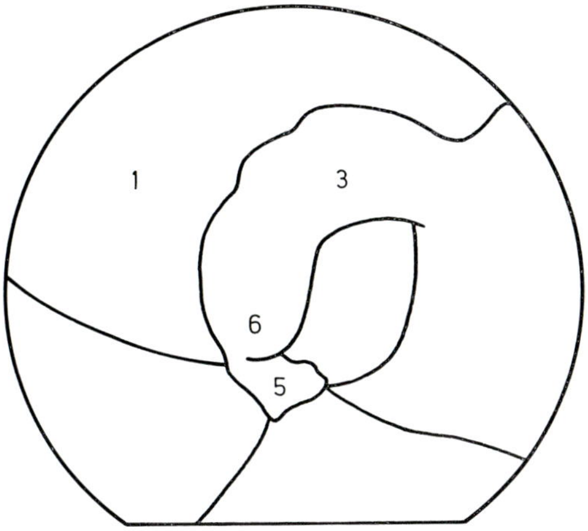
1
3
6
5

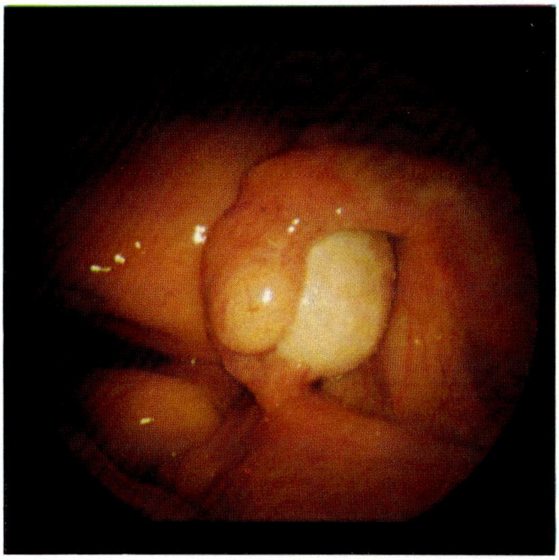

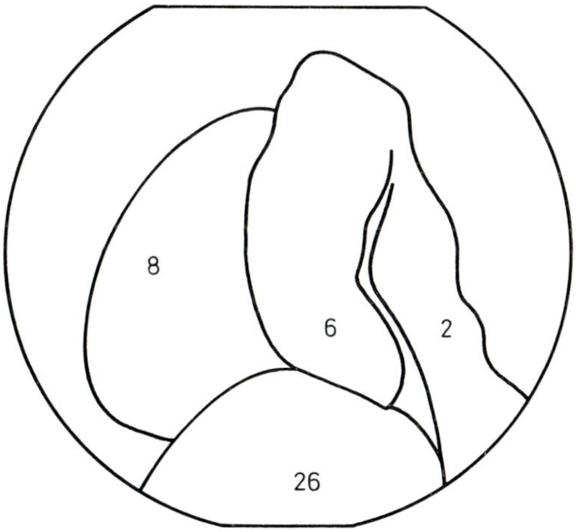
8
6
2
26

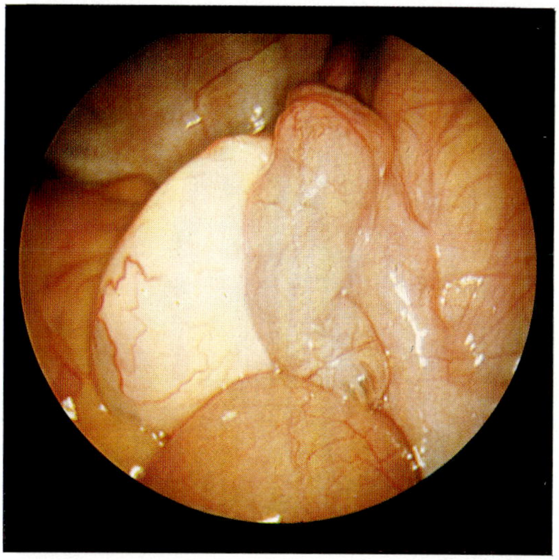

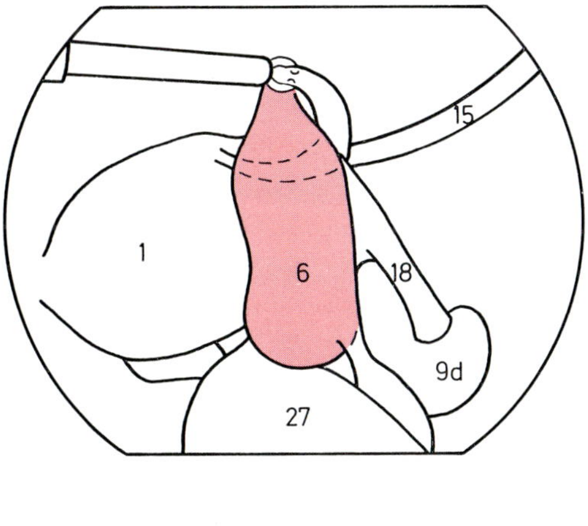
15
1
6
18
9d
27

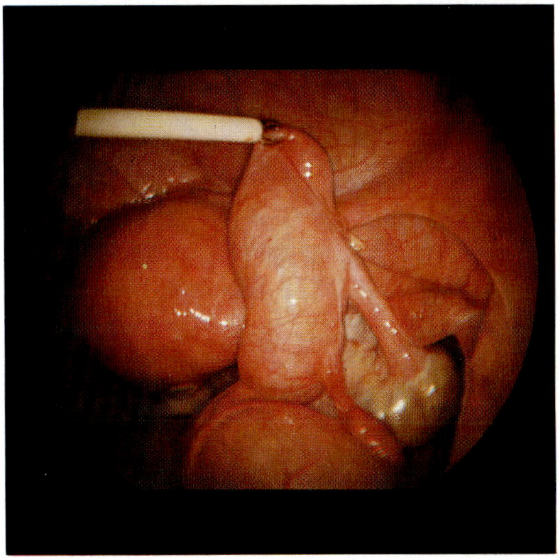

(i) Acute or Subacute Lower Abdominal Disease—Suspicion of Extrauterine Pregnancy

Fig. 245. From the perspective of the navel, a large amount of blood usually is seen in the cul-de-sac in cases of ectopic pregnancy. This blood, however, can be distinguished by differential diagnosis from blood coming from ruptured "chocolate cysts" in cases of endometriosis (Fig. 212), follicular bleeding (Fig. 253), etc. Arrow (→) shows a tubal abortion.

Fig. 246. In a case of tubal pregnancy, blood is found also in the upper abdomen above the omentum, spreading as far as the liver and the diaphragm. This also is true if, as in the present case of extrauterine pregnancy (see Fig. 247), it is only a matter of an incipient tubal abortion, and a relatively small amount of blood has seeped into the abdomen.

Fig. 247. Only after elevation of the uterus with the aid of the suction intrauterine cannula does the ectopic pregnancy situated in the ampullar part of the left tube become clearly visible. In differential diagnosis between intrauterine and tubal pregnancy, the suction intrauterine cannula is *not* used at first. In most cases it suffices if a swab-holder is introduced into the vagina or rectal ampulla in order to elevate the uterus slightly out of the pelvis. In cases of doubt, the uterus is elevated through a second puncture with the aid of atraumatic forceps (see Figs. 64–67). The cause of this tubal pregnancy might be traceable to the numerous endometrial implants in the region of the left broad ligament.

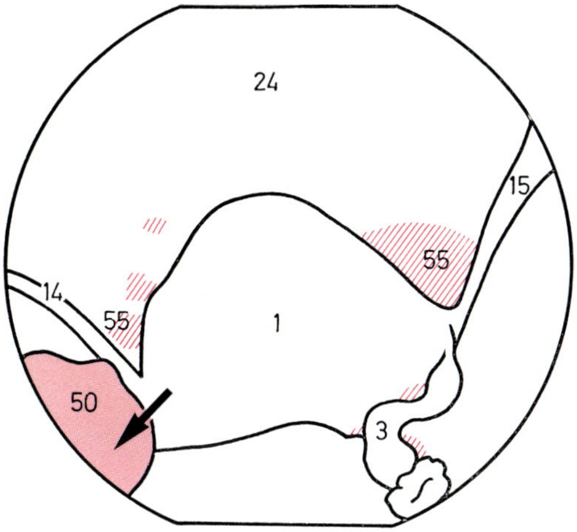
24
15
55
14
55
1
50
3

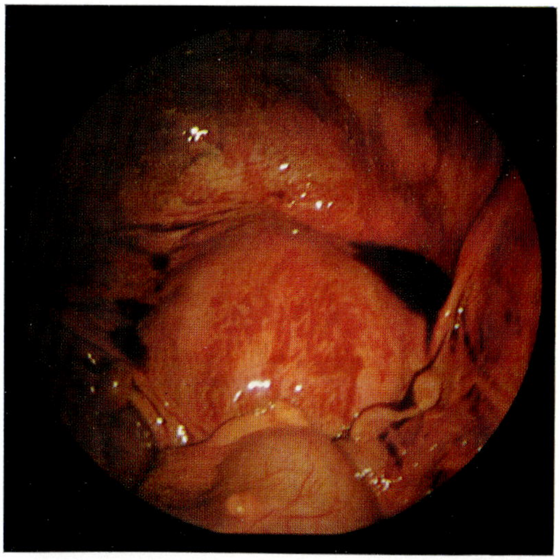

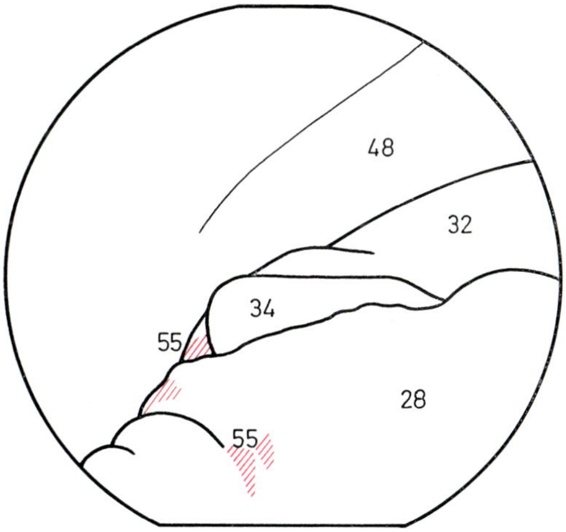
48
32
34
55
28
55

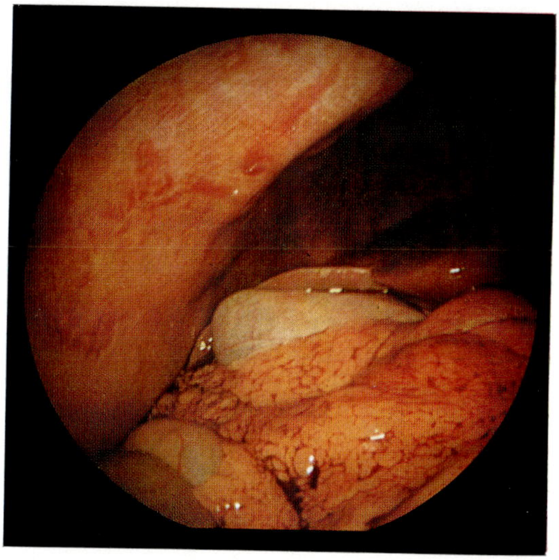

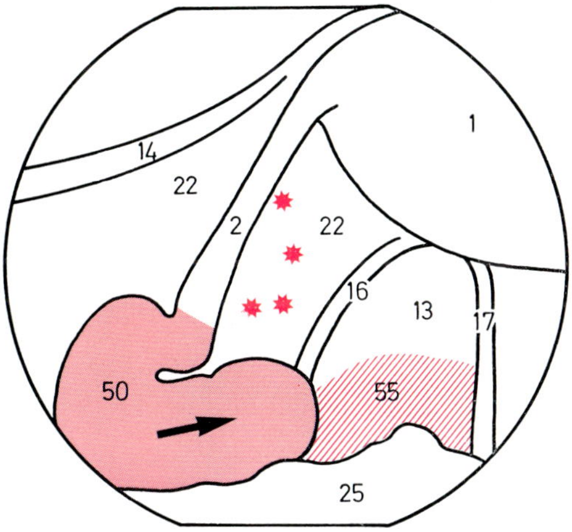
14
1
22
2
22
16
13
17
50
55
25

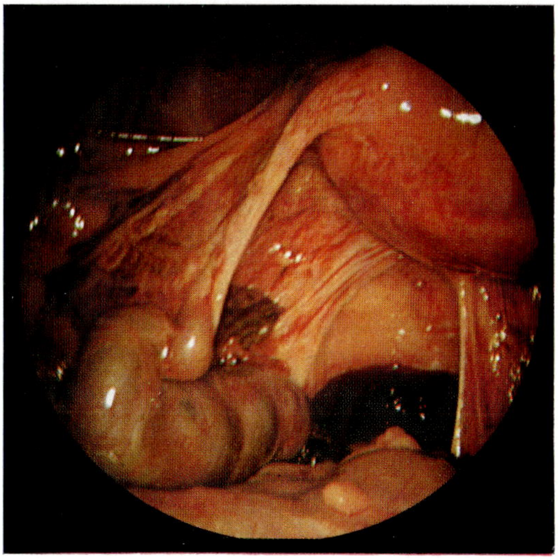

The value of a conservative operative technique in tubal pregnancy may be demonstrated in Figures 248–250.

Fig. 248. This shows a tube after tubal pregnancy in which only the tubal ampulla was removed. The stump shown here, which (as proved by tubal dye insufflation) is still distally patent, affords the possibility of a tuboplasty.

Fig. 249. In this instance too, there was a history of a conservative operation for tubal pregnancy four years previously. The ampulla is occluded in the form of a sac. The chance of refertilization by a tuboplasty is very favorable in this case, but if routine salpingectomy had been performed there would have been no such chance. Here, too, the cause of the tubal pregnancy may be traceable to the endometriosis in the region of the uterosacral ligaments.

Fig. 250. This conservative tubal surgery performed in conjunction with a left adnexectomy, leaving a stump about 2 cm long, technically offers a very slight chance of restoration of tubal patency. The chance of refertilization is extremely slim, since on this side the ovary also is missing.

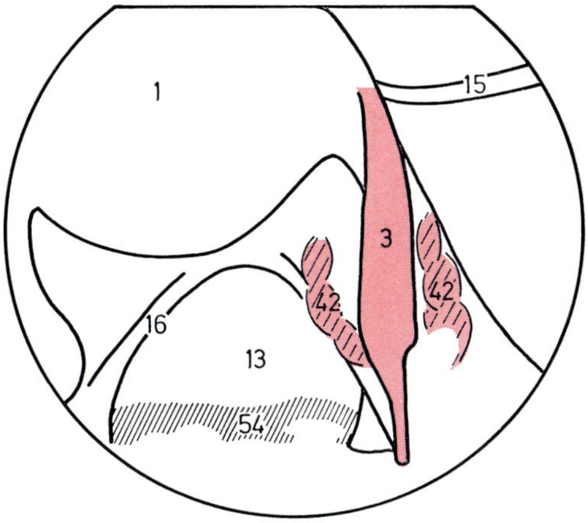
1
15
3
42
42
16
13
54

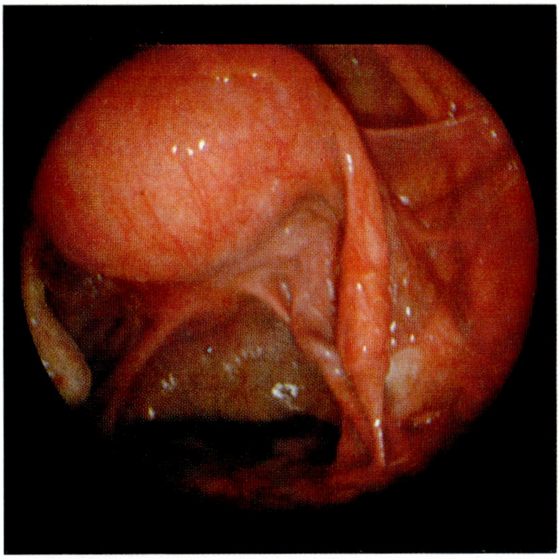

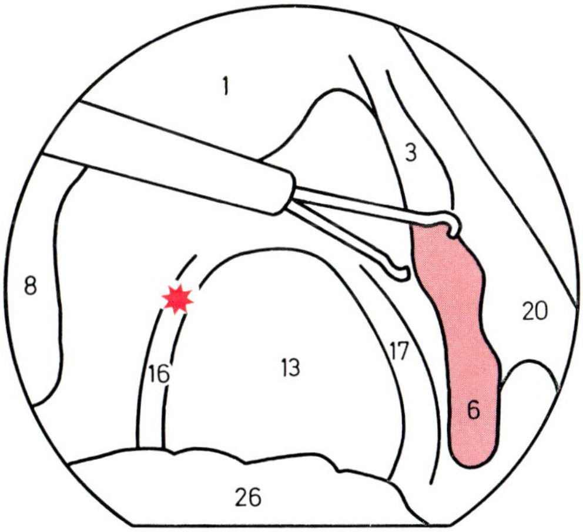
1
3
8
20
16
13
17
6
26

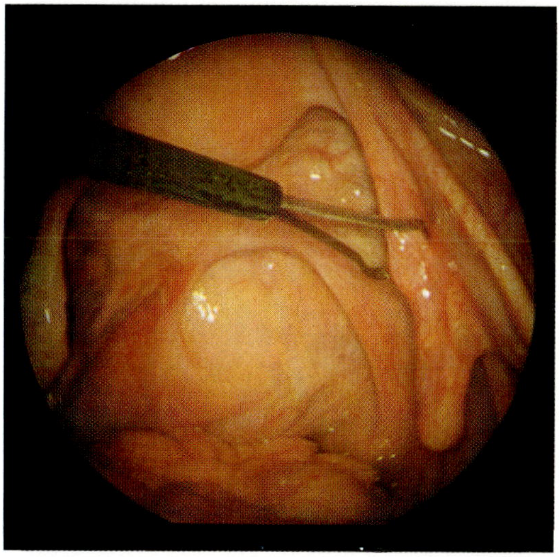

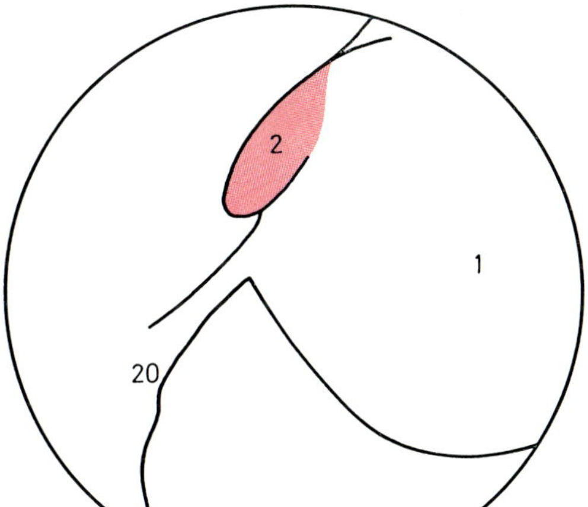
2
1
20

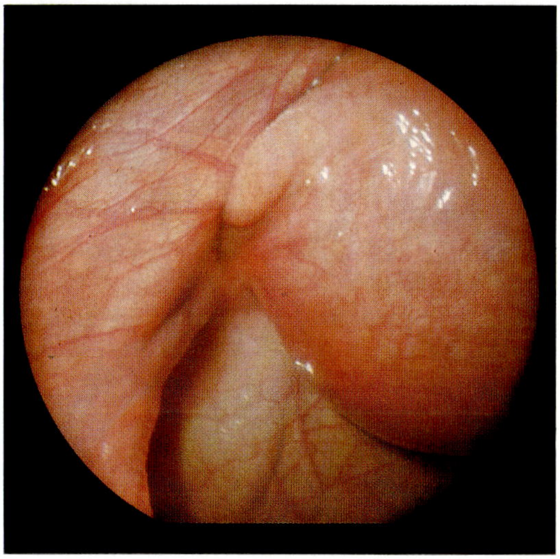

(k) Corpus Luteum Bleeding

Fig. 251. Just before the elevation of the uterus seen here, the tubal ampulla resting over the mature follicle was removed with atraumatic forceps. This picture may be taken as proof that the ampulla actively claps itself over the erupting follicle as an ovum is extruded.

Fig. 252. The ovary is being elevated in this picture with the aid of atraumatic forceps. The corpus luteum of pregnancy at the lower pole is revealed. At some points the tunica albuginea is distinctly ruptured.

Fig. 253. Sometimes the eruption of a follicle leads to massive ovarian bleeding. A tubal pregnancy is then clinically a matter for differential diagnosis. The ruptured follicle on the right tube has led to massive intra-abdominal bleeding in this case. The blood was successfully aspirated at laparoscopy, and the follicular bleeding was stemmed by coagulation. Laparotomy was not necessary.

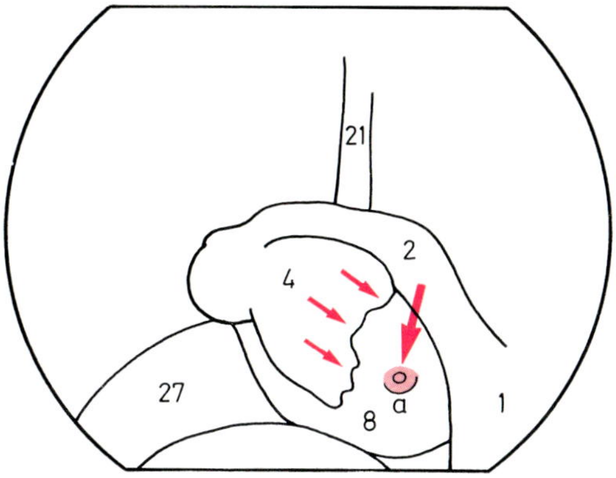
21
2
4
27
a
8
1

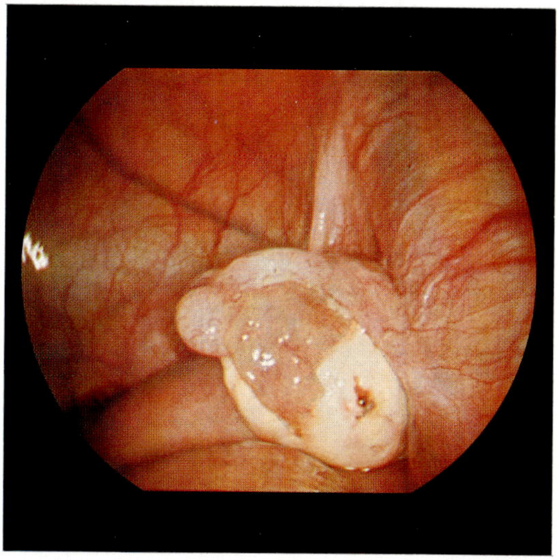

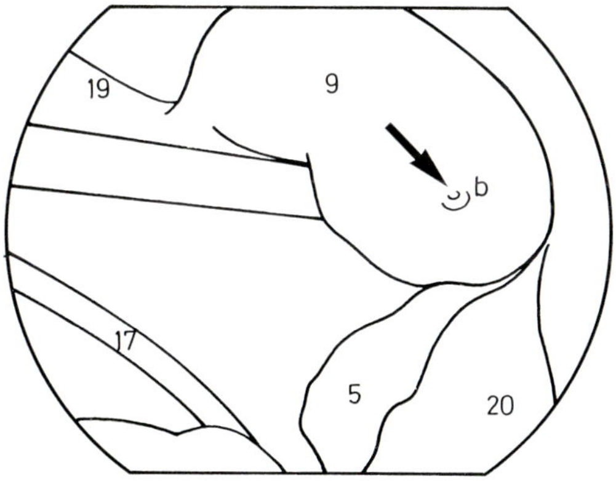
19
9
b
17
5
20

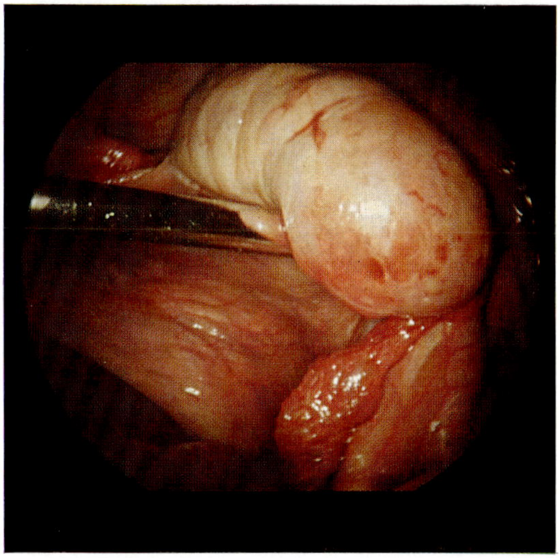

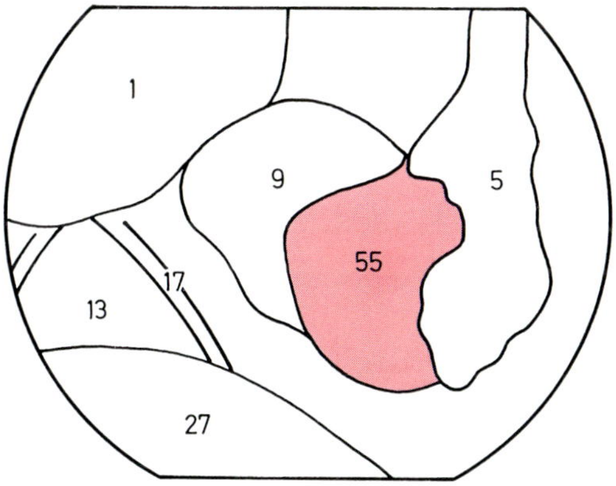
1
9
5
55
17
13
27

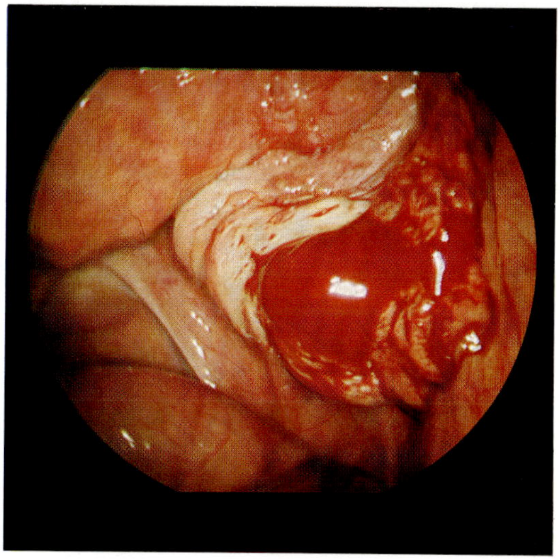

(l) *Differential Diagnosis Between Ovarian Vs. Adnexal Tumors and Myomas*

Fig. 254. This picture shows a fist-sized myomatous uterus with intramural myomas, some of them developing subserosally. It is interesting that a picture of a myomatous uterus is always associated with changes in both ovaries.

Fig. 255. This myomatous uterus bears at the left cornu of the fundus a subserosal myoma as large as the distal segment of a human thumb. The situation shown is after left adnexectomy.

As a result of the postoperative adhesions from omentum to the fundus, the right adnexa are not visible without the aid of atraumatic forceps.

Fig. 256. Multilocular subserosal myomas of this type, some of them borne on pedicles, create difficulties in the differential diagnosis of ovarian tumors. Here laparoscopy can provide immediate clarity. With correspondingly difficult coexisting conditions, the patient is spared the laparotomy that would have been absolutely indicated on suspicion of an ovarian tumor.

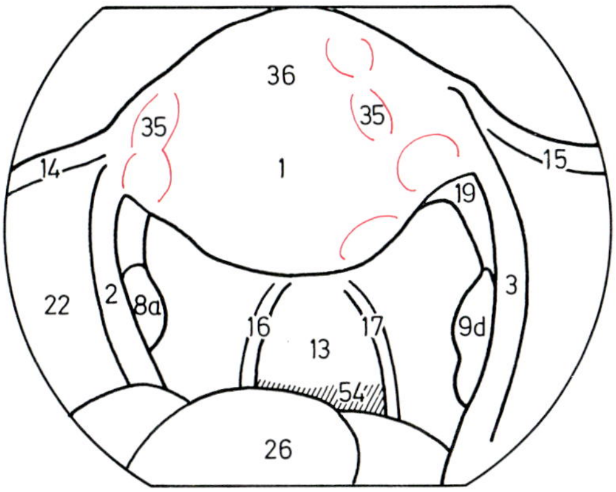
36
35
35
1
14
15
19
22
2
8a
16
13
17
9d
3
54
26

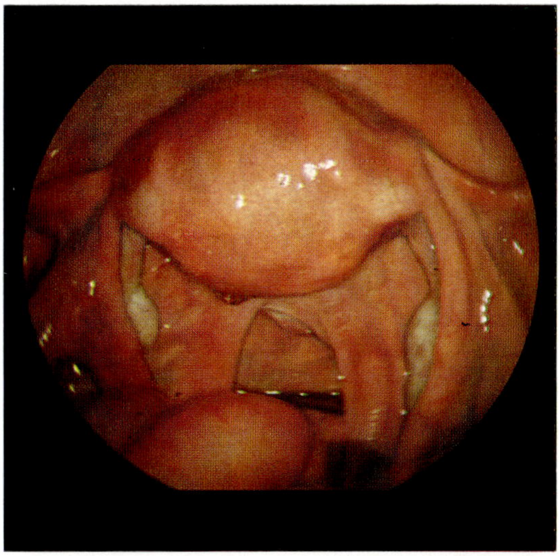

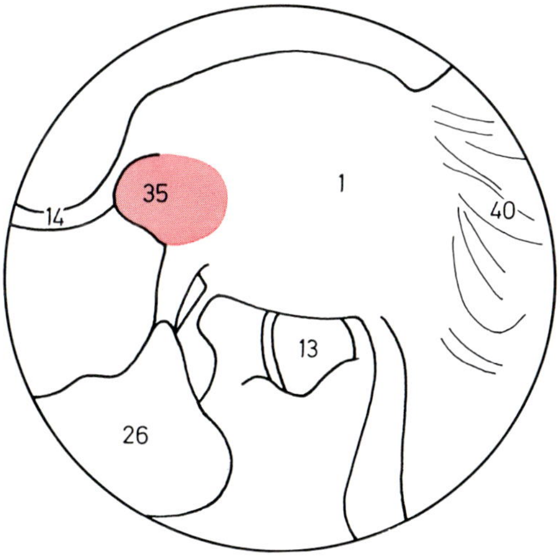
35
1
14
40
13
26

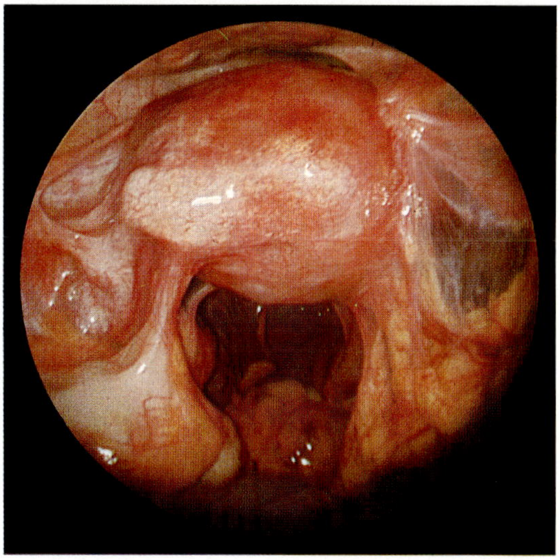

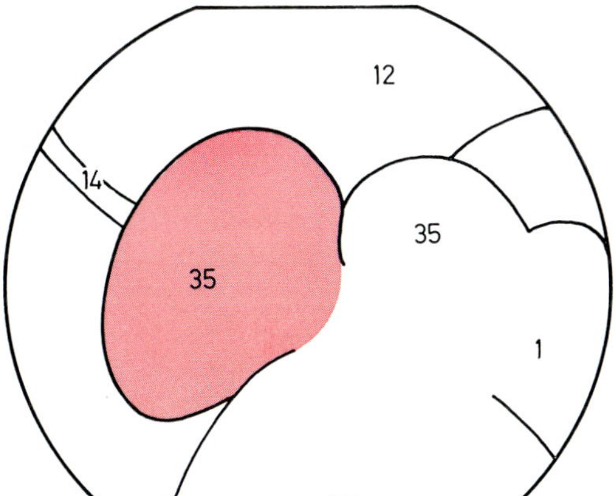
12
14
35
35
1
35

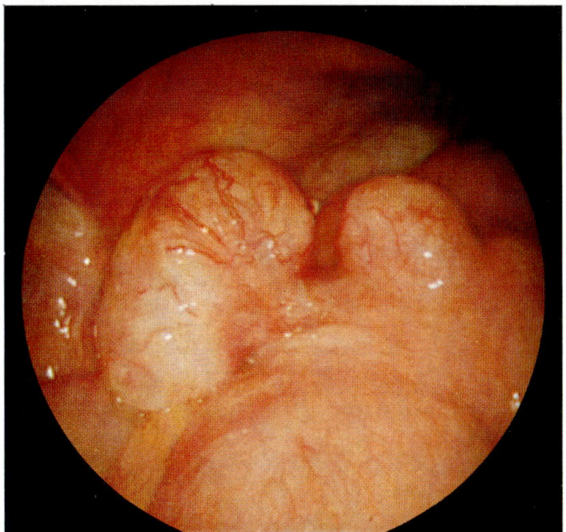

Fig. 257. In connection with the cystically altered ovaries, this small subserosal myoma on the posterior wall of the uterus of a postmenopausal woman made differential diagnosis difficult. Laparoscopy rendered laparotomy unnecessary.

Fig. 258. A subserosal myoma is grafted to this uterus in its anterior wall. The right ovary is the size of a plum and has a convoluted surface, the left ovary being polycystic.

Fig. 259. In this picture a subserosal myoma the size of an egg, borne on a pedicle and arising from the posterior wall of the uterus, simulates a left side ovarian tumor. The knobby nature of the regressively altered myoma is an indication for laparotomy because of a suspicion of a malignant ovarian tumor in the postmenopausal patient. In aged patients who are poor operative risks the laparoscopic finding is sufficient.

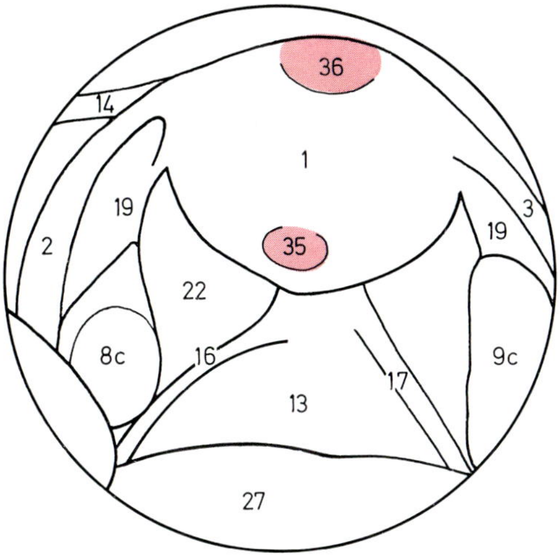
36
14
1
19
3
2
35
19
22
8c
16
9c
17
13
27

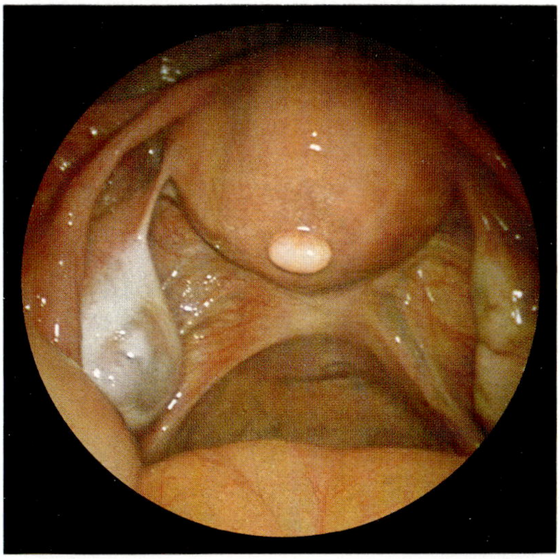

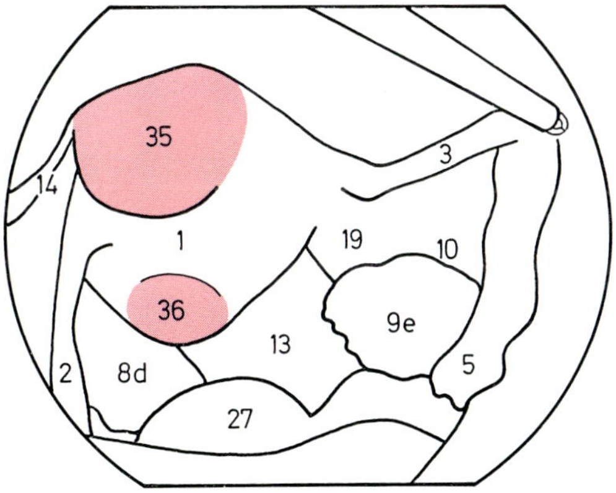
35
3
14
1
19
10
36
9e
13
2
8d
5
27

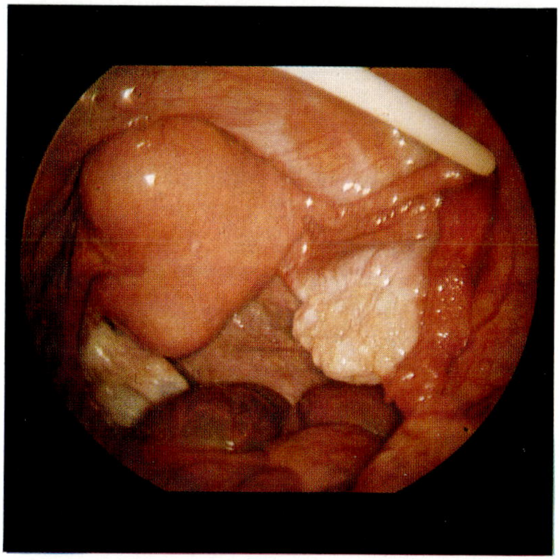

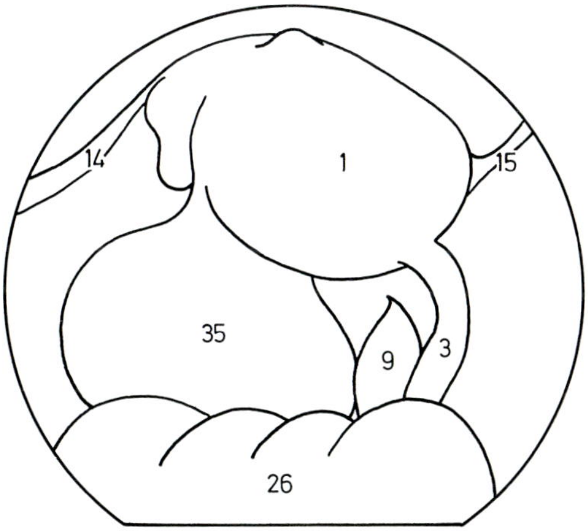
14
1
15
35
3
9
26

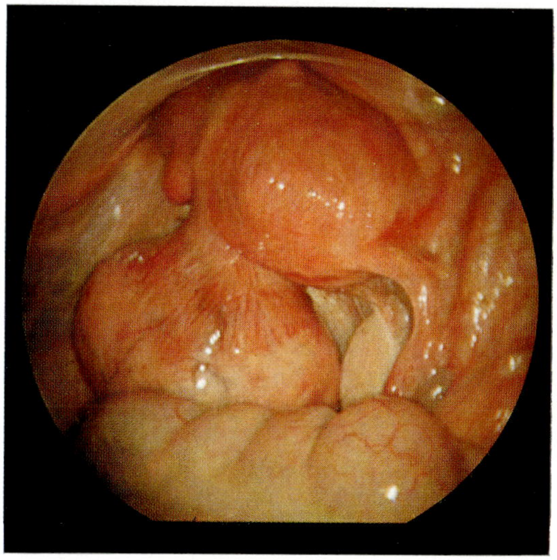

(m) Differential Diagnosis: Bicornuate Uterus or Ovarian Tumor?

Fig. 260. In the presence of normally formed external genitalia, the second uterus (uterus bicornis unicollis) generally would have been diagnosed as an ovarian tumor. At laparoscopy the uterus bicornis unicollis can be diagnosed instantly. The probability of being able to elevate both cornua of the uterus with one cervical forceps is remarkable. The chronic lower abdominal distress of this patient, manifested for years as disease of the adnexa through palpation of the swelling, was "eliminated" in the course of this laparoscopy.

Fig. 261. This patient, scheduled for laparotomy, had acute abdominal symptoms and a positive pregnancy test on the basis of two missed menstrual periods and a fist-sized tumor on the right side. At laparoscopy, a uterus bicornis unicollis with a pregnancy in the right cornu was diagnosed. The acute abdominal symptoms apparently were caused by a transient gastrointestinal disturbance. The pregnancy proceeded normally to term. The illustration shows the nonpregnant uterine cornu at left and the pregnant one at the right.

Fig. 262. This illustration demonstrates the unilateral absence of the uterus and adnexum (müllerian duct). The ovary is also missing on the left side. The atraumatic forceps are elevating the otherwise normal right cornu.

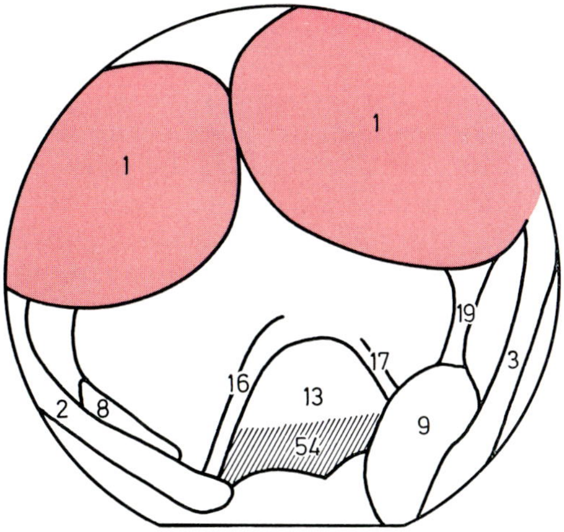
1
1
19
17
16
13
3
2
8
54
9

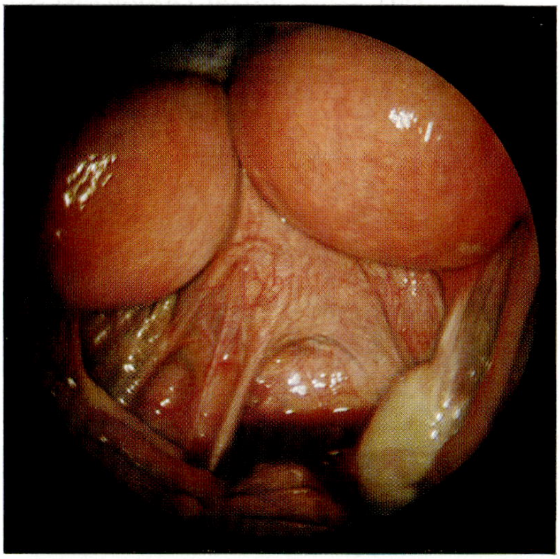

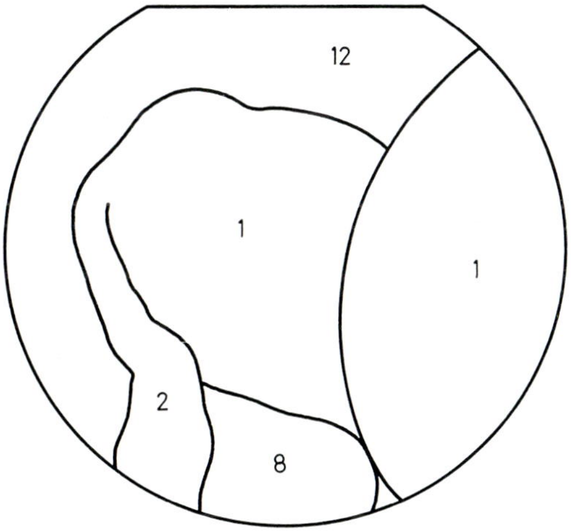
12
1
1
2
8

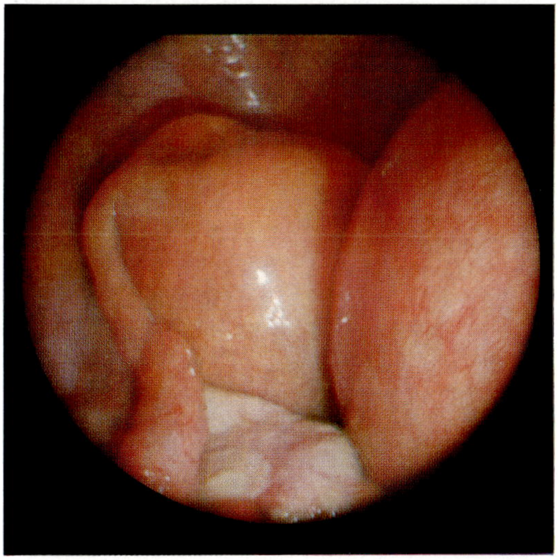

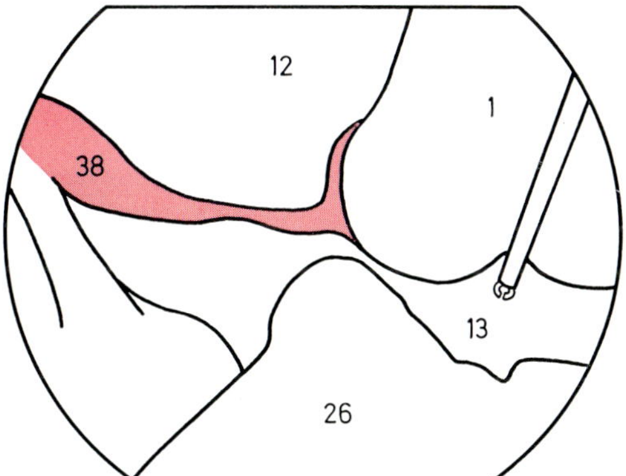
12
1
38
13
26

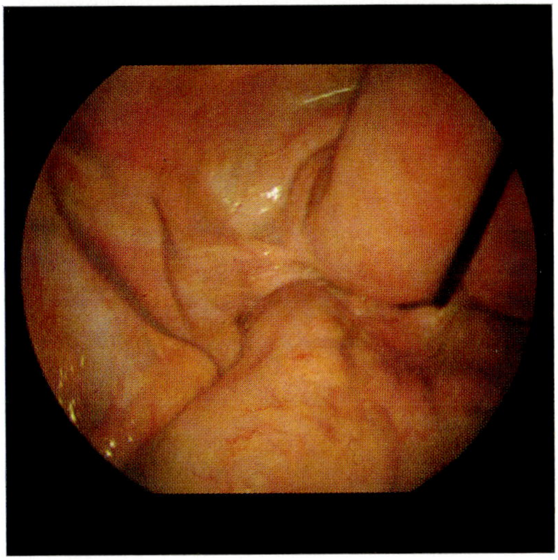

(n) Differential Diagnosis: Adnexitis or Appendicitis?

Fig. 263. A differential diagnosis between acute or chronic adnexitis and acute or chronic appendicitis most often requires consultation between surgeons and gynecologists. Endoscopic monitoring of this trouble spot in the lower abdomen enables rapid, accurate evaluation of the problem. In this instance, it is a matter of a retrograde elevated appendix adherent to the cecum by numerous fine adhesions. The ascending colon in addition is attached velamentously to the parietal peritoneum.

Fig. 264. This appendix shows a U-shaped kink, somewhat congested toward the end, and also a small focus of bleeding at the U-bend. The veins also are distended in the region of the mesoappendix (see under Fig. 265).

Fig. 265. Upon touching the appendix in Figure 264, the cause of the fixed U-shaped kink is seen to be a bleeding endometrial implant. This extragenital endometriosis was associated also with endometriosis in the pelvis.

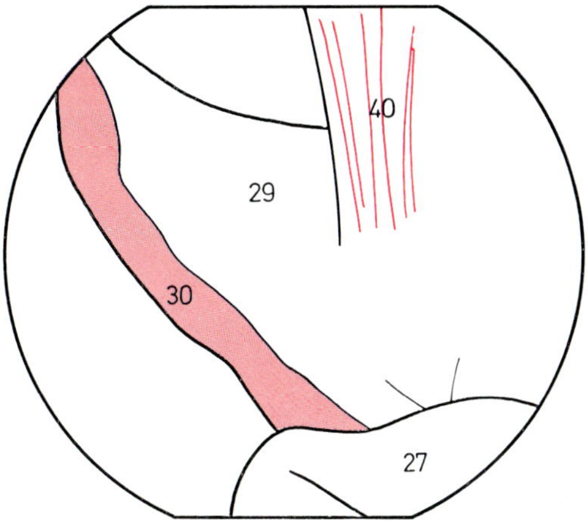
40
29
30
27

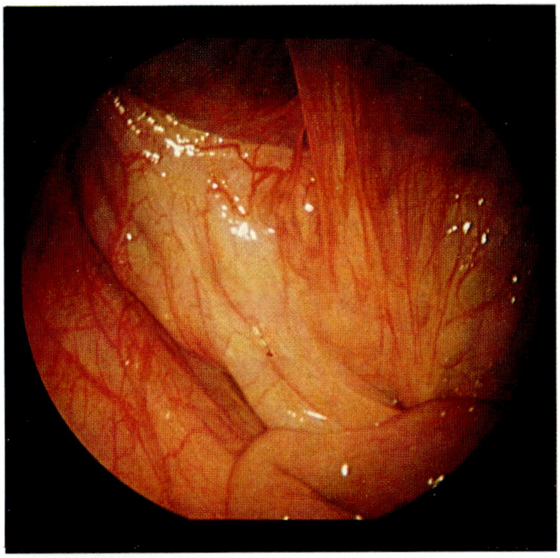

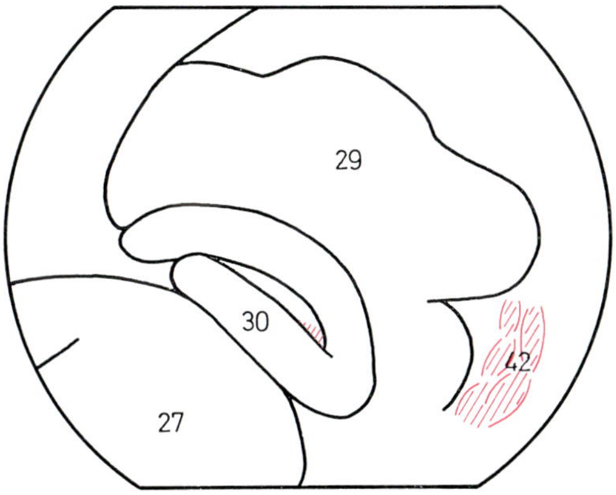
29
30
42
27

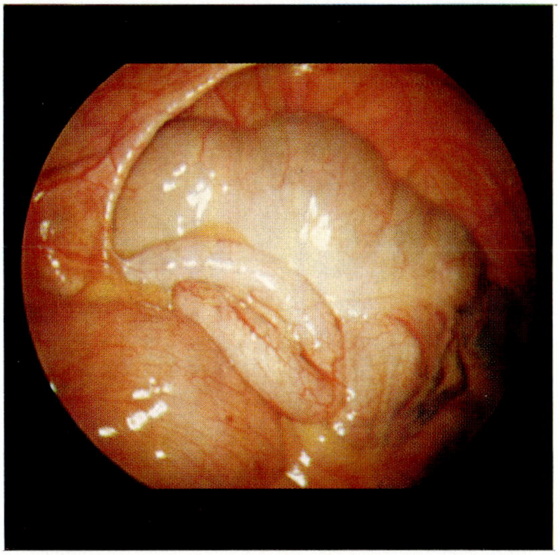

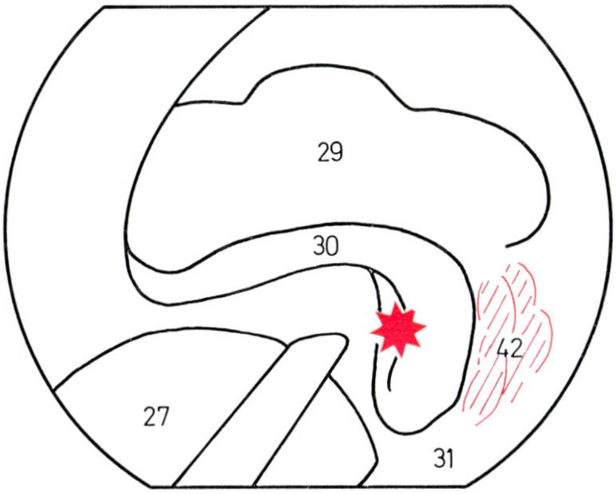
29
30
42
27
31

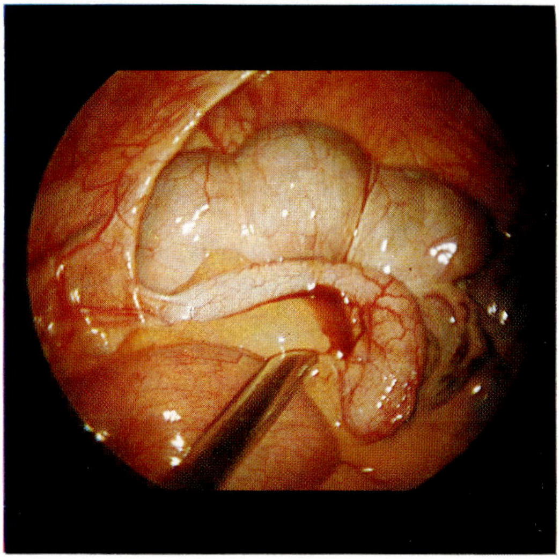

Fig. 266. The appendix was elevated out of the colonic niche with a suction probe and extended to a straight line by suction. The appendix and its epiploica are clearly visible. The suction probe produces no trauma to the intestine (Figs. 64–67).

Fig. 267. Even during the puerperium there is no reason to shun laparoscopy for purposes of differential diagnosis. Here on the fourth puerperal day (after manual loosening of an adherent placenta) the patient became acutely febrile and developed lower abdominal localized pain, especially on the right side. The clinical diagnosis was appendicitis in puerperium.

At laparoscopy, however, an incipient parametritis was revealed with marked swelling of the right utero-ovarian ligament and the broad ligament with new inflammatory peritubal exudation of fibrin. But see below, Figure 268.

Fig. 268. The appendix, however, is shown to be completely free of inflammation and in correct anatomic position. In the present instance an appendectomy would have constituted an additional tax upon the puerpera, and at the same time would have spread the incipient parametritis, which had not yet even been diagnosed.

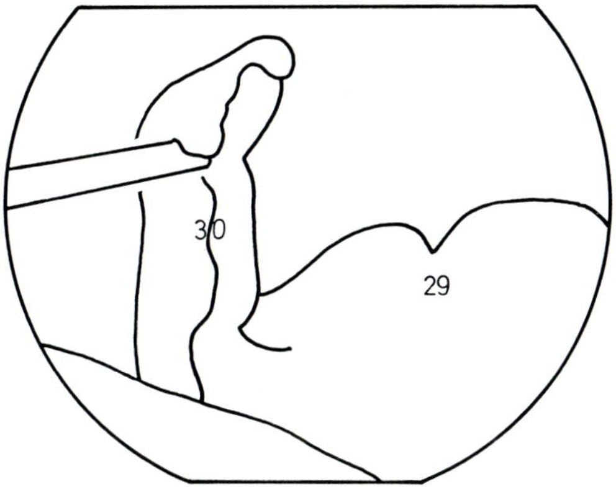
30
29
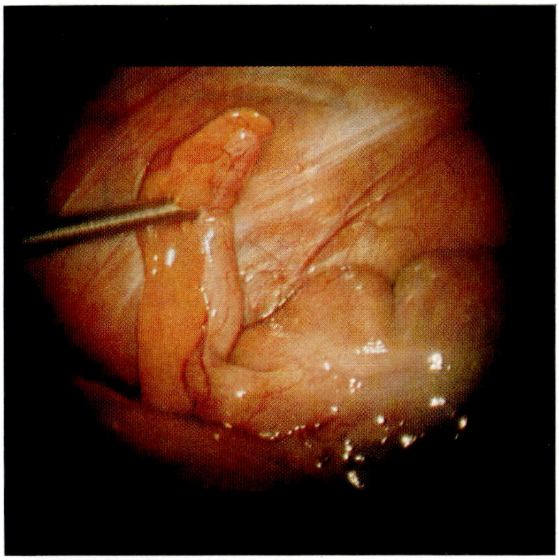
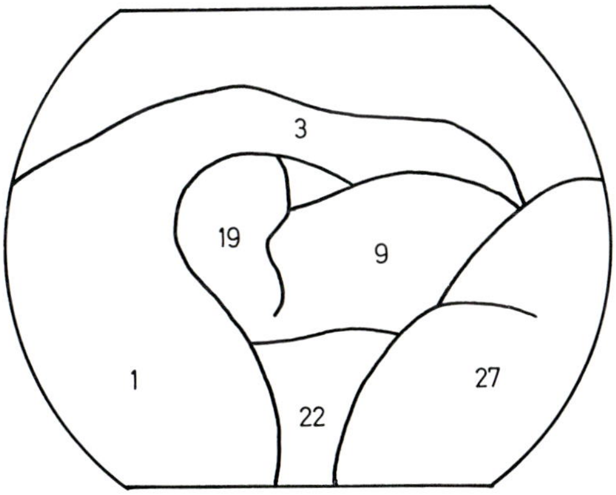
3
19
9
1
22
27
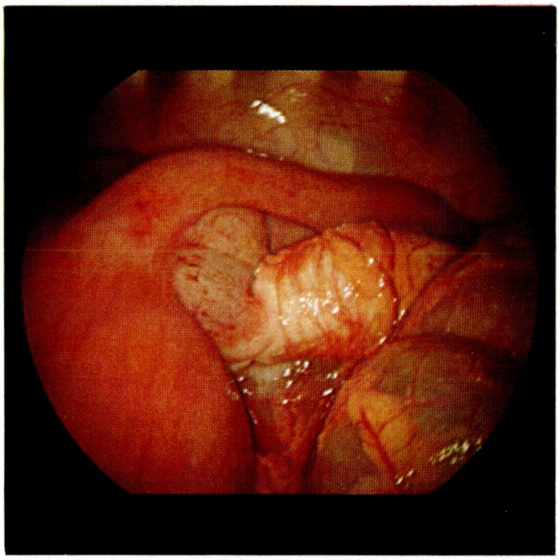
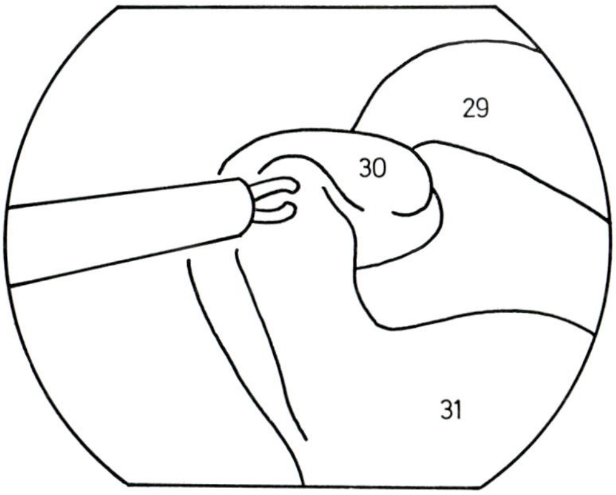
29
30
31
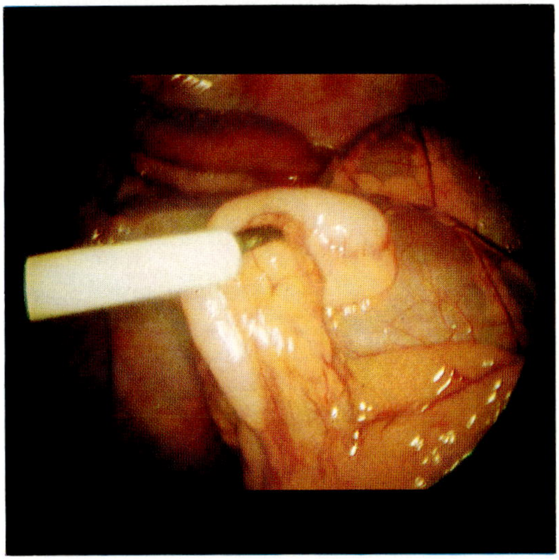

(o) Genital Hypoplasia and Aplasia

Fig. 269. This genital hypoplasia is characterized by the hypoplastic uterus in which the length of the corpus relative to that of the cervix is 2:1. That ratio distinguishes this uterus from an infantile one, where we find the ratio of corpus to cervix is 1:2. The ligaments are hypoplastic on both sides. The ovaries are small and can be considered the morphologic consequence of genital hypoplasia with resultant ovarian insufficiency. The differential diagnosis between infantile uterus and genital hypoplasia is of great importance in judging the chances for fertility. In infantile uterus we must reckon with only a slight (4 per cent) possibility of conception. Since the infantile uterus also usually has a tricornuate cavity, the performance of a hysteroscopy or a hysterogram is of diagnostic value. On the basis of the collected data we distinguish between a primary hypoplasia and an acquired or secondary one—for example, after prolonged ovarian insufficiency or in exaggerated puerperal involution.

Fig. 270. This hypoplastic uterus is associated with a general genital hypoplasia. In such cases it is recommended to biopsy one ovary in order to distinguish between primary and secondary hypoplasia. In primary hypoplasia of the ovaries we find a striking reduction in the content of primary follicles as a result of a deficiency of primordium, whereas in secondary hypoplasia the ovary, although too small, does contain sufficient germ parenchyma.

These fallopian tubes are normally placed and have merely failed to develop. The differential diagnosis between primordial anomaly (primary hypoplasia) and developmental anomaly (secondary hypoplasia) is of importance for the assessment of the chances of success for fertility treatment, and can be resolved only at laparoscopy plus histology in combination with an endocrine evaluation.

Fig. 271. Primary ovarian hypoplasia can be diagnosed merely macroscopically at laparoscopy if the ovaries show the typical "button-hole" or "streak" appearance. This configuration of the ovaries is possible only in the primary form of ovarian hypoplasia.

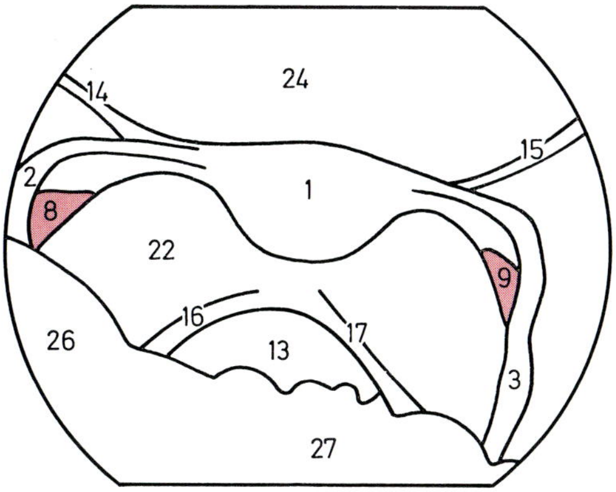
24
14
15
2
1
8
22
9
16
17
26
13
3
27

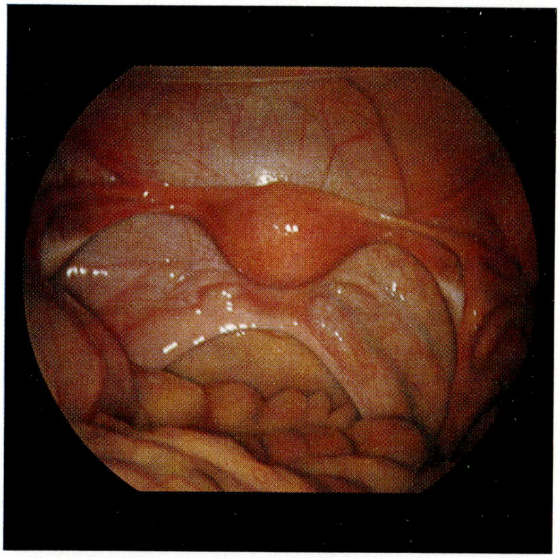

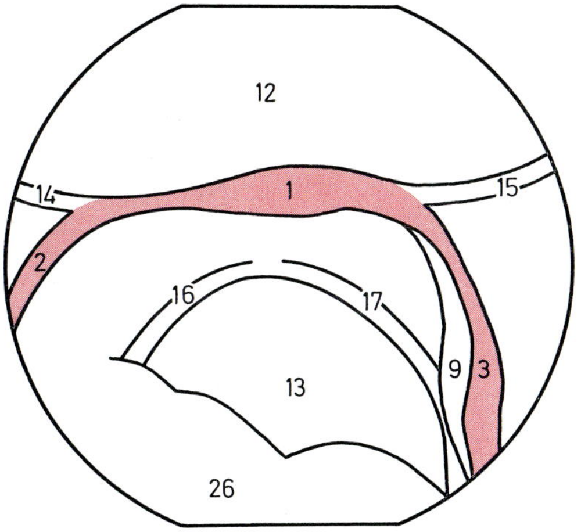
12
14
1
15
2
16
17
9
3
13
26

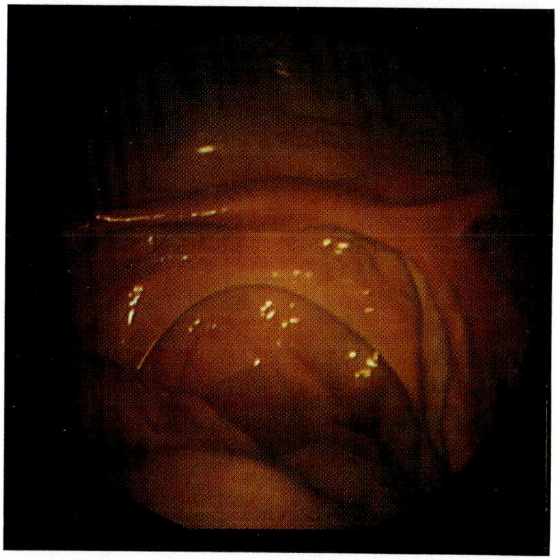

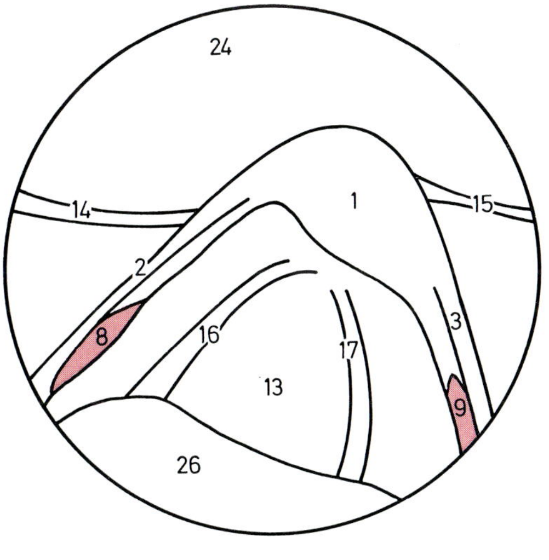
24
14
1
15
2
8
16
3
17
13
9
26

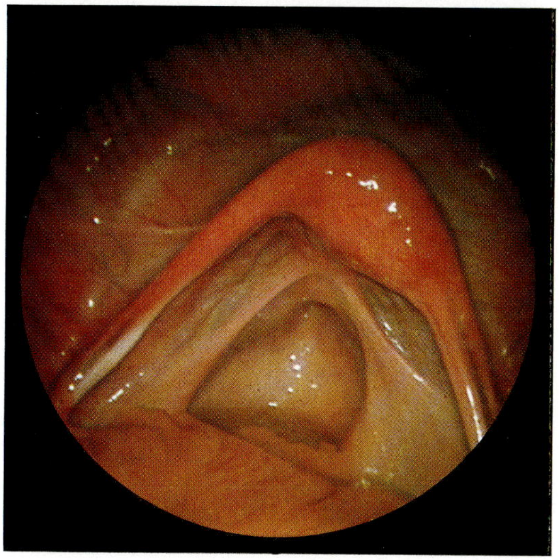

Fig. 272. Here also it is indubitably a case of so-called "streak" ovary. However, the uterus and especially the tubal portion are relatively well developed in comparison to Figure 270.

Fig. 273. This small supernumerary ovary represents a functionally, as well as morphologically, unimportant auxiliary finding. In the cul-de-sac there is also about 10 ml of bloody serous fluid, a relatively commonplace finding, especially in the middle of the cycle.

Fig. 274. This almost cherry-sized supernumerary ovary shows the same surface condition as the normal-shaped ovary, and did not differ histologically from normal ovarian tissue.

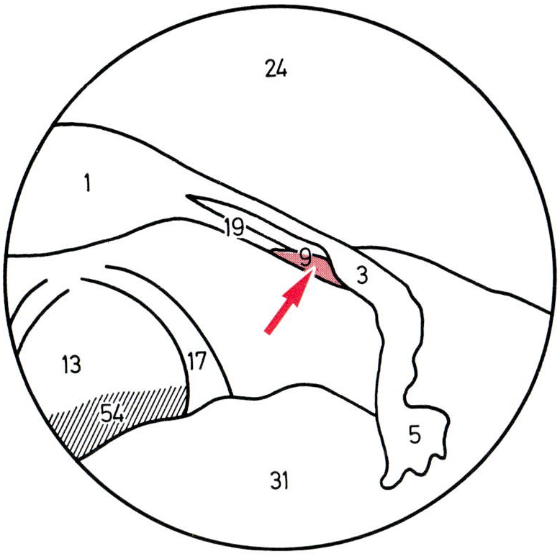
24
1
19
9
3
13
17
54
5
31

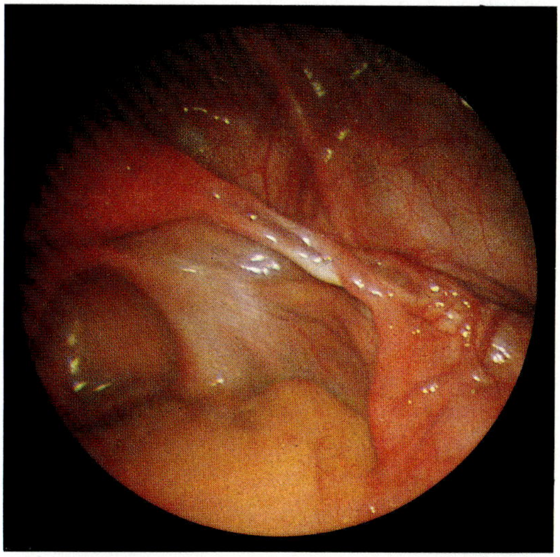

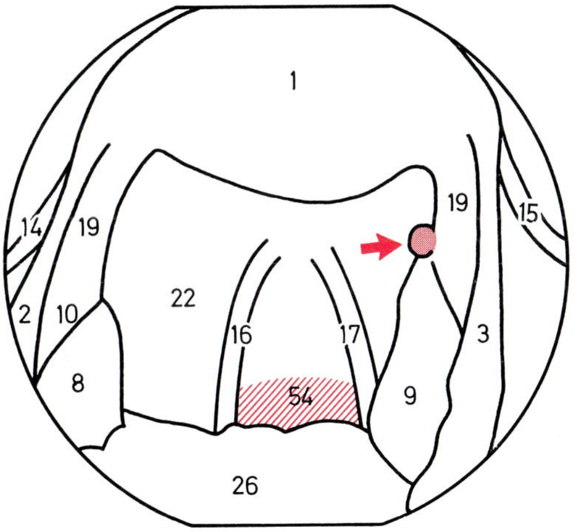
1
14
19
19
15
22
2
10
16
17
3
8
54
9
26

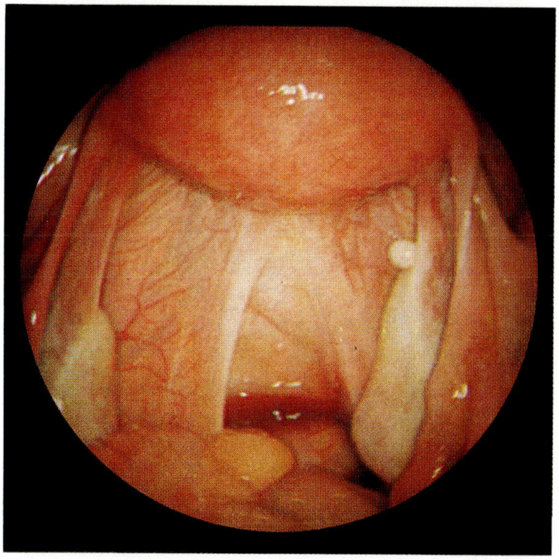

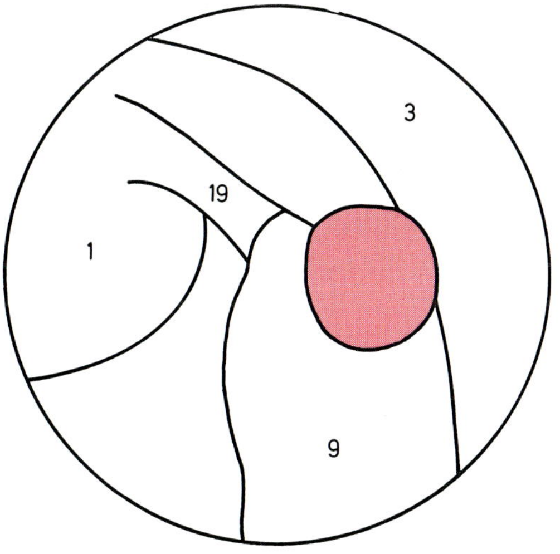
3
19
1
9

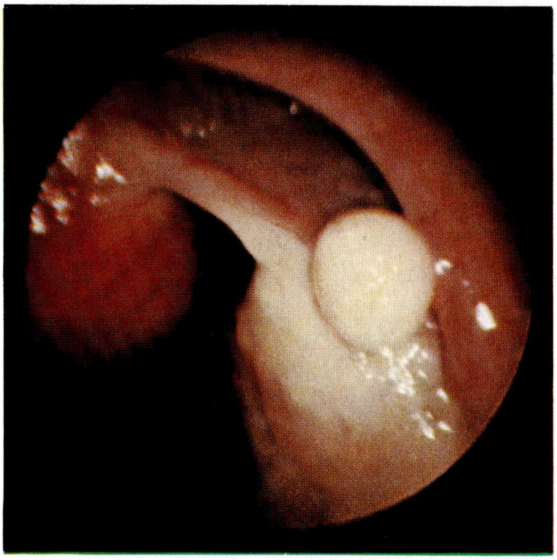

Fig. 275. In this case there is aplasia of the left ovary and marked atrophy of the left tubes beginning 2 cm distal from the fundus.

Fig. 276. Aplasia of the left urogenital fold occurred in this patient, who had borne nine healthy children and was examined at laparoscopy in the course of sterilization. Instead of the left adnexum there is only a hint of a peritoneal cord. We are dealing here with complete aplasia of the urogenital fold, a defect that must have originated in the third or fourth embryonic week. In the ensuing time the gonadal cells arising from the primordial kidney, as well as the part of the tube and uterus developing from the müllerian duct were never formed. The uterus, formed exclusively from the right müllerian duct (cervix plus uterine corpus), is here in the 11th week of pregnancy.

Fig. 277. The same situation as in Figure 276, showing the right tube which is just being sterilized by coagulation with the aid of the atraumatic coagulation forceps and high-frequency current. Notice once more the uterus, at this time pregnant in the 11th week, which had been formed exclusively from the right müllerian duct and which subsequently was emptied by means of suction curettage after nine spontaneous births because of medical indication on the part of the mother.

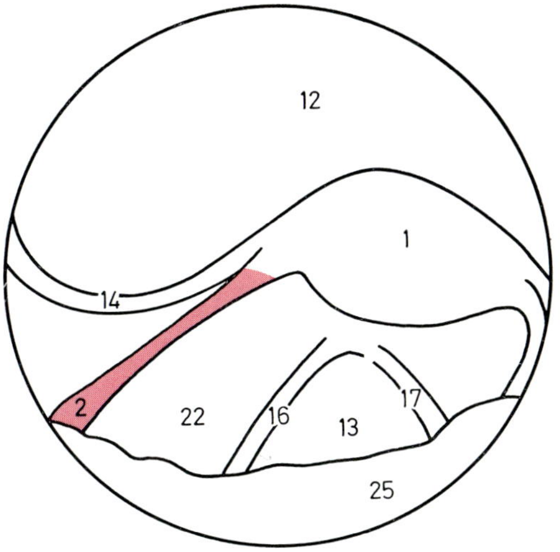
12
1
14
2
22
16
13
17
25

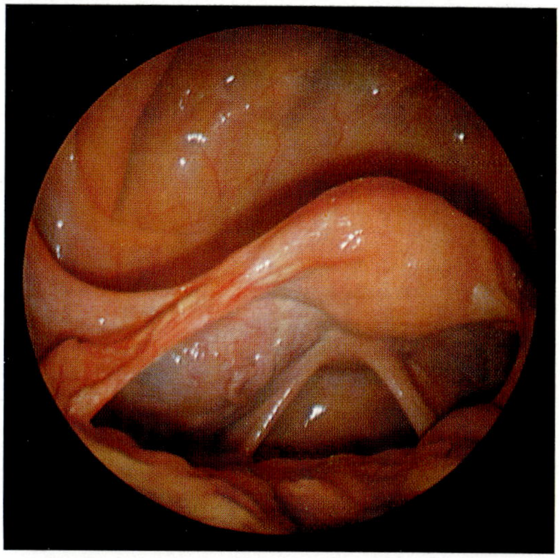

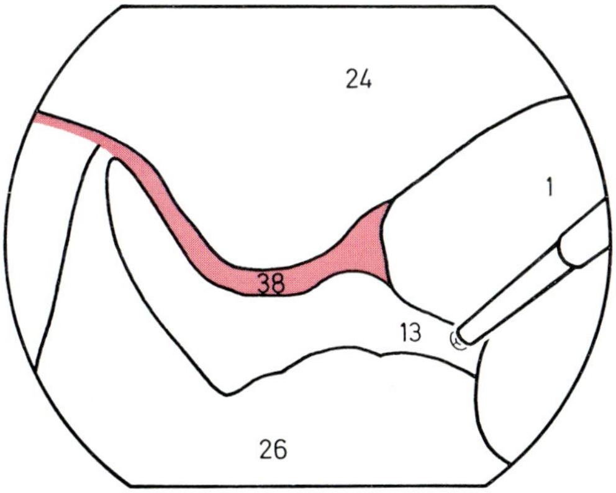
24
1
38
13
26

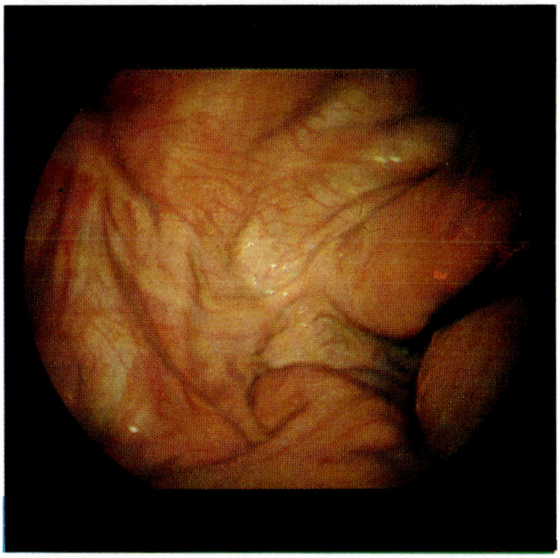

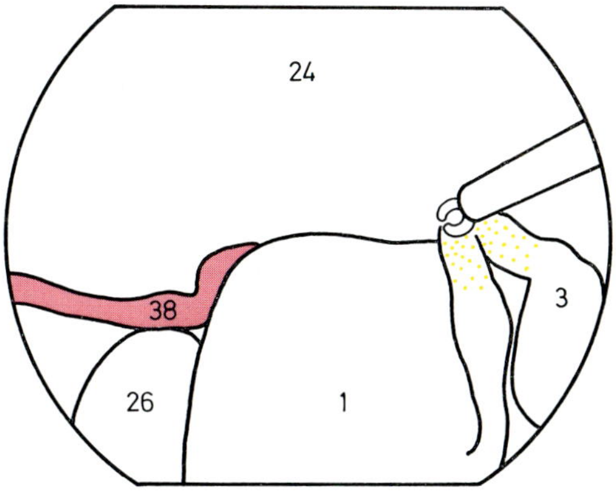
24
38
3
26
1

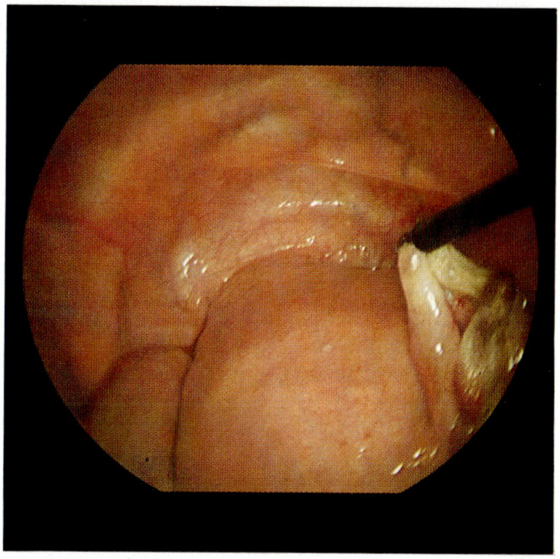

Fig. 278. This patient was laparoscoped because of a Rokitansky-Küster-Hauser (also known as "Mayer-Rokitansky-Küster" or "Mayer-Rokitansky-Küster-Hauser") syndrome with vaginal aplasia and a rudimentary uterus. In the region of the uterus we recognize only a somewhat profiled genital ridge. At the base of the left uterosacral ligament lies a uterine bud about as thick as the little finger. An almost normally developed adnexal bundle follows it. The dome of the bladder is marked by an inserted catheter at the arrow.

Fig. 279. In the enlarged detail view we can clearly recognize the left uterine bud. The patient herself had completely female secondary sexual characteristics.

Fig. 280. The uterine bud on the right side appears more as a body 3 to 4 cm long, cylindric, and as thick as a lead pencil; the location can best be spotted by the base of the right round ligament. Ovary and tube are of almost normal size and configuration.

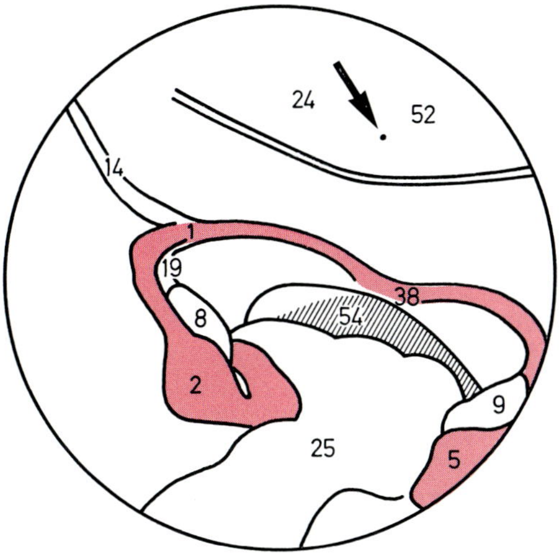

24
52
14
1
19
38
8
54
2
9
25
5

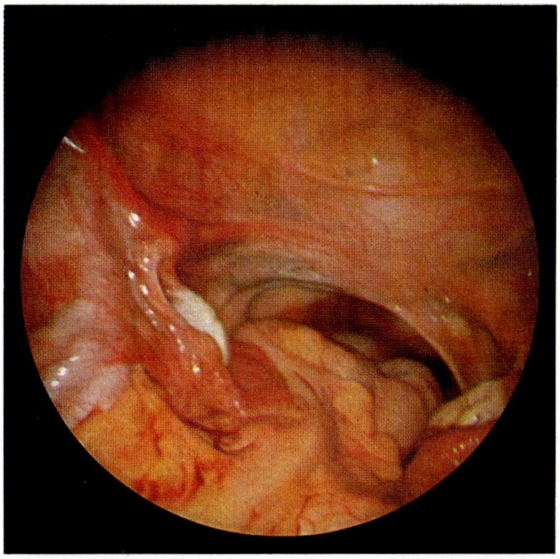

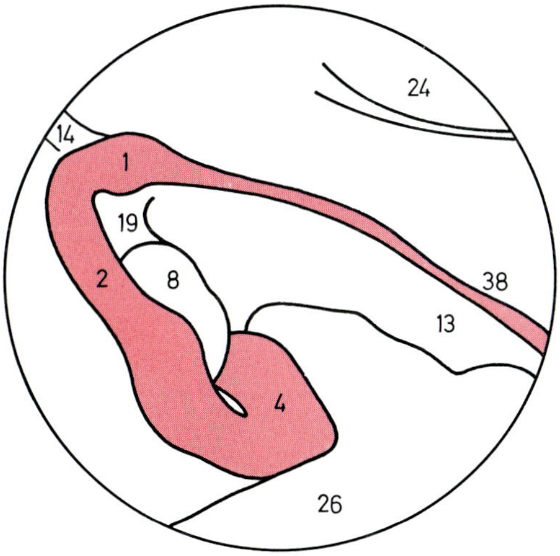

24
14
1
19
2
8
38
13
4
26

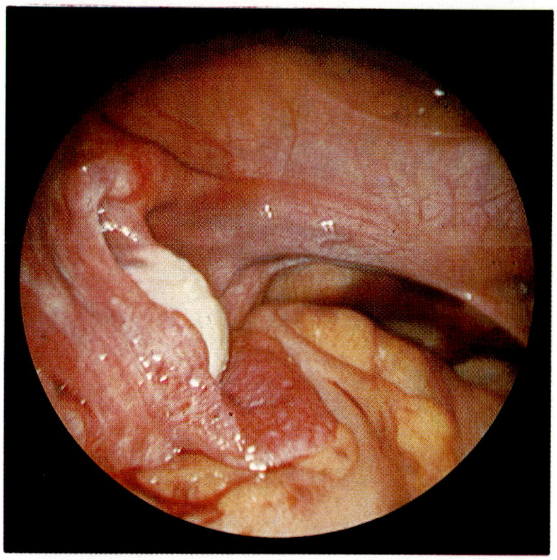

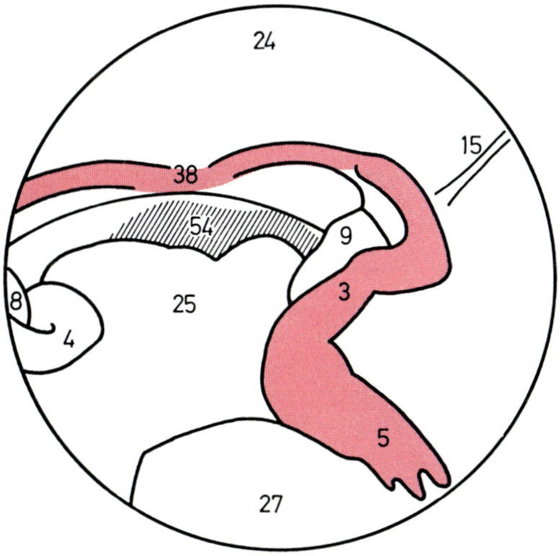

24
15
38
54
9
8
3
25
4
5
27

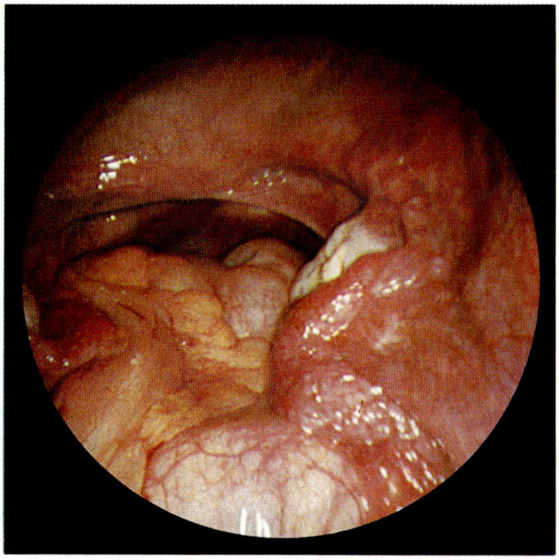

Fig. 281. In all forms of genital hypoplasia it is recommended to perform an endometrial biopsy in addition to the ovarian biopsy described in Chapter VII, Section 2a. The suction biopsy curet is well suited for obtaining cylindric mucosal samples from the anterior and posterior walls of the uterine cavity. These endometrial specimens may then be examined by routine histology and by research techniques for progesterone receptors in the endometrium.

The suction biopsy curet (1) consists of two hollow tubes that freely rotate about each other and have a wide sidewall opening near the distal end. After grasping the anterior lip of the cervix (2), the instrument is gently inserted into the uterine cavity. Both 3- and 5-mm diameter instruments are available to facilitate ready passage of the cervical canal. A guide shows the direction of the opening on the outer tube. After a 180° turn (3), the opening lies on the endometrial surface. A vacuum is produced by withdrawing the plunger of a 10-ml suction syringe (4), which draws the tissue into the lumen of the tube. By rotating the inner tube (5), the endometrial specimen is sharply cut away from the basal endometrium. The lumen is again closed and the entire instrument is removed (6), containing a cylinder of endometrium in the distal chamber.

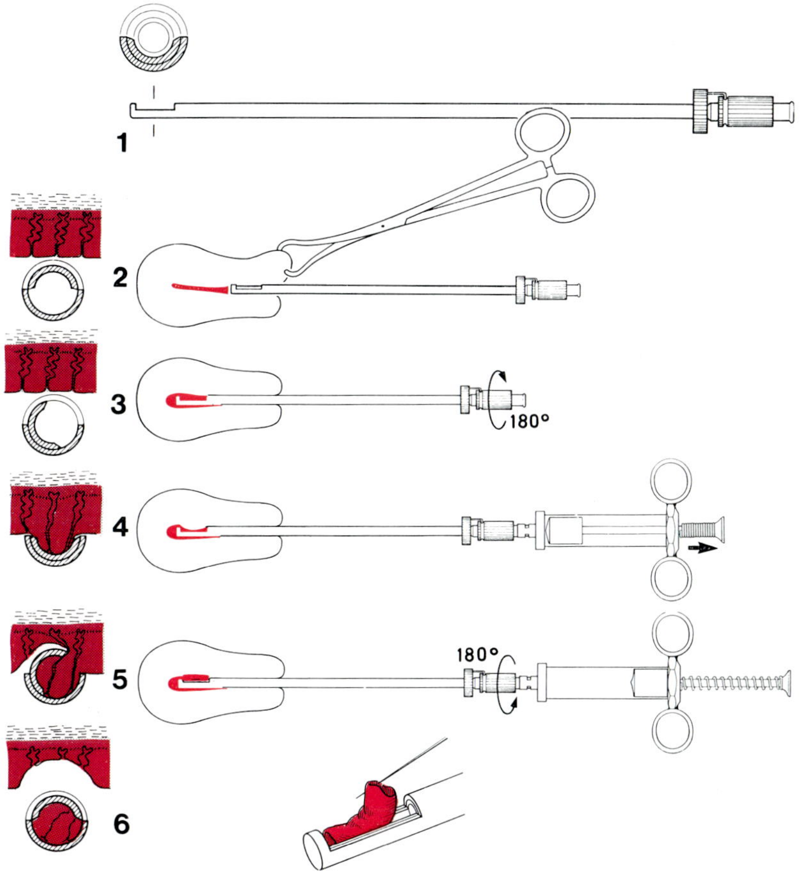

Figure 281

(p) Therapy-Resistant Abdominal Distress

Fig. 282. Interestingly, in the course of laparoscopy in a patient without previous surgery or history of inflammation, we sometimes find an abdomen filled with adhesions usually seen only after laparotomy or severe peritonitis. These adhesions in the region of the ascending colon explain the chronic lower abdominal distress for which no cause can be found. Through the advanced techniques made possible with the low-frequency electrocoagulation system, many of these adhesions can be safely lysed during a therapeutic laparoscopy.

Fig. 283. These adhesions between omentum and parietal peritoneum on the right side of the lower abdomen are typical of peritoneal scars after appendectomy. Lysis of these adhesions is accomplished by cutting through the blood vessel-free spaces and coagulating bleeding sites as needed.

Fig. 284. These omental adhesions with the parietal peritoneum in the upper right abdomen were found in a patient who showed no surgical history of them.

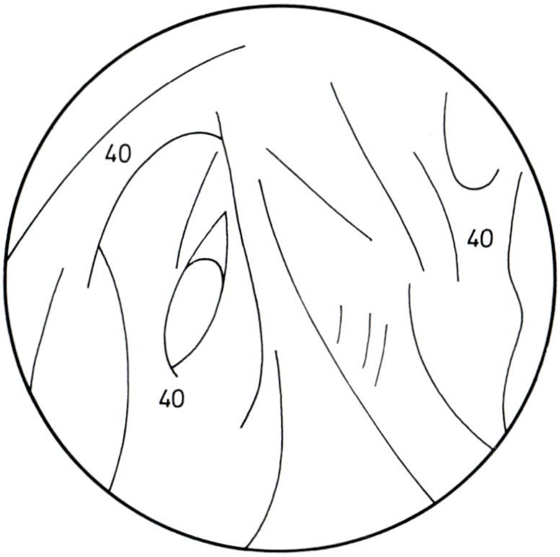
40
40
40

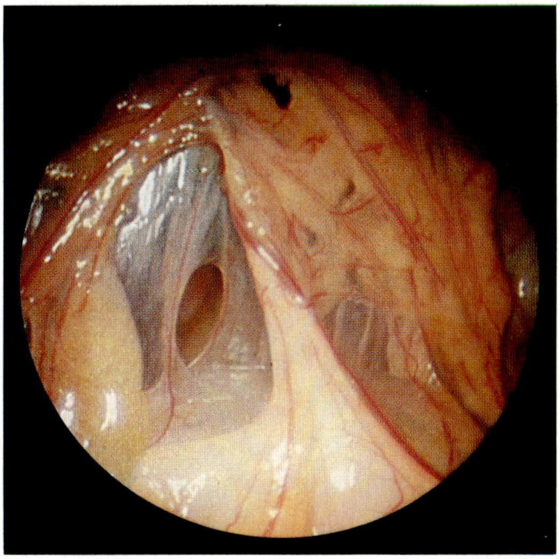

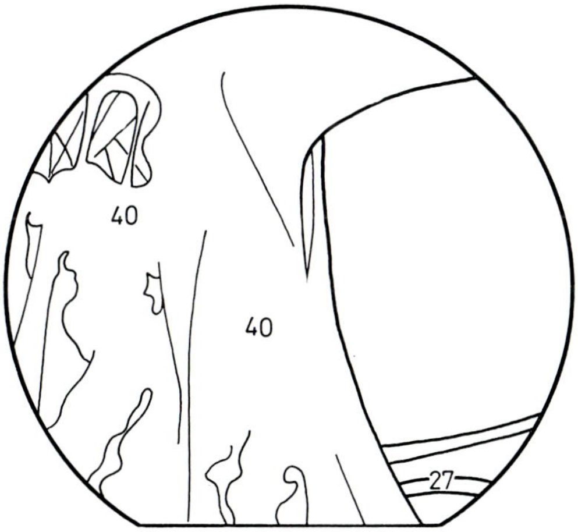
40
40
27

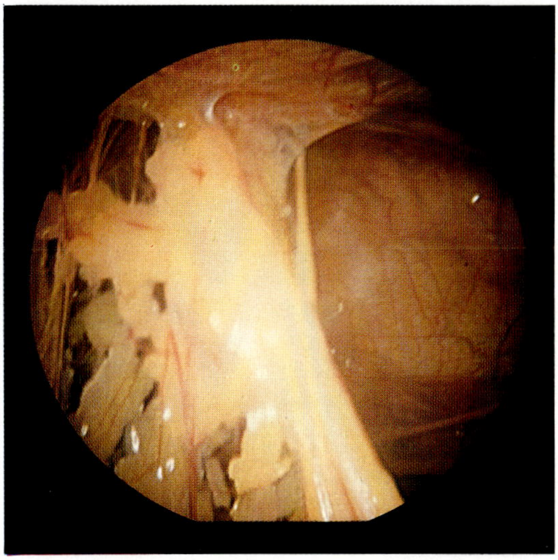

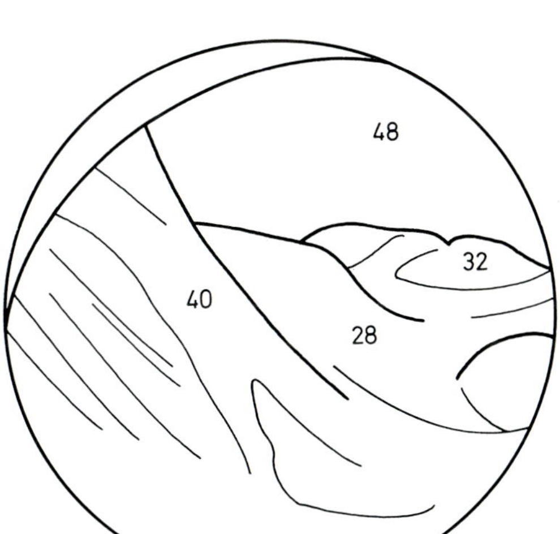
48
32
40
28

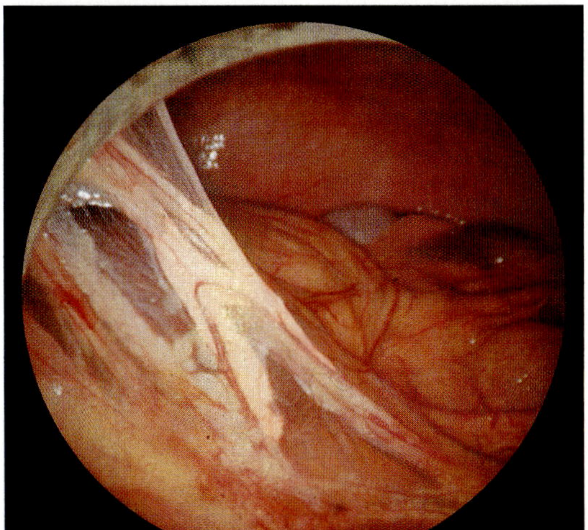

Fig. 285. This sort of intestinal loop attached to the parietal peritoneum represents a particular risk for the laparoscopic puncture. Therefore, before every laparoscopy, these safety tests should be carried out religiously: (1) needle test: testing the resistance of the insufflation needle; (2) aspiration test: instillation of 5 ml of sterile saline solution after the puncture, and attempting to reaspirate same; (3) probe test: feeling out the pneumoperitoneal cavity with a needle 0.8 mm thick and 15 cm long (see Fig. 161). This will ensure that an adherent loop of intestine is not perforated. This small intestinal loop has become adherent after a cholecystectomy.

With the crocodile forceps the adhesive band is coagulated, and the uninjured bowel falls free of the peritoneal cavity wall and back into the abdominal cavity. Using high-frequency coagulation, lysis of such adhesions is impossible. The current travels through the bowel rich in electrolytes rather than through the electrolyte-poor subperitoneal fat. This may lead unavoidably to a local bowel wall burn and subsequent necrosis.

Fig. 286. View into a lower abdomen with massive omental and intestinal adhesions resulting from a cesarean section.

Fig. 287. Especially dense adhesions are regularly found after operations on the adnexa. Here, for example, the cranial portion of the sigmoid loop can be seen broadly attached to the cornu of the uterus after adnexectomy, causing pain. With the modern Endotherm-coagulation technique these omental adhesions can easily be detached from the round ligament and the cornu.

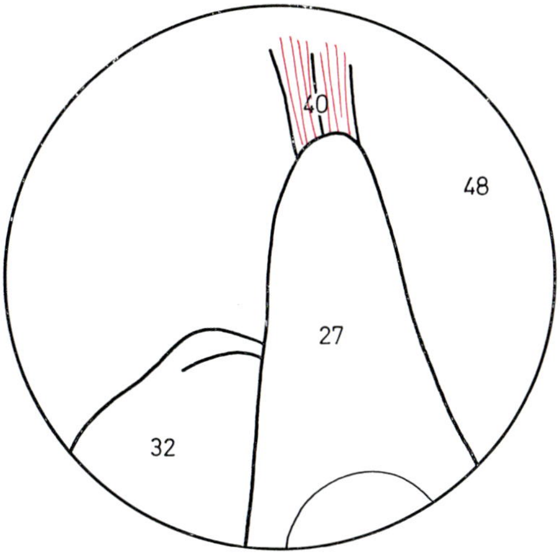
40
48
27
32

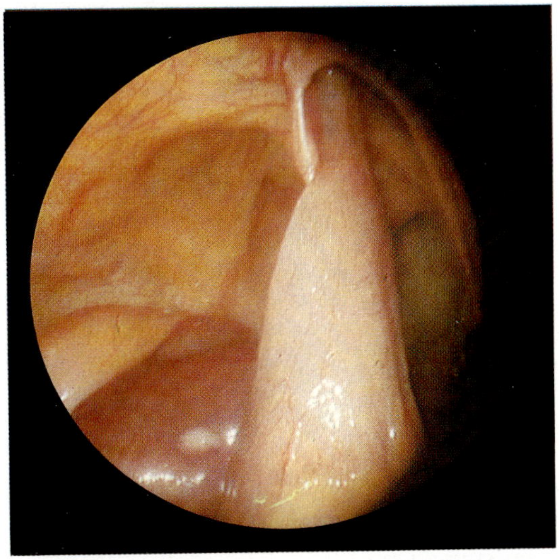

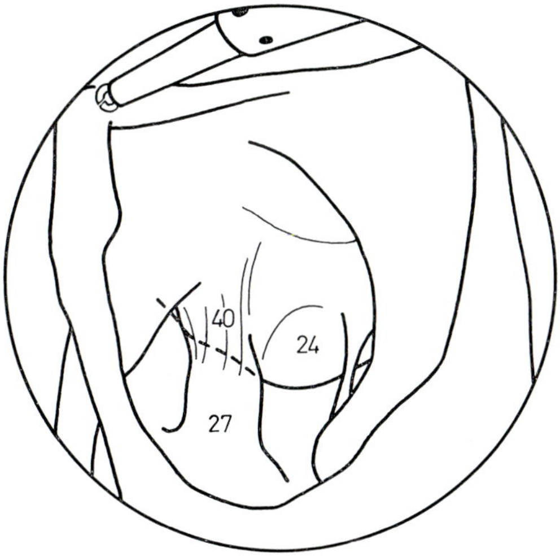
40
24
27

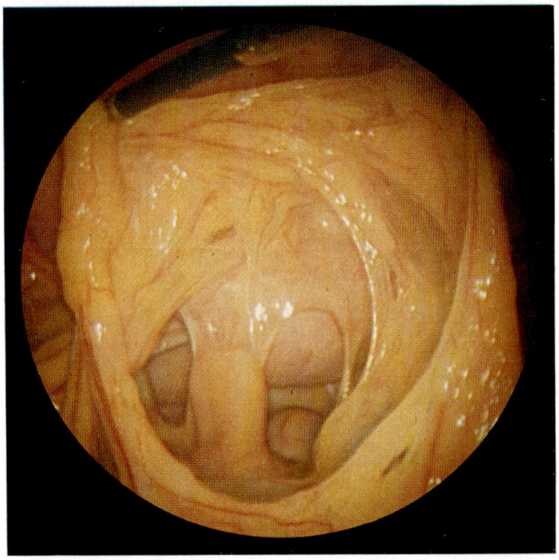

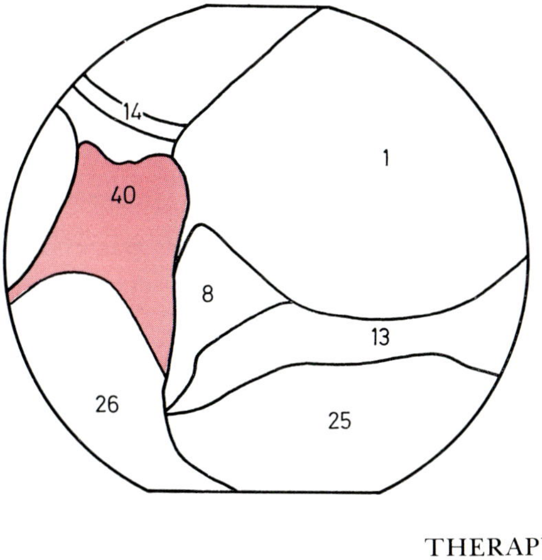
14
1
40
8
13
26
25

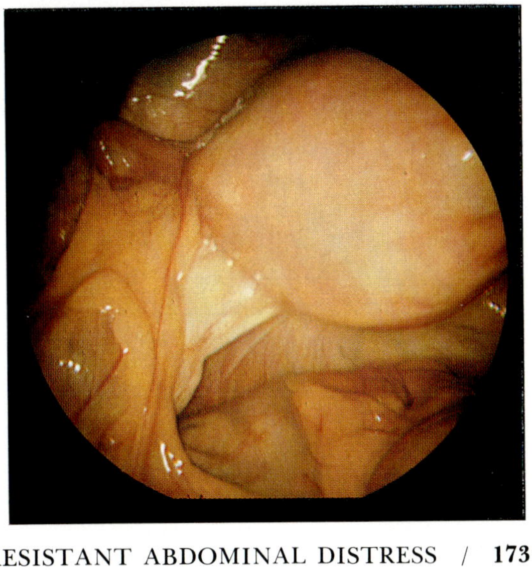

Fig. 288. This situation after a left adnexectomy shows clearly how the infundibulopelvic ligament is broadly adherent to the left wall of the uterus as a consequence of large-scale peritoneization. Pain in the lower abdomen, especially upon displacement of the uterus, is readily understandable.

Fig. 289. These broad adhesions without any particular history led to years of diagnostic consultations about chronic adnexitis on the right and chronic appendicitis. After elimination of these velamentous omental adhesions at laparoscopy, the patient was free of pain.

Fig. 290. Distress in the upper abdomen often is reflected into the lower abdomen, and vice versa, so that a glance at the upper abdomen is routine during laparoscopy. Here there are massive adhesions between the surface of the liver and the diaphragm. The patient had no past hepatic illness. The obscure distress in the middle and lower abdomen is attributable to these linear adhesions. Since such adhesions are of no consequence for the function of the liver and are of no other therapeutic consequence, the diagnosis is sufficient to rule out completely the idea of a "chronic illness" and the specter of cancer.

When a patient is prone to such fears, an explanatory chat after laparoscopy, by removing the mentally taxing "condition," is often enough to help her become clinically well despite the continued existence of the morphologic situation.

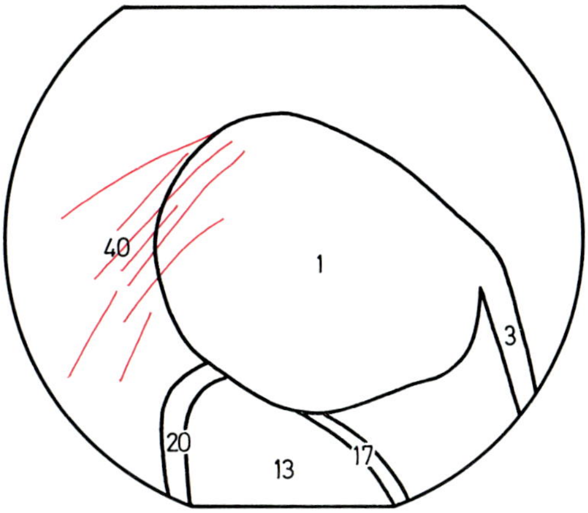
40
1
3
20
13
17

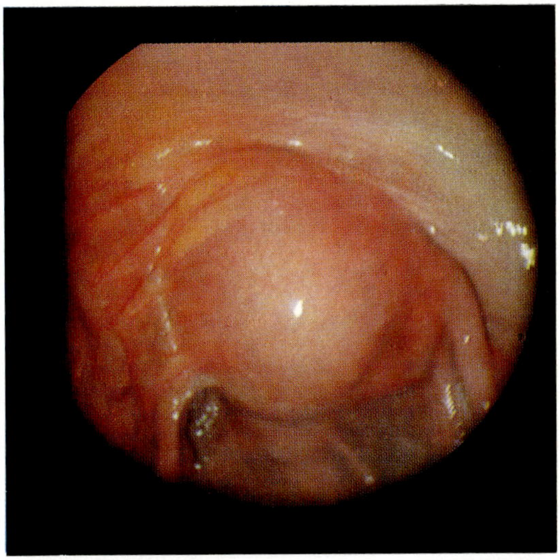

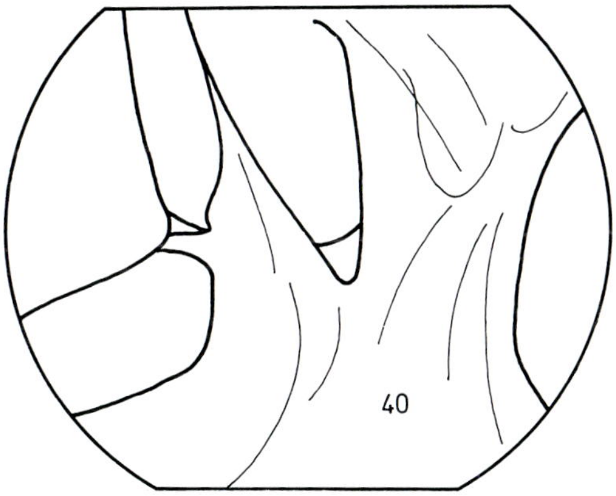
40

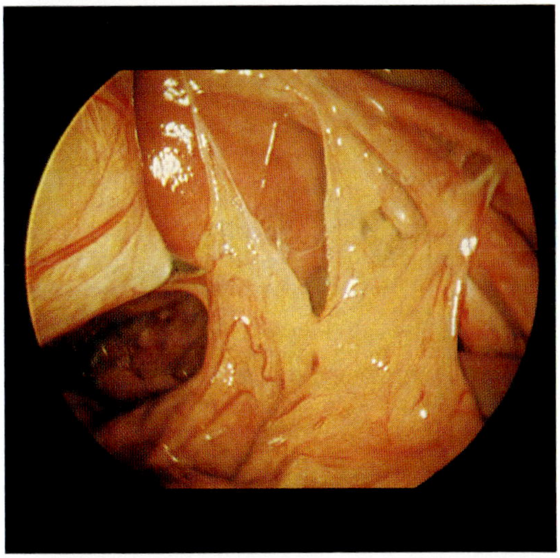

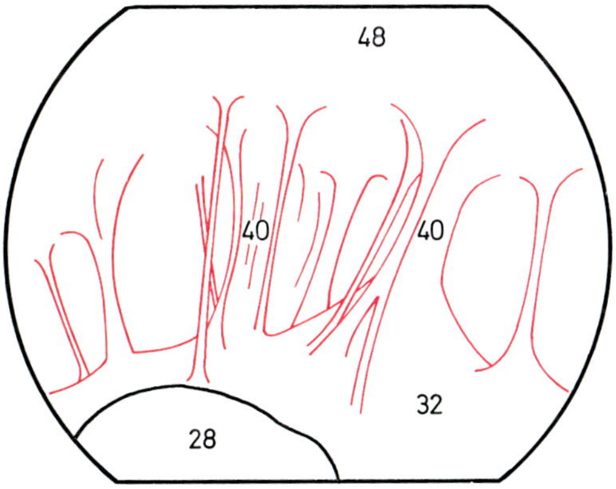
48
40
40
32
28

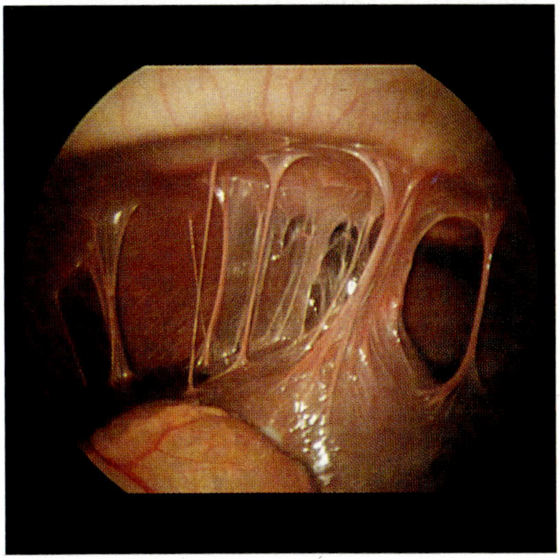

Fig. 291. Perihepatic adhesions between the surface of the liver and the diaphragm often are diagnosed at laparoscopy although the patient may be unable to give any specific history of them.

Fig. 292. Such perihepatic adhesions, with no known hepatitis, are often the cause of complaints of obscure abdominal pain which frequently are referred into the lower abdomen in conjunction with the menstrual periods.

Fig. 293. Here, beneath the elevated lobe of the liver, we see a gallbladder packed full of stones. This patient was advised to seek medical and/or surgical treatment. The chronic obscure abdominal distress, formerly blamed on a prior right-side adnexitis, is now explained.

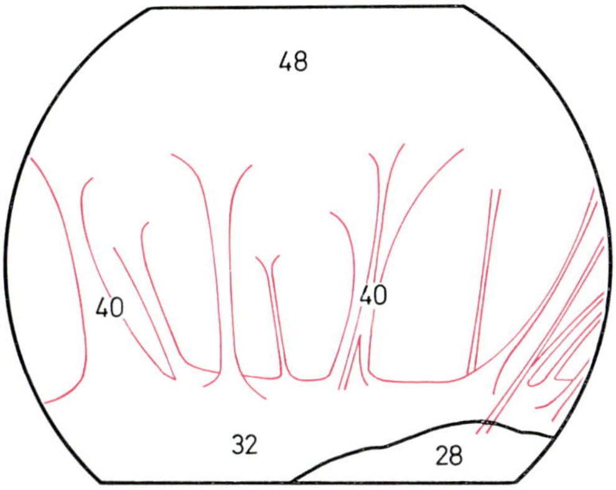
48
40
40
32
28

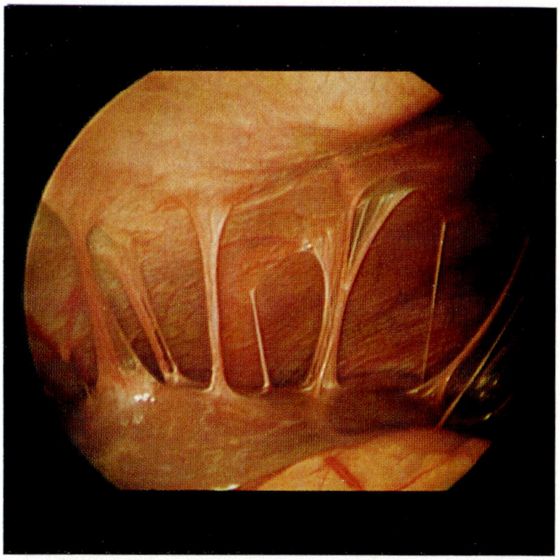

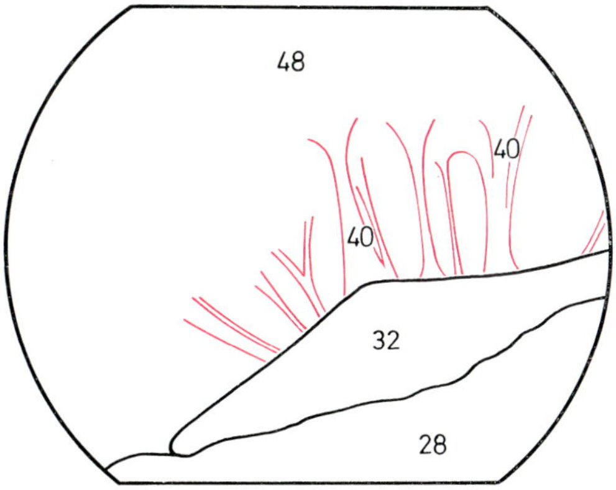
48
40
40
32
28

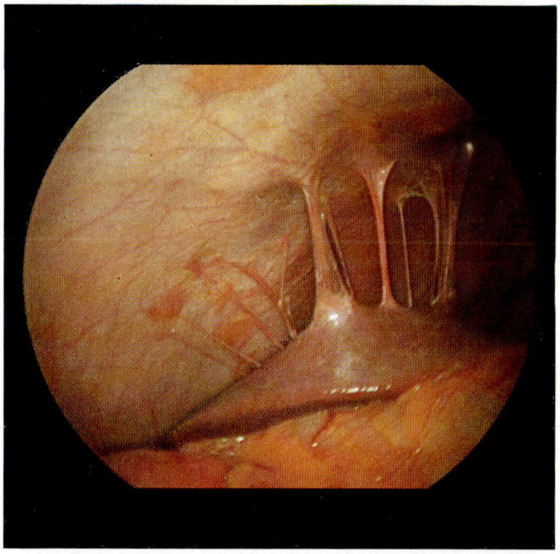

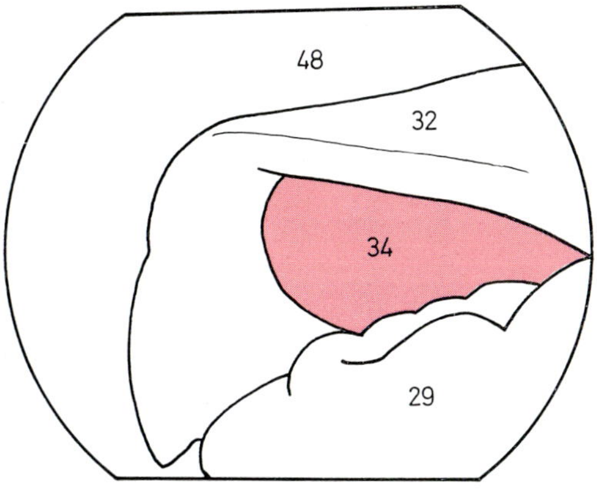
48
32
34
29

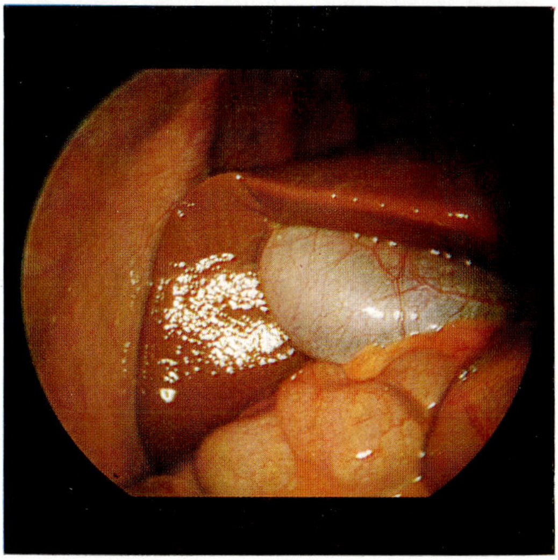

2

Surgical Diagnostic Laparoscopy

(a) Ovarian and Tubal Sterility: Biopsy and Tubal Dye Insufflation

Fig. 294. Since a pronounced arcuate uterus or bicornuate uterus often is associated with primary ovarian hypoplasia, a test biopsy in the right ovary was performed here in a case of secondary amenorrhea accompanied by a desire for a child. The arrow shows the biopsy site.

Fig. 295. Here, in addition to a clubbed tube filled with blue dye following dye insufflation, we can recognize the biopsy wound in the right ovary. The picture shows clearly the large, deep pit resulting from the biopsy and the subsequent punch technique with the trocar sleeve (see also Fig. 70). The arrow shows the biopsy site.

Fig. 296. In secondary sterility, the second puncture in the left side of the lower abdomen for a planned subsequent biopsy of the right ovary is demonstrated here. In selecting the location, it should always be borne in mind that the second puncture should be made *opposite* to the site of the intended procedure. This provides considerable freedom of motion for the operating instrument and at the same time affords good spatial orientation (see also Fig. 37). Moreover, the biopsy forceps can grasp the ovarian tissue most advantageously when the approach is at a right angle. If this is not successful in the position shown here, one should proceed as follows. Move the uterus as far into the cul-de-sac as possible so that the ovary comes to lie on its anterior wall. Here the ovary is sufficiently steadied against the lateral wall of the pelvis so that it can be grasped with the biopsy forceps (see also Figs. 383–385).

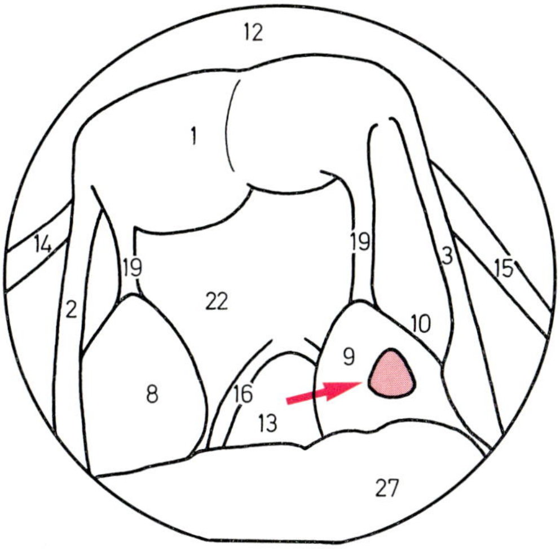
12
1
14
19
19
3
15
2
22
10
9
8
16
13
27

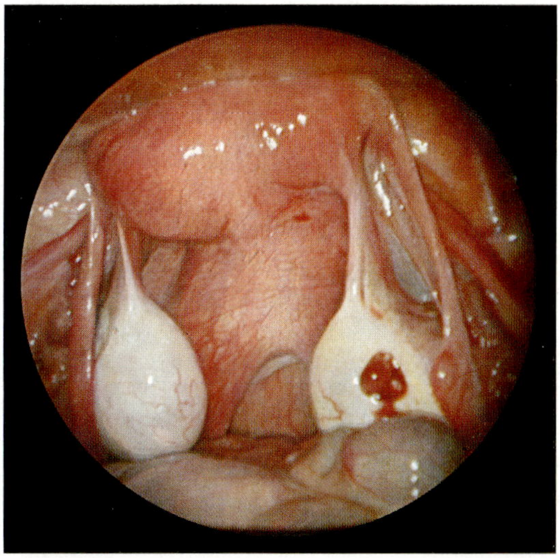

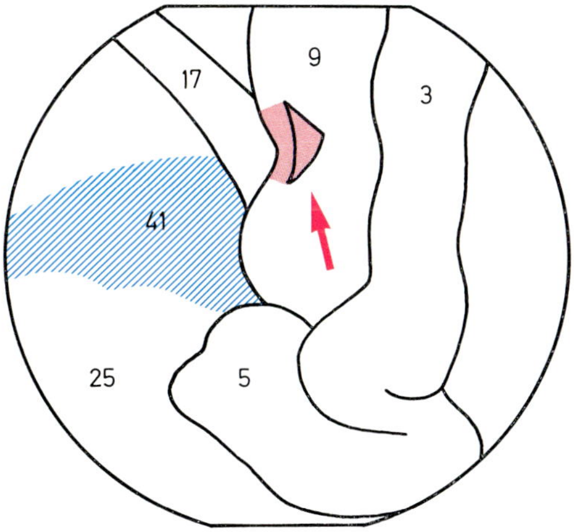
9
17
3
41
25
5

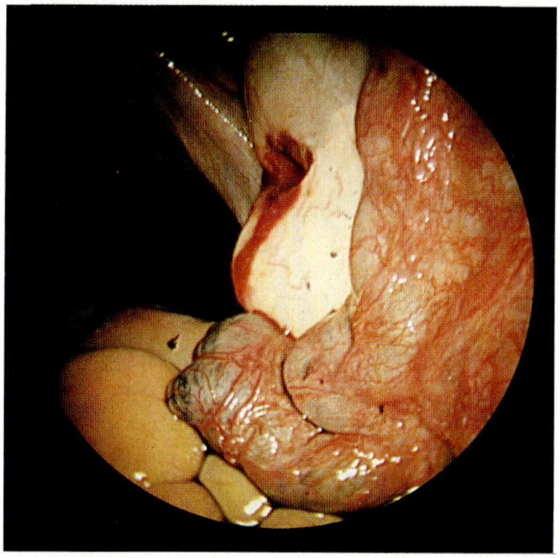

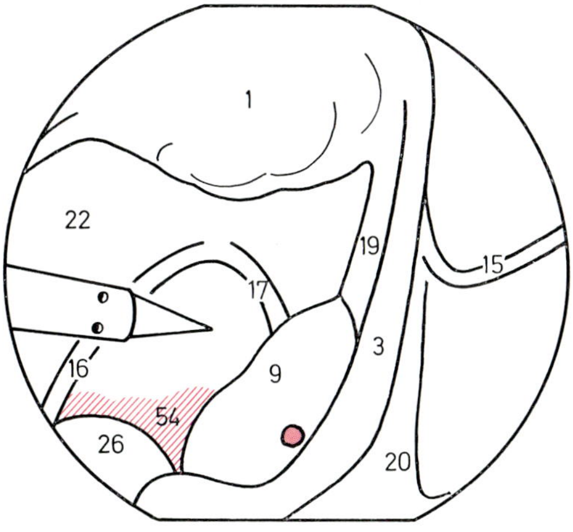
1
22
19
15
17
16
3
9
54
26
20

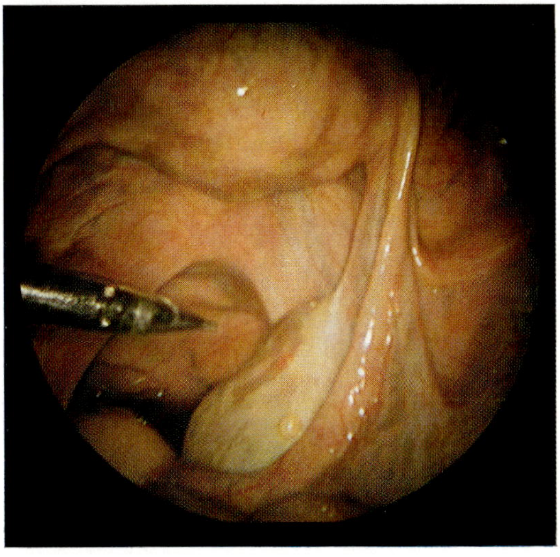

(b) Chromopertubation

As a test for tubal patency, laparoscopy is far superior to both instrument-guided pneumatic insufflation and hysterosalpingography. With the aid of the former it is possible to gain a primary orientation as to patency. Fikentscher and Semm grade the tubal patency according to time and pressure of the CO_2-gas insufflation as follows: (1) normal patency; (2) poor patency; (3) highly stenosed tube. If, by this insufflation technique, we do not get clear-cut Grade 1 patency, laparoscopy is indicated. For the last ten years, we have been performing hysterosalpingography only in individual cases in the sense of hysterography. The estimation of tubal patency on the basis of salpingography with a contrast medium is no longer the method of choice today. As shown by the following tubal dye insufflation diagrams, tubal patency all too often is falsely indicated by hysterosalpingography, and even though the tube actually may be patent, this does not necessarily mean that an ovum will be accepted. The contrast medium does pass out into the free abdominal cavity, but only through splits or ruptures, which are of no importance in the mechanism of acceptance of ova.

Figure 297 shows the principle of dye insufflation at laparoscopy. After placement of the suction intrauterine cannula, the blue dye is pumped under mechanical pressure control out of the intermediate container hanging from the patient's thigh into the uterine cavity. The instillation must be accomplished under constant, uniform pressure, which requires an insufflation pump.

Fig. 298. The common practice of blowing in the dye by hand is contraindicated, since the tremor of the thumb when instilling the liquid leads to mechanical stimulation of the uterine musculature, followed by an intramural tubal spasm. It also leads to an incorrect negative test if this procedure is prolonged.

The 20 ml of dye solution within the container, the rubber tubing, and the uterine vacuum sound are filled as follows:

15 ml	instillation of fluid as described in the text
5 ml	indigo carmine (sterile injection)
= 20 ml	insufflation solution

Fig. 299. Even with the insufflation of the dye under machine-controlled CO_2-gas pressure, intravascular absorption of the fluid may occur. Such aberrations are unknown to us with tubal insufflation using gas (tubal insufflation with air has sometimes led to fatal air emboli) and hysterosalpingography using x-ray contrast medium, widely demonstrated in other atlases. Since the insufflated dye solution consists of intravenously acceptable medications (streptomycin, hydrocortisone, alpha-chymotrypsin, procaine, and physiologic saline solution), such absorption in the course of the procedure is not dangerous. If blue discoloration is detected in the uterus, mesosalpinx, or parametria, insufflation should be stopped.

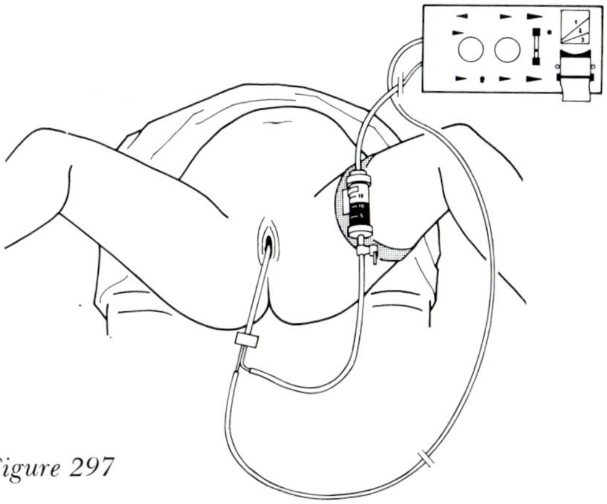

Figure 297

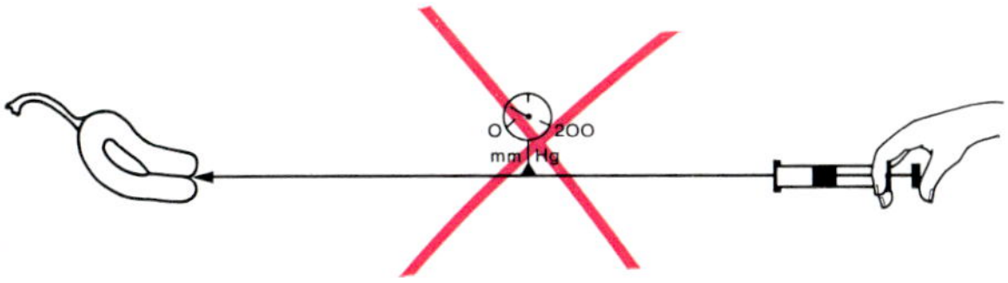

Figure 298

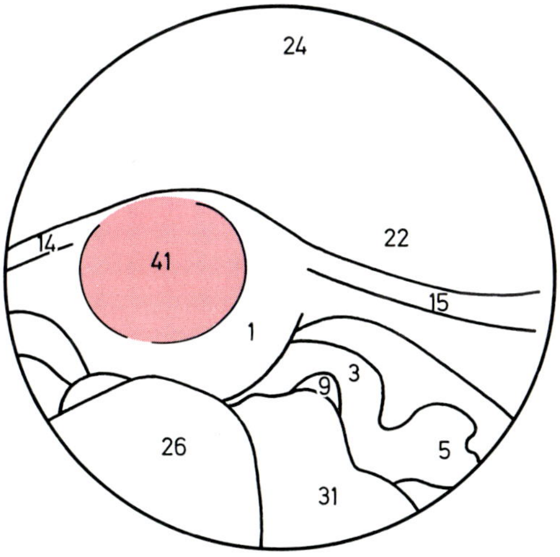

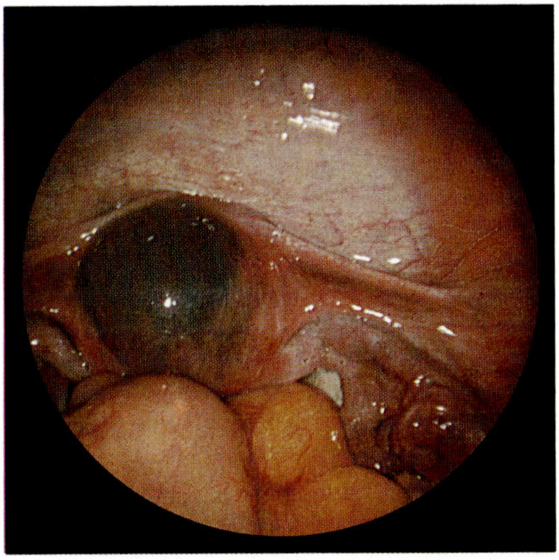

Fig. 300. In tubal dye insufflation done at a pressure-range of from 100 to a maximum of 300 mm Hg, we distinguish four possibilities.

(*A*) Normal configuration of the tubes, and full patency: the dye flows out freely into the cul-de-sac without causing blue coloration of the tube.

(*B*) The tubes are patent, but there are stenoses in them, before which the tube bulges out sharply from the insufflation pressure. We then note the blue dye emerging in drops or a thin stream, and the tube engorged and bluish before the stenoses. This is of great diagnostic importance and can be detected only visually at laparoscopy. In such cases hysterosalpingography gives an incorrect positive test result.

(*C*) The tubes are occluded in the ampullar region. The tube is engorged under the pressure of insufflation. The blue color shows through the tubal wall more or less clearly, depending on the degree of atrophy of the tubal or ampullar musculature. These conclusions are of decisive importance in the prognosis for subsequent salpingolysis or neotubostomy.

(*D*) The occlusion of the fallopian tubes is intramural. Despite the use of a pressure of 300 mm Hg, no change becomes noticeable in the tubes. Sometimes a whitish color change can be seen in the cornua, where the tubes are attached to the uterus, when high pressures are used. This can be explained by the fact that the fluid is forced under a pressure of 300 mm Hg as far as the obstructed lumen of the tubes in the area of the uterine musculature. This leads to an ischemia that is clearly visible on the surface of the cornua.

Fig. 301. In extensive endometriosis in the region of the cul-de-sac as well as the right ovary, the tube can be seen here filled with blue dye all the way to the ampulla. In considering an operation for restoration of fertility in this sterile patient, a salpingolysis or neotubostomy would offer a good prognosis for operative success.

However, a complete cure of the endometriosis is an absolute prerequisite before attempting surgery.

The cure begins with the coagulation of the visible implants of endometriosis in the area of both the cul-de-sac and the ovary, to be performed at laparoscopy with low voltage from the Endotherm. Then follows six to nine months of hormone treatment. A subsequent laparoscopic examination enables the chances for success from the operation to be estimated. *Only if the endometriosis is completely cured can a sterility operation for restoration of tubal patency to the ampulla be considered wise.*

Fig. 302. The right oviduct here is elevated and attached above the linea terminalis by the pull of a scar after a previous appendectomy. The lumen of the tube is perfectly patent to the passage of the dye and CO_2 gas. The tubal ampulla, however, is severely limited in its motility, and the physiologic mechanism for acceptance of the ovum is disturbed.

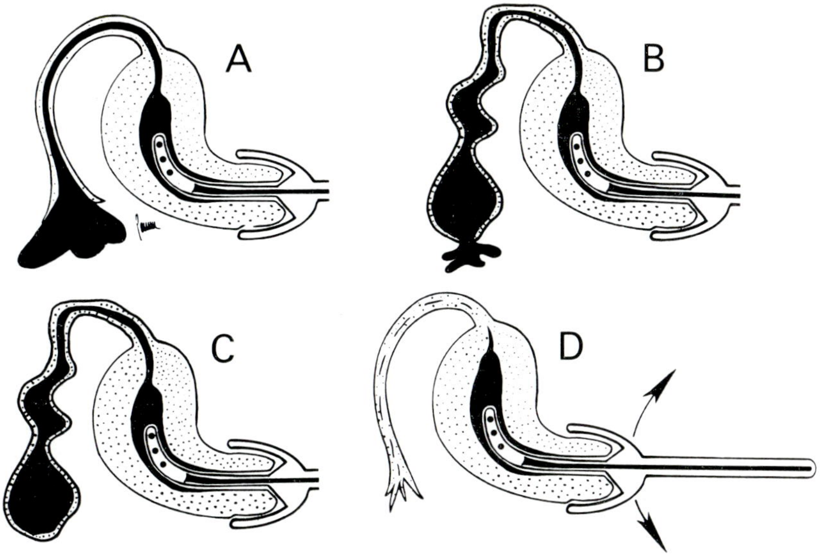
A
B
C
D

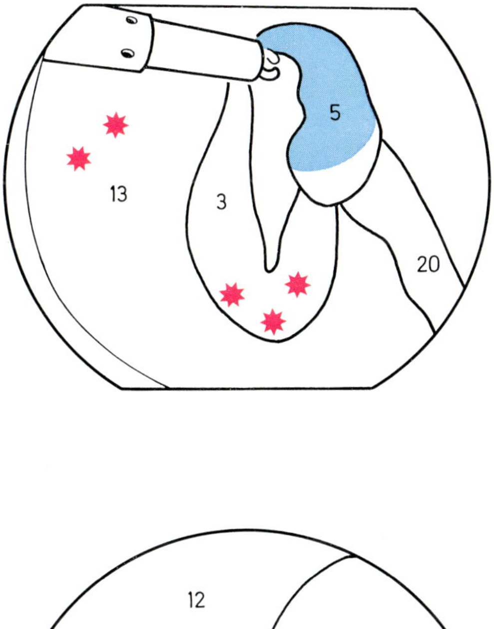
5
13
3
20

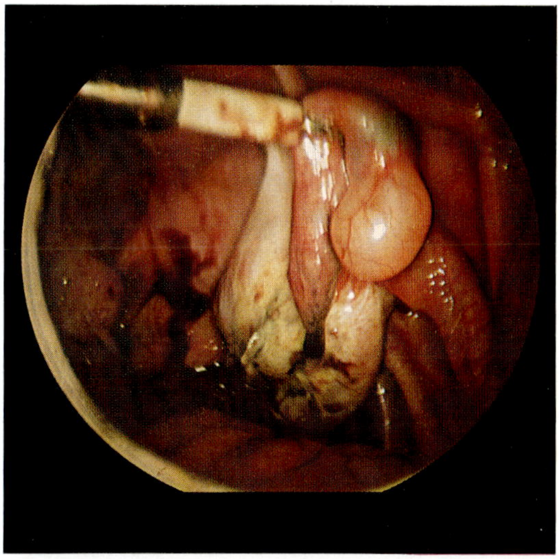

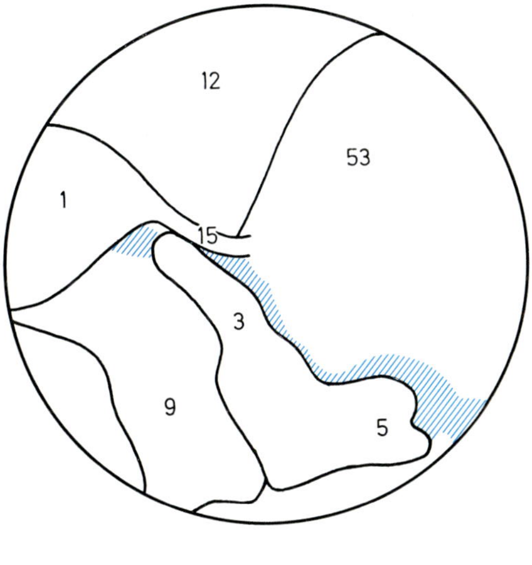
12
53
1
15
3
9
5

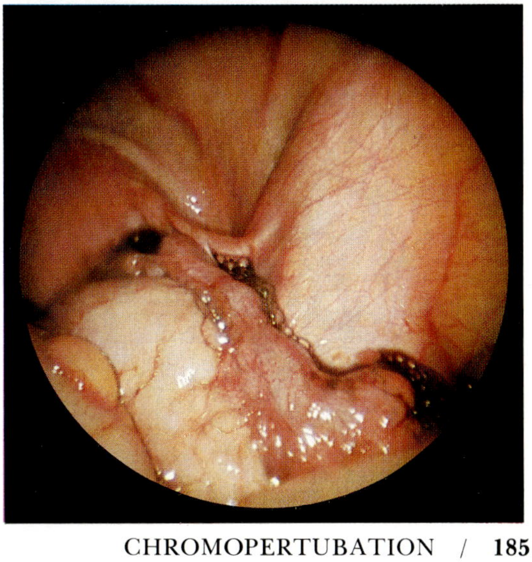

Fig. 303. As a consequence of ampullar stenosis, the left tube is engorged under a pressure of 250 mm Hg. The fimbriae are not completely occluded, however. The blue dye appears very slowly between the intestinal loops. The stricture can be located through subsequent elevation of this tube.

Fig. 304. Under a pressure of 300 mm Hg, the blue dye has emerged subperitoneally at a peritubal stenosis. A rupture of the wall then occurred (*arrow*), and the dye emerged mixed with carbon dioxide gas into the free abdominal cavity. This artificial emergence is diagnosed without difficulty at laparoscopy, whereas hysterosalpingography would have led to an incorrect finding through false interpretation.

Fig. 305. In this enlarged photo we can see clearly the subperitoneal emergence of the blue dye in the region of the left tubal stricture (from Fig. 304). There is a tertiary follicle (*arrow*) on the ovary.

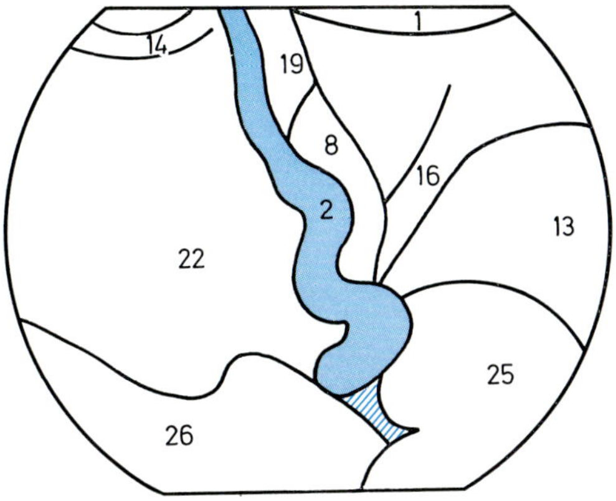
1
14
19
8
16
2
13
22
25
26

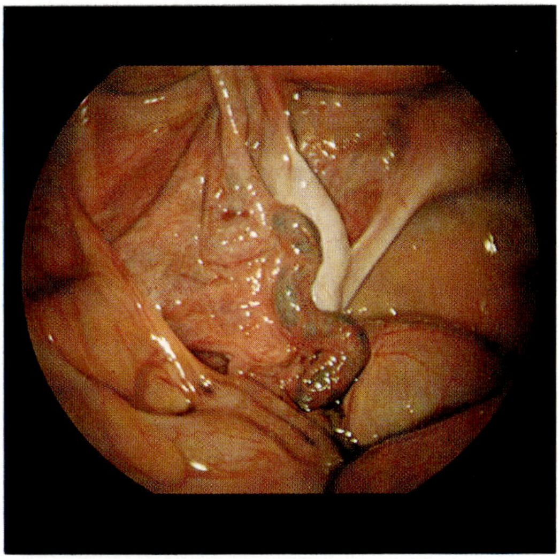

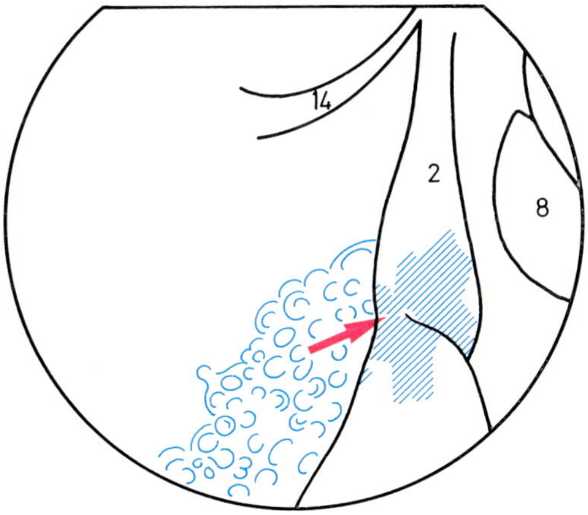
14
2
8

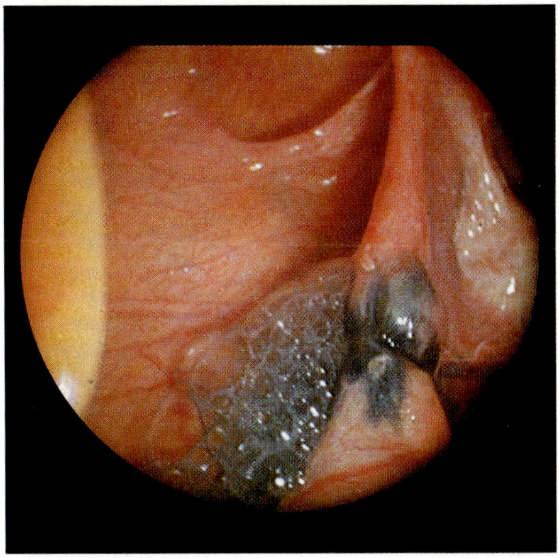

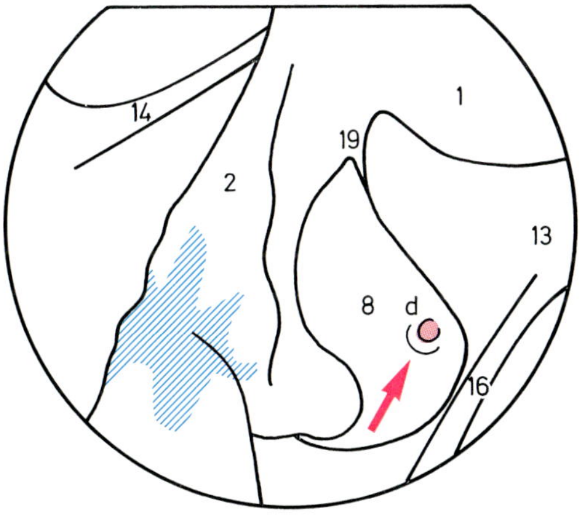
1
14
19
2
13
8
d
16

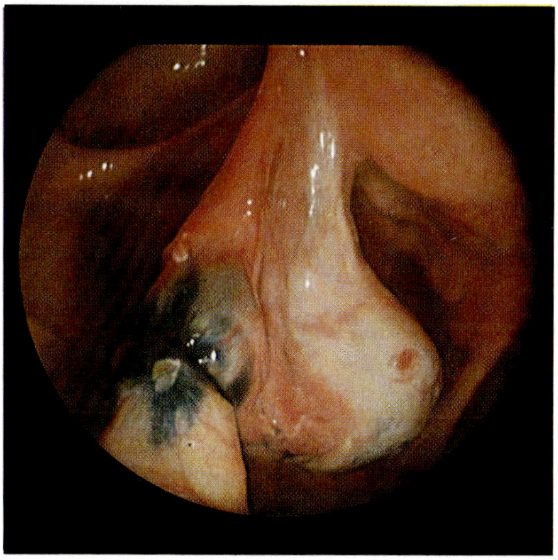

Fig. 306. With elevation of the uterus and an intrauterine pressure of 250 mm Hg, we can see here a demonstration of an occluded hypoplastic tube filled to the tubal ampulla with blue dye. The ovary also is hypoplastic and can already be seen macroscopically from its "streaked" shape as a pronounced case of primary ovarian hypoplasia.

In addition, there are some small endometrial implants on the left tube and in the vicinity of the uterosacral ligaments. In genital hypoplasia the course of the ureter usually is very clearly visible. When performing coagulation of implants one must always take care not to confuse the uterosacral ligament with a prominent ureter, which might lead to catastrophic consequences (see also Fig. 376).

Fig. 307. Under a pressure of 250 mm Hg the right tube is seen here engorged with blue dye all the way to its scarred ampullar end. The blue color shows through especially in the area of the U-bend in the scarred tube: this is a sure sign that the musculature is seriously atrophied in this portion of the tube. It must be regarded as a negative factor for later motility after neotubostomy in calculating the chances for ultimate fertility.

Fig. 308. The right tube, here under an intrauterine pressure of 300 mm Hg, is filled with blue dye all the way to its badly scarred and massively engorged ampullar end. After elevation in the area of the infundibulo-ovarian ligament, the tube can be seen clearly.

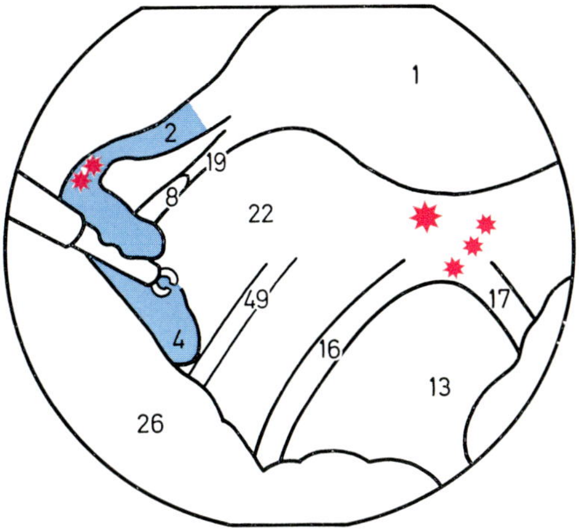
1
2
19
8
22
49
4
17
16
13
26

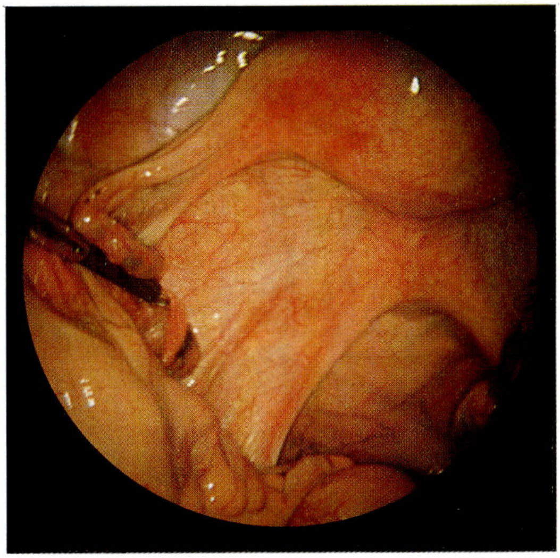

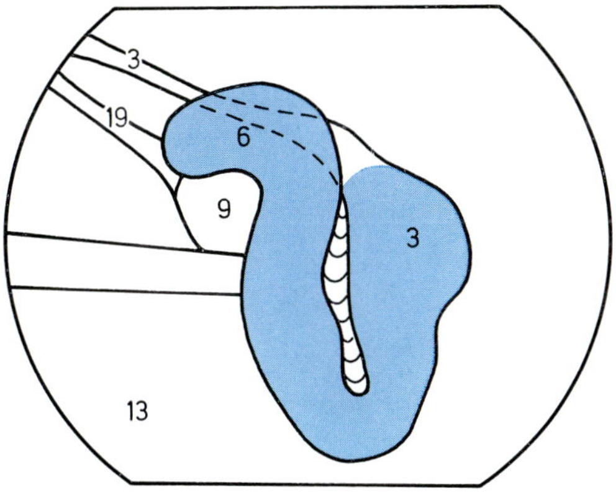
3
19
6
9
3
13

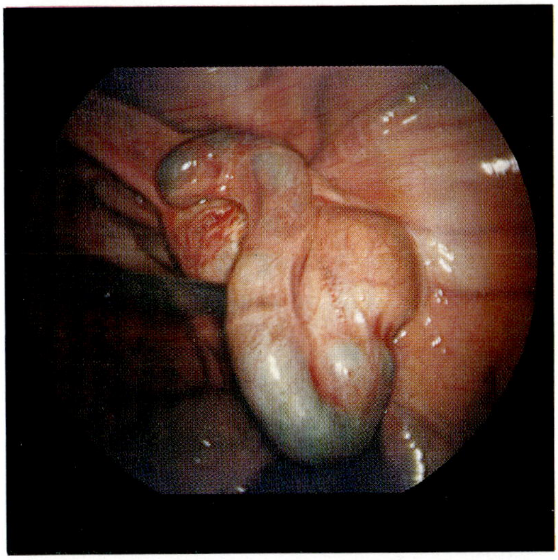

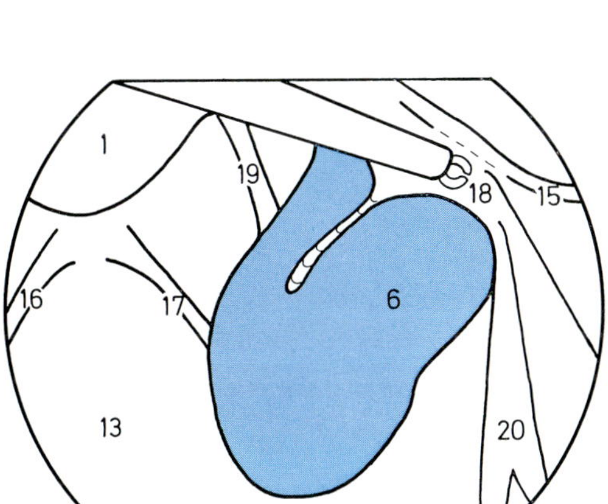
1
19
18
15
16
17
6
13
20

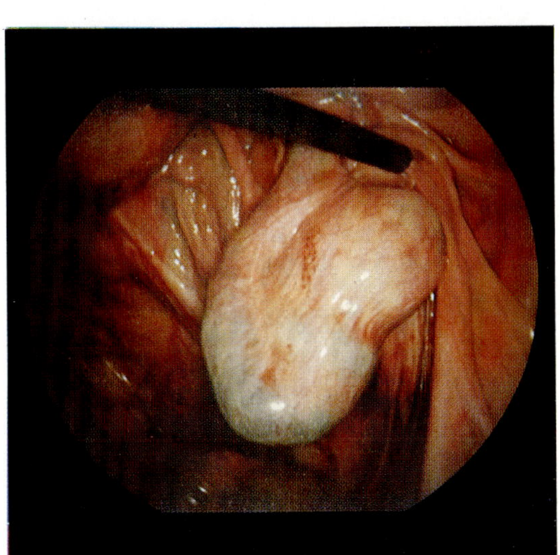

Fig. 309. Typical picture of a hydrosalpinx shaped like a cow's horn in a situation resulting from a left adnexectomy. The horn-shaped right tube is seen almost as thick as a banana with numerous peritubal adhesions running into the cul-de-sac. It is under a pressure of 250 mm Hg and engorged to the bursting point with blue dye, which also is visible in the cul-de-sac. The dye is emerging through a perforation caused by the pressure. In this case, too, one might have diagnosed an incorrect positive finding on the basis of hysterosalpingography.

Fig. 310. The right tube is massively filled with dye, especially the ampulla, under an insufflation pressure of 200 mm Hg. The dye combined with carbon dioxide gas is seen emerging through a medium-grade stenosis near the ampulla. The peritubal adhesions are connected with the endometriosis in the vicinity of the cul-de-sac. A long series of hydropertubations is indicated here as a therapeutic measure.

Fig. 311. This tube remained unchanged even under a pressure of 300 mm Hg, indicating that the occlusion is in the intramural part of the tube. Cherry-sized hydatids were visible upon mobilization of the tubal ampulla, which is badly scarred.

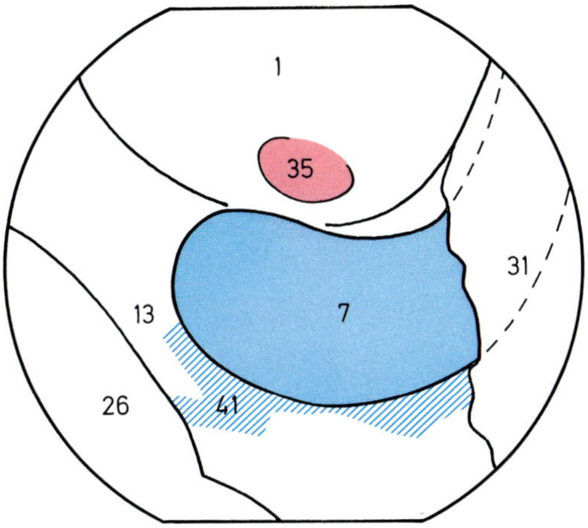
1
35
31
13
7
26
41

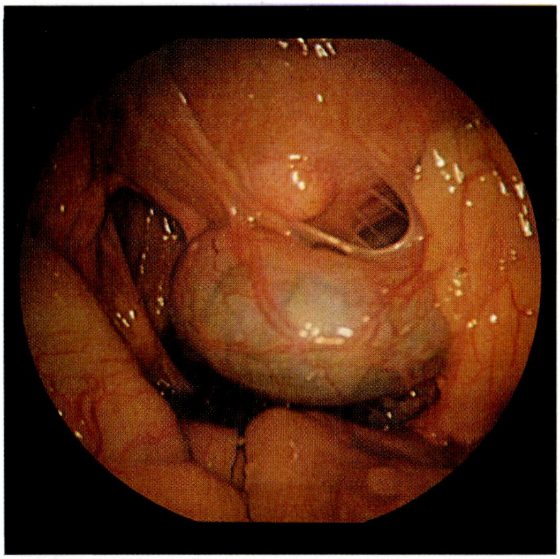

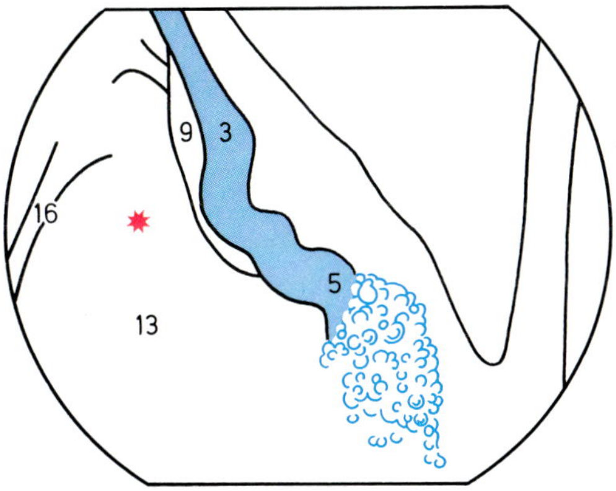
9
3
16
13
5

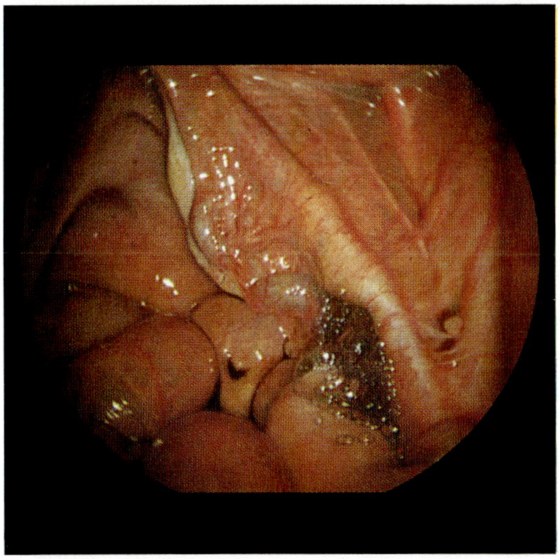

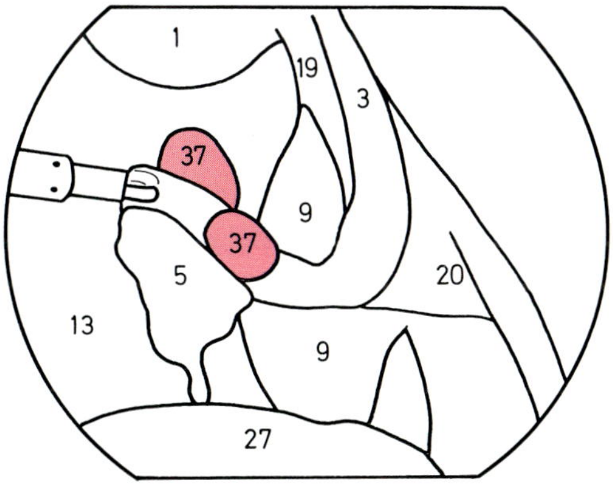
1
19
3
37
9
37
5
20
13
9
27

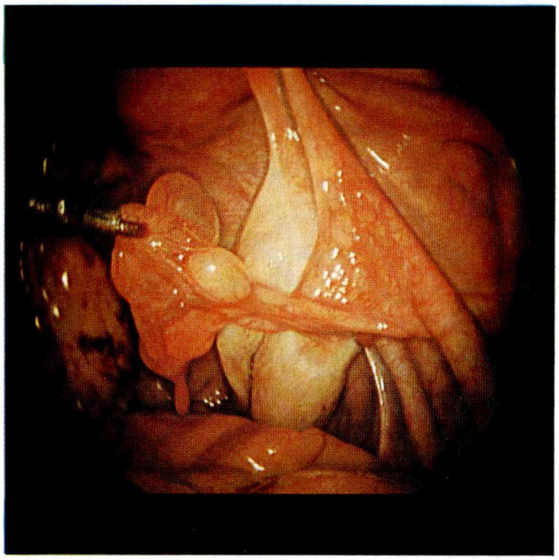

Fig. 312. Upon elevation of the left tube onto the infundibulo-ovarian ligament, a severe ampullar stenosis is revealed. The tube, under a pressure of 300 mm Hg, is maximally engorged as far as just before the ampulla. Beyond this stenosis the dye is dripping out sparingly. The endometriosis, clearly seen here on the left ovary, can be regarded as the cause of this ampullar stenosis.

Fig. 313. A further elevation of the tube in Figure 312 at the mesosalpinx reveals even more closely the stenosis in the ampullar vicinity. The fimbriae are not scarred. A severe intra-ampullar stenosis must be present proximal to the ampulla, and it has led to the massive retrograde engorgement of the tube. Although the carbon dioxide gas is emerging freely, such a tubal stenosis requires at least a conservative oviduct treatment, e.g., a prolonged series of hydropertubations.

At best it should be possible to enter the ampullar lumen with an atraumatic forceps and burst the de facto minor adhesions. Reattachment of the adhesions will be prevented by the subsequent series of hydropertubations (see also Figs. 315, 361, 382).

Fig. 314. The sketch shows once more that, when elevating the fallopian tube, we should avoid direct grasping of the tube as much as possible. Usually it is possible to elevate the ampulla out of the cul-de-sac by grasping the mesosalpinx and bringing it within range of the lens. The jaws of the atraumatic forceps are shaped in such a way that they do not injure the peritoneum if they are manipulated carefully. If the tube is indeed grasped with the forceps, care must be taken that the arched jaws completely encompass the tube so as not to crush the endosalpinx. Optimal mobilization of the tubal ampulla may be accomplished with the suction probe (Figs. 64–67), and is demonstrated in Figures 315–317.

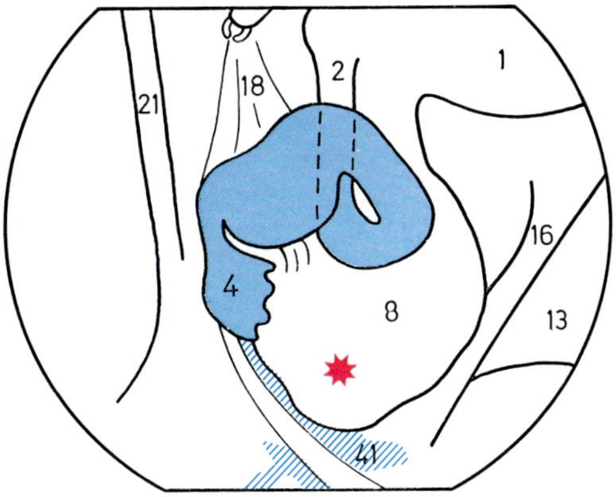
1
2
18
21
16
4
8
13
41

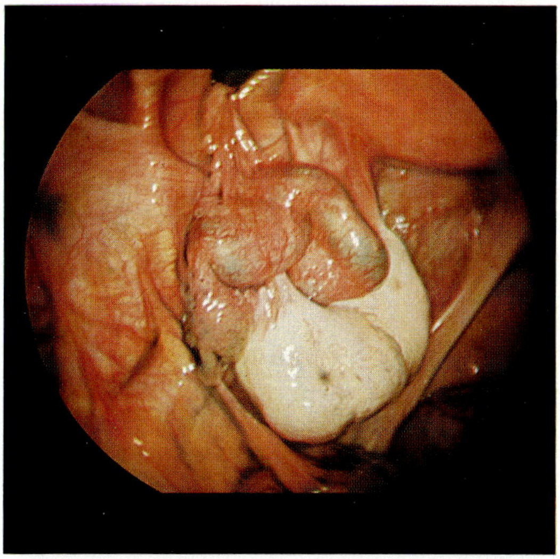

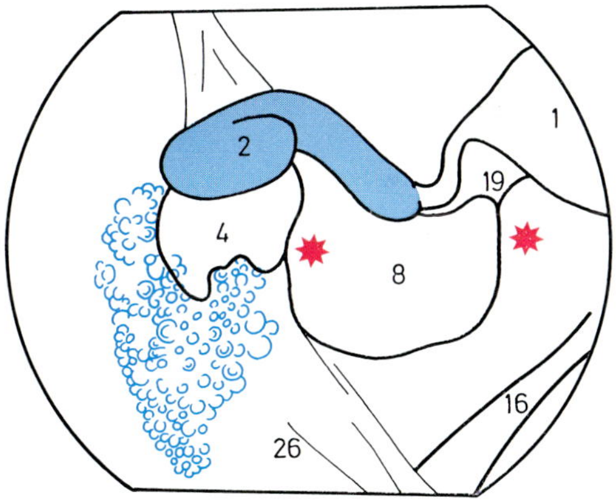
1
2
19
4
8
16
26

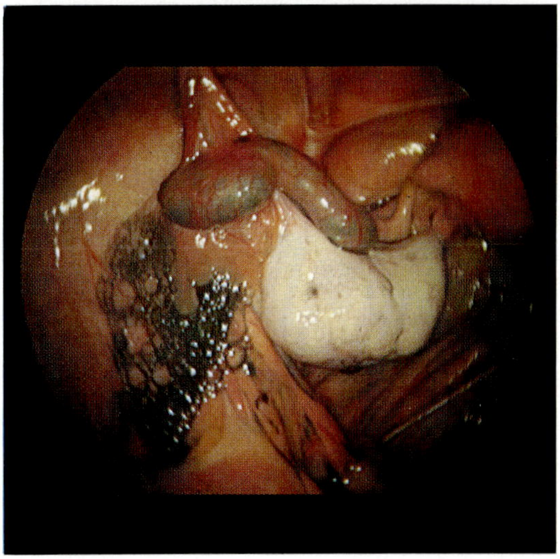

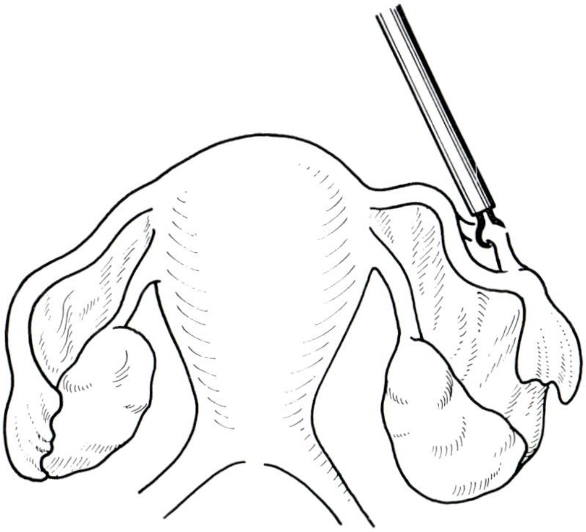

Fig. 315. Here, in order to show the ampulla, it has been elevated out of the lesser pelvis with the 3-mm suction probe while blue dye is being pumped in under a pressure of 250 mm Hg. The tube is dilated and kinked by this high pressure. The fluid is emerging from the stenosed end of the ampulla mixed with gas bubbles. As a consequence of endometriosis (clearly visible on the right ovary) fimbrial adhesions have occurred, which on one side have led to a narrowing of the ampulla and on the other side are drawn to the left as far as the sigmoid loop.

Fig. 316. To remove the fimbrial adhesions described in Figure 315 and caused by the endometriosis, the ampullar end is elevated by means of the 3-mm suction probe. After entry of the atraumatic forceps, its jaws are opened and it is withdrawn (see illustration). This detaches the ampullar adhesions in the fimbriae. Thus, the stenosis can be relieved at laparoscopy through combined use of suction probe and atraumatic forceps.

Fig. 317. The preampullar section of the right tube is shown being elevated with the aid of the 3-mm suction probe. Without reducing the tubal lumen, the fimbriae are brought within range of the lens. The blue dye is emerging mixed with bubbles of gas. The massive distention of the tube, in no way caused by elevation with the suction probe, is sufficient reason for the diagnosis of a preampullar stenosis.

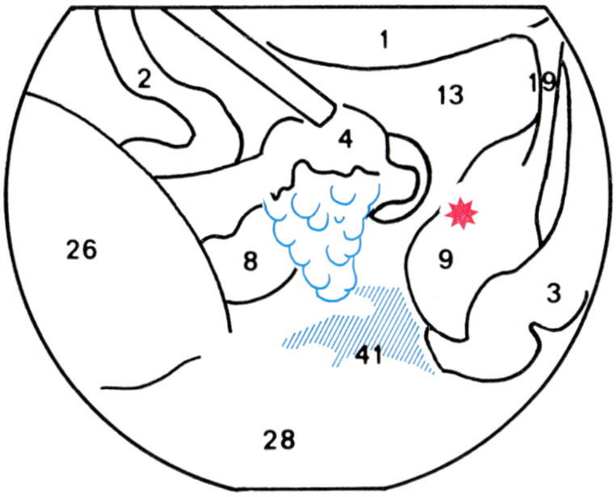
1
2
13
19
4
26
8
9
3
41
28

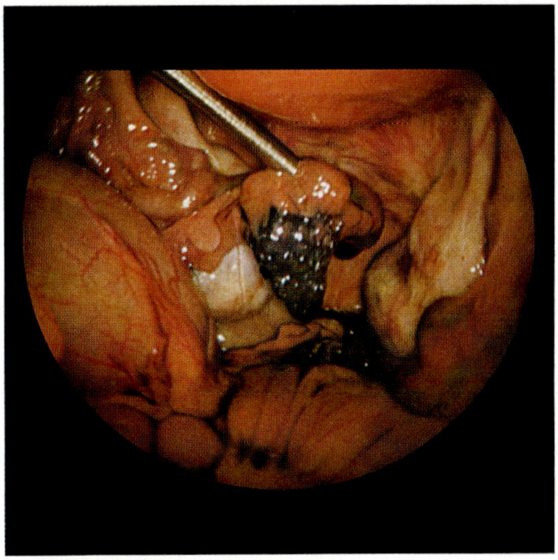

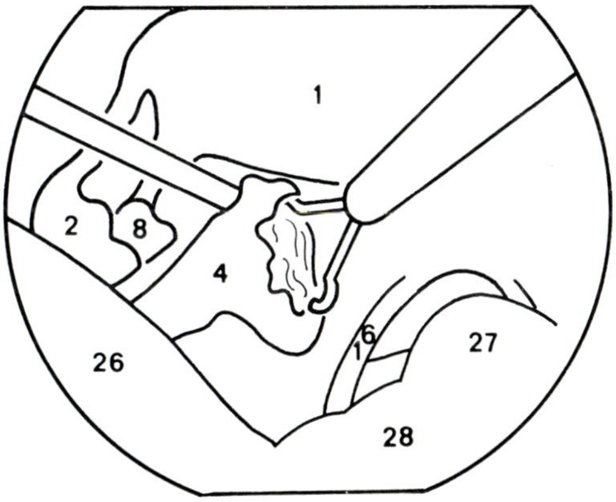
1
2
8
4
6
1
27
26
28

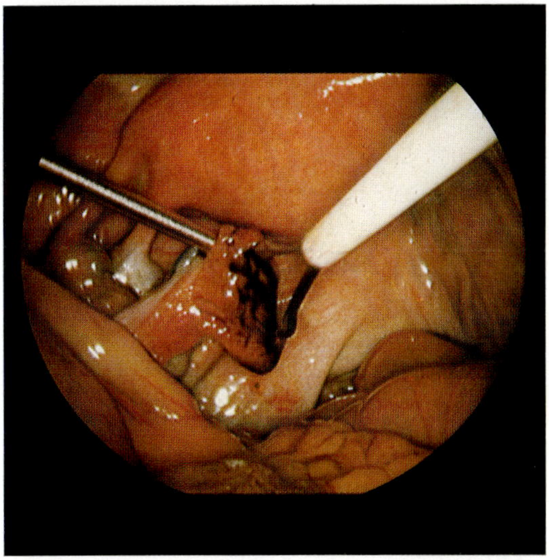

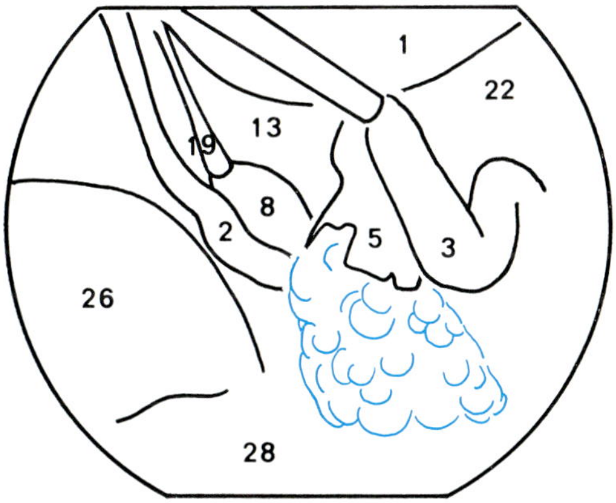
1
22
13
19
8
2
5
3
26
28

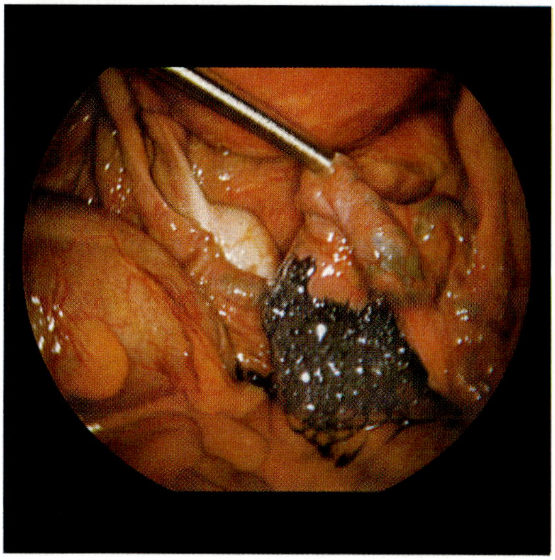

(c) Cytology of the Cul-de-Sac

Fig. 318. In principle, ovarian biopsy serves only in selected cases for a diagnosis of whether ovarian carcinoma is or is not present. In its early stages, even ovarian carcinoma grows discretely at various points in the ovary, and these are under no circumstances 100 per cent detectable at laparoscopy. Even an already advanced malignant process can escape the biopsy forceps, which actually can reach only about 40 per cent of the ovarian surface. Therefore laparoscopy must not be relied on too heavily in making a diagnosis of ovarian carcinoma. In all cases of uncertain ovarian findings at laparoscopy, the secretion always present in the cul-de-sac should be extracted for cytologic examination. Here bloody serous secretion is being extracted from the cul-de-sac for cytologic study in a case of uterine leiomyomata in a postmenopausal patient (extraction device, see Figs. 67 and 320).

Fig. 319. The extracted contents of even a juvenile cyst after puncture should be subjected as a matter of course to histologic and cytologic examination. The pointed puncture cannula serves for the extraction (see Fig. 72).

Fig. 320. The sketch shows the instruments for collecting the extracted fluid. The vacuum produced by an ordinary aspirator or anesthesia apparatus is coupled to the aspirate-collecting jar. The speed of suction is regulated by intermittent pressure of a finger as shown, or by lifting the tip of the cannula free of the tissue being aspirated. The basic rule should be: *any fluid aspirated from the pelvic cavity should be examined cytologically.*

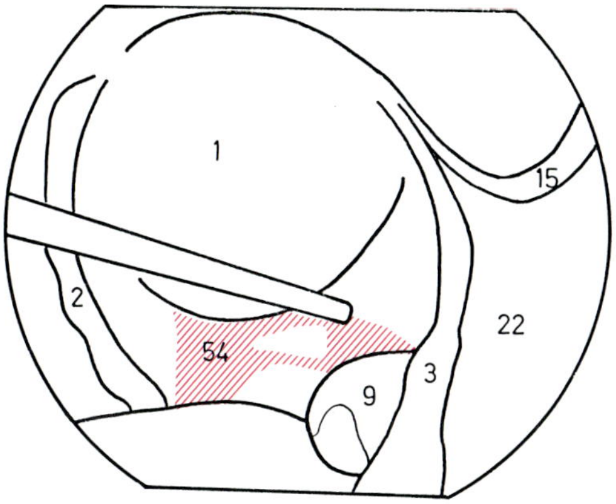
1
15
2
22
54
3
9

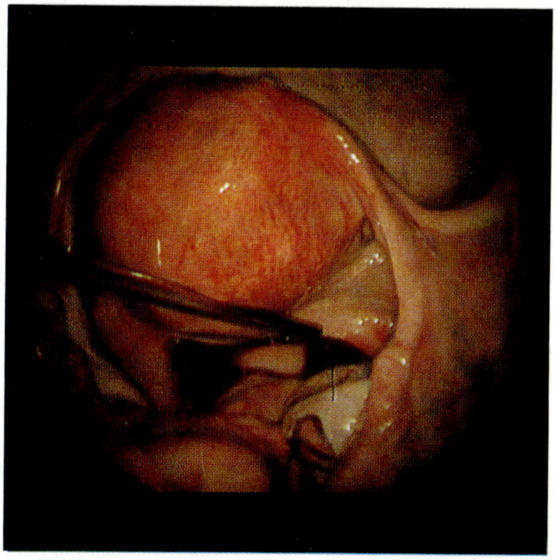

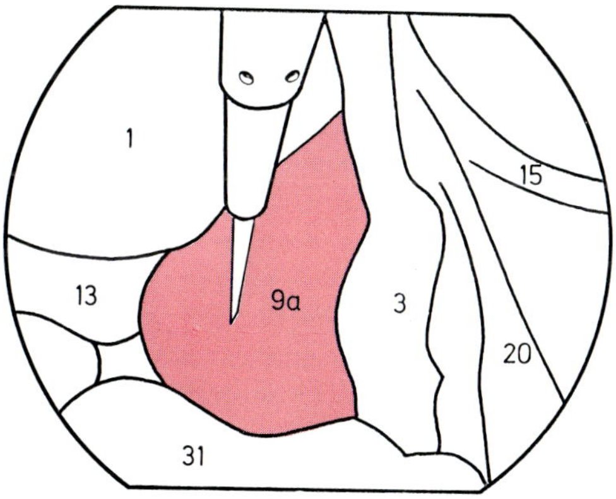
1
15
13
9a
3
20
31

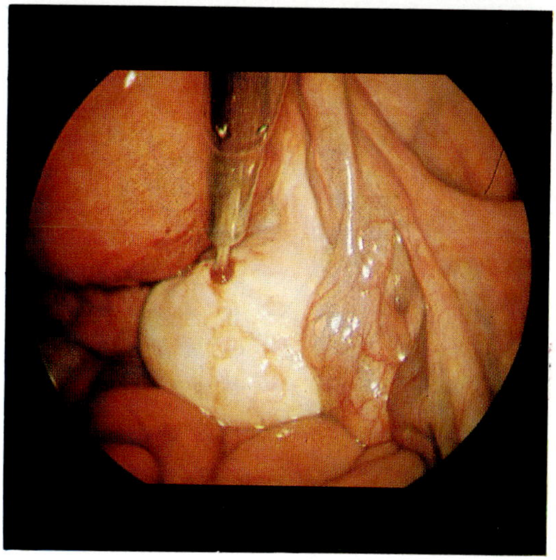

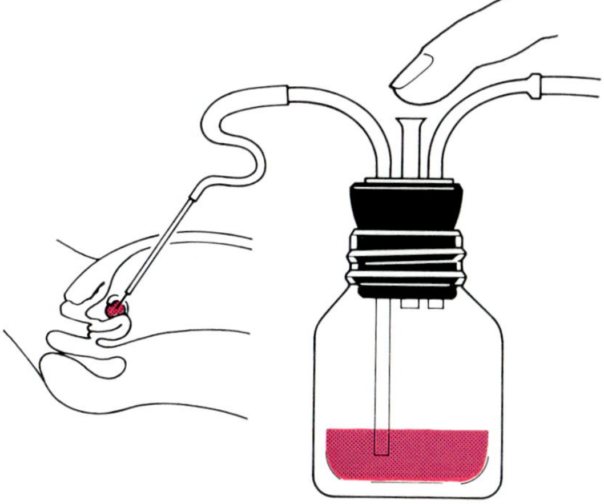

(d) *Biopsy of the Gonads for Sex Determination in Aplasia of the Uterus*

Fig. 321. In a Rokitansky-Küster-Hauser syndrome a laparoscopy with ovarian biopsy was performed for gonadal diagnosis. The illustration shows the insertion of the trocar from the left, since it had been decided to take a biopsy from the right gonad. The genital ridge is only faintly apparent. A catheter introduced into the urethra demonstrates the topography of the dome of the bladder. The vagina is totally absent. The external female genitals are normal. About 15 ml of turbid, bloody, serous fluid is present in the cul-de-sac.

Fig. 322. From the smooth-walled gonad, which is being elevated along with the superimposed fallopian tube above the linea terminalis on the right wall of the pelvis, a large biopsy is being excised. The histologic finding from the biopsy was "undifferentiated testicular tissue."

The laparoscopic gonadal biopsy renders superfluous the exploratory laparotomy that once would have been necessary, and which would be taxing to the "female" patient and not justifiable in relation to its diagnostic value.

Fig. 323. Picture of the situation after biopsy from the right gonad performed at laparoscopy, the histologic diagnosis being gonadal dysgenesis.

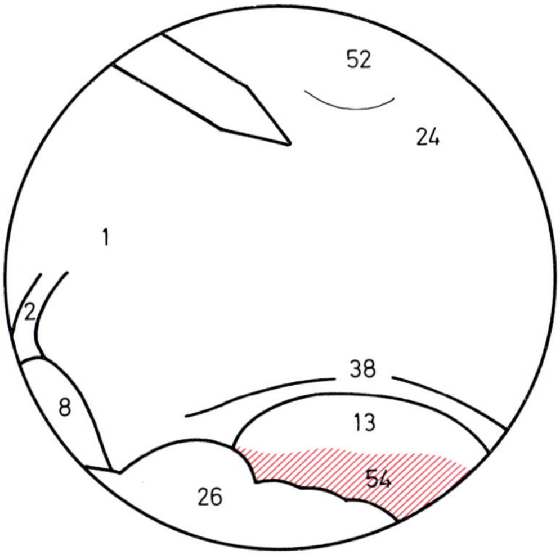
52
24
1
2
38
8
13
54
26

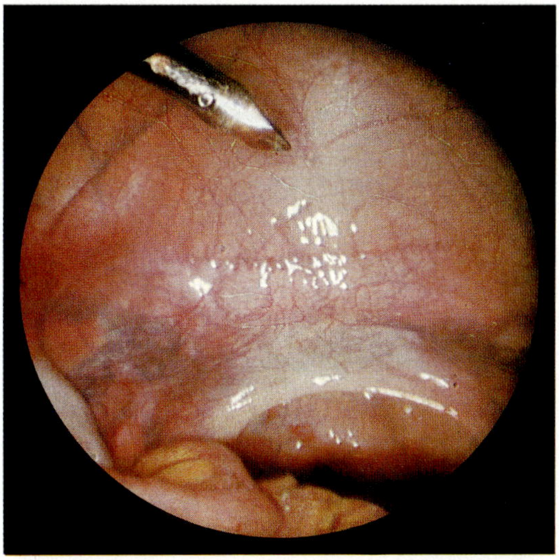

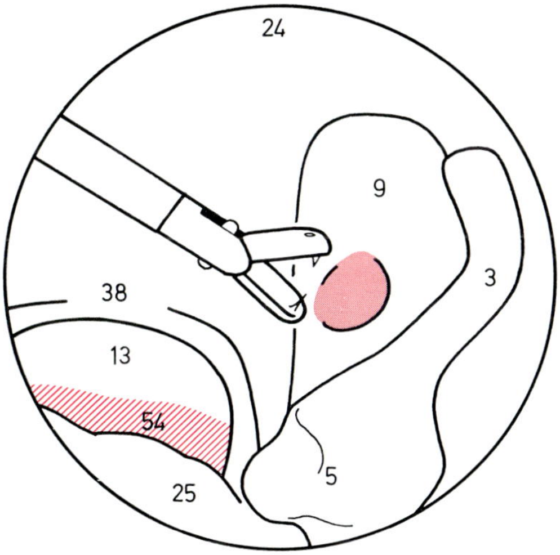
24
9
3
38
13
54
5
25

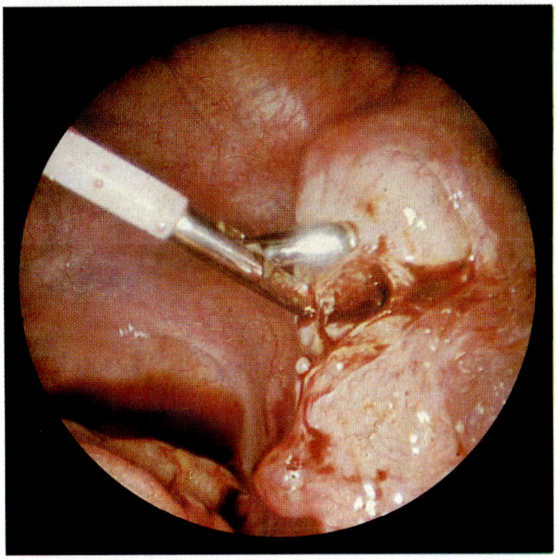

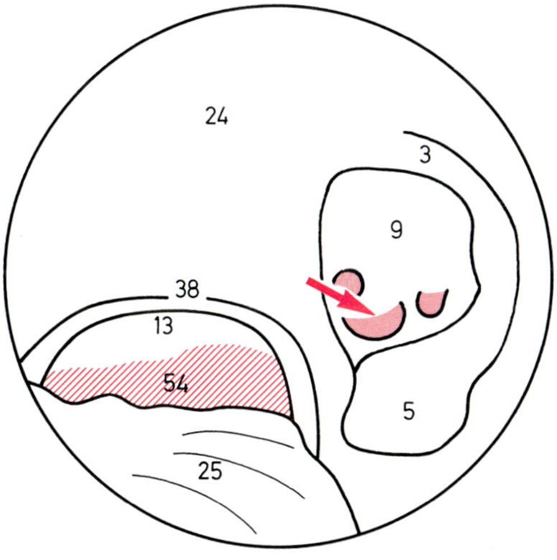
24
3
9
38
13
54
5
25

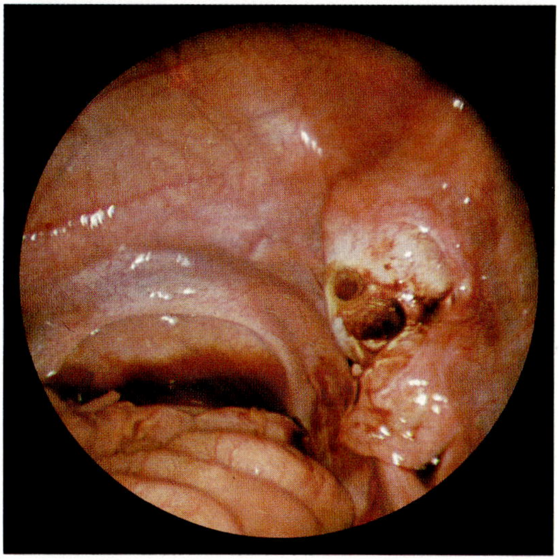

(e) Ovarian Carcinoma and Substitution of Laparoscopy for Exploratory Laparotomy

Fig. 324. When ovarian carcinoma is suspected, laparoscopy in many cases may replace exploratory laparotomy. Instead of the latter undertaking, which is very taxing to the patient and in many cases therapeutically superfluous, it is possible today to make an unequivocal diagnosis at laparoscopy and to decide whether this particular ovarian carcinoma is primarily still operable or whether chemotherapy must precede an operative approach.

Upon scanning the cul-de-sac we usually find extensive ascites, which is aspirated and subjected to cytologic study. Biopsies are possible from the metastatic peritoneal dispersion.

Fig. 325. This metastasizing ovarian carcinoma has led to extensive peritoneal seeding with broad adherence of small intestinal loops to the peritoneum.

Fig. 326. The descending colon is broadly adherent to the parietal peritoneum by metastatic proliferations. A primary operation is ruled out in such cases. Chemotherapy is instituted immediately in connection with the laparoscopy. Subject to the result of this, laparoscopy is repeated after two to six months as a "second-look" operation instead of the second laparotomy usually recommended in ovarian carcinoma. In the course of this procedure we often are surprised at the therapeutic success of the chemotherapy and it often is possible at the same time to remove the ovarian carcinoma, which has now become operable.

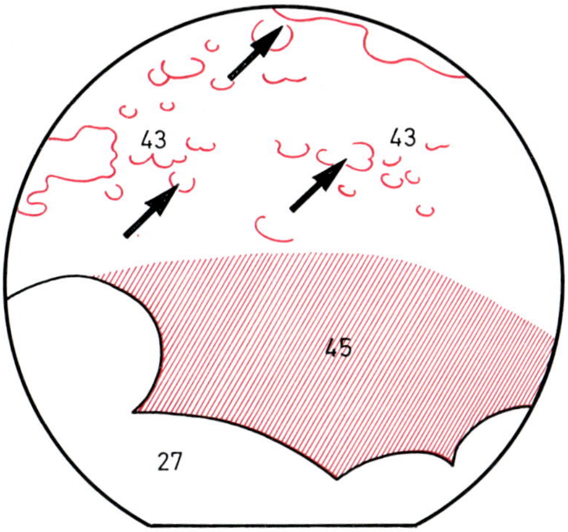
43
43
45
27

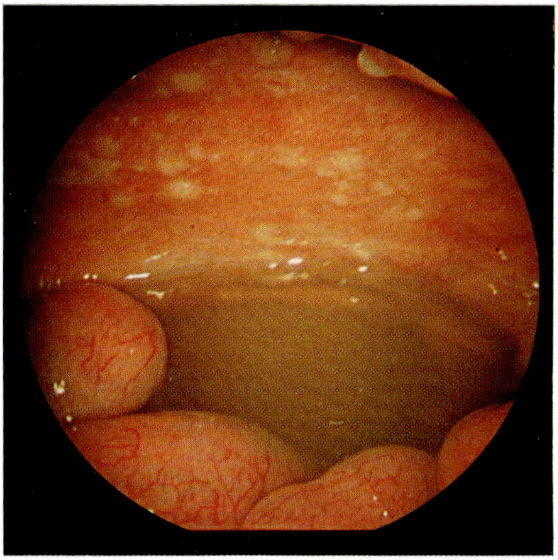

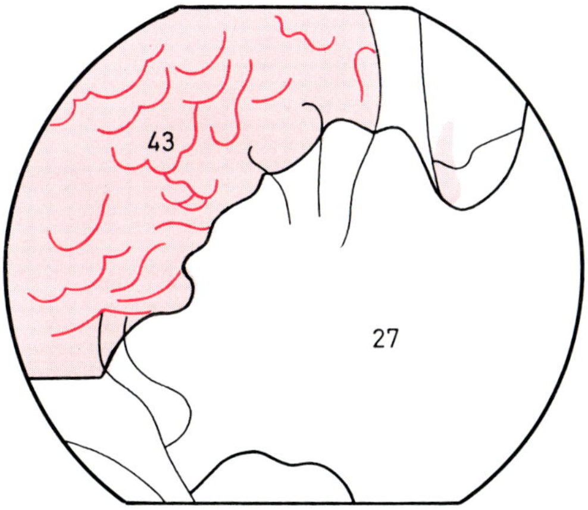
43
27

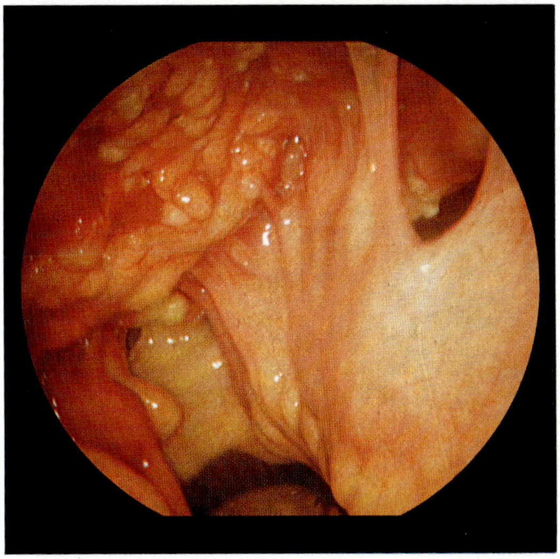

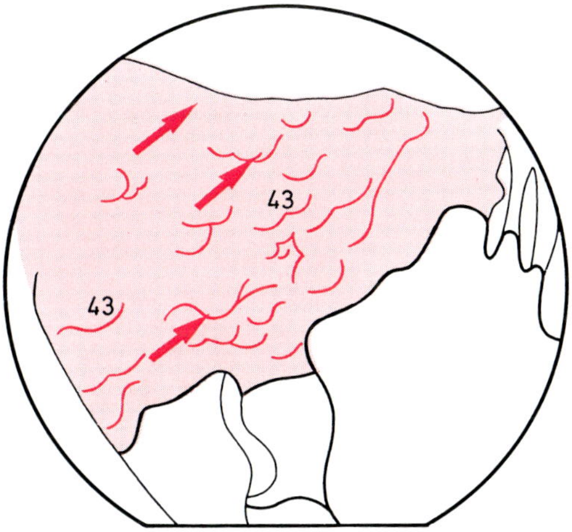
43
43

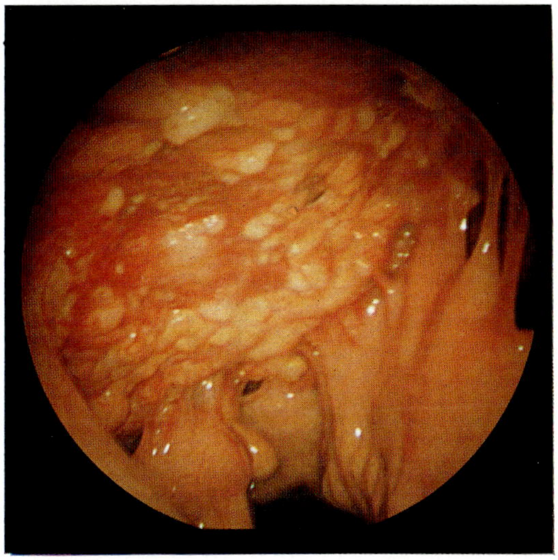

(f) Genital or Abdominal Tuberculosis

Fig. 327. Genital tuberculosis with the classic presentation of the miliary tubercle in the genital region of the peritoneum has almost disappeared today. At endoscopy we sometimes find merely a picture of rigid, immobile tubes, very firm to the touch. This macroscopic diagnosis, however, cannot be made with certainty. This illustration shows a tubercular tube. The diagnosis could be histologically confirmed only at laparotomy, however. The clear amber exudate in the cul-de-sac gave a negative reading in an animal experiment. Nevertheless, the classic tubercle was found histologically in the endosalpinx and endometrium.

Unfortunately, it is technically impossible to obtain sample excisions from the tubes at laparoscopy because of the excessive risk of hemorrhage. Thus, today, the diagnostic procedure in tuberculosis of the fallopian tubes is limited to the diagnosis of stiff, thick-walled, firm tubes. In connection with this, the classic diagnostic measures in genital tuberculosis must be taken: collection of menstrual blood; biopsy of the endometrium; etc.

Fig. 328. After elevation of the uterus, we see here the typical picture of cured genital tuberculosis with sclerotic, immobile, stiff-walled tubes showing Grade 3 patency to dye insufflation and CO_2 gas.

Fig. 329. To obtain menstrual blood, the Semm menstrual-blood adapter is recommended. Using negative pressure, a clear plastic bell (Fig. 330) is placed by suction to the cervix. The menstrual blood then runs under sterile conditions out of the cavity through a plastic hose into a rubber finger-cot dangling from the vulva (Fig. 331). As soon as sufficient blood has been collected, the finger-cot is detached and sent to the laboratory for bacteriologic examination.

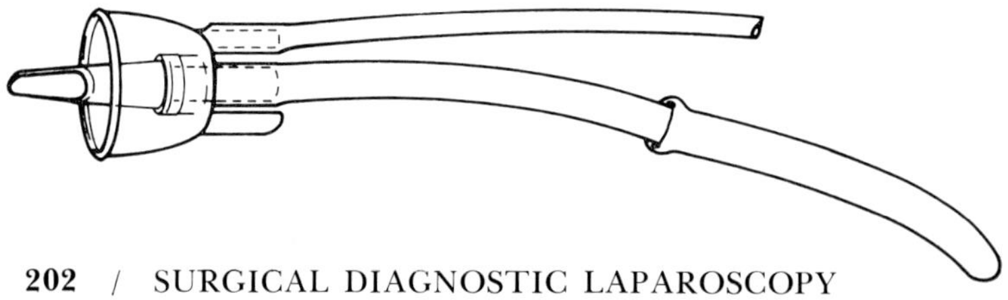

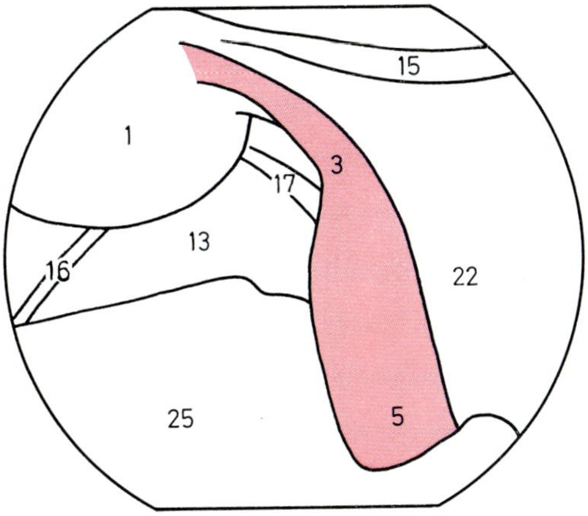

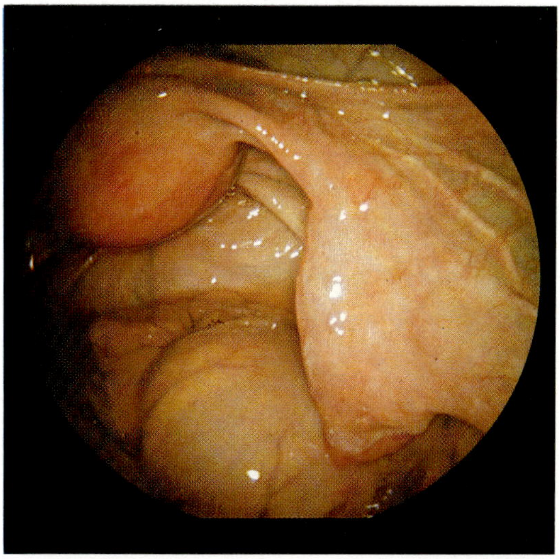

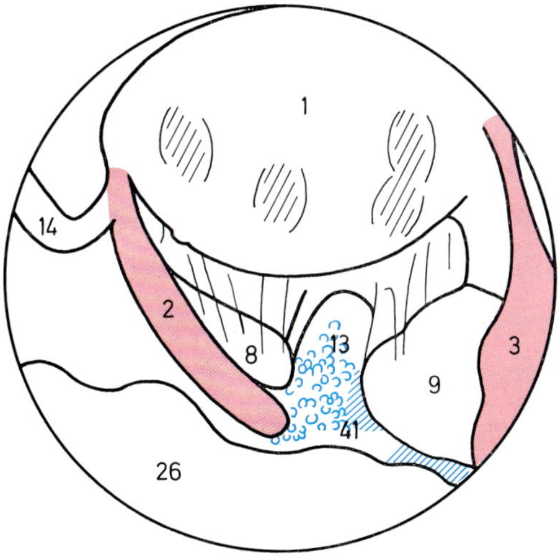

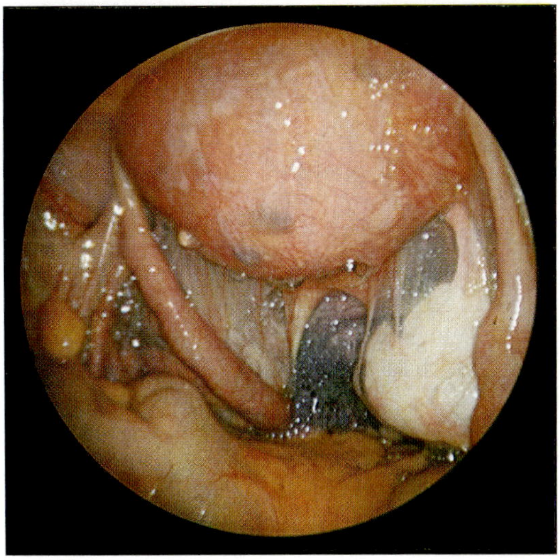

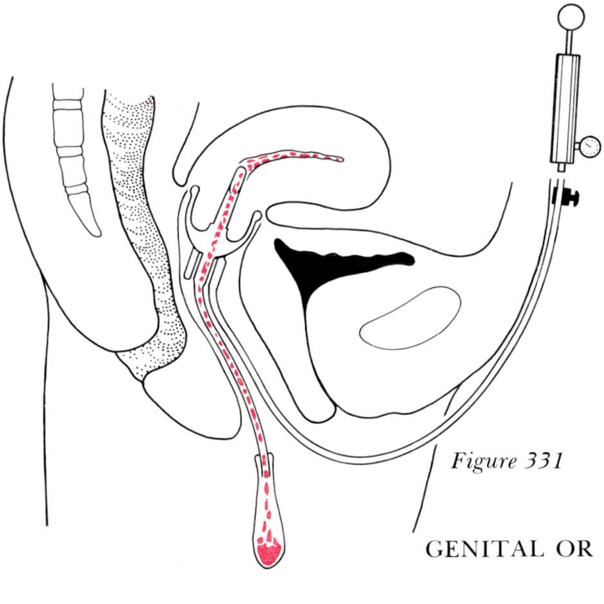

Figure 331

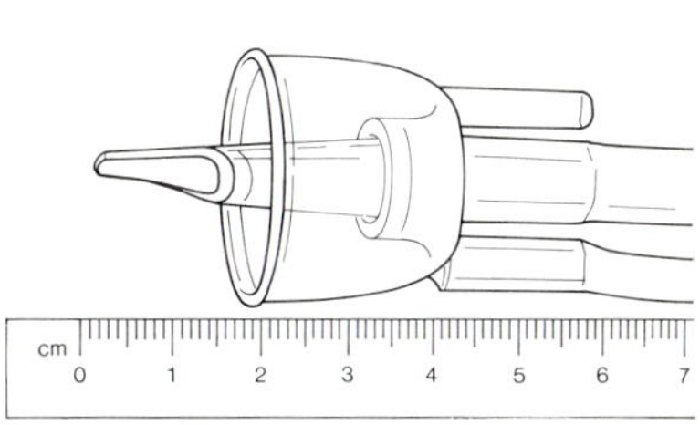

Figure 330

3

Surgical Therapeutic Laparoscopy

(a) Tubal Sterilization by Coagulation with High-Frequency and Low Voltage Current in the Nonpregnant Uterus in Puerperium and Following Abortion

Fig. 332. After grasping the tube about 3 cm distally from the uterus with atraumatic forceps, it was slowly coagulated at about 50 watts for 20 seconds. The whitish color change shows clearly how the high-frequency electricity flowed partly from the region of the corpus, but especially from the highly vascular mesosalpinx to the atraumatic forceps. The tube was coagulated at two points *(arrows a* and *b*). In the mesosalpinx of the left adnexum, finger-thick varicosities are noticeable.

Fig. 333. In consequence of the marked vascularity of the mesosalpinx, the current flowed less from the region of the fundus, as seen in Figure 332, but rather almost exclusively from the broad ligament and mesosalpinx. Worthy of note is the coagulation extending as far as the ampulla of the tube, which lies some 5 cm away from the coagulation forceps. This emphasizes how uncontrollably the high-frequency current flows to the forceps in tubal sterilization.

In the left infundibulopelvic ligament, pencil-thick varicosities predominate.

Fig. 334. Coagulation with high-frequency current is especially risky in the vicinity of the great venous complexes in the ligaments lying close to the tubes. Here there is danger of coagulation of the venous walls, which may not rupture, however, until several hours or days later. This picture demonstrates once more the variability of the course taken by the high-frequency current. Because of the good conductivity of the blood vessels, the high-frequency current flowed via the venous convolution from the mesosalpinx into the vicinity of the forceps in the tube. The two points of coagulation *(arrows a* and *b)* can be clearly identified.

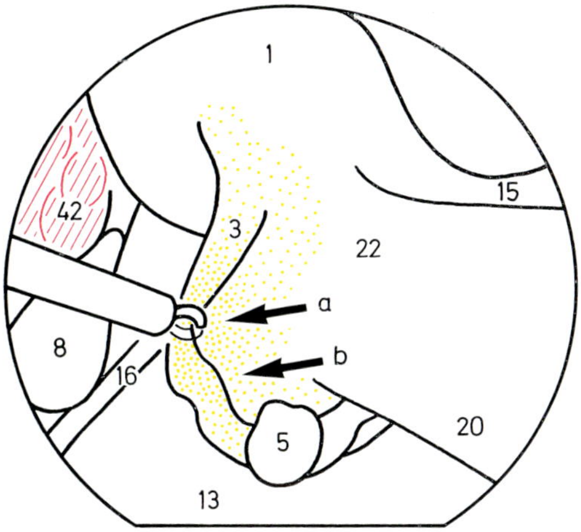
1
15
42
3
22
a
8
b
16
20
5
13

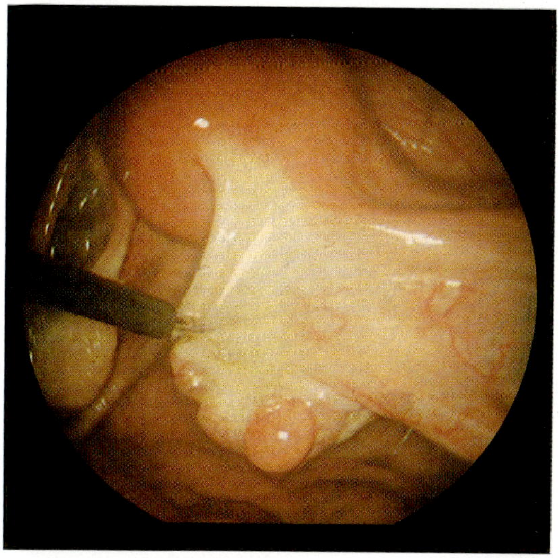

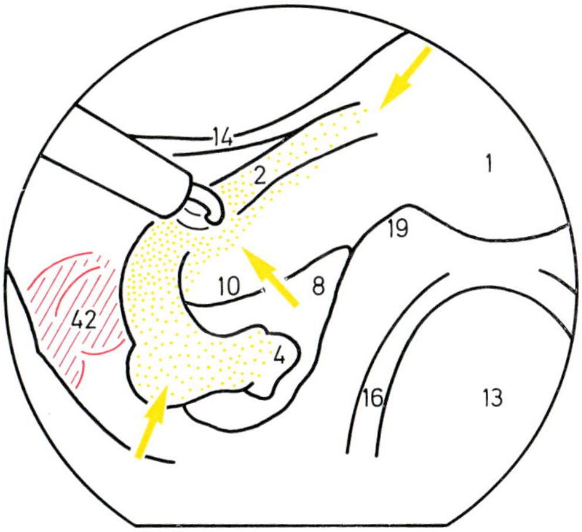
14
1
2
19
10
8
42
4
16
13

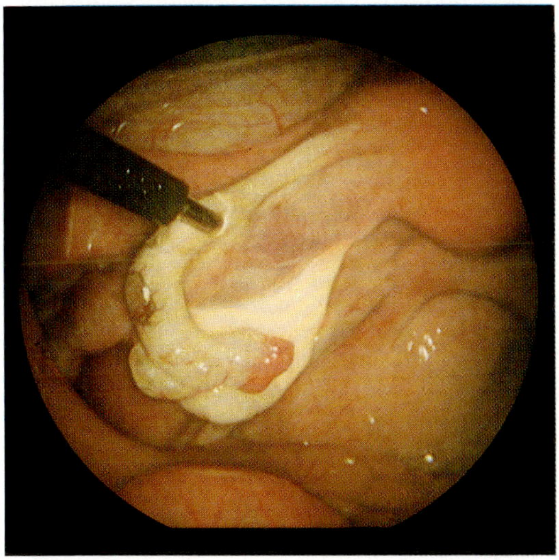

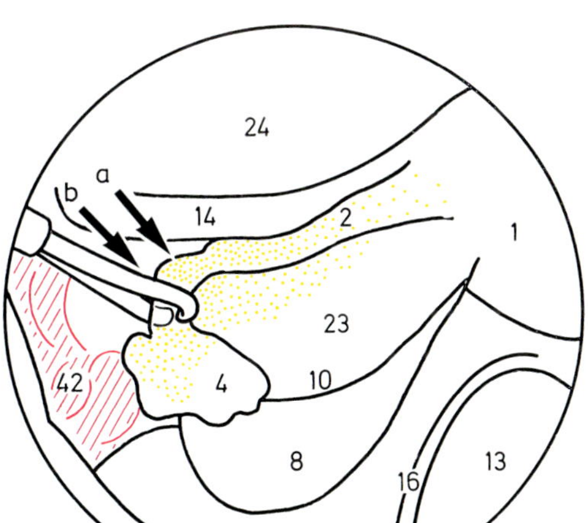
24
a
b
14
2
1
23
42
4
10
8
16
13

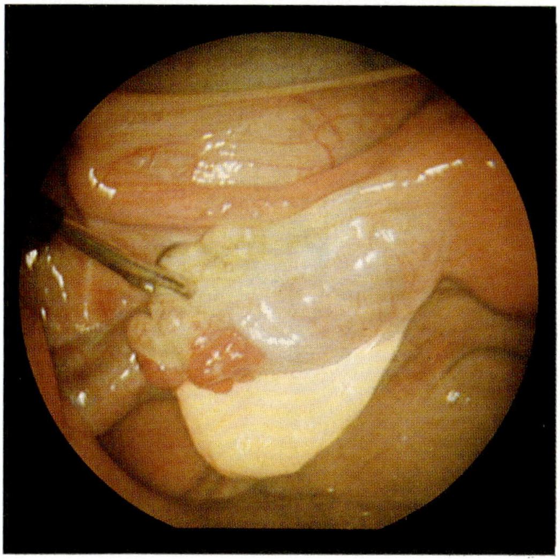

Fig. 335. The difference between the uncontrollable high-frequency coagulation and that achieved at low voltage by the Tubal or Endo-Coagulator is documented by this picture. While the mesosalpinx is burned along with the tube as far as a point deep in the infundibulopelvic ligament when high-frequency current is used, the point of coagulation with low voltage is sharply defined and limited to the tube itself.

Fig. 336. The tube has been grasped about 3 cm away from the cornu with the low-voltage Endotherm coagulation forceps and coagulated for 30 seconds at 120° C. The whitened area indicates that portion of tissue in which biologic death has occurred. In the broad ligament, almost finger-thick varicose complexes predominate.

Fig. 337. Four months after sterilization this patient had to undergo an abdominal hysterectomy because of Stage 0 carcinoma of the cervix, diagnosed in the course of a conization. This picture taken during the operation shows the point of coagulation free of any adhesions after low voltage coagulation. The tube has been converted into a whitish strand of connective tissue 2 cm from the cornu. Only connective tissue was histologically present at this time. (In this instance the tube had not been severed.)

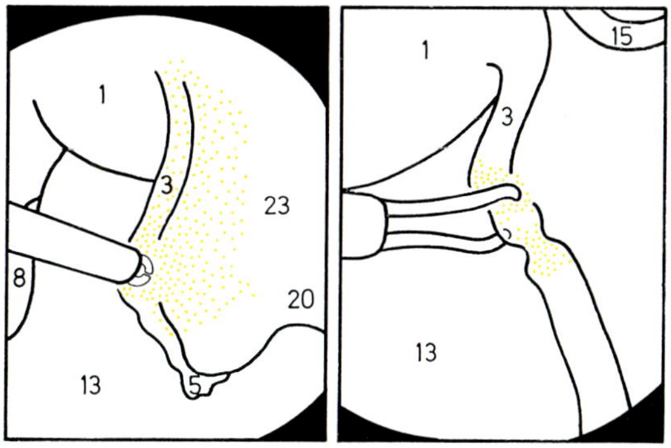
1
3
23
8
20
13
5
1
15
3
13

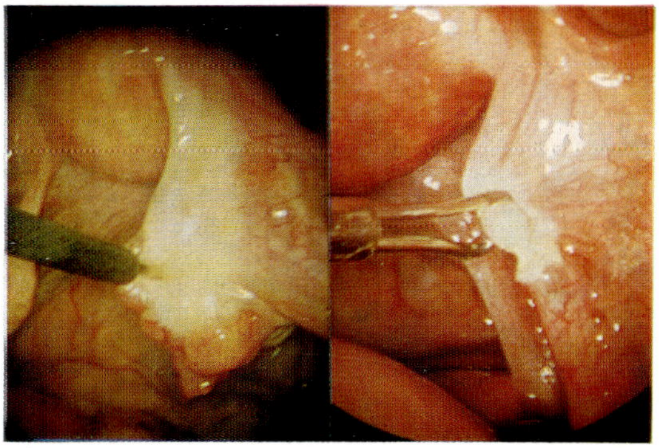

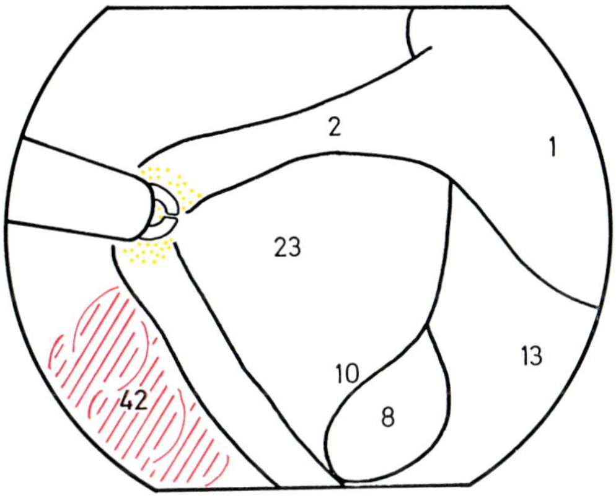
2
1
23
13
10
8
42

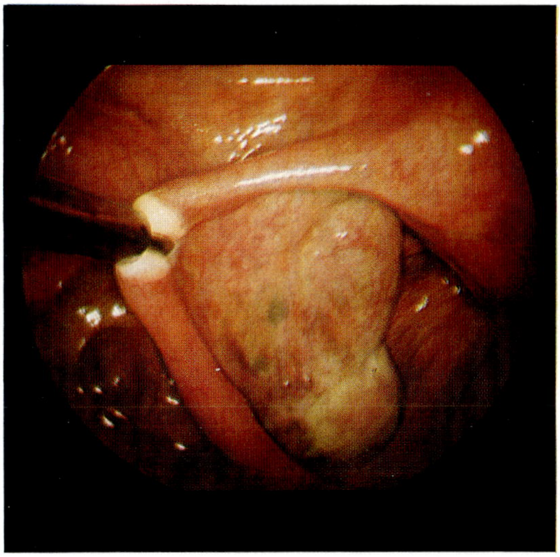

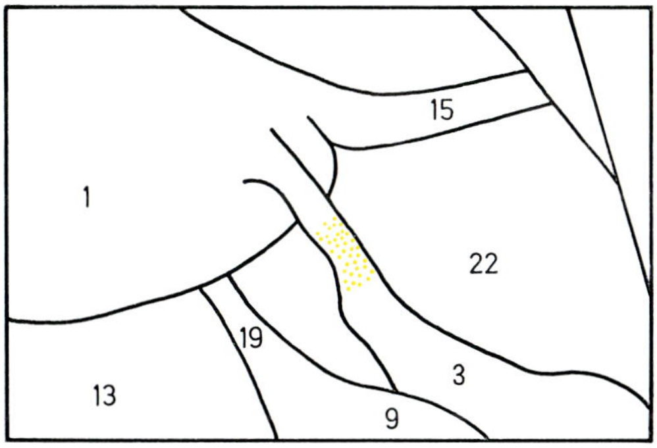
15
1
22
19
13
3
9

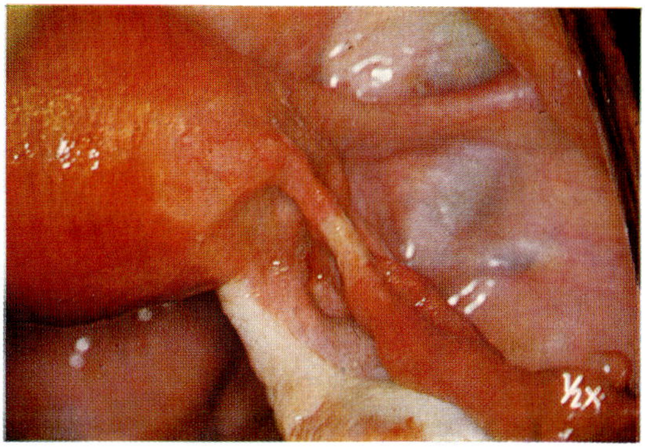
½x

Figures 338–340 show the technique of low voltage coagulation with atraumatic forceps in conjunction with the Tubal or Endo-Coagulator.

Fig. 338. Grasping the tube. Note that the atraumatic forceps is correctly placed and completely encircles the tube with its heated jaws. There is a possibility of error if the tube is not completely grasped when the jaws are closed. The operator, therefore, should always make certain laparoscopically when elevating the forceps that the jaws lie well within the mesosalpinx.

Fig. 339. After 20 seconds of burn at 120° C the coagulation of the first portion of the tube is complete. The biologic killing of tubal tissue is limited to the tube and does not, as is usual with high-frequency current, extend to the mesosalpinx.

Fig. 340. Completion of sterilization of the right oviduct at low voltage: the two points of contact for the coagulation *(arrows a* and *b)* can be clearly seen. The points of coagulation should lie so close to one another that the zones of coagulation overlap, so that subsequent severance of the tube with scissors involves absolutely no bleeding (Fig. 341).

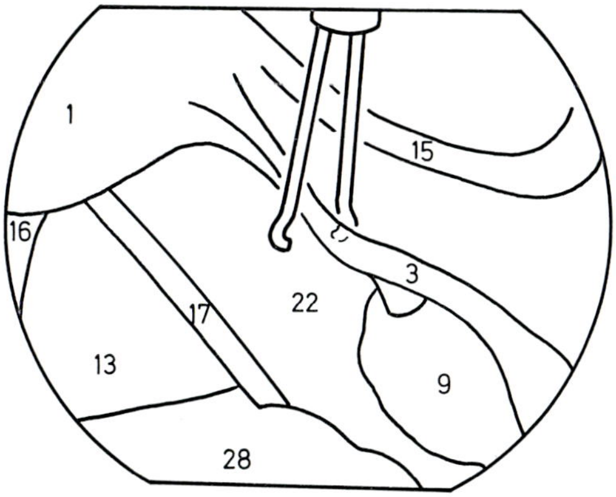
1
15
16
3
22
17
13
9
28

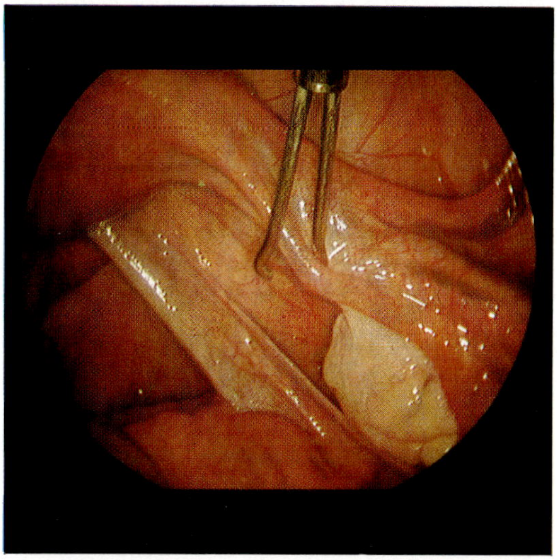

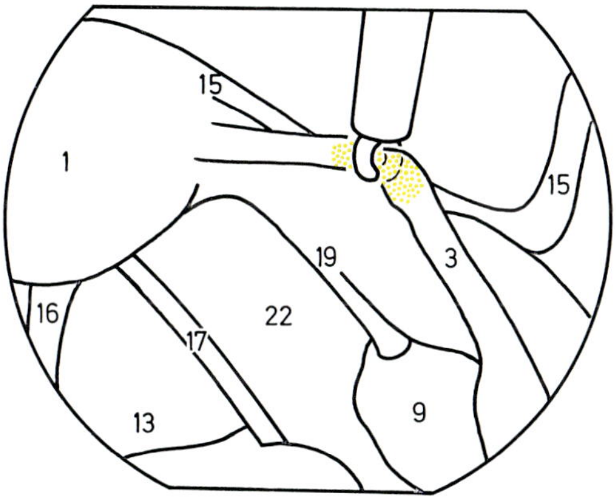
15
1
15
19
3
16
22
17
13
9

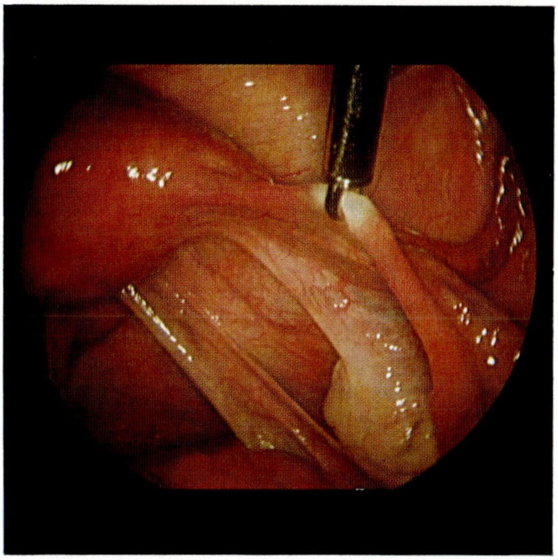

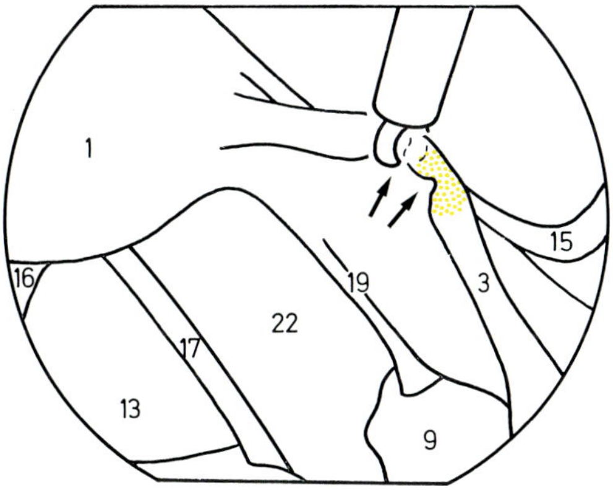
1
15
16
19
3
22
17
13
9

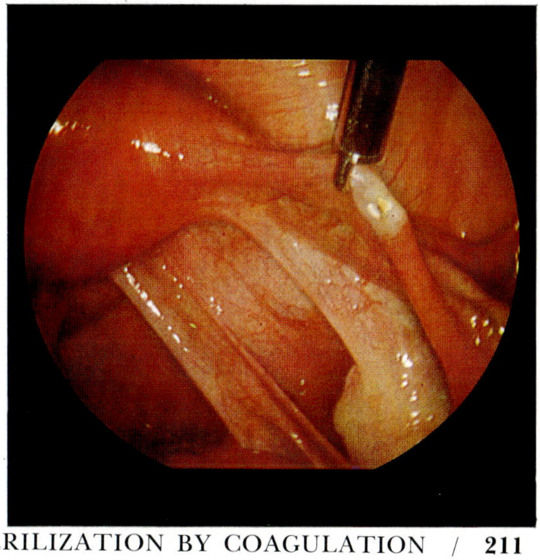

Fig. 341. After coagulation of the right tube in two places at low voltage (Figs. 338–340), the hooked Frangenheim scissors are inserted and the tube severed under direct vision in the middle of the coagulated area.

Fig. 342. The right oviduct is coagulated twice about 3 cm away from the uterus, and severed bloodlessly.

Fig. 343. Coagulation and cutting have to be done in two steps when low voltage current is used for coagulation. Whereas with the high-frequency technique one always coagulates the tissue area down to the mesosalpinx (see Figs. 332–335), the low voltage current coagulates only the tube. Even under optical endoscopic control, one can easily grasp not only the tube but its underlying parallel vascular bundle. If the coagulation forceps is combined with a cutting device, transection follows coagulation without control, and this may lead to undesirable bleeding. Therefore, one should always carefully inspect the coagulated site prior to cutting. If it is desired actually to transect the coagulated site, the hook scissors are especially suited for this since they divide only the muscular layer of the tube.

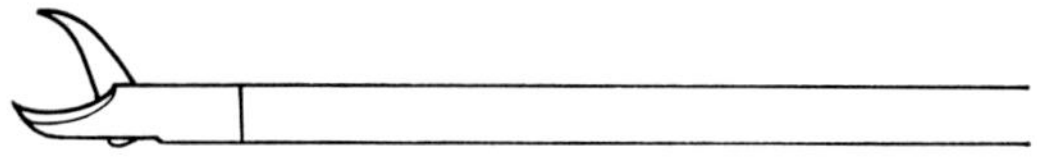

Fig. 344. Three months after the coagulation of the tube only a thin strand about 2 cm long can be seen in place of the original tubal musculature, showing no adhesions whatsoever with the surroundings *(arrow).* To date, adhesions have never been observed after low voltage coagulation.

Sterilization on the puerperal uterus is sometimes more difficult: the uterus cannot be elevated and the tubes are directed posteriorly. Elevation of a puerperal uterus is not advisable because of the danger of infection via the vagina, but it is a simple matter to mobilize the tubes ventrally with atraumatic forceps. Here again the guide-line is:

The tubes can be identified by the ampullae at their ends.

Performing coagulation without identifying the ampulla may result in a peritoneal fold being coagulated instead of the tube.

This picture shows the end of the first coagulation point about 3 cm away from the point of attachment of the left tube to the cornu.

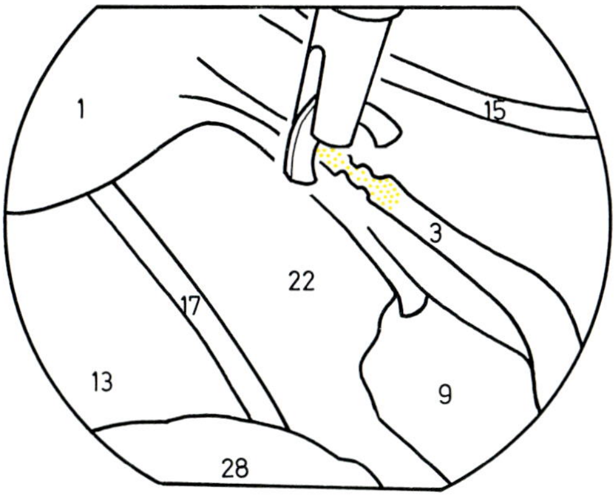
1
15
3
22
17
13
9
28

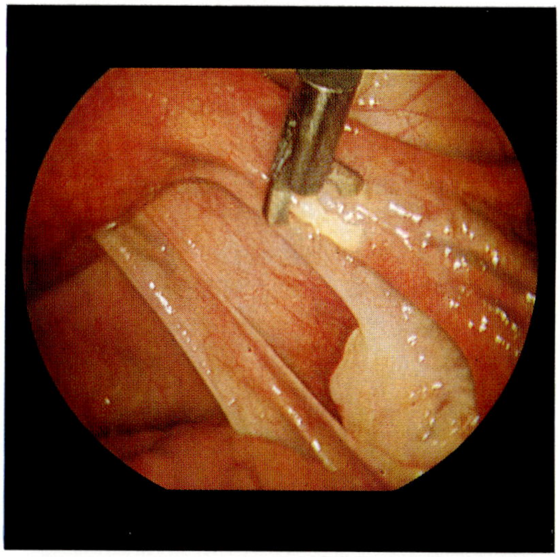

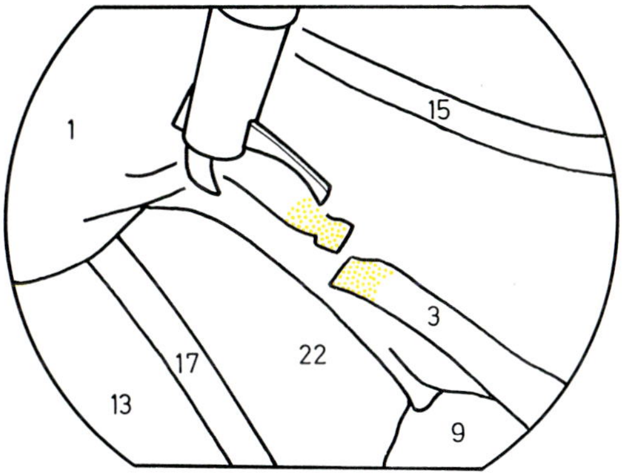
1
15
3
22
17
13
9

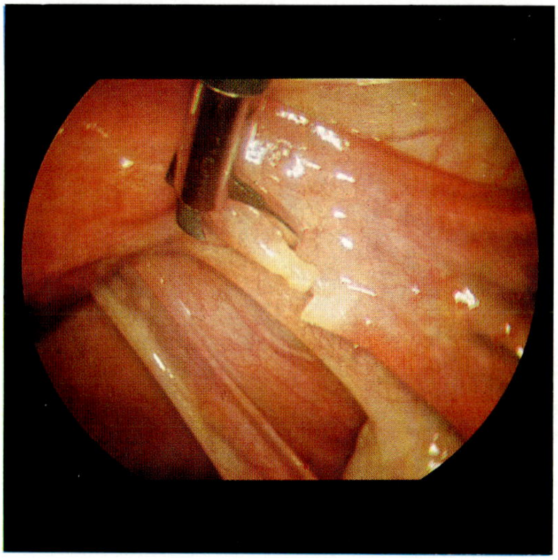

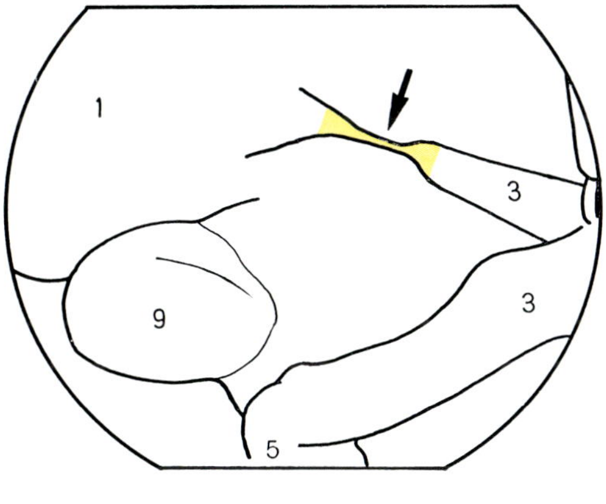
1
3
9
3
5

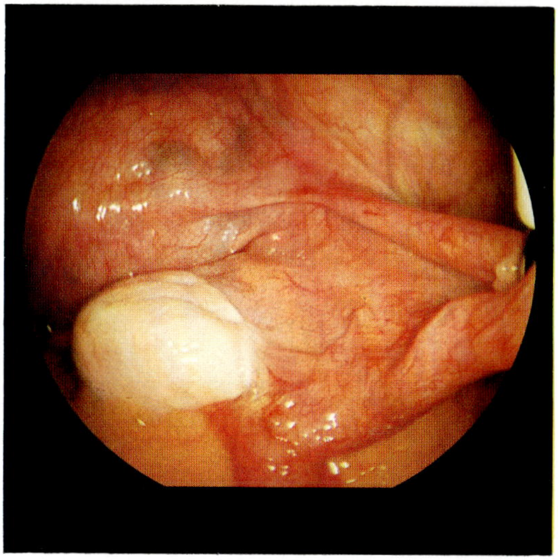

Figures 345–347 demonstrate tubal sterilization with the Semm low voltage technique. The tubal tissue is heated with an electric device such as the crocodile forceps (Fig. 348) to its boiling point, and coagulated for a few seconds. The Tubal or Endo-Coagulator monitors the heating acoustically and shows the coagulation temperature on a large dial in both Celsius and Fahrenheit.

Fig. 345. After 20 seconds' coagulation at about 120° C using the Endo-Coagulator (Fig. 105), one opens the jaws of the forceps. The yellow coagulation point can be recognized readily. Since the heating of the tubal tissue proceeds from below, the whitish discoloration on the visible surface confirms complete coagulation.

Fig. 346. About 1 cm beyond the area coagulated in Figure 345, the crocodile forceps is once more applied and coagulation is repeated for 20 seconds. This picture clearly shows that the area of coagulation is exclusively limited to the tissue within the grasp of the instrument. With this low voltage technique, coagulation of the tissue beyond the tip of the forceps does not occur as it does with high-frequency current (Fig. 333).

Fig. 347. After double coagulation of the right tube, 1 cm apart, the coagulated ischemic end of the tubal muscle is being separated by the hooked scissors. One sees the gaping lumen of the tube and notes that the underlying vascular bundle has not been grasped.

The question whether one definitely should transect the tube after coagulation has not yet been answered. We do either three coagulations side-by-side without transection, or transect with the hooked scissors between two coagulated areas produced by the crocodile forceps.

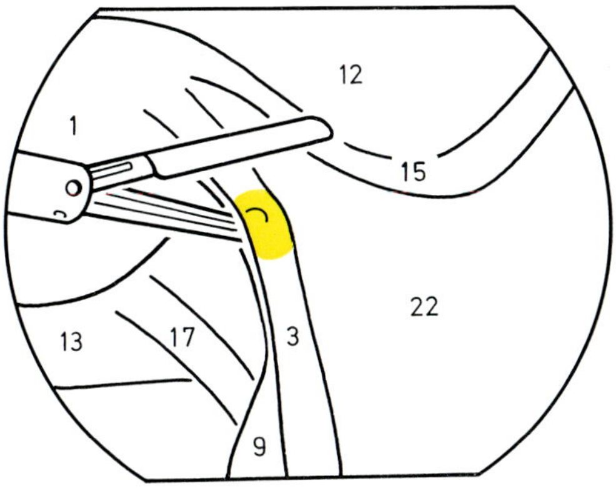
12
1
15
22
13
17
3
9

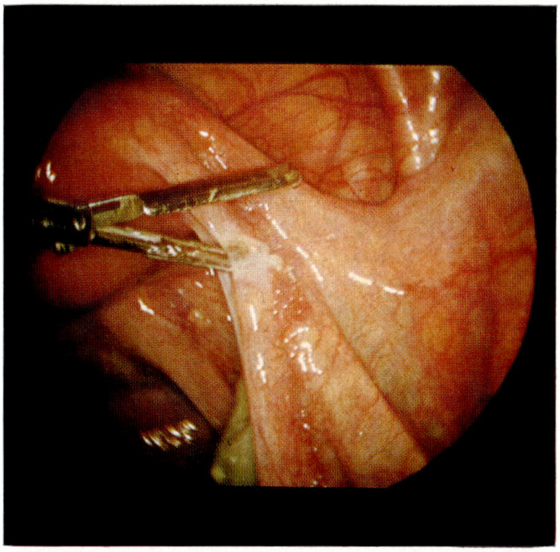

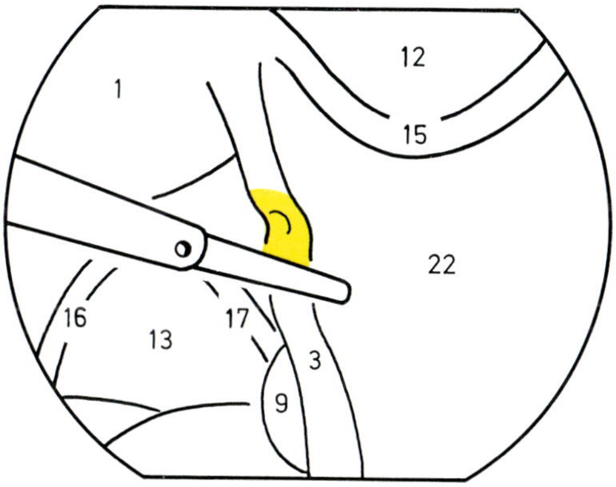
12
1
15
22
16
13
17
3
9

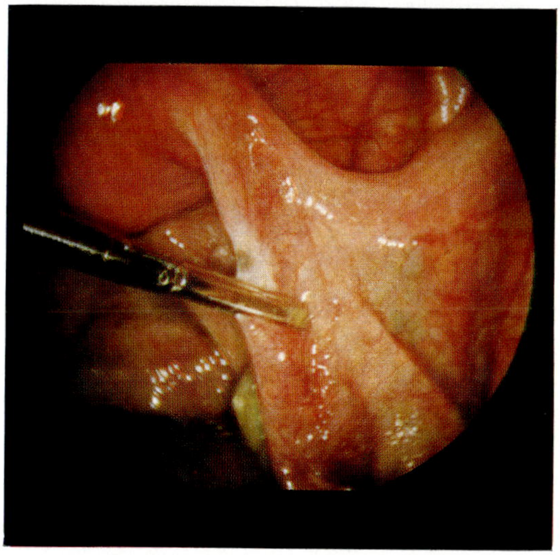

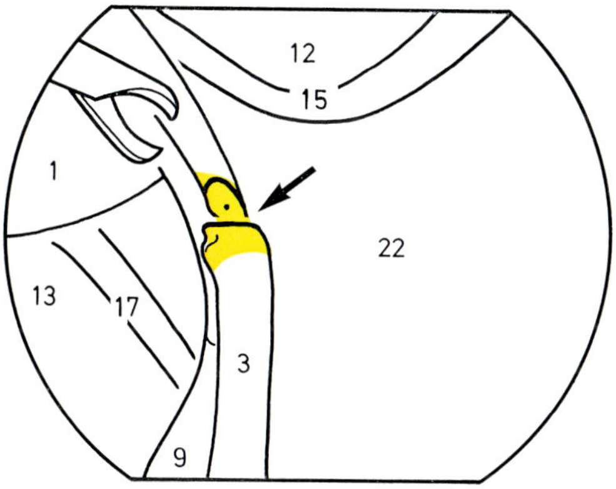
12
15
1
22
13
17
3
9

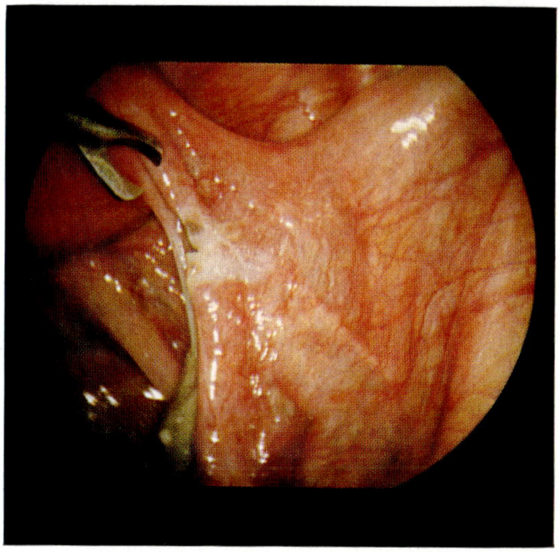

Fig. 348. This figure gives an overview of the possible uses of the crocodile forceps. The Tubal or Endo-Coagulator provides the low voltage electric current. The jaws of the forceps perform two movements: (1) as the forceps is opened, the upper jaw moves forward 5 mm, opening to an angle of 70°. This large opening facilitates grasping and coagulation of tissues, especially adhesions. Complete visualization (2) of the abdomen must always precede any laparoscopic operative procedure.

In cases of tubal sterilization (3), the tubal tissue is firmly grasped while the jaws close and the upper jaw recedes into the coagulation position. After the coagulation process is finished, the trocar sleeve is pushed forward a short distance over the closed jaws. Multiple back-and-forth motions (4) of the unopened forceps additionally crush the coagulated tissue. The trocar sleeve then is withdrawn a short way, the jaws are opened, and the tube is grasped again immediately next to the coagulated site (5). After the coagulation process is completed, the instrument is withdrawn and the tube is severed with the hooked scissors if desired (6). One should ensure: (1) that the tube has actually been coagulated; and (2) that the vascular bundle has not been severed.

The Wisap crocodile forceps is heated by the Tubal or Endo-Coagulator to any temperature between 50° and 200° C. Independent of the quantity of tissue grasped or its thermal conduction, the jaws reach the boiling point (100° C) in about five seconds. As soon as the tissue water evaporates, the forceps temperature rises to that preselected on the dial. Simultaneously, the audio signal indicates by tone that this temperature has been reached. The surgeon thereby knows the temperature of the forceps without having to look away from the operative field.

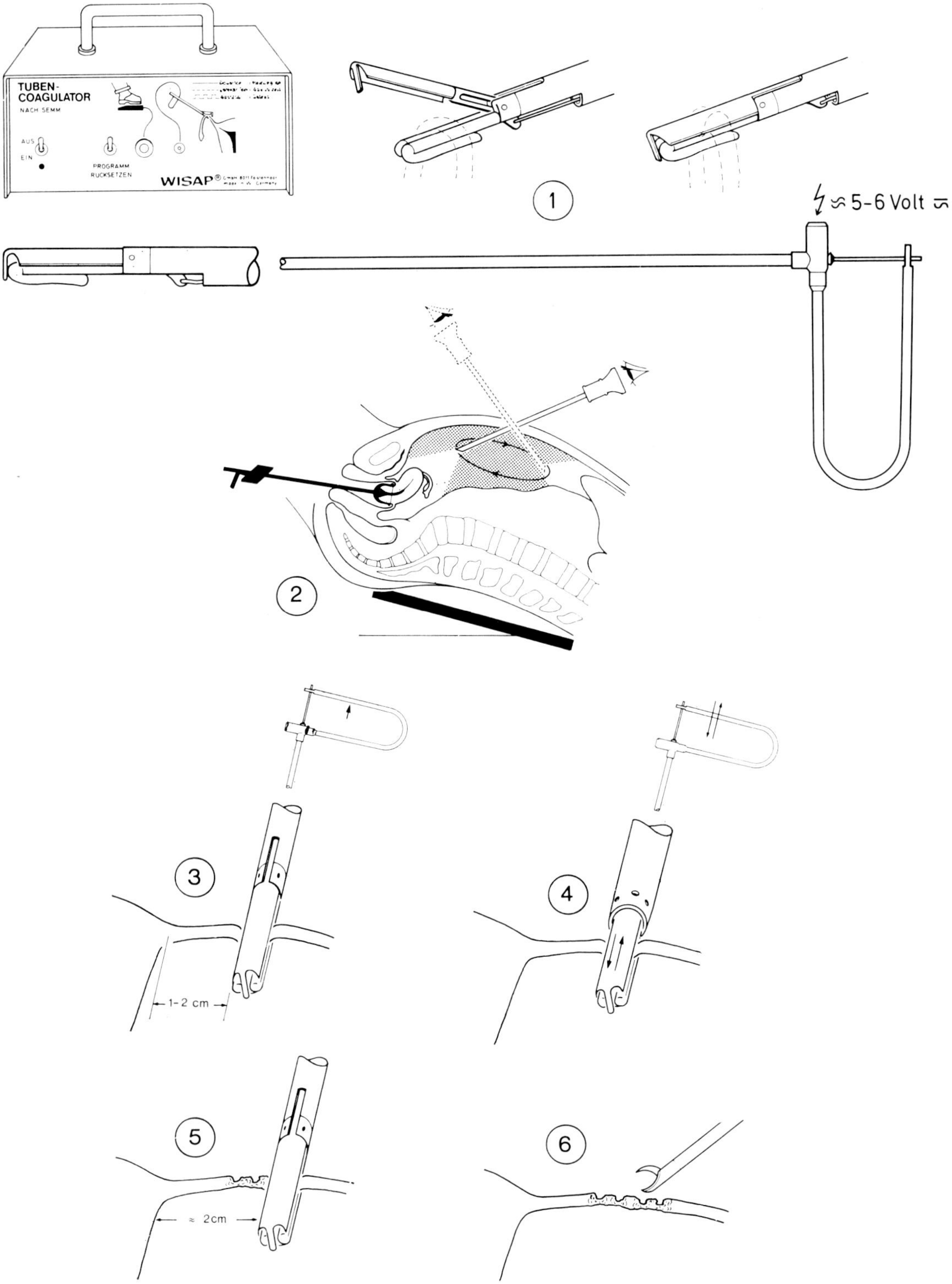
TUBEN-
COAGULATOR
NACH SEMM
AUS
EIN
PROGRAMM
RUCKSETZEN
WISAP®
1
5-6 Volt
2
3
1-2 cm
4
5
≈ 2cm
6

Figure 348

(b) Tubal Sterilization with Tantalum Clips

Figures 349–351 clearly demonstrate the problems involved in interrupting tubal patency with a metal clip. Despite a suitable location as determined by both endoscopy and x-ray, intrauterine pregnancy ensued in this case five months later.

Fig. 349. Sterilization by use of tantalum clips has been tried experimentally for several years. Here we see two tantulum clips that have been in place on the right tube for eight months, partially obscured by puffiness of the peritoneum. The uterus also is visible—12 weeks pregnant.

Fig. 350. After moving the pregnant uterus aside with the aid of atraumatic forceps, the proper positioning of the two tantalum clips on the right oviduct is visible. Despite the correct position and full closure of the clips, pregnancy occurred five months after they had been placed. The correct placement of the clips and closure of the tubal lumen were even monitored by x-ray.

Fig. 351. On the left side also the tantalum clips were properly in place near the point of attachment of the tubes and totally embracing the oviduct. The pregnant uterus here is crowding the adnexum beyond the terminal line of the pelvis. Pregnancies have been observed in a number of cases after placement of tantalum clips.

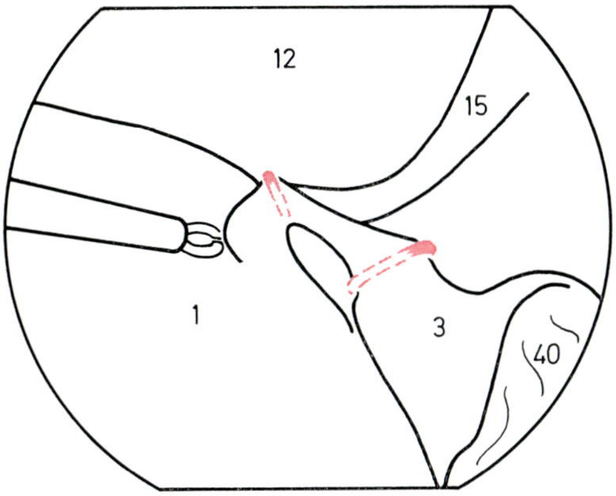
12
15
1
3
40

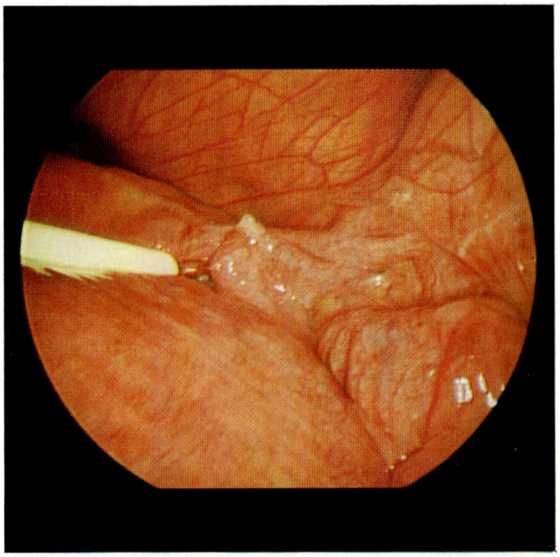

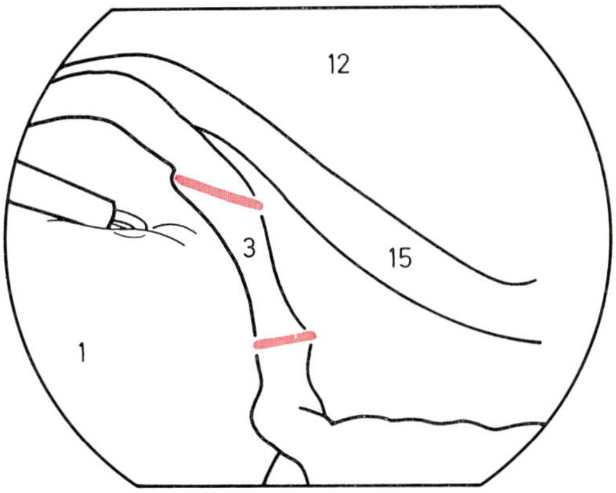
12
3
15
1

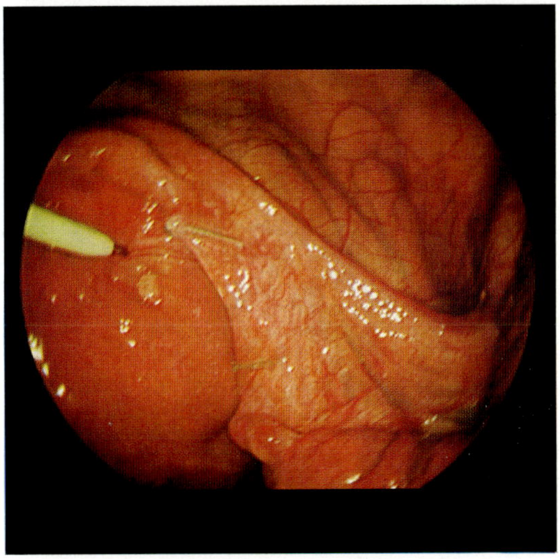

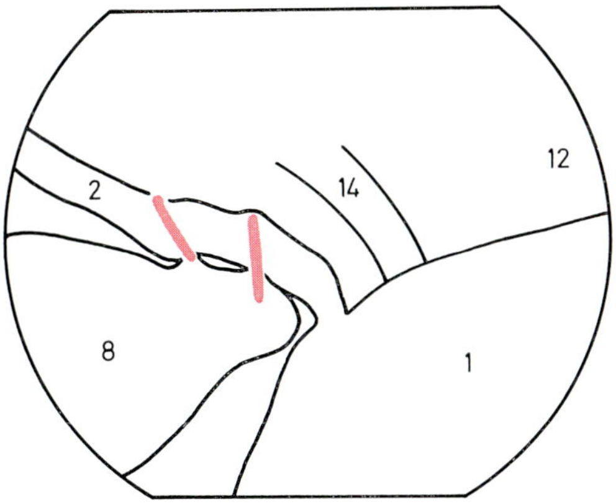
2
14
12
8
1

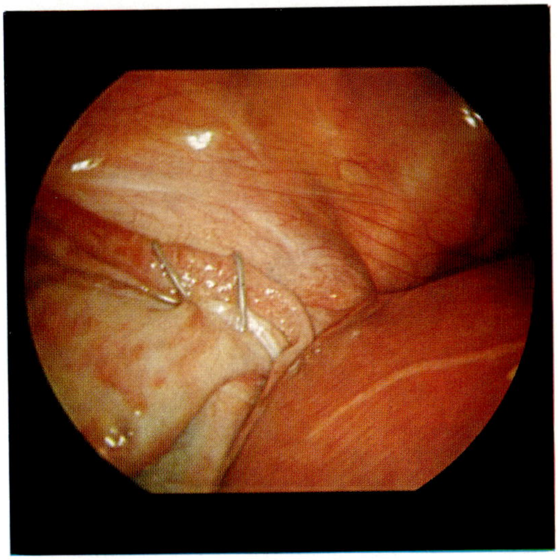

Fig. 352. A specially designed 11-mm diameter applicator is used to apply tantalum clips. The difficulty lies in grasping the entire tube when it is not completely stabilized with another instrument. This problem is readily seen in the figure demonstrating the Weck hemoclip. The diagram shows clearly how pregnancy still may result despite good compression of the tube.

Fig. 353. Because of the disappointing results with the tantalum clips, plastic clips have been developed to improve the occlusion of the lumen. The closing mechanism is shown in diagrams *a* through *d.* This clip presents the same problems as the tantalum clip because of the narrow opening angle. Instruments are currently being developed for laparoscopic application of this and other types of mechanical devices, and will be available for either single or double puncture procedures.

Fig. 354. This endoscopic photograph shows plastic clips in place three weeks after application through a posterior colpotomy incision.

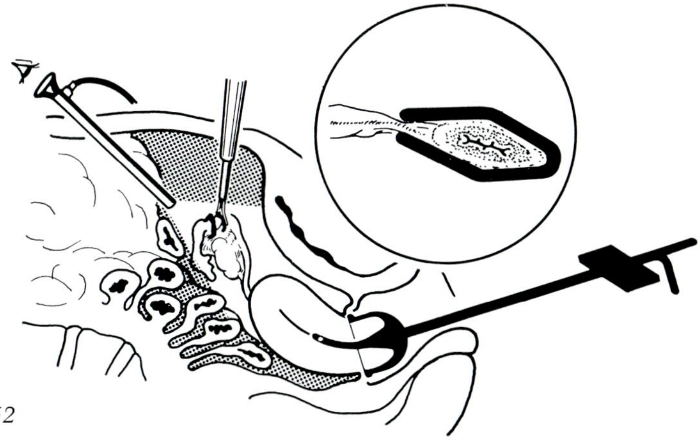

Figure 352

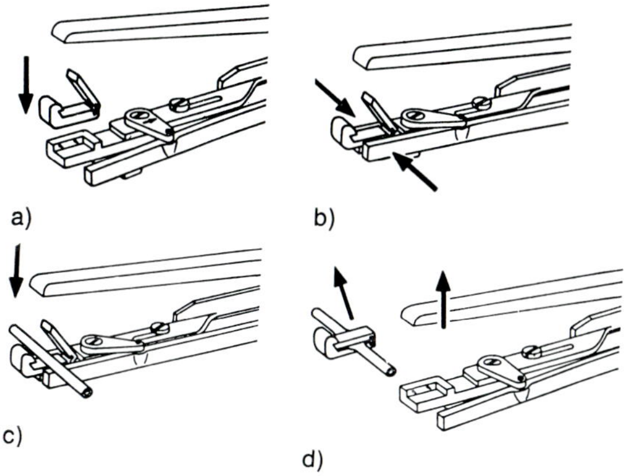

Figure 353

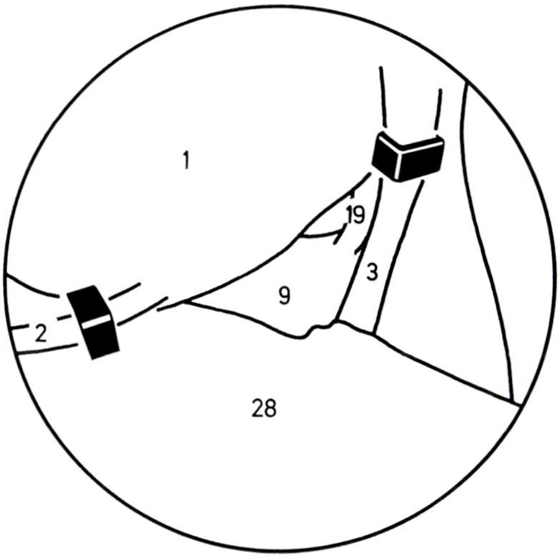

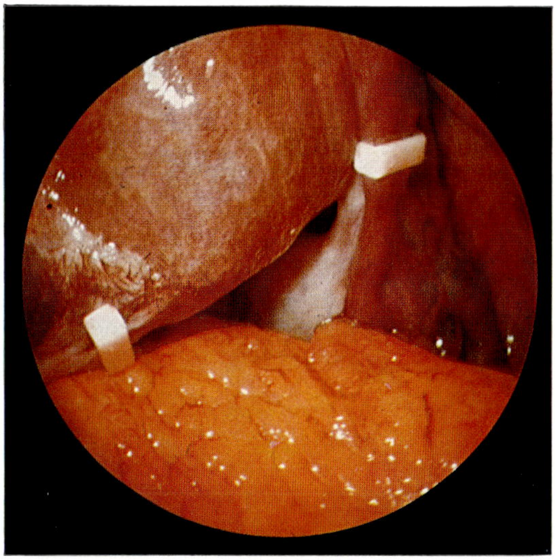

(c) Findings Following Pomeroy and Madlener Sterilization Procedures

Figures 355–357 show the situation following Pomeroy abdominal sterilization.

Fig. 355. With the uterus elevated, the resection site in the right tube is clearly visible. Either before or after sterilization, ampullar tubal occlusion occurred, so that a hydrosalpinx is now hanging from the mesosalpinx. In the left uterosacral ligament an endometrial implant is visible *(arrow),* which apparently is responsible for the ampullar tubal occlusion on both sides.

Fig. 356. Grasping the hydrosalpinx and medially displacing it demonstrates the sterilizing effect of Pomeroy's method.

Fig. 357. On the left side, the tube is almost invisible. A tongue of omentum has become adherent at the site of the operation and blocks the view of the tube.

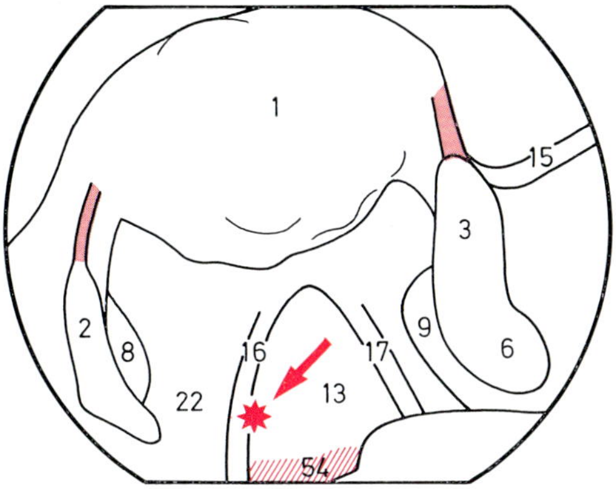
1
15
3
2
8
16
17
9
6
22
13
54

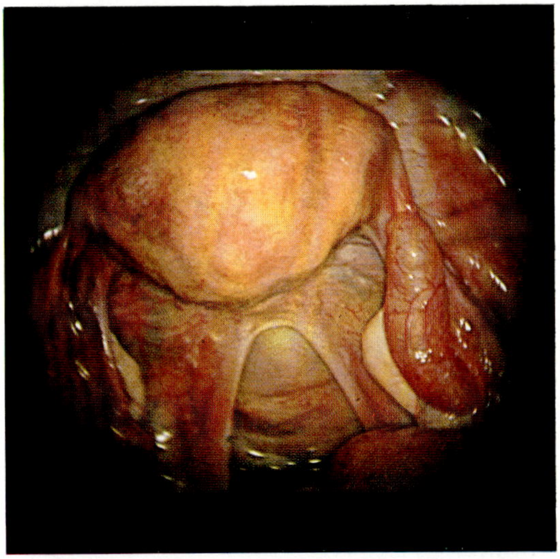

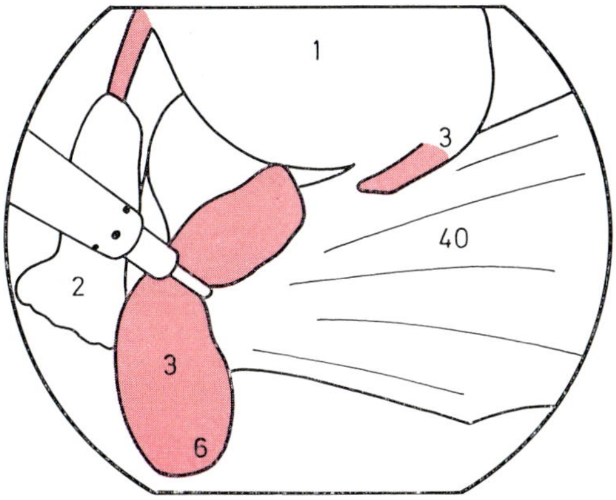
1
3
40
2
3
6

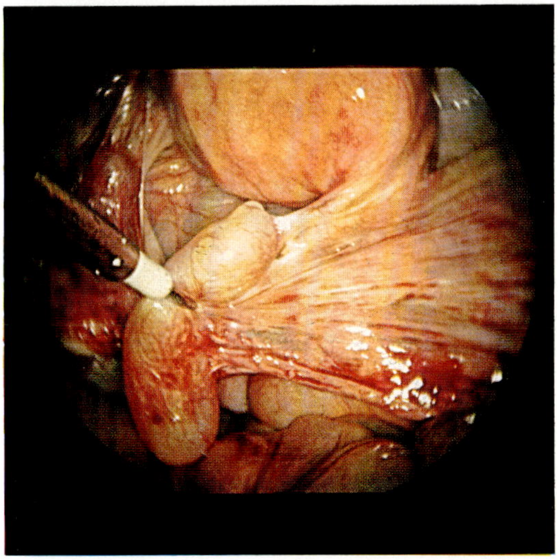

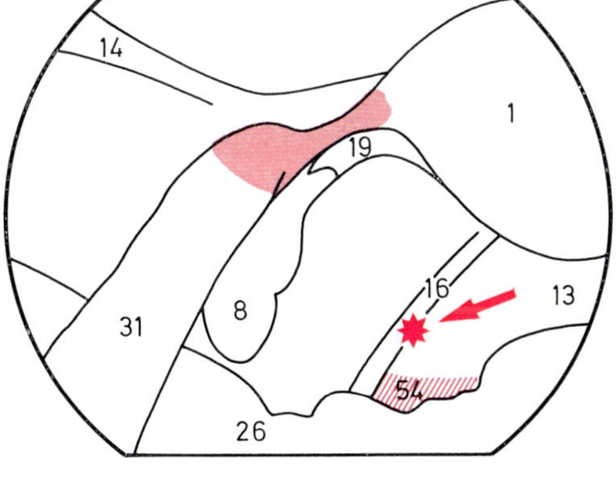
14
1
19
16
13
8
31
54
26

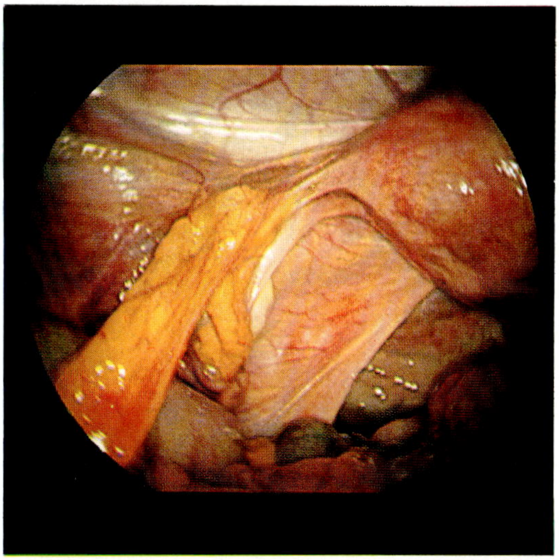

Fig. 358. Only after dislodging the adherent omental tongue at the operation site can the situation produced by the Pomeroy operation for sterilization on the left tube be demonstrated.

Fig. 359. This is a case of a sterilization performed nine years previously by the Madlener procedure. On both sides an atrophic tubal stump about 2 to 3 cm long can be seen. Pelvic congestion dominates the scene in the right broad ligament.

Fig. 360. Two months after sterilization with atraumatic forceps in conjunction with the Endotherm, the left tube shows a ribbon-like band about 1 cm long. Beside it lies the fundus of a three- to four-month pregnant uterus grown above the terminal line of the pelvis. The patient had been sterilized during the first or second month of pregnancy.

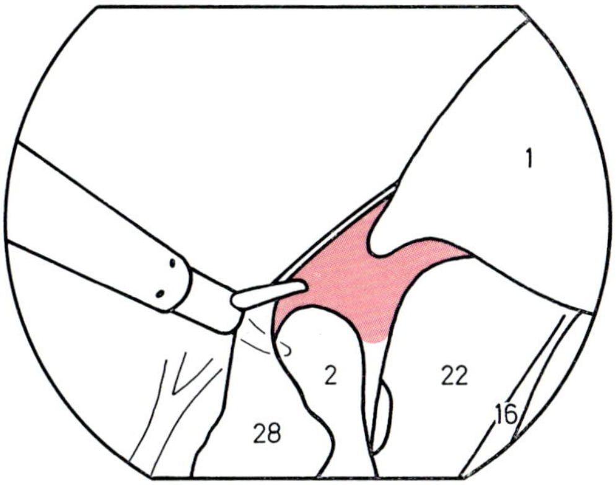
1
2
22
16
28

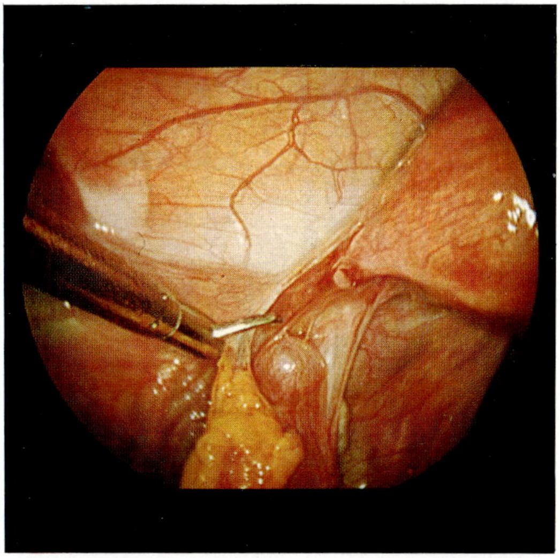

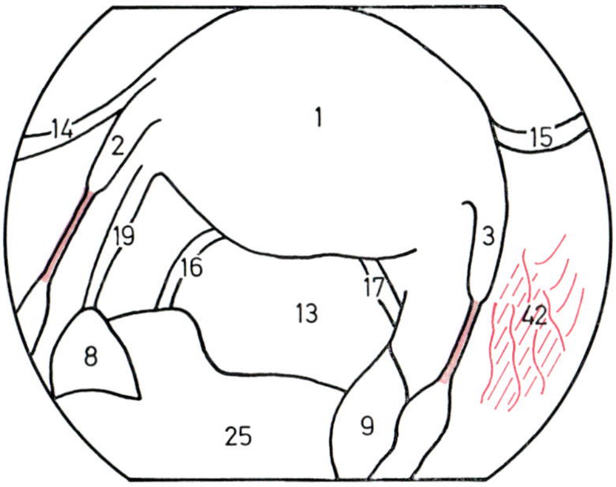
14
2
1
15
19
16
13
17
3
42
8
25
9

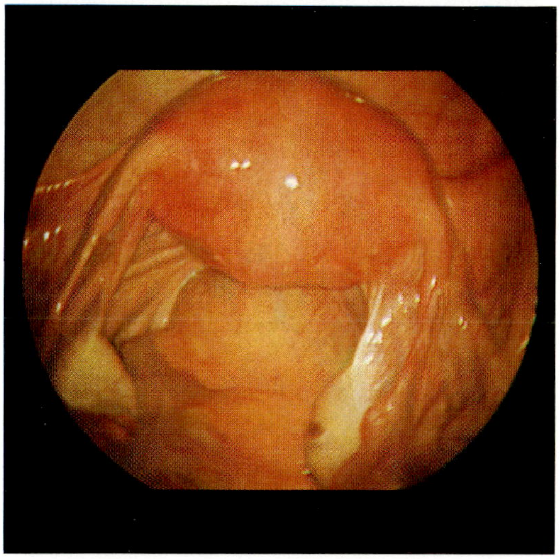

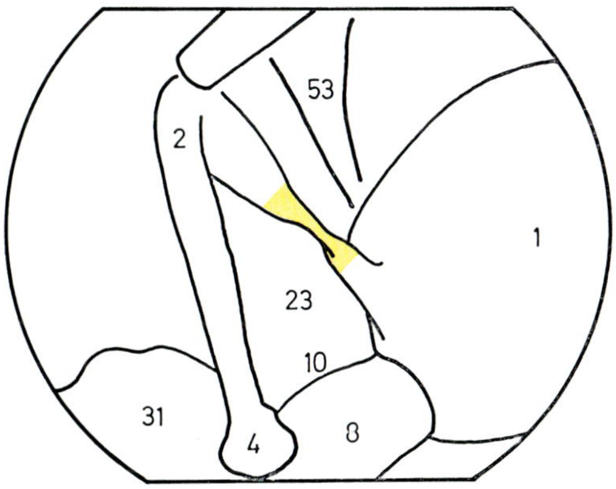
53
2
1
23
10
31
4
8

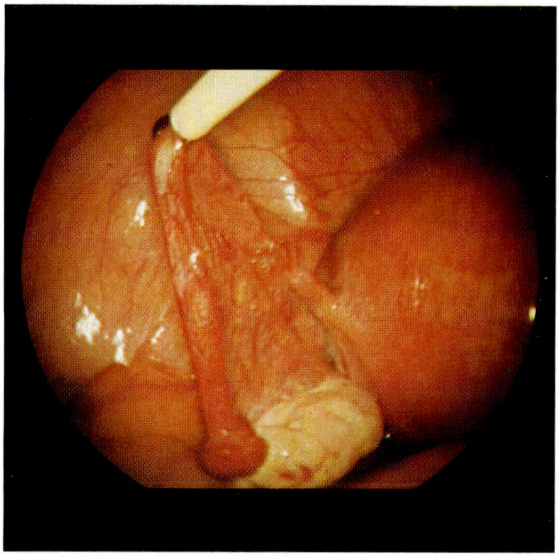

(d) Elimination of Ampullar Stenoses by Dilation

Fig. 361. Elevation of the left tube in the region of the mesosalpinx reveals the whole length of the tube. The ampulla has normal configuration and a knobby thickening is evident at its central ampullar portion. In the left uterosacral ligament a previously coagulated endometrial implant can be seen.

Fig. 362. Tubal dye insufflation makes it evident that, apparently as a consequence of inflammation, the fimbriae are far removed from the point where the blue dye is emerging. There is a rupture of an ampullar stenosis, apparently freshly caused by the high intrauterine pressure of 250 mm Hg.

Fig. 363. The ampullar stenosis demonstrated in Figures 361 and 362 is here being dilated with the aid of atraumatic forceps. The closed jaws of the forceps are introduced into the funnel of the ampulla, then opened and slowly withdrawn in an open position. In this way minor but functionally absolute obstructions causing sterility can readily be eliminated at laparoscopy. Renewed adhesion formation is discouraged by hydropertubating the patient for five successive days after the laparoscopy and five to seven additional times later on (see Figs. 366, 382).

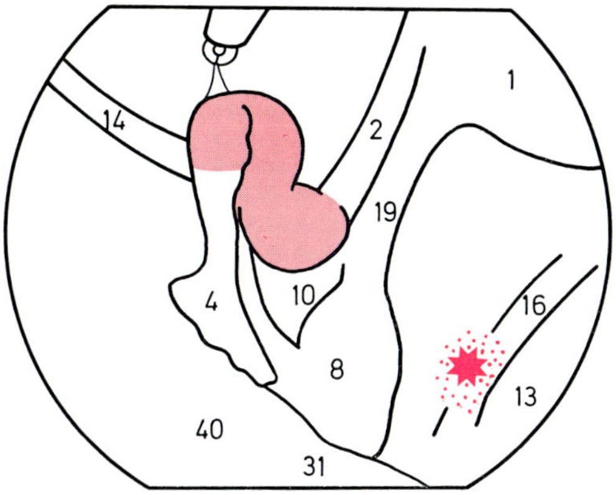
14
1
2
19
10
4
16
8
13
40
31

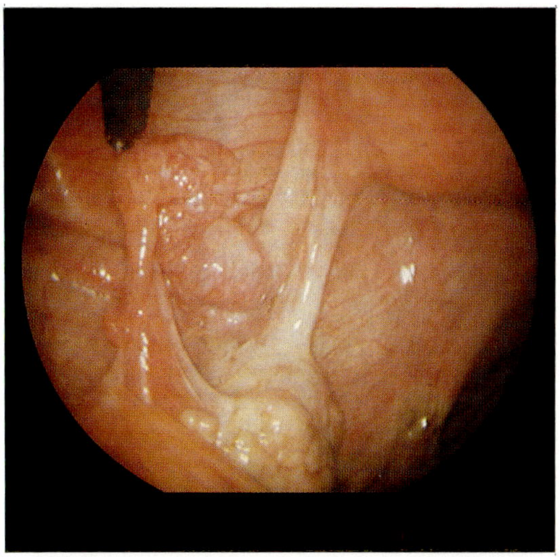

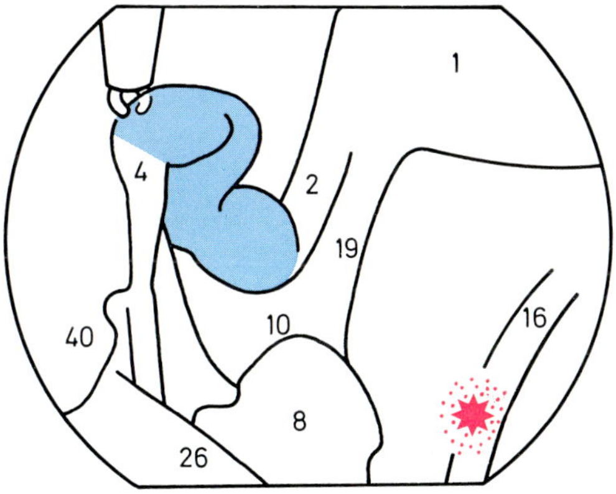
1
4
2
19
10
40
16
8
26

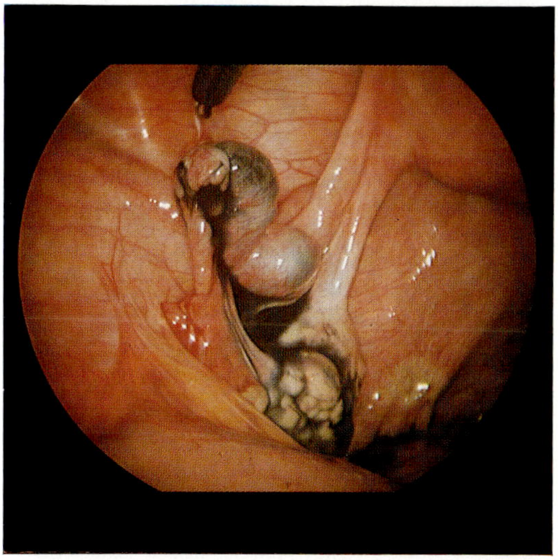

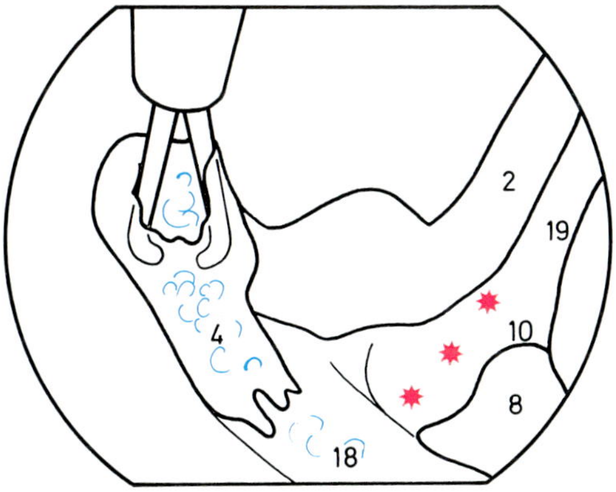
2
19
4
10
8
18

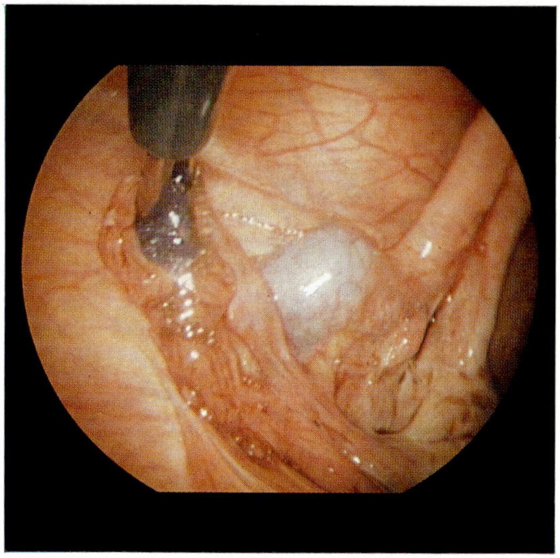

(e) Adnexal Corrections after Infertility Operations

Figures 364–366 show the correction of bilateral adnexal adhesions arising after an infertility operation with implantation of both tubes.

Fig. 364. The uterus elevated with the aid of the suction intrauterine cannula shows massive adhesions on its posterior wall between the reimplanted tubes and the sigmoid colon. The arrows indicate the points of reimplantation. At first the case was diagnosed as hopeless.

Fig. 365. Under pressure of 300 mm Hg the blue dye is emerging, after manipulation with the atraumatic forceps, from the left tube at a place visible through the adhesions.

Fig. 366. Through further surgical procedure with atraumatic scissors after coagulation at low voltage, adhesions surrounding the left reimplanted tube can be detached and displaced.

After painstaking coagulation at low voltage, a linear adhesion between the left round ligament and the sigmoid loop is being severed. Coagulation in such a situation is impossible at high frequency because the heat generated in the jaws of the forceps would spread simultaneously to the base of the adhesion on the intestine and result in a dime-sized necrotic area.

After severance of this adhesion and further mobilization of the tube, the pelvis was rinsed free of blood with saline solution. To obviate further adhesions, 500 mg of hydrocortisone was instilled, dissolved in 500 ml of physiologic saline solution warmed to body temperature. In the course of the series of hydropertubations carried out in connection with the above, the patient was given hydrocortisone in decreasing dosage: 50 mg cortisone four times a day at six-hour intervals on the first and second postoperative days; 50 mg three times at eight-hour intervals on the third day; and 50 mg twice on the fourth day at 12-hour intervals. The patient subsequently established an intrauterine pregnancy and delivered a full-term, live child.

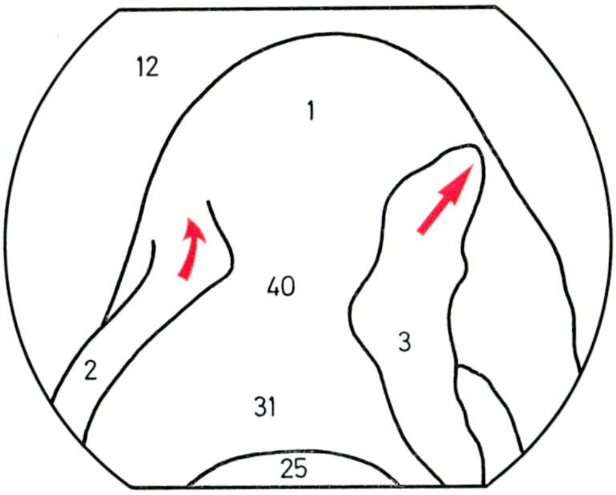
12
1
40
3
2
31
25

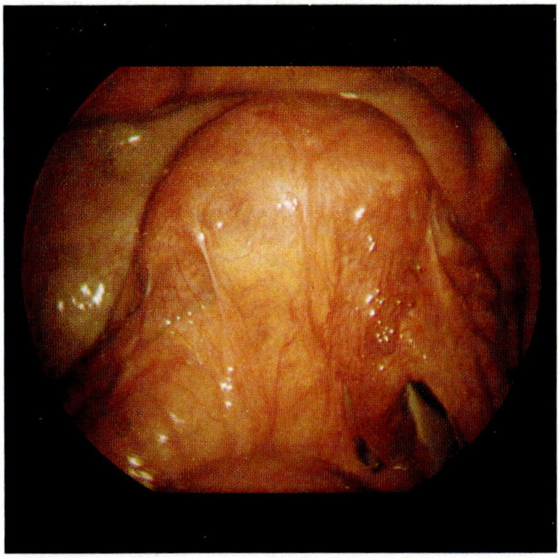

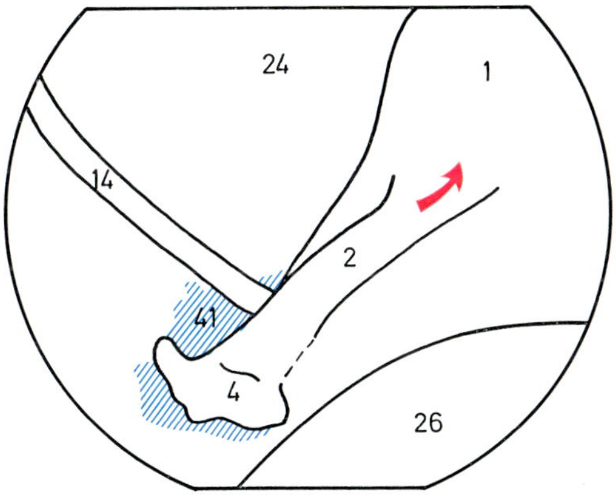
24
1
14
2
41
4
26

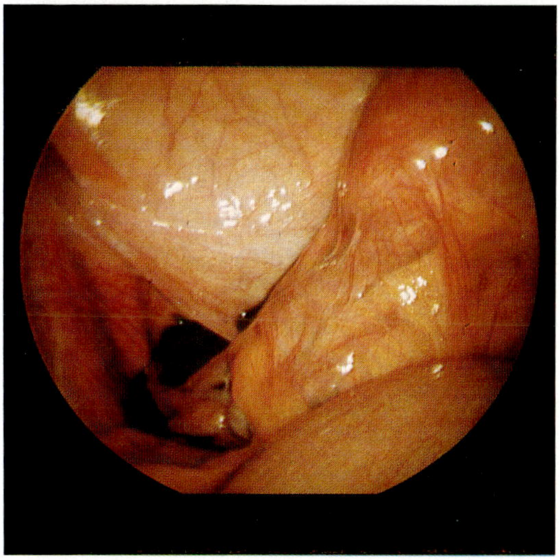

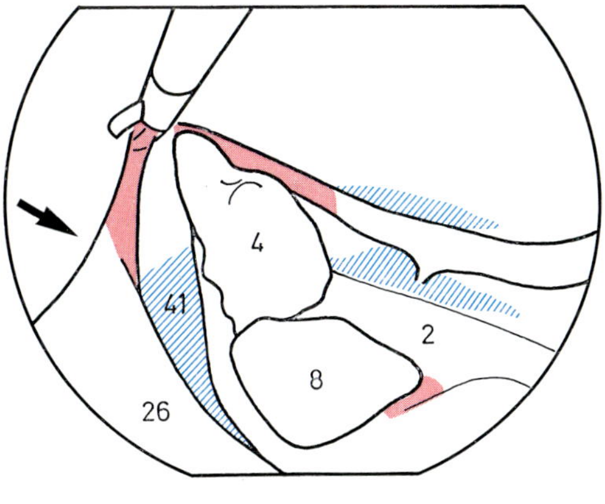
4
41
2
8
26

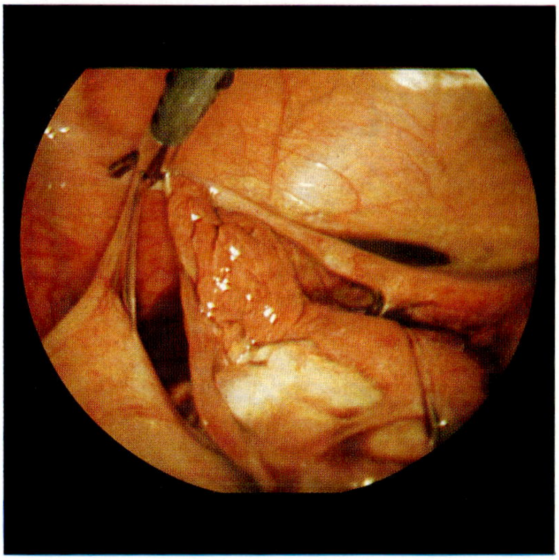

In order to maintain therapeutic success in restoring tubal patency at laparoscopy, whether by means of the pressure of the insufflation solution alone (e.g., in minor adherence of the fimbriae) or by instrumental manipulation (e.g., in dilation of the ampullae, see Figs. 315 and 363), it is necessary to institute a series of hydropertubations immediately after laparoscopy. We recommend a mixture of streptomycin, hydrocortisone, procaine, and alpha-chymotrypsin as the solution of choice for hydropertubation, which has proved its value in more than 6000 insufflations.

The instillation solution is always freshly prepared from a stock solution as follows: procaine hydrochloricum, 0.4 gm; streptomycin sulfate, 0.4 gm; hydrocortisone acetate, 0.1 gm; distilled water add to 100 ml, prepared under sterile conditions, stored in the refrigerator, and shaken before use. This can be kept for about one week.

Twenty ml of this stock solution is withdrawn under sterile conditions for each instillation, 5 ml of it being used to dissolve 5 mg of alpha-chymotrypsin in dry powder form. The resulting solution is used for the instillation.

For the painless use of this solution, which remains in the tubes for about six to eight hours after instillation (see Fig. 382), the following instruments have been employed:

Fig. 367. Cervical adapter by Fikentscher and Semm, made from clear plastic for atraumatic sealing of the cervix for gas insufflation, hysterosalpingography, and especially hydropertubation.

Fig. 368. By means of negative pressure (produced by the Universal Pertubation Apparatus (see Fig. 182) or manually with a hand pump as shown in this sketch), the cervical adapter with its flexible hoses is placed by suction to the cervix. The hydropertubation solution is injected slowly under controlled pressure produced by the apparatus. The duration and pressure of injection (recorded graphically) permit simultaneous reading of the tubal patency and its improvement.

Fig. 369. The Semm duckbill speculum permits completely painless placement of the adapter. This three-part speculum has its fulcrum within the vulva so that wide opening of the blades causes no pain, unlike specula with the fulcrum located outside the vulva. This speculum makes possible the painless use of sizes A or B adapters (Fig. 370).

Fig. 371. The cervical adapter is attached to the adapter forceps for placement on the portio, and guided to the latter by means of the duckbill speculum. The roller clips on the hose prevent the pertubation solution from flowing out, and also maintain the vacuum for holding the adapter fast to the cervix.

Fig. 372. In cases of secondary infertility, the cervix often is deformed as a result of previous deliveries, and this reduces the ability of the adapter to achieve the required seal. For this reason the double-balloon catheter (Fikentscher and Semm) is inserted atraumatically into the cervical canal and attached with the aid of ball-tipped forceps.

Fig. 373. The double-balloon catheter (Fikentscher and Semm) also is applicable for cervices in which suction attachment of the adapter is not practicable because of traumatic malformation.

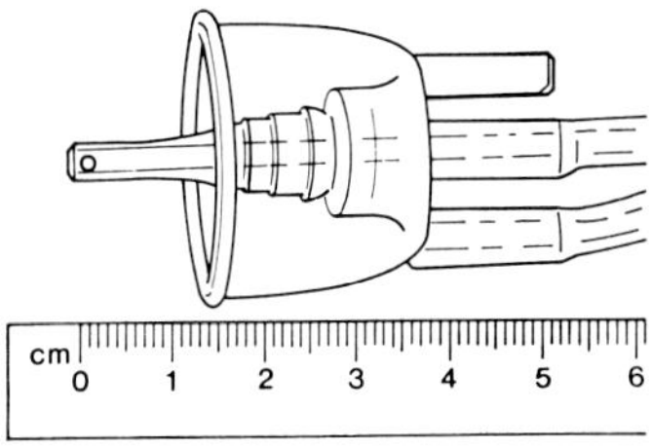

Figure 367

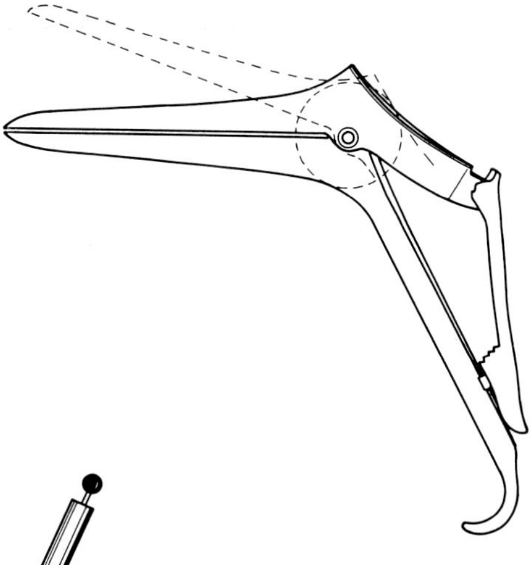

Figure 369

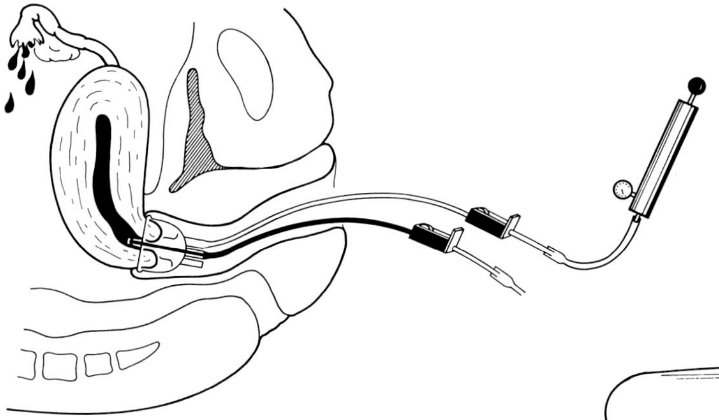

Figure 368

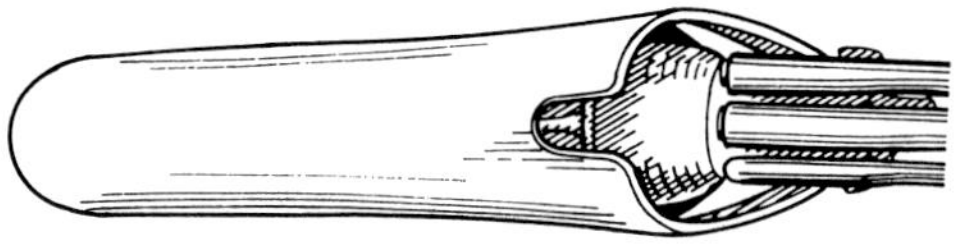

Figure 370

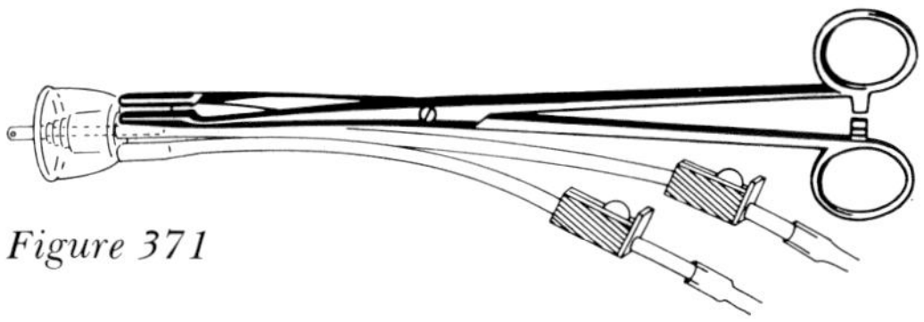

Figure 371

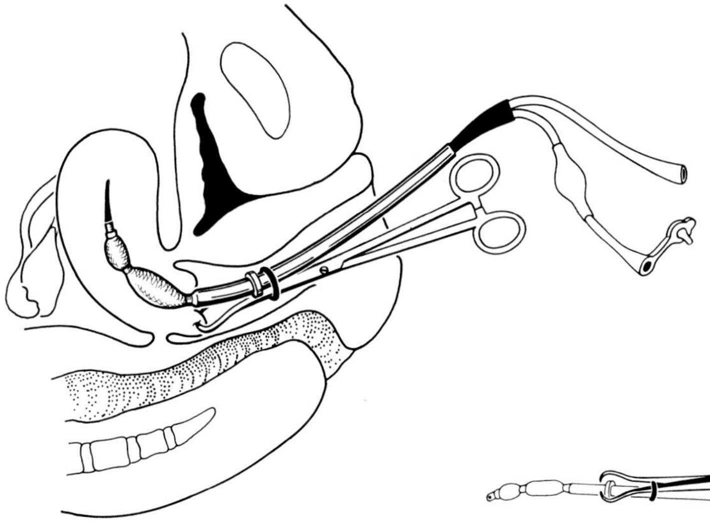

Figure 372

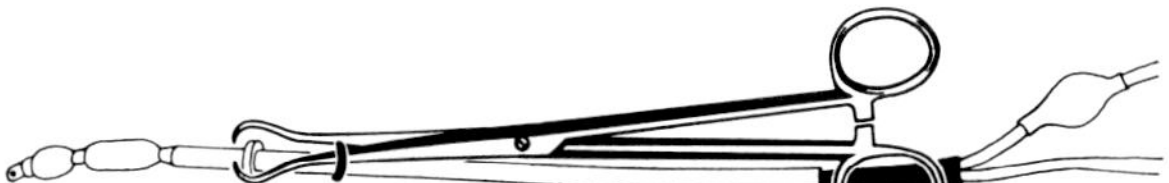

Figure 373

(f) Coagulation of Endometrial Implants

Fig. 374. Chronic lower abdominal distress in many instances is characterized by inaccessible endometrial implants, and these can be spotted at laparoscopy far better than at laparotomy. The sharp lower abdominal pains occurring intermittently in the case shown here were caused in part by a linear adhesion pulling from the broad ligament on the right to the ovary, which undoubtedly arose from an implant of endometriosis. The arrow demonstrates a well-formed scar from a previous laceration in the left broad ligament, interpreted as the consequence of peritoneal tears during delivery (Allen–Masters syndrome).

Fig. 375. When the lens is brought closer, the subperitoneal and multilocular topography of the implants becomes clearly evident. The peritoneal opening at the left below the implant, appearing as though made with a punch, is to be attributed to peritoneal tears during delivery.

Fig. 376. Chronic lower abdominal distress of many years' standing can be relieved by successful coagulation of endometrial implants. Since there is an ever-present danger that not all the existing implants are detectable, it is recommended that, in conjunction with coagulation, a continuous six- to nine-month treatment with progestogens be instituted. The following rule should be observed: In the presence of implants of endometriosis, sterility operations have little prospect of success. First the implants must be coagulated at laparoscopy, and then completely healed through medical treatment as described above.

In coagulating implants of endometriosis, it is vital that pains be taken to *identify the ureter carefully.* It is clearly visible in this picture. The confusion of a uterosacral ligament with a ureter could have dire consequences.

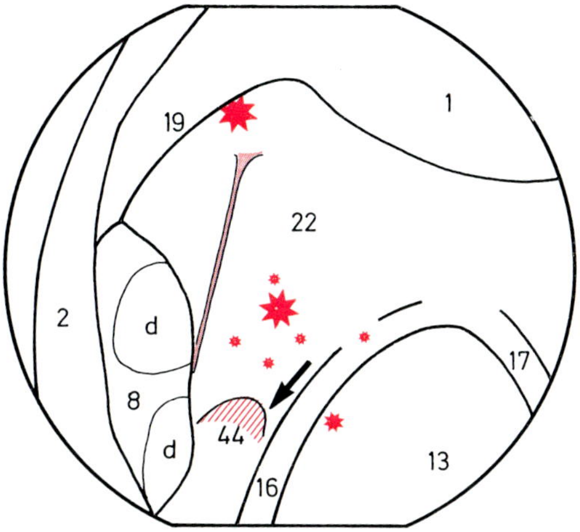
19
1
22
2
d
8
d
44
16
17
13

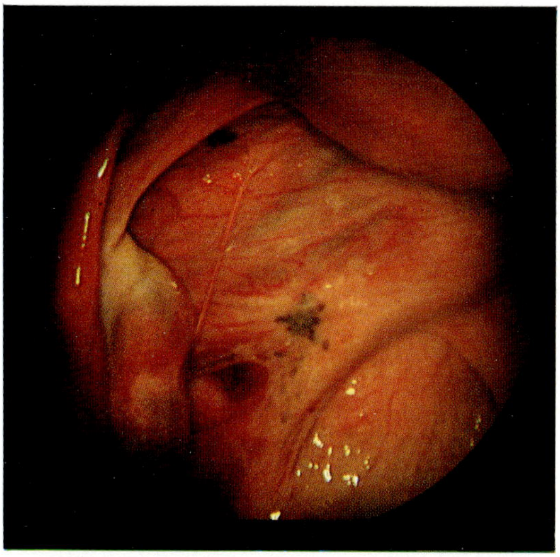

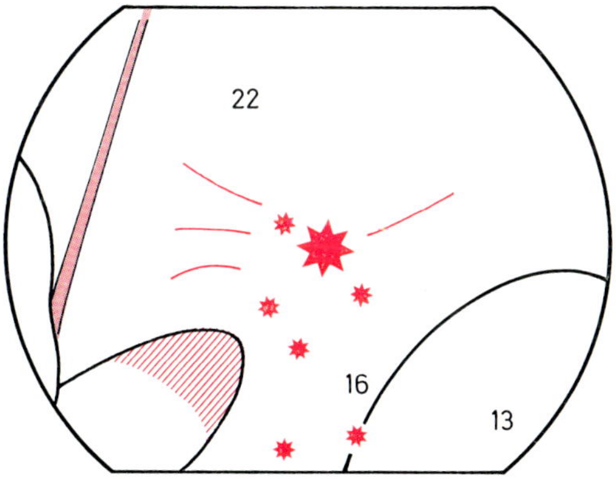
22
16
13

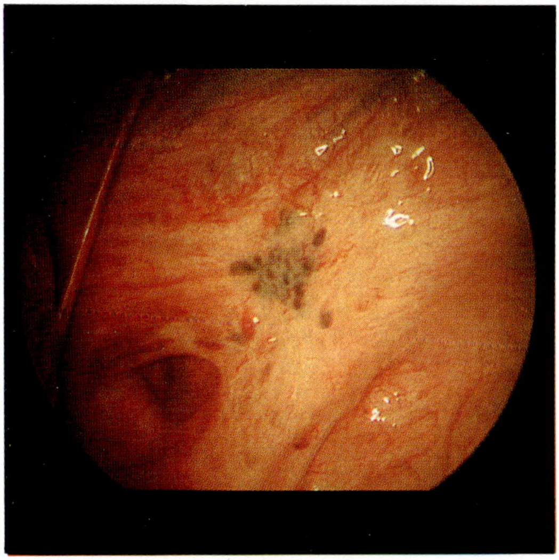

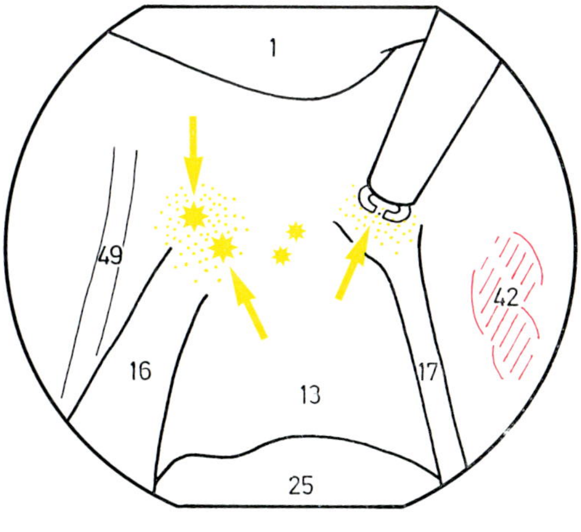
1
49
42
16
13
17
25

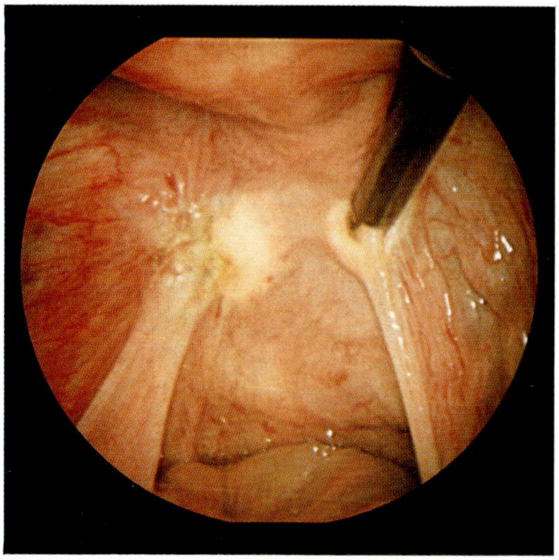

Fig. 377. Because of primary infertility in this patient, a culdoscopy had been performed three months prior to the laparoscopy. The point of perforation by the culdoscope is marked by the larger arrow. It was not possible to diagnose the implants of endometriosis located in the cul-de-sac with the culdoscope, which does not offer sufficient opportunity to look back into the area of its own puncture. Since most implants are located in the cul-de-sac, it is easy to understand why culdoscopy, especially in the diagnosis of the causes of sterility, is no longer of any value today.

From the vantage point of laparoscopy, the implants lie well within the range of vision. The star-shaped perforation wound caused by the culdoscope is closed by velamentous peritoneal adhesions. There is about 10 ml of bloody serous fluid in the cul-de-sac. Note the ureter passing to the right of the uterosacral ligament. It shows a peristaltic wave in its upper portion *(red arrow).* The right uterosacral ligament shows severe hypertrophy suggestive of chronic spasm, probably caused by the endometriosis, which is especially pronounced in this ligament. (Note that the ureter is incorrectly numbered 40 in this Figure. The correct identification number is 49.)

Fig. 378. Under subsequent tubal dye insufflation, the ampullar part of the right tube is massively engorged under a pressure of 300 mm Hg. The musculature is thin-walled and the blue shows through clearly. The dye is emerging from the left tube, but only with severe distention of the ampullar part of the tube, caused by an ampullar stenosis. Endometriosis again is a possible cause for this tubal feature. The patient gives no other history of inflammation.

Fig. 379. After the coagulation of the endometrial implants demonstrated in Figures 377 and 378, it can be seen that the implants in the right uterosacral ligament had riddled the entire ligament. This is probably also the reason why the trocar of the culdoscope was deflected downward on encountering this resistance.

A series of five to seven hydropertubations in conjunction with a six- to nine-month course of progestogen treatment follows as an additional therapeutic measure. Then laparoscopy is repeated in order further to monitor the situation in the pelvis if the prior control pertubation does not produce tubal patency of Grade 1. The star and arrow again mark the point of perforation by the culdoscope.

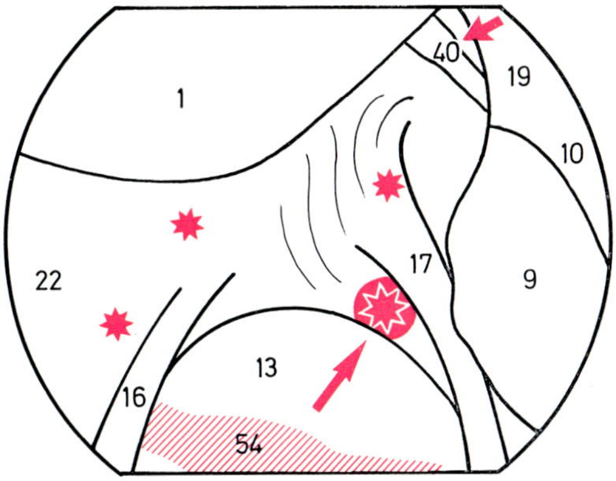
40
19
1
10
22
17
9
13
16
54

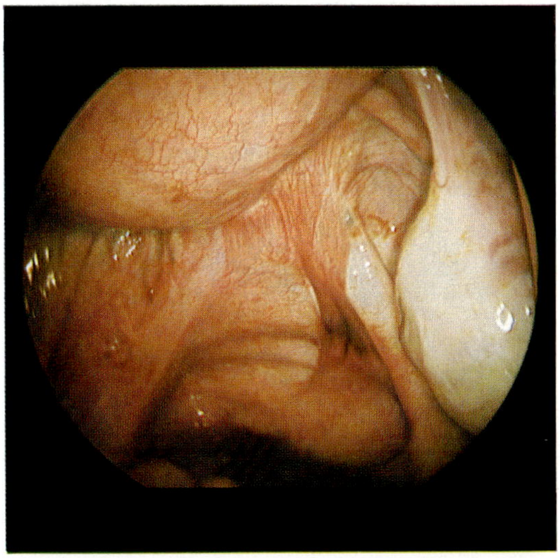

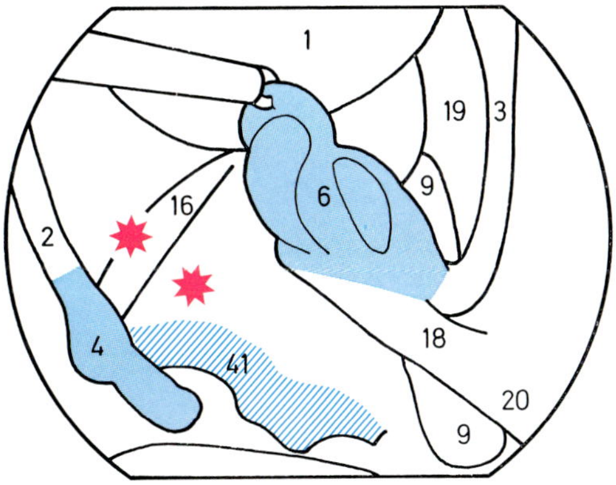
1
19
3
9
6
16
2
18
4
41
20
9

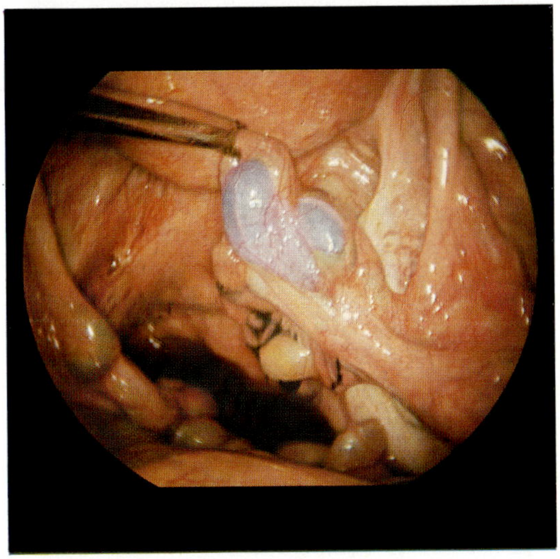

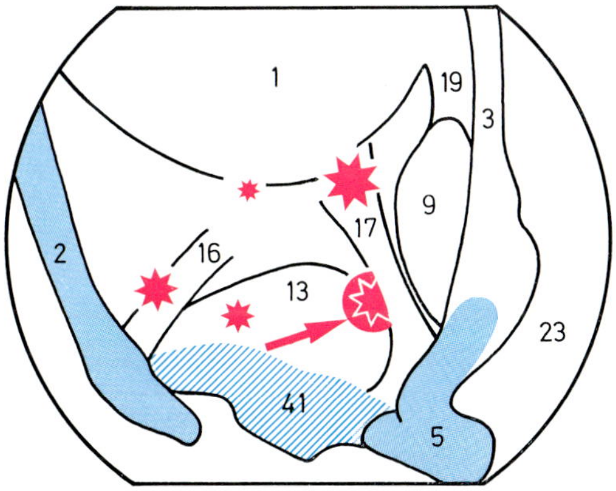
1
19
3
9
17
16
2
13
23
41
5

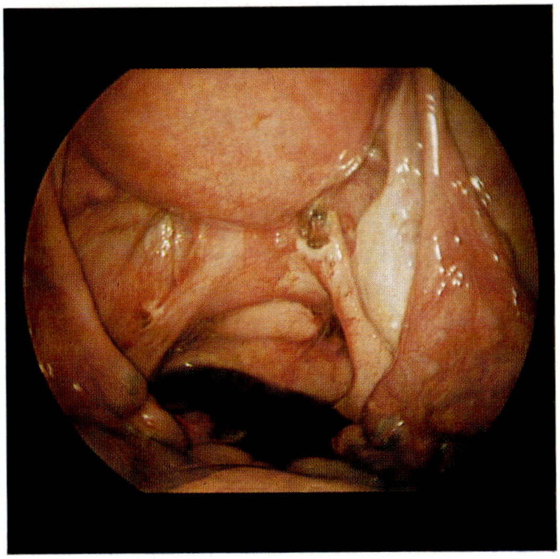

Fig. 380. Endometriosis plays a special role in primary and secondary infertility. Often even small implants, as in this case, suffice to give rise to a severe ampullar stenosis. Here we see at first only the grain-of-rice-sized implants in the left uterosacral ligament. After the latter is moved aside, however (see Fig. 381), the chief implant becomes visible in the region of the cul-de-sac.

Fig. 381. Elevation of the left uterosacral ligament reveals another, still larger implant in the cul-de-sac. In this picture it has already been coagulated with low voltage forceps. The coagulation brings out the chocolate-colored hematomas with added clarity.

Fig. 382. In endometriosis, tubal blockages usually are present only in the form of thin-walled adhesions. These can readily be eliminated by means of repeated and prolonged hydropertubation. The same is true of adhesions arising immediately after an infertility operation.

The principle of repeated hydropertubations is that they should be started immediately after menstruation ceases and repeated on six or seven successive days.

(1) With a mechanically controlled pressure of no more than 300 mm Hg, the hydropertubation solution (for formula, see descriptive text, Fig. 366) is instilled. The solution spreads as far as the tubal obstruction.

(2) By the third day some adhesions have been eliminated and additional solution can be instilled.

(3) The fluid does not emerge from the tubes until the fifth to seventh day, and then only if the series gives positive results.

The cervical adapter (Fikentscher and Semm, Figs. 367–371) is always left on the cervix for six to eight hours after instillation in order to prevent the fluid from running out immediately and to assure a six- to eight-hour local effect.

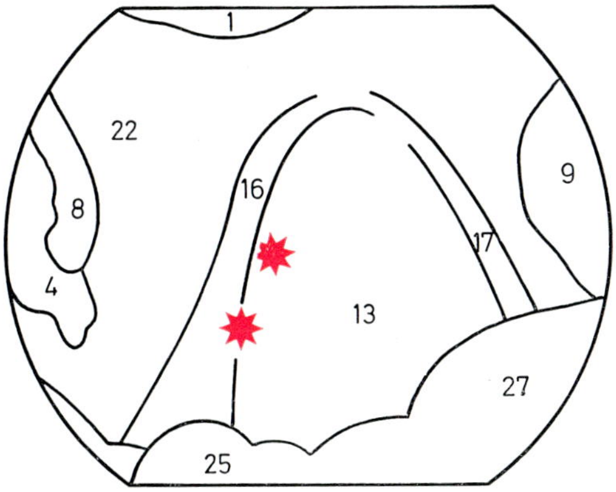
1
22
8
4
16
17
9
13
27
25

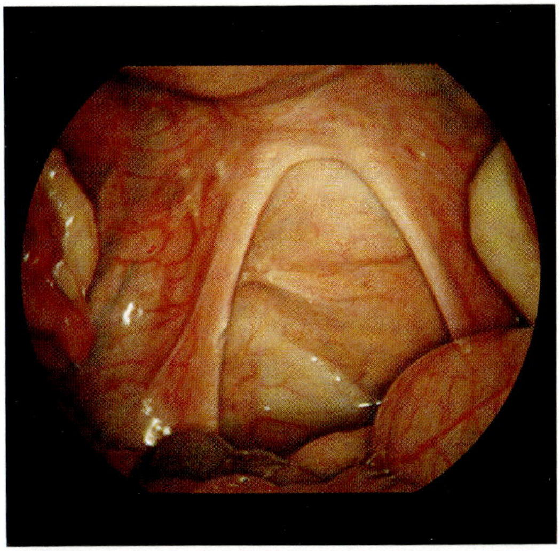

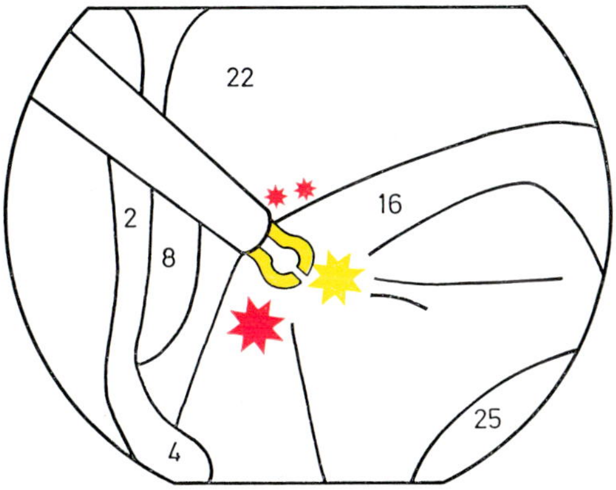
22
16
2
8
4
25

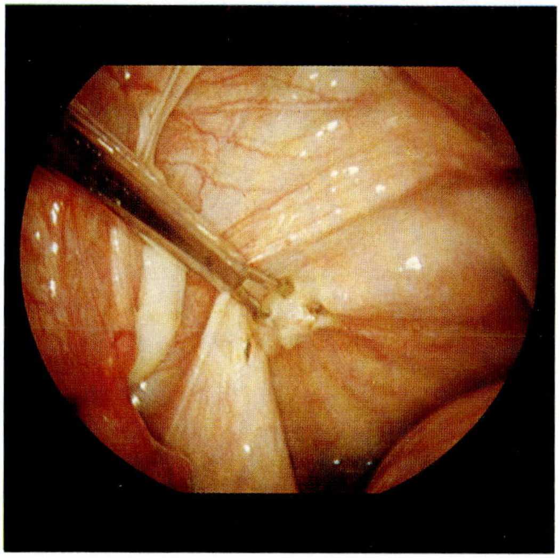

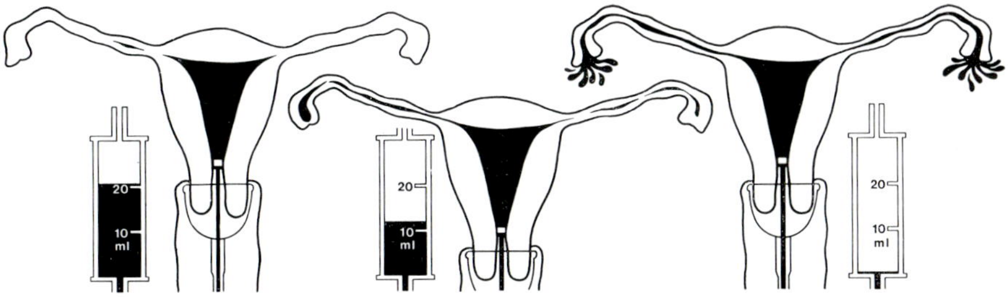
20
10
ml
20
10
ml
20
10
ml

(g) *Puncture of Juvenile Ovarian or "Chocolate" Cysts with Resection of the Cyst Wall*

A basic rule to remember is that laparoscopy is insufficient as a method of eliminating benign or malignant ovarian tumors. Nevertheless, benign, usually juvenile, tumors are a broad area of indication for laparoscopy. Puncture with resection of the cyst wall at laparoscopy spares the young patient a laparotomy. This method has been most effective especially during early pregnancy and in overstimulation by HMG–HCG treatment.

Fig. 383. Sometimes the extreme mobility of the cystic ovary, supported by the utero-ovarian and infundibulopelvic ligaments, makes puncture difficult. This can be overcome by displacing the uterus as far as possible into the cul-de-sac, as shown in the illustration, and thus wedging the ovarian cyst between the fundus and the lateral wall of the pelvis. The puncture at an angle of 90° is now possible without increased risk. The aspiration is done intermittently with the device shown in Figure 74. It is mandatory that the aspirated material be evaluated histologically and cytologically.

Fig. 384. A simple puncture of the cyst, however, usually leads quickly to fluid reaccumulation. The puncture of an ovarian cyst, consequently, is meaningful only if a partial resection of the cyst wall is done at the same time. Therefore, after removal of the contents of the cyst with biopsy forceps aided by the trocar sleeve (grasp the cyst wall with the biopsy forceps and punch out the tissue by a rotation of the sleeve as in Fig. 70), a large hole is punched in the cystic sac through step-by-step resection of the cyst wall. The red line marks the edge of the punched-out cyst wall. Within this line the endothelium of the retention cyst can be seen.

Fig. 385. When sufficient cyst wall has been resected, we start coagulating the free edge of the cyst bit by bit with atraumatic forceps (if using high-frequency current), or atraumatic coagulation forceps (if using the low voltage Endotherm), or crocodile forceps (with the Sterilization Unit for control). Recently the crocodile forceps, not shown here (Fig. 348), has been used to special advantage in coagulation. At the conclusion of the coagulation there usually remains an ovarian body only the size of a large cherry. After some months this cyst, emptied and resected at laparoscopy, will have been converted into a somewhat scarified ovary such as we are accustomed to seeing after spontaneous rupture of ovarian cysts. In our own statistics 85 per cent of such cysts do not recur.

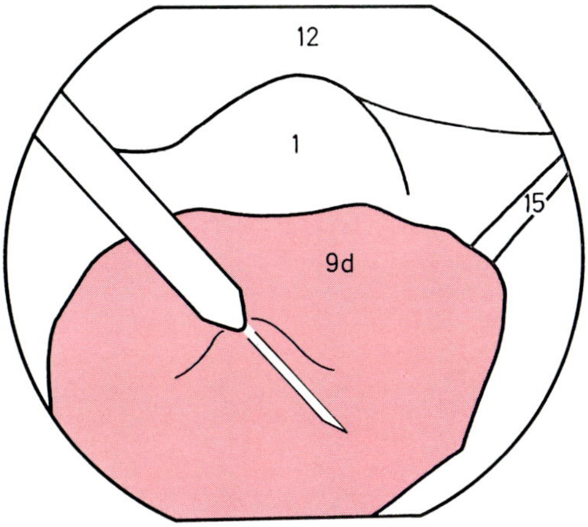
12
1
15
9d

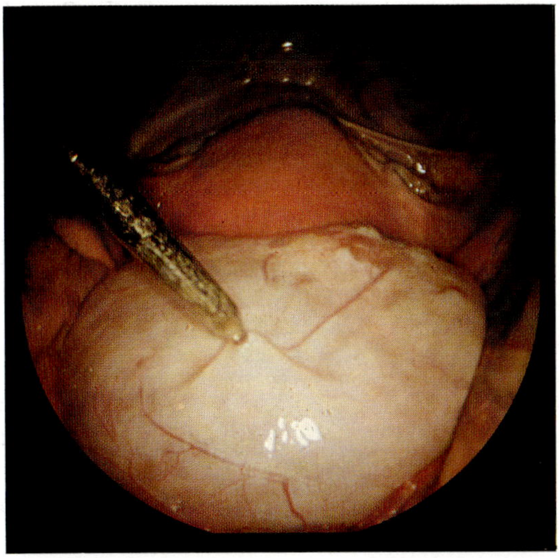

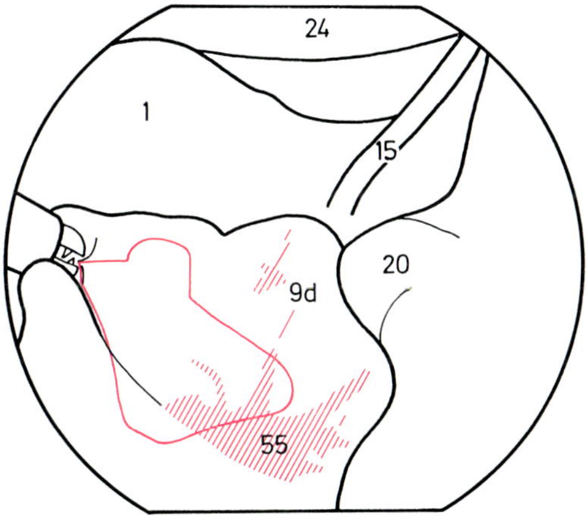
24
1
15
20
9d
55

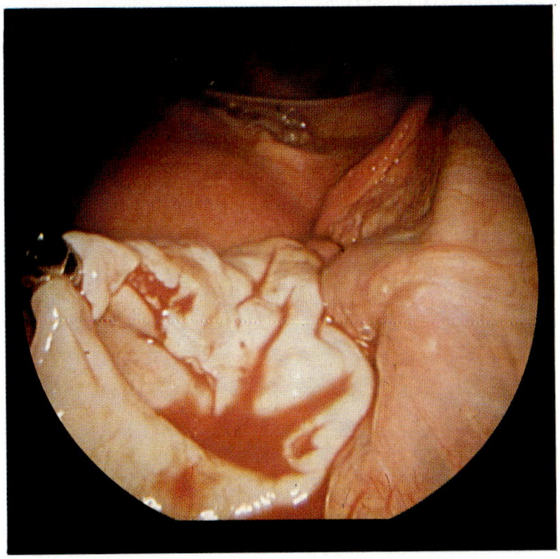

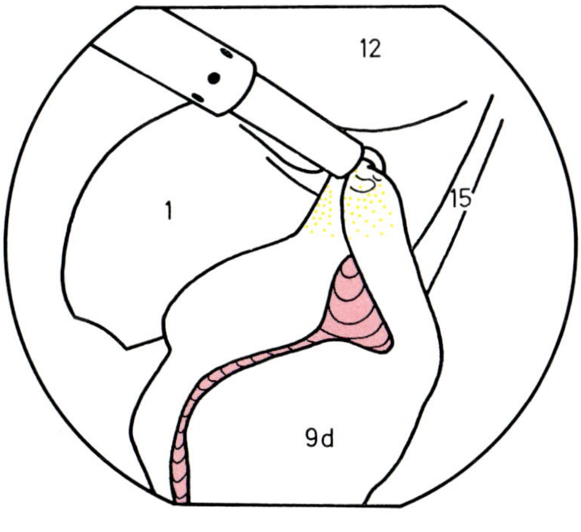
12
1
15
9d

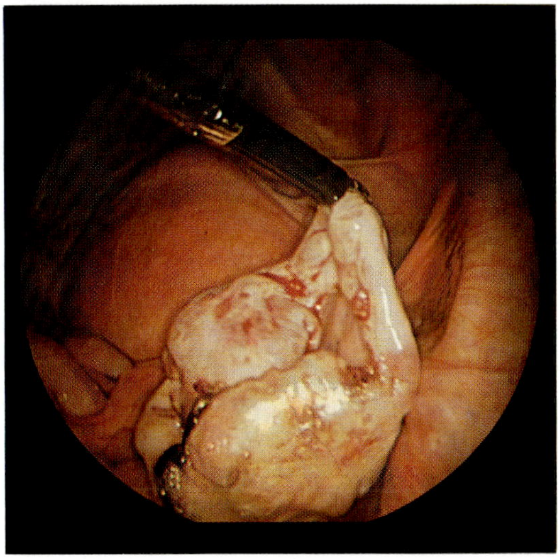

Figures 386–394 show the laparoscopic operative technique in bilateral "chocolate cysts."

In young patients, we often are faced with a difficult decision in the therapy of bilateral ovarian cysts associated with endometriosis. At laparotomy we can perform either total extirpation of the ovaries or their partial resection. With any degree of skill the latter technique is fully practicable at laparoscopy, and has the advantage that the procedure is minimally taxing for the patient and leaves no postoperative adhesions. This contrasts sharply with the healing phase after techniques in which the abdomen is opened. After laparotomy for endometriosis, the usual result is an abdomen filled with adhesions.

Fig. 386. In the puncture of a chocolate cyst we always make certain that the cyst has steadying support and that the needle perforates it at an angle of 90°.

Fig. 387. After aspiration, the capsule wall can be laid open with the aid of the injection needle. We are looking into the cavity of the cyst. Most of the cyst contents have spilled out into the cul-de-sac.

Fig. 388. After a large part of the cyst wall has been punched out with the biopsy forceps, aided by the trocar cannula, we now proceed to the stepwise coagulation of the remaining cyst wall at low voltage (Sterilization Unit or Endotherm), or, if neither is available, cautiously by means of high-frequency coagulation. The arrow is pointing into the cavity of what was the "chocolate cyst."

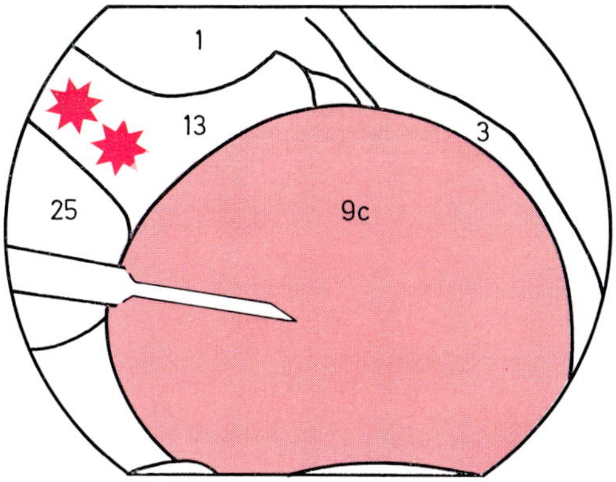
1
13
3
25
9c

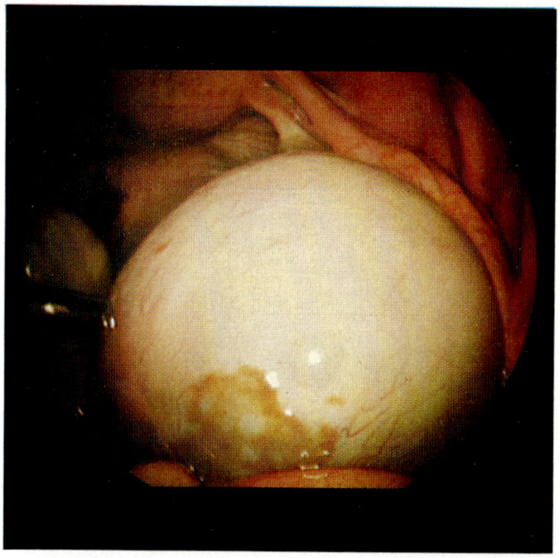

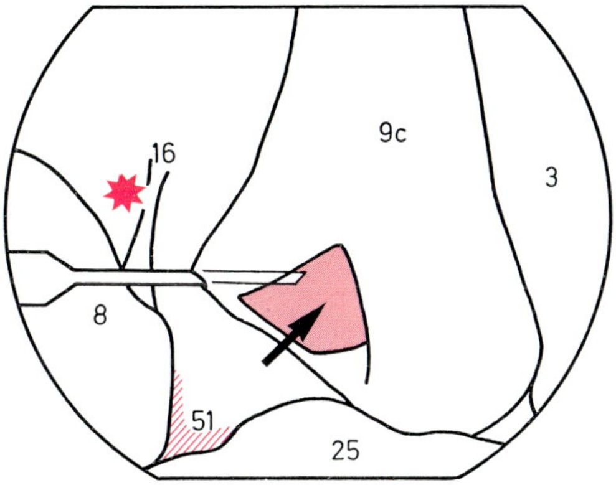
16
9c
3
8
51
25

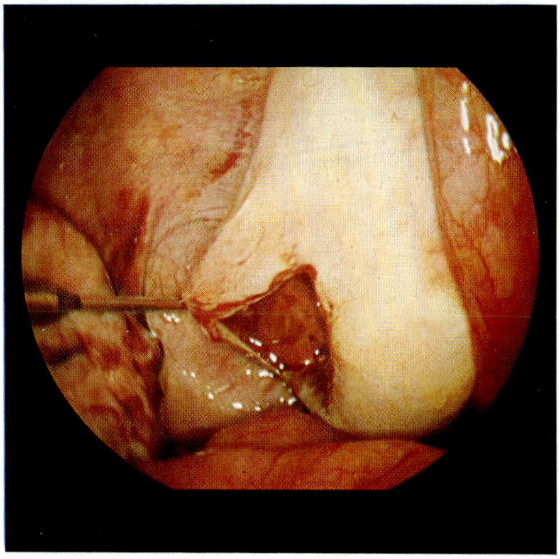

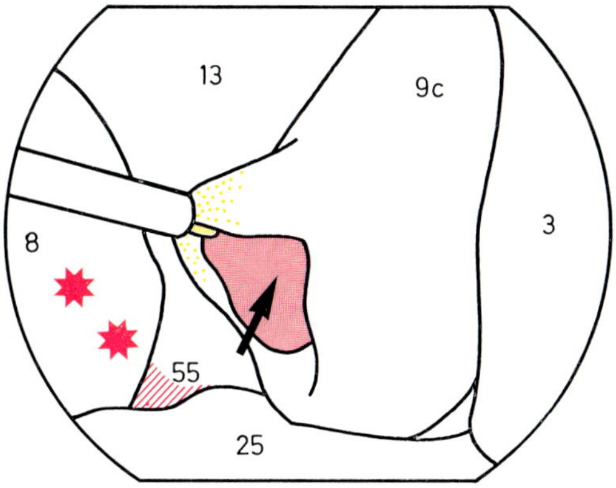
13
9c
8
3
55
25

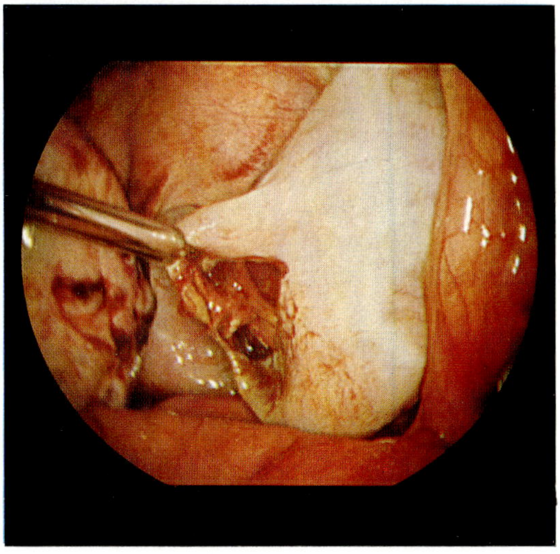

Fig. 389. Even this multiloculated left ovary filled with "chocolate cysts" can be reduced through multiple punctures to the size of a pingpong ball or a cherry. Numerous punctures are needed for this. It is inevitable that the contents of the "chocolate cysts" run out past the puncture needle into the cul-de-sac. The arrows point to the coagulated edge of the cyst wall of the right ovary, which was originally as big as a large hen's egg. In the left ovary the arrows point to the three coagulated puncture sites.

Fig. 390. When both ovaries have been emptied and the cystic endothelium at the bottom, as well as all visible implants of endometriosis in the vicinity of the cul-de-sac, have been coagulated, we begin cleaning up the cul-de-sac by alternate instillation and aspiration of about 500 to 1000 ml of sterile physiologic saline solution warmed to body temperature, using the large aspiration cannula.

Fig. 391. The final situation after aspiration and coagulation of large bilateral "chocolate cysts". Both ovaries have been reduced to one-quarter of their original size. The edges of the cysts are partially resected or coagulated. The cul-de-sac is cleansed by rinsing. This laparoscopic procedure is followed by nine months of progestogen therapy as hormonal treatment for the endometriosis.

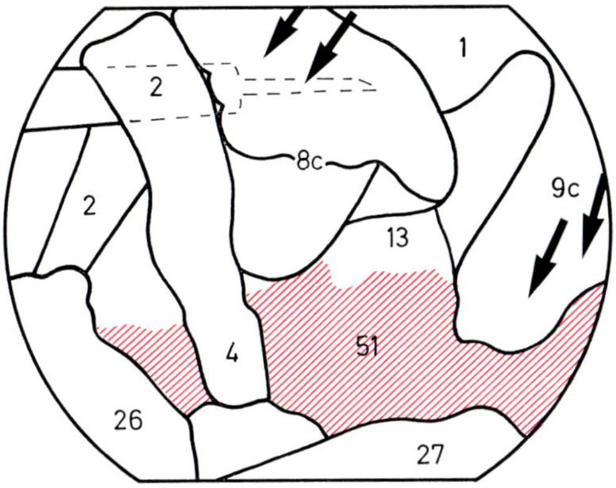
1
2
2
8c
9c
13
4
51
26
27

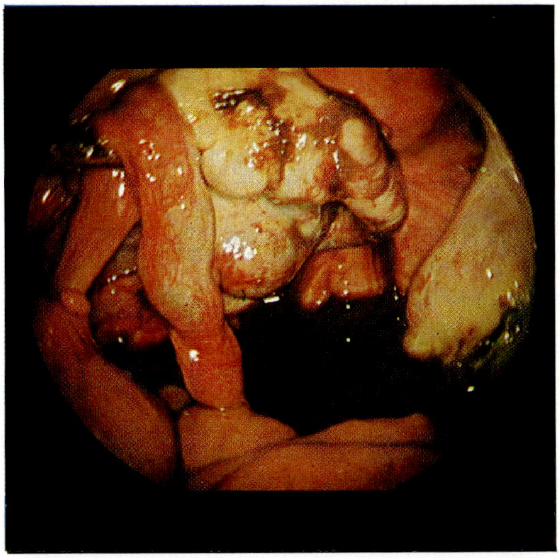

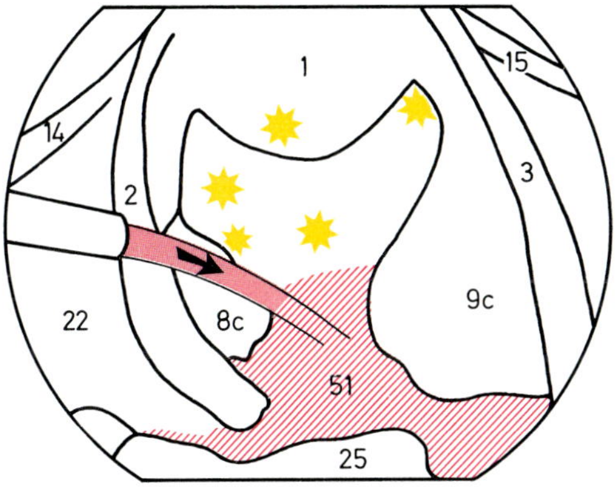
1
15
14
2
3
22
8c
9c
51
25

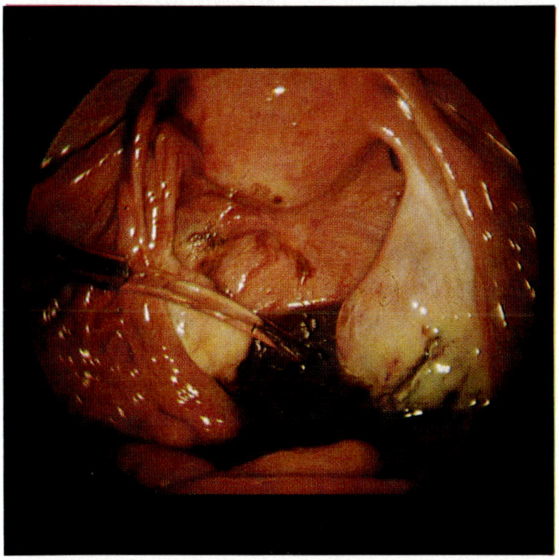

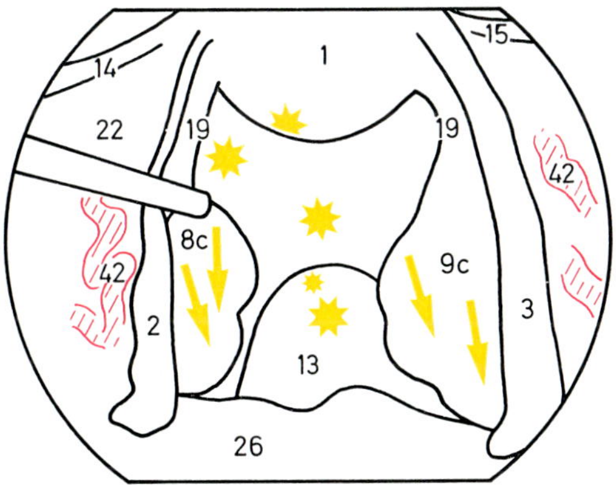
1
15
14
22
19
19
42
42
8c
9c
2
3
13
26

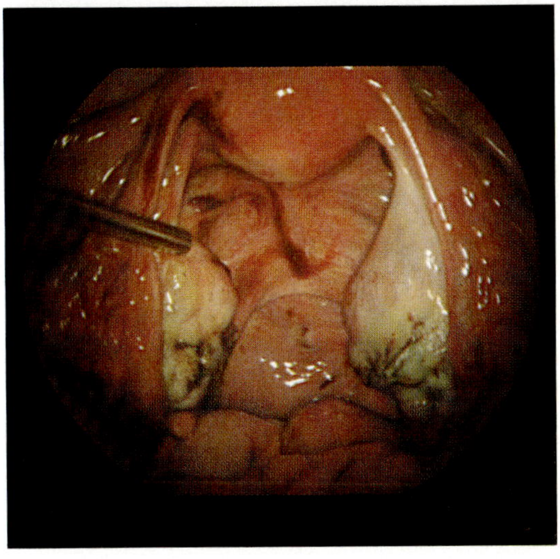

Fig. 392. These two ovaries, smooth-walled and somewhat brownish in color, demonstrate a case of bilateral "chocolate cysts." The arrows point to the thin-walled parts of the cysts, which are on the verge of spontaneous rupture.

Fig. 393. Since the thick chocolate-like mass could not be removed even with two punctures (see arrows), a hole is being cut into the cyst with the biopsy forceps. We grasp the ovarian cyst with the biopsy forceps before perforating it by advancing the trocar sleeve, as demonstrated in Figure 394.

Fig. 394. Here we see the cyst wall grasped in the biopsy forceps being drawn into the trocar sleeve in order to punch out the cyst wall over a large area.

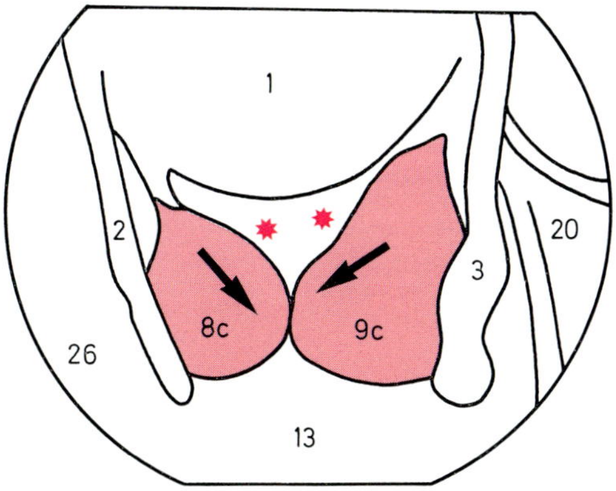
1
2
20
3
8c
9c
26
13

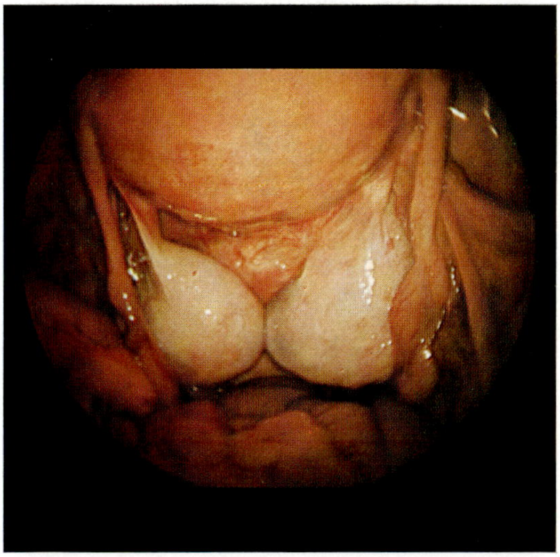

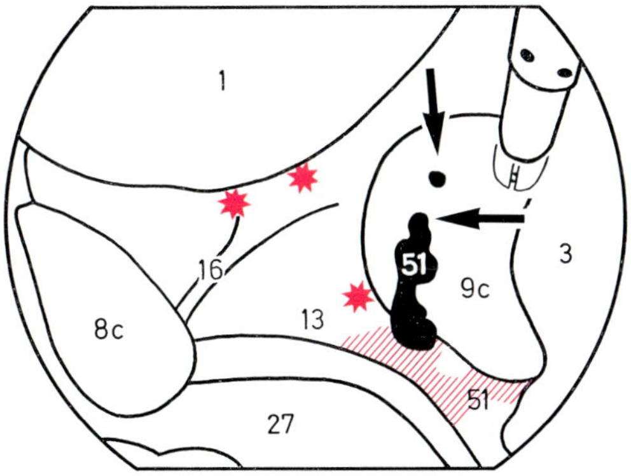
1
16
8c
13
51
9c
3
51
27

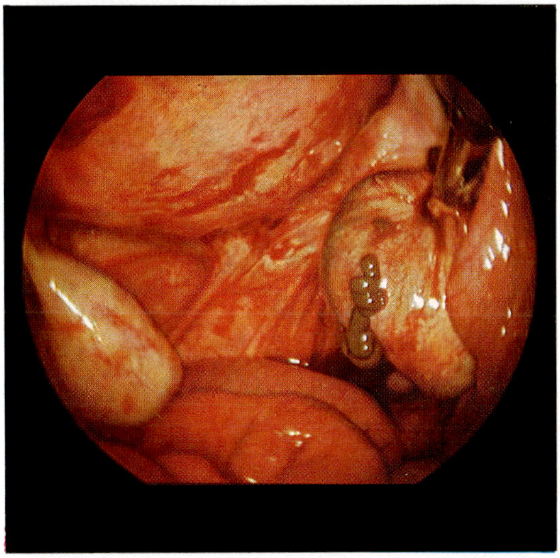

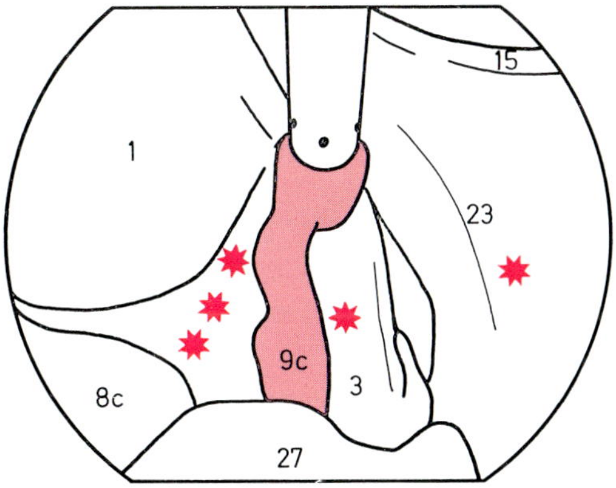
15
1
23
9c
3
8c
27

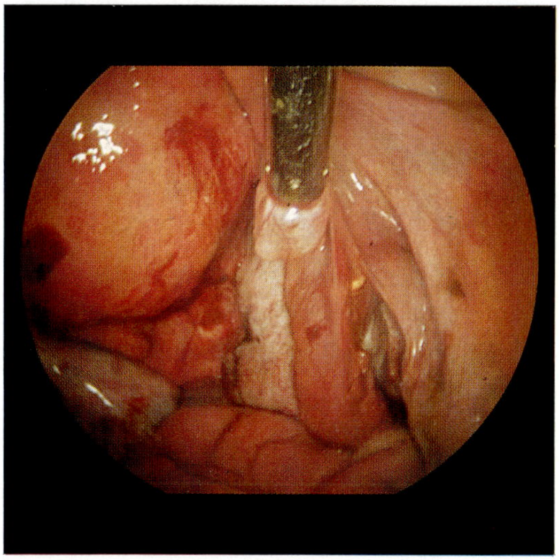

Figures 395–400 show the operative technique for puncturing a juvenile ovarian cyst.

Fig. 395. This juvenile retention cyst on the right side is being elevated out of the cul-de-sac with the aid of the atraumatic forceps. At the same time we lower the uterus in order to steady the cyst against its anterior wall.

Fig. 396. The needle puncture into the right ovarian cyst is made at right angles against the firm surface of the fundus and lateral pelvic wall. The uterus is being steadied in the cul-de-sac by the suction intrauterine cannula.

Fig. 397. After aspiration of the clear serous contents of the cyst collected in the intermediate container (see Fig. 74), it is subjected to cytologic examination. The thin-walled part of the cystic sac is then punched out. For this purpose the empty cyst is grasped with the biopsy forceps, and the first hole is punched into it by pushing down the trocar sleeve.

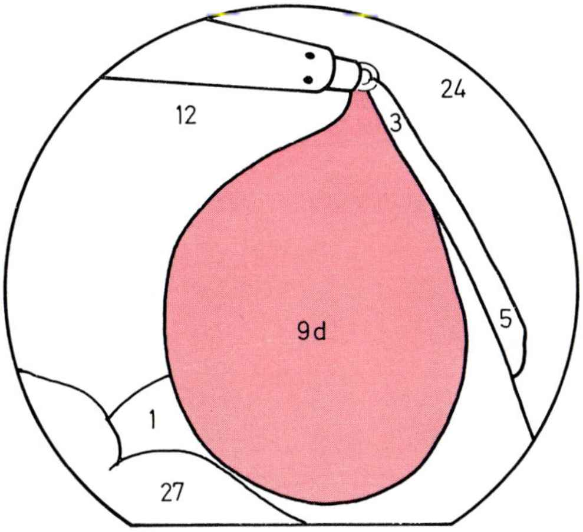
24
12
3
9d
5
1
27

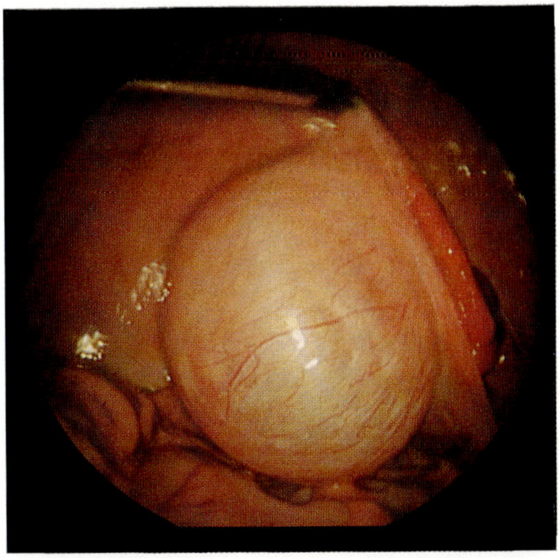

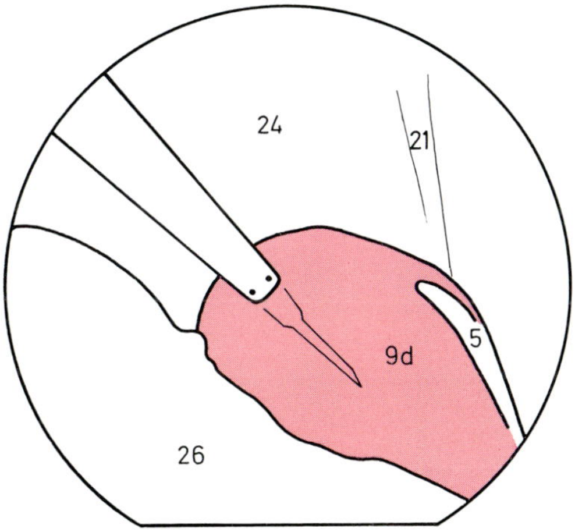
24
21
5
9d
26

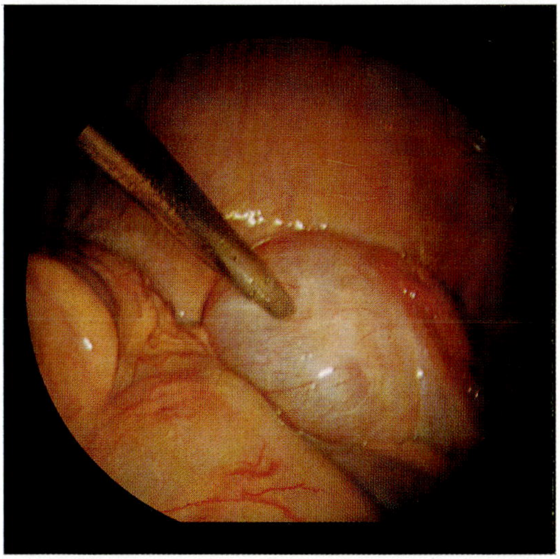

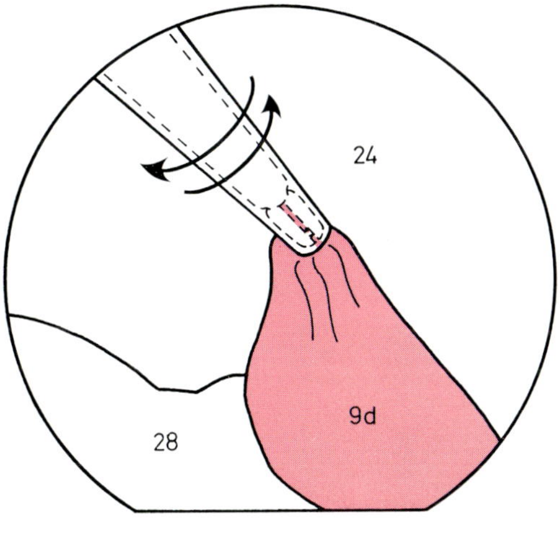
24
28
9d

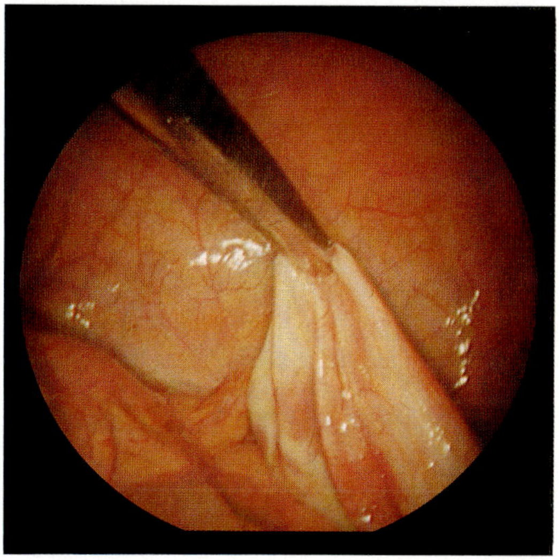

Fig. 398. After the first rather large perforation of the cyst wall, its contents are spilling out.

Through multiple biopsies with the forceps, the major part of the thin-walled cyst is removed step by step. The thick-walled parts, which still contain germinal epithelium, are allowed to remain.

Fig. 399. By means of continued, stepwise, endoscopically monitored biopsy, all the thin-walled parts of the ovarian cyst are removed.

Fig. 400. When enough of the cyst wall has been resected, coagulate the edges of the wall that may be bleeding, carefully using the high-frequency coagulator or (with greater safety) the low voltage Endotherm or Sterilization Unit. The rate of recurrence for cysts punctured and resected is less than 15 per cent.

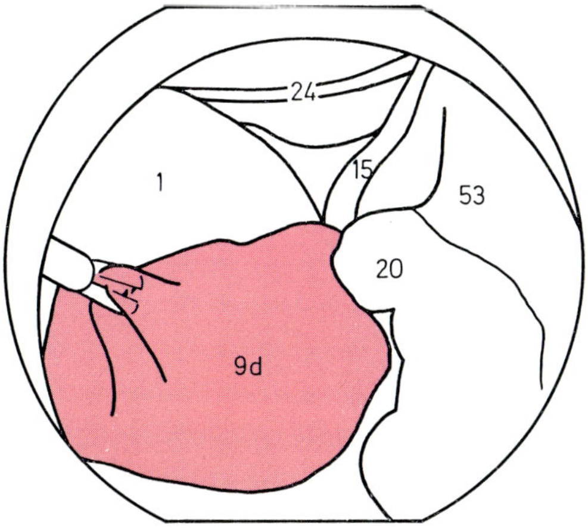
24
1
15
53
20
9d

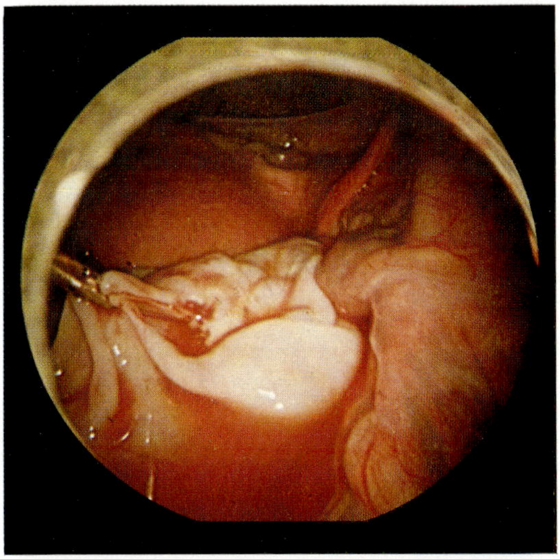

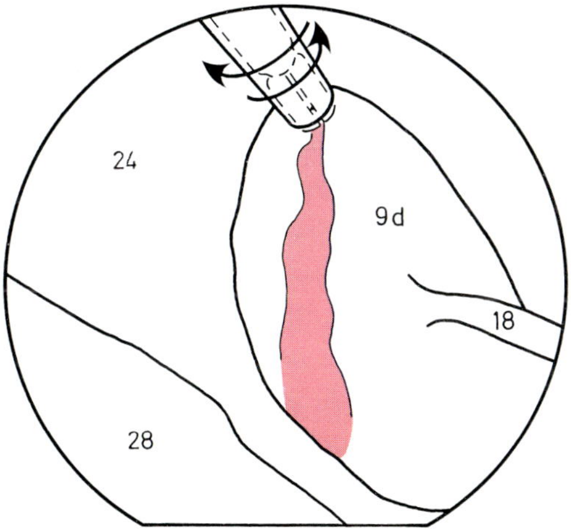
24
9d
18
28

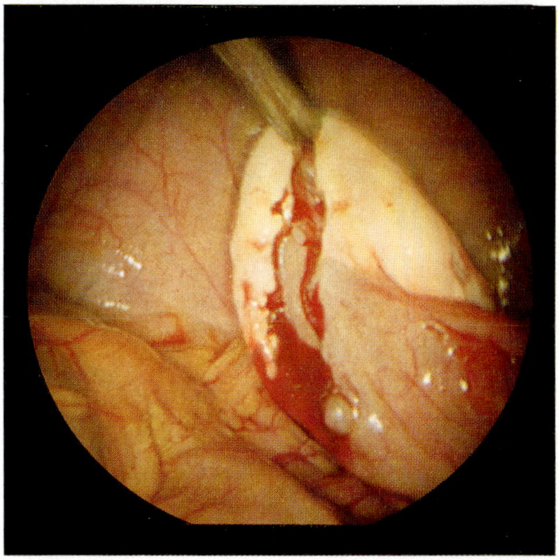

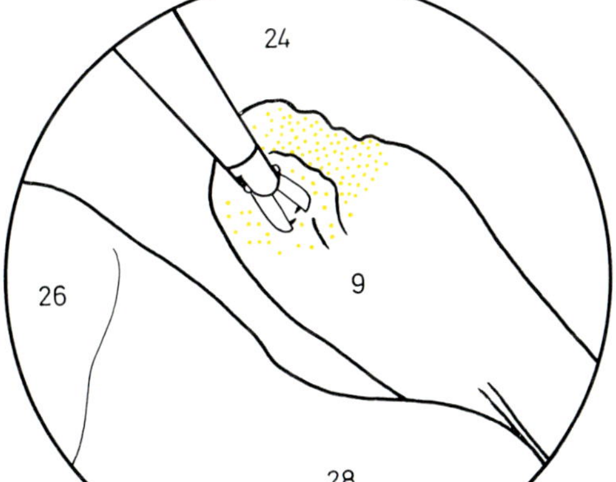
24
26
9
28

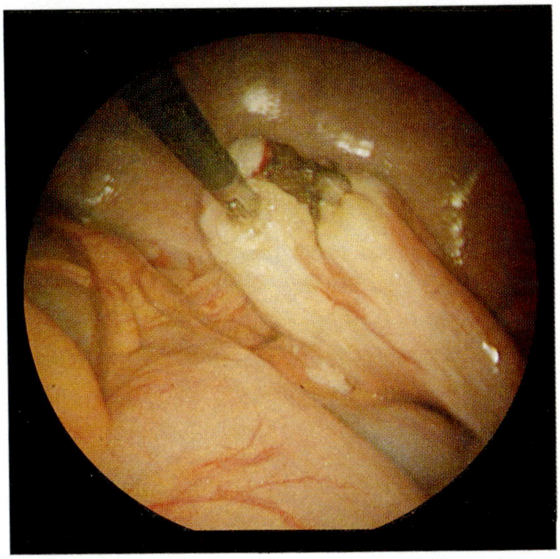

(h) Correction of Postoperative Adhesions

Fig. 401. These typical adhesions resulting from an appendectomy often give rise to obscure abdominal distress. When discovered at laparoscopy they can be cleanly severed with scissors, provided they are avascular. Here the hook scissors (Fig. 71) are starting to shear away the omental adhesions close to the parietal peritoneum.

Fig. 402. In severing such omental adhesions, a precise topographic orientation is essential. It is all too easy to slit the raised velamentous parietal peritoneum at the same time if the adhesions run too far laterally. Therefore, when dealing with such adhesions, the operator should maintain a margin of safety of at least 1 to 2 cm from the lateral abdominal wall.

Fig. 403. Postoperative adhesions on the tubes or ovaries, running between the lateral wall of the uterus and the sigmoid loop, are very common and can be severed at laparoscopy if they are nonvascular. In doing so, however, the laparoscope must be brought very close in order to monitor the topography as precisely as possible and thus obviate injury to any organs.

It must again be emphasized that such procedures should never be undertaken except with the aid of a second puncture: only in this way does the instrument have sufficient freedom of motion (see Fig. 182). With endoscopes carrying a working tube parallel to the optical system, such surgical laparoscopic manipulations are impossible for lack of three-dimensional vision and spatial control.

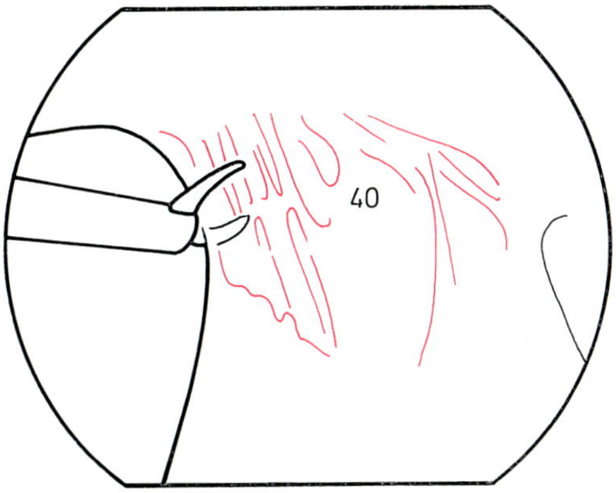
40

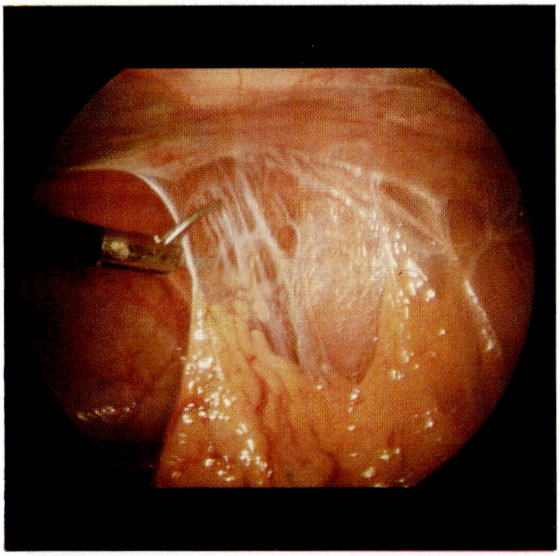

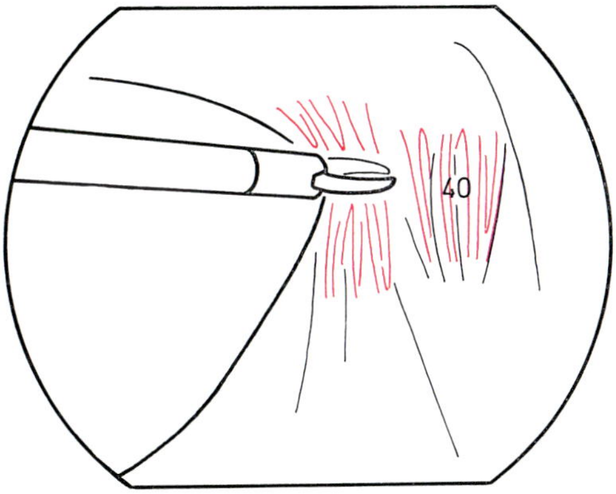
40

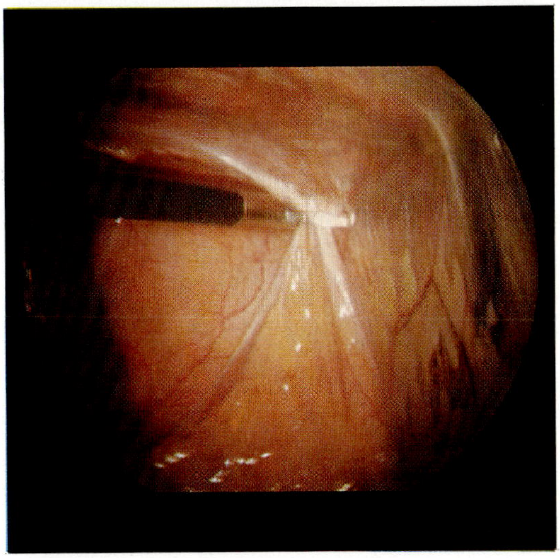

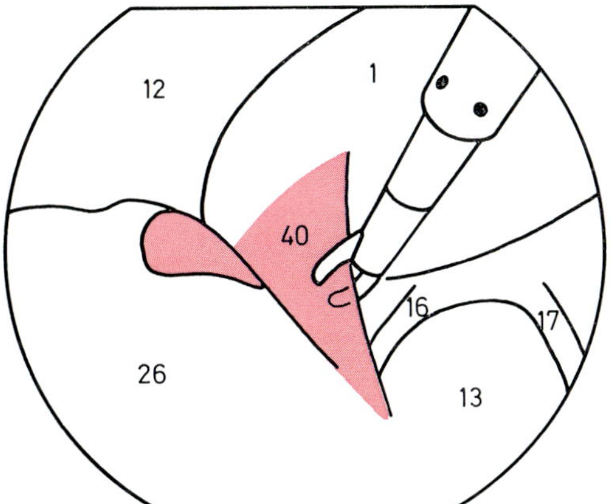
12
1
40
16
17
26
13

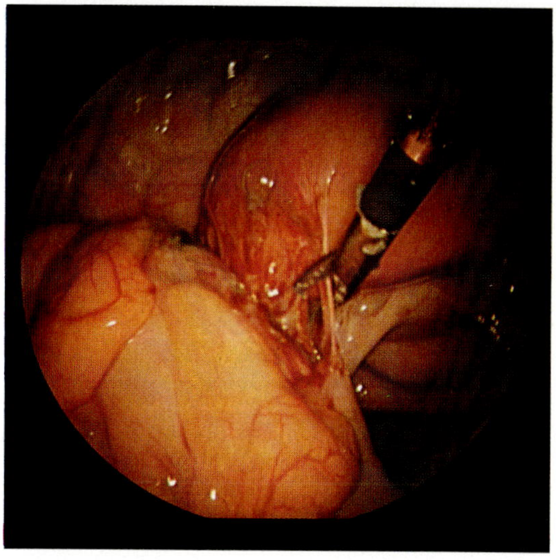

Fig. 404. Fine adhesions resulting from perisalpingitis in the adnexal region are usually nonvascular. They can be severed sharply with a snip of the hook scissors. It should be mentioned once more that these scissors (Fig. 71) are particularly well adapted by their curved jaws for the removal of fine tissue since they prevent the adhesion from sliding out when the jaws are closed.

Fig. 405. This vascular linear adhesion between the small intestine and lateral abdominal wall, almost as thick as a pencil, must not be cut until after broad coagulation in order to prevent bleeding. It must be borne in mind that high-frequency current flows along the adhesion *toward* the coagulating forceps, and naturally heats up the spot on the intestine where the adhesion is attached in addition to the adhesion itself; therefore, it is very dangerous to coagulate such adhesions by high-frequency (Figs. 97 and 98)—only low voltage should be used for coagulation, since the low voltage forceps (Fig. 345) heats up only that portion of tissue being grasped.

Fig. 406. The linear adhesion shown in Figure 405, which is vascular, is not snipped apart with the scissors until it is sufficiently coagulated. Complete hemostasis in the blood vessels of the adhesion must be monitored visually and guaranteed *before* it is severed with the hook scissors.

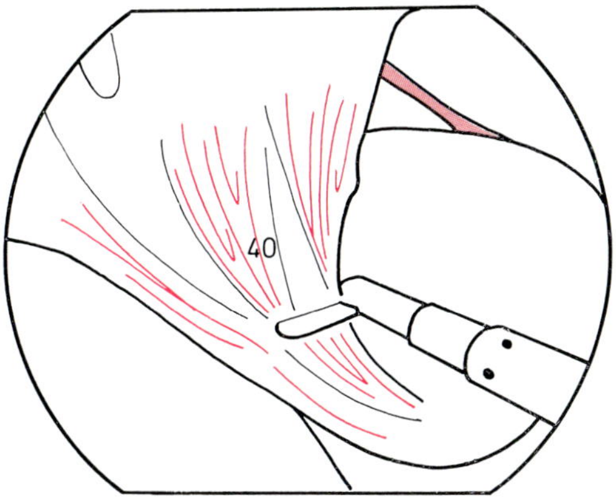
40

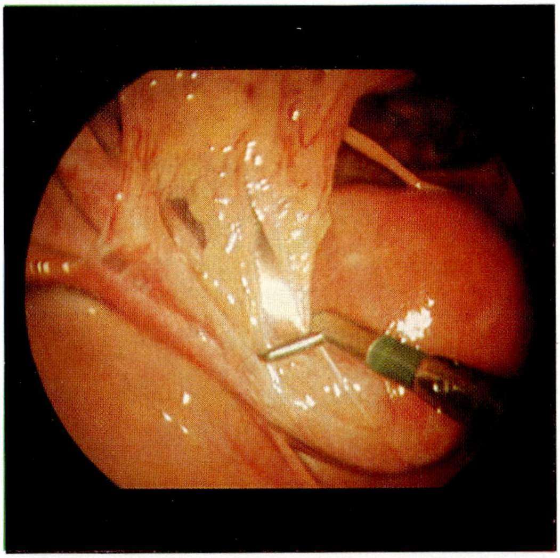

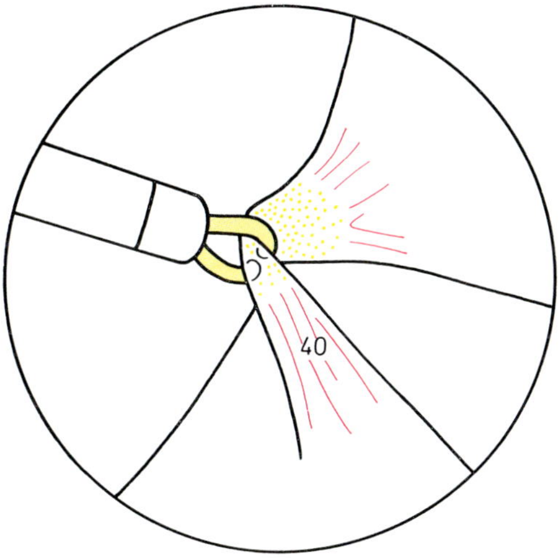
40

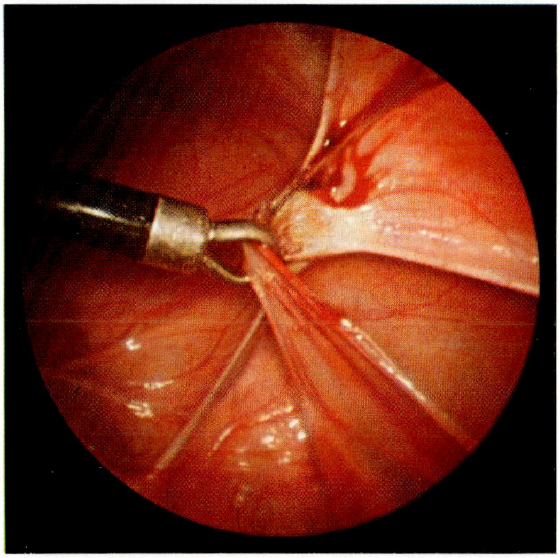

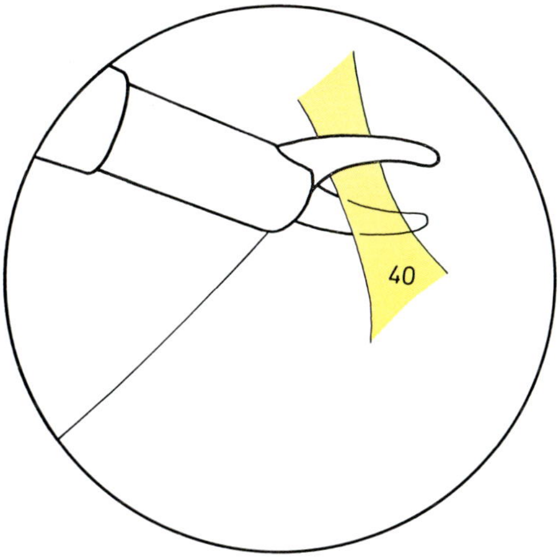
40

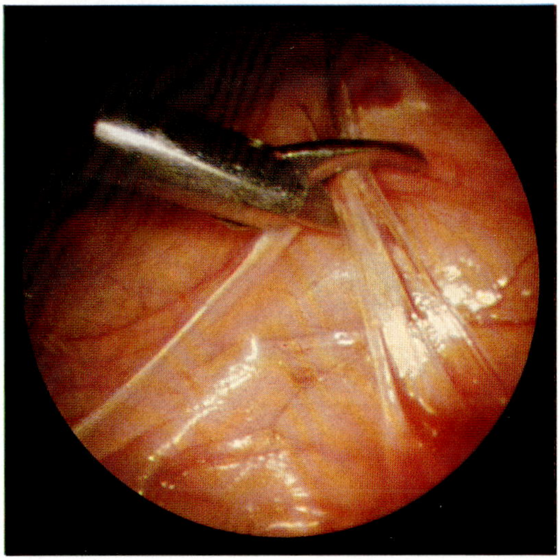

(i) Puncture of a Mature Follicle to Obtain an Ovum

Fig. 407. Upon elevation of the fallopian tube by the mesosalpinx with the atraumatic forceps, a mature follicle is revealed here on the left ovary. For diagnostic purposes regarding the tube, the latter was insufflated with blue dye.

Fig. 408. By retroflexing the uterus into the cul-de-sac with the aid of the suction intrauterine cannula, the left adnexa are well steadied between the anterior wall of the uterus and the lateral pelvic wall in the area of the pelvic brim. The puncture into the mature follicle thus is readily achieved. The ovum is extracted with the device shown in Figure 75.

Fig. 409. Sometimes there is difficulty in keeping the mature follicle in the same position long enough to puncture it and obtain the ovum. In such cases we resort to grasping the ovary with the biopsy forceps in order to aim the follicle at an angle of 90° to the insertion of the extraction cannula.

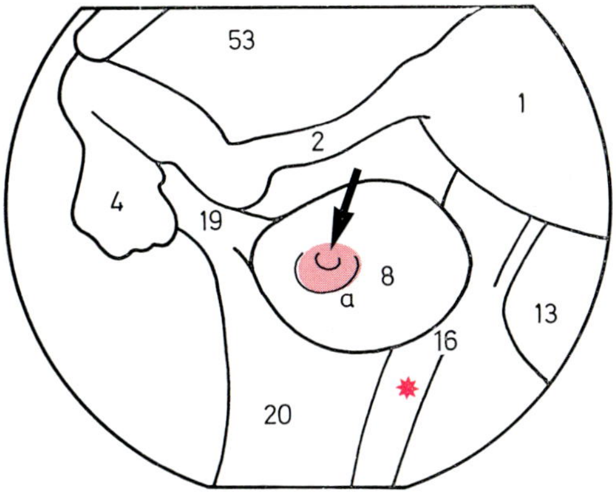
53
1
2
4
19
8
a
13
16
20

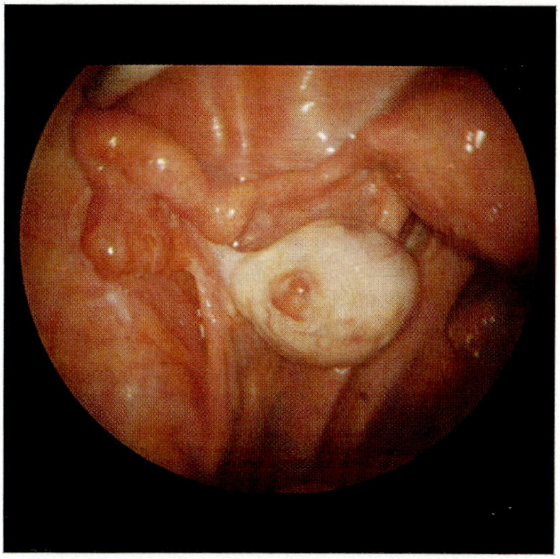

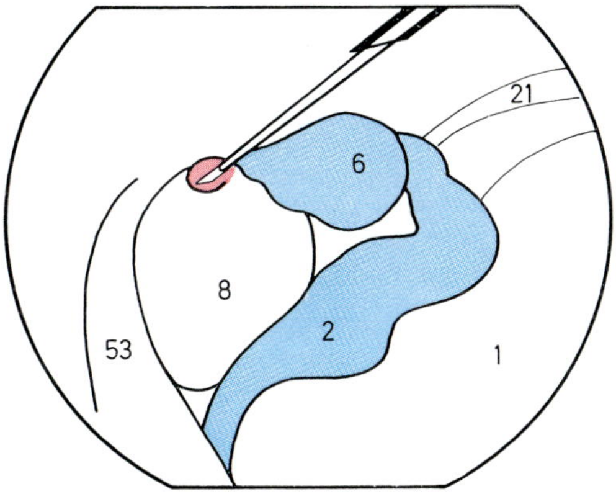
21
6
8
2
53
1

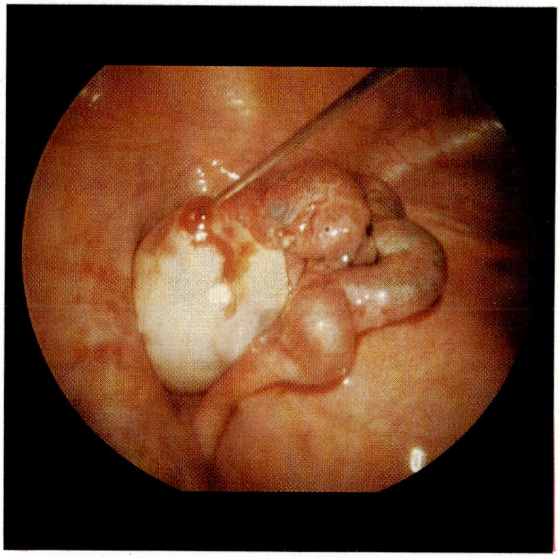

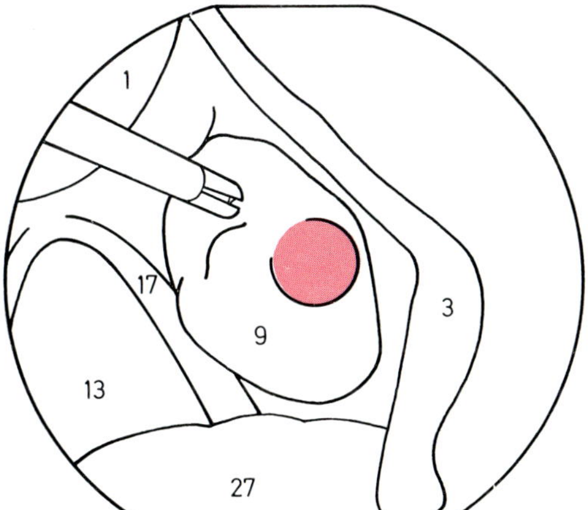
1
17
3
9
13
27

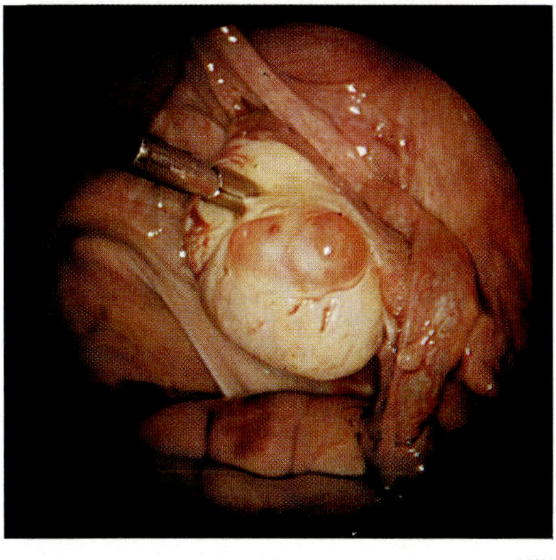

Figures 410–412 demonstrate the simultaneous extraction of two mature ova from a patient's ovary. This constitutes endoscopic proof, incidentally, of a genuine instance of double ovulation. We were able to retrieve one mature ovum from each aspirate for scientific use in research on the human ovum.

Fig. 410. Here the atraumatic forceps is taking hold of the mesosalpinx of the ovary at right angles to the puncture needle in conjunction with the lateral inclination of the uterus effected by the suction intrauterine cannula.

Fig. 411. In the same patient seen in Figure 410, the atraumatic forceps is bringing the mature follicle on the left ovary likewise into a 90° position relative to the puncture needle.

Fig. 412. The bleeding that sometimes occurs after the puncture of a mature follicle is stopped by coagulation at low voltage (see Fig. 80) or, if that is not available, high-frequency current.

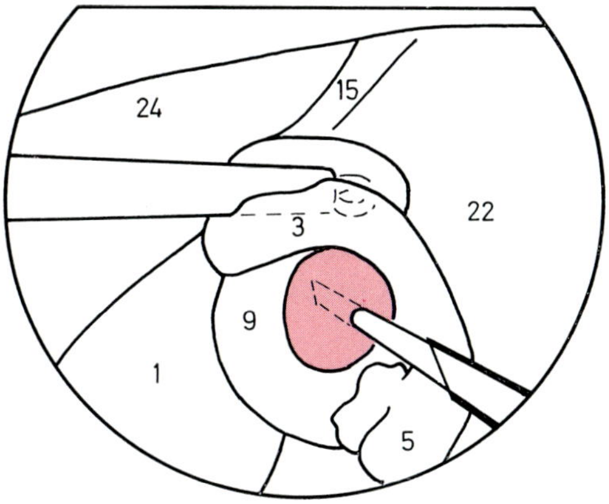
24
15
22
3
9
1
5

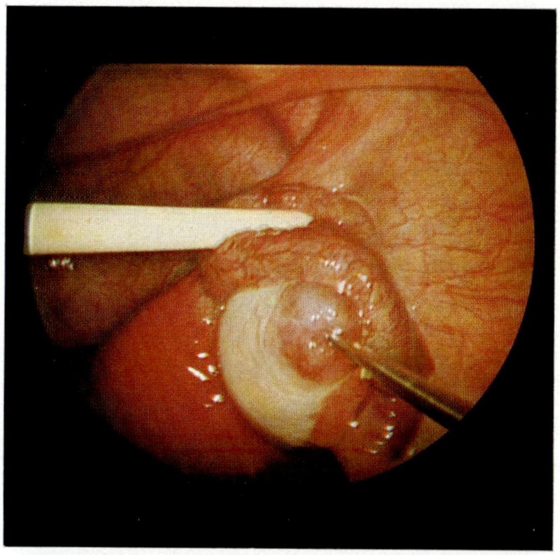

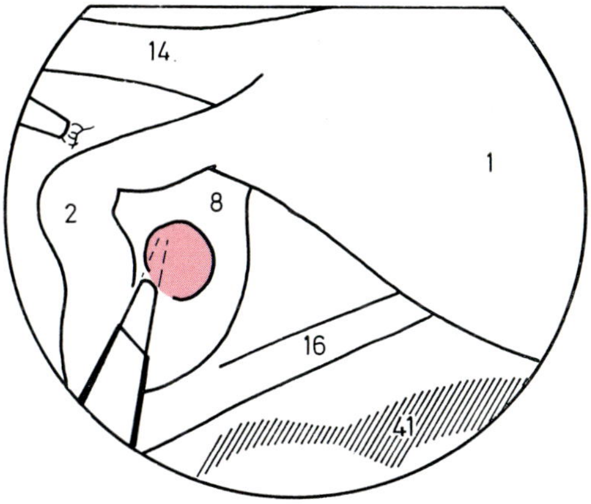
14
1
2
8
16
41

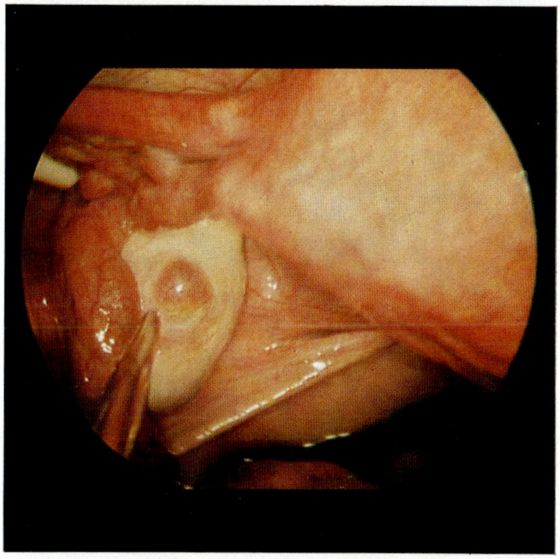

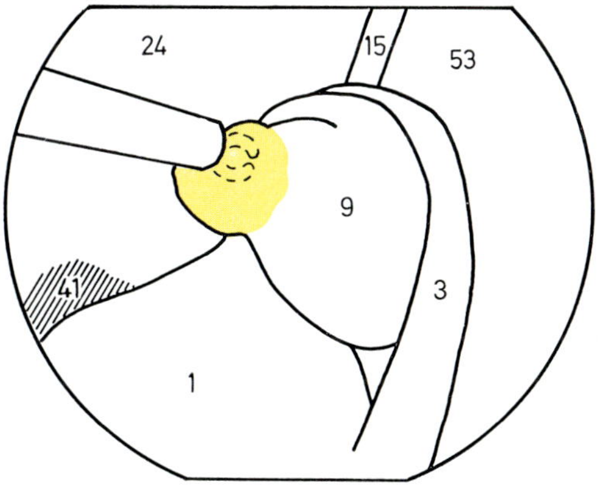
24
15
53
9
41
3
1

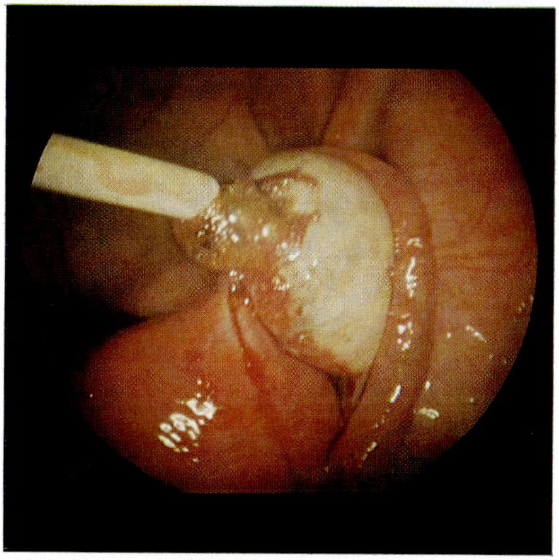

(k) *Puncture of Cysts and Aspiration of Ascites after HMG/HCG Treatment*

Fig. 413. After the administration of 2025 units of the human menopausal gonadotropin Humegon (FSH/LH) from the third to the 14th day of the menstrual cycle and 25,000 units of the human chorionic gonadotropin Predalone (LH) from the 14th to the 16th day (estrogens on the 14th day 96 μg/24 hr, on the 22nd day 2000 μg/24 hr) this excessive follicular maturation with simultaneous formation of ascites was observable in both ovaries on the 22nd day of treatment.

Fig. 414. In this patient, after administration of 1350 units of Humegon (FSH/LH) from the third to the 11th day of the menstrual cycle, and 10,000 units of Predalone (LH) on the 14th day (estrogens on the 14th day 74 μg/24 hr and on the 27th day 530 μg/24 hr), all signs of acute abdominal distress were visible 27 days after the start of treatment as a result of overstimulation of the right ovary to fist size. The left ovary remained almost unaffected by this overstimulation.

Fig. 415. The overstimulated right ovary of the patient in Figure 414 was successfully reduced to one-half its size by means of numerous punctures. The ascites and the blood were aspirated, and the acute abdominal symptoms disappeared after laparoscopy. The patient was released after four more days of observation.

The puncture at laparoscopy of ovaries overstimulated by HMG/HCG treatment and removal of the ascites is regarded by us as the method of choice when such hormone therapy produces acute abdominal distress.

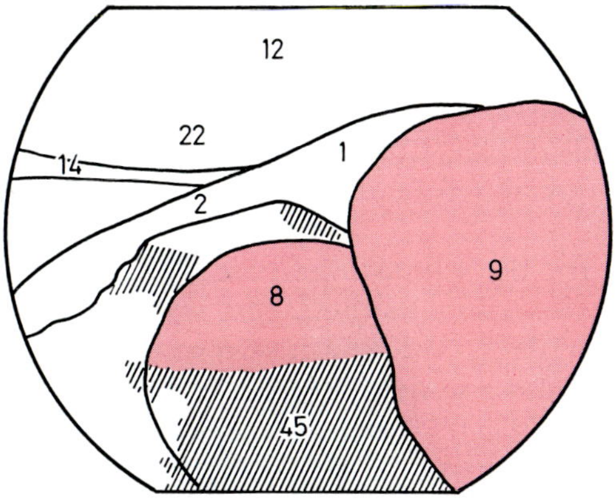
12
22
14
1
2
9
8
45

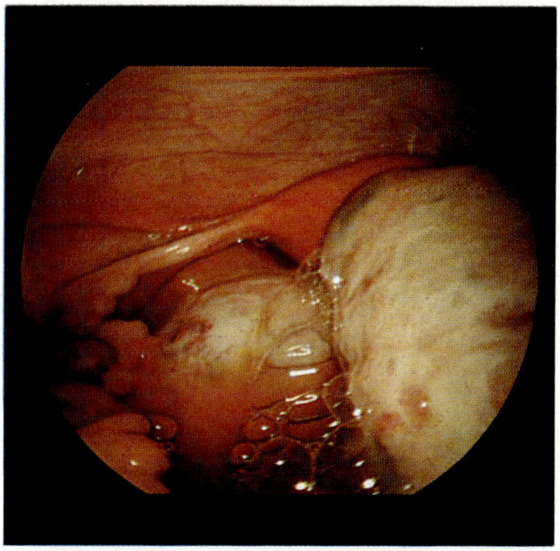

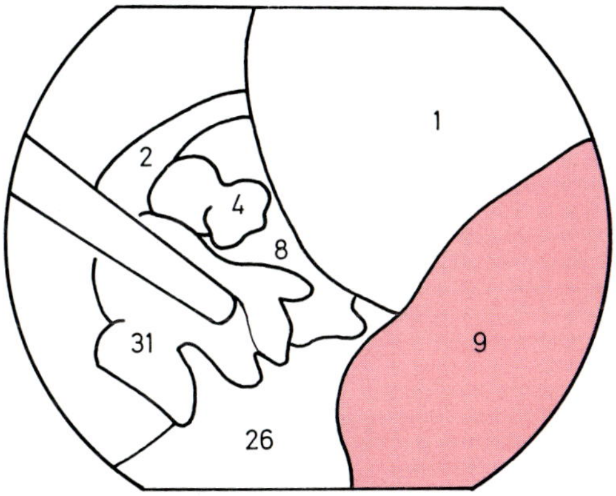
1
2
4
8
9
31
26

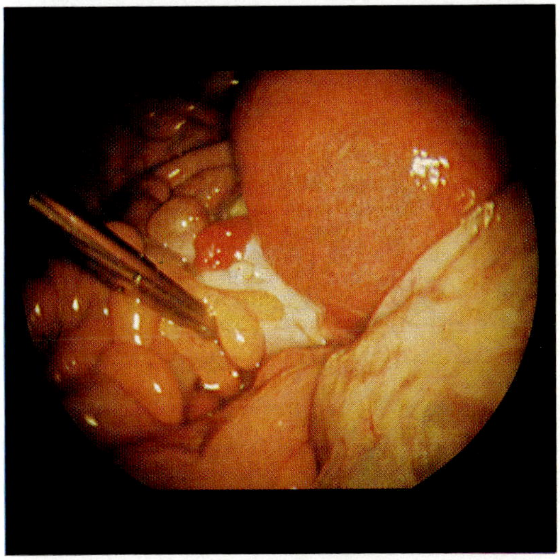

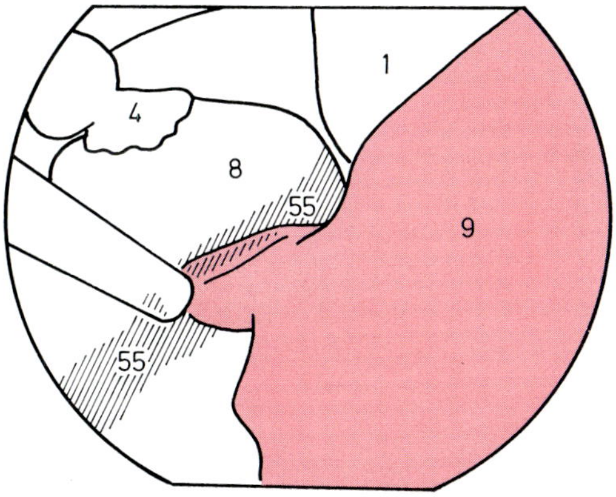
1
4
8
55
9
55

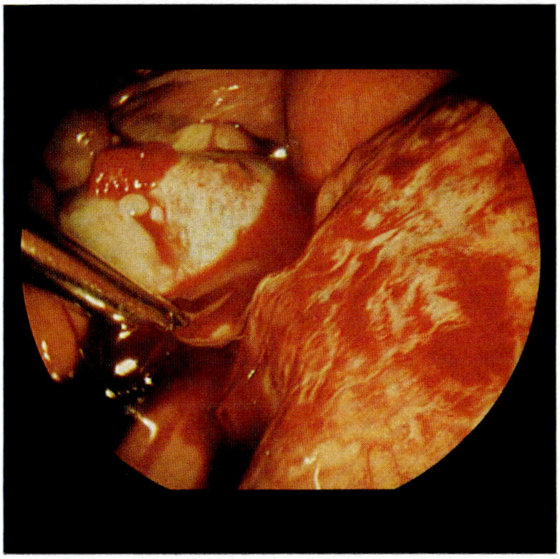

(l) Repositioning of Herniated Omentum after Laparoscopy

Fig. 416. As mentioned several times above, if the trocar is inserted in the area of the linea alba below the navel, it is possible for the non-elastic fascia to remain in an oval gap after the trocar is withdrawn. Coughing or straining can easily force the omentum or bowel into this fascial defect, and this usually leads to adhesions without clinical symptoms.

In the present case the 11 mm trocar for the cinematographic laparoscope was not inserted according to the Z-track insertion method, but was pushed through the fascia directly below the navel. On the second day the skin suture below the navel was routinely removed. Four hours later a somewhat engorged tongue of omentum larger than the distal end of a human thumb was found lying on the outside surface of the abdomen. The diagnosis was herniation of the omentum through the trocar wound located medially in the fascial region.

Fig. 417. After the diagnosis of omental herniation, a laparoscopy was performed through the second puncture in the left side of the lower abdomen (Fig. 180). This showed that the omentum was herniated out through the perforation wound made by the trocar. With the aid of the atraumatic forceps and external assistance it proved possible to reinsert the prolapsed fat. With a visually monitored penetrating suture (Fig. 181), the wound was closed. The postoperative course was free of complications.

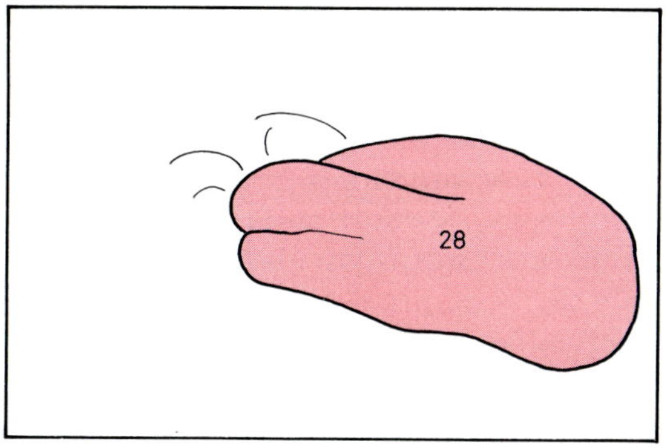
28

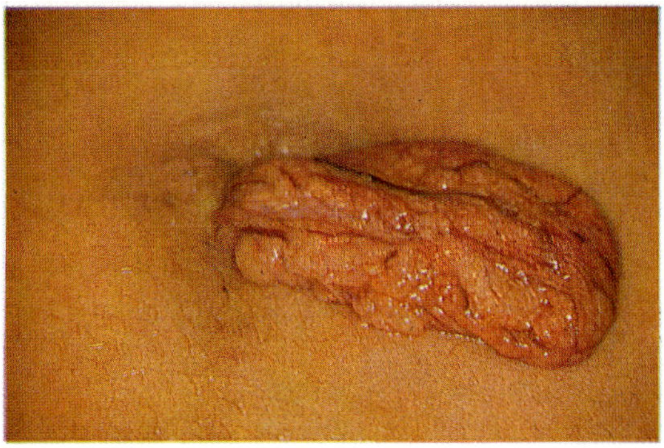

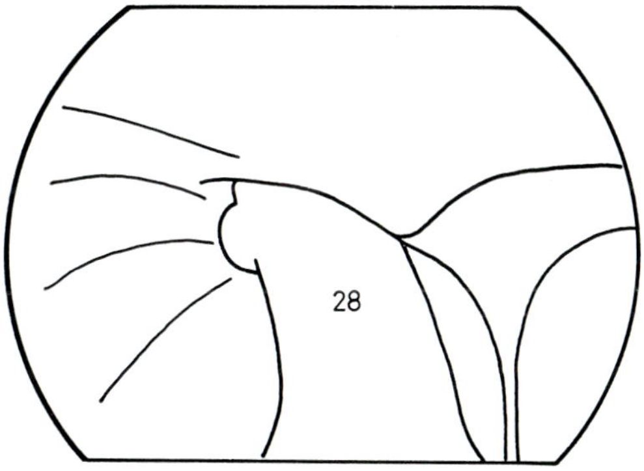
28

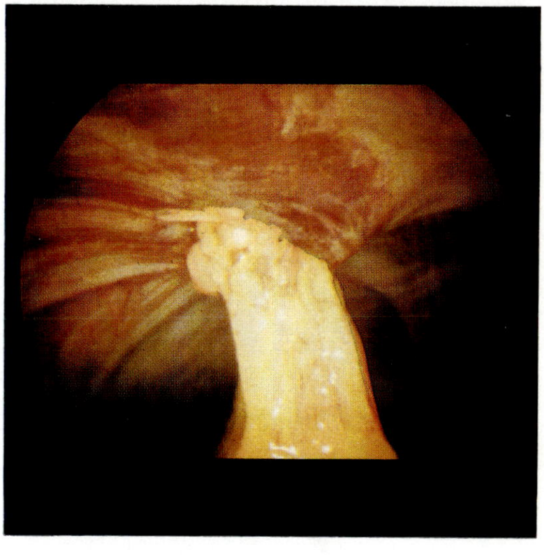

(m) *Celiotonometry*

In the early days of laparoscopy the abdomen was inflated with a volume of gas estimated according to body size. The laparoscopic procedure was then instituted by a mechanically automated insufflation of gas whose limit was set not by volume but by intra-abdominal gas pressure. Gas insufflators in use up to the present time measure simultaneously the insufflation pressure and that of the gas-bubble while the abdomen is being inflated. In other words, the "body-cavity-pressure" gauge (Fig. 54, 3) measures primarily the static pressure in the insufflation hose during inflation as long as the gas emerges from the Verres needle at 0 mm Hg. Secondarily the intra-abdominal pressure is added to this in a partially potentiating way. The measurement of static pressure is here of elementary importance since it tells at once if insufflation is encountering some resistance (e.g., vascular pressure, omental emphysema, intestinal pressure, etc.). We can read the actual intra-abdominal pressure via the manometer test (Fig. 154). This, however, requires an additional manipulation, that is, shutting off the gas, whereupon the gauge falls back to the actual pressure in the gas-bubble thus far achieved.

A reliable reading of the actual pressure at the tip of the needle, the point of introduction of the gas, is afforded by the Celiotonometer or "via falsa indicator" (Fig. 417a) in conjunction with the Semm Y-insufflation needle (Fig. 417b). The "CO_2-insufflation" gauge of the Semm insufflator (CO_2-Pneu-Automatik) (Fig. 54, 3) meanwhile shows the actual inflation pressure, while the gauge on the celiotonometer (Fig. 417a) registers the gas pressure at the point of emission from the needle. From the difference between these two pressures can be calculated the force necessary to drive the gas from the insufflator to the tip of the needle. By means of a three-way valve (Fig. 417c), the operator controls the reading and insufflation procedure. The celiotonometer affords an unbroken reading of the intra-abdominal pressure actually achieved.

The Y-insufflation needle should in future supplant the monofilar technique of measurement, since bifilar measurement at the point of emission of the gas is the optimal method of recognizing at once a false insufflation route ("via falsa"). A celiotonometer can be added to any insufflator now in use. Verres needles now in use can be equipped with an attachable three-way valve (Fig. 417c); that is, they can be adapted for its use.

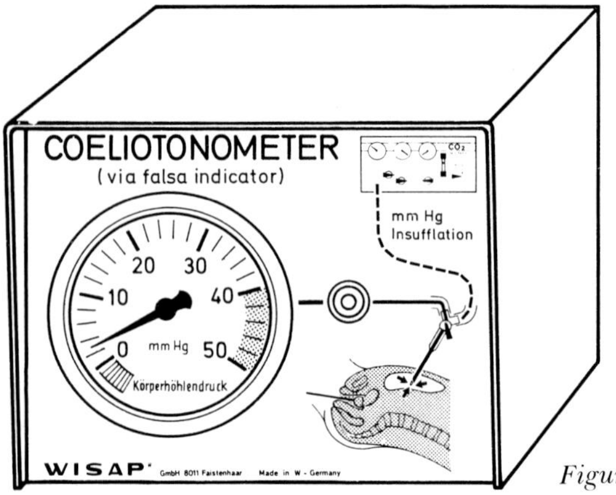

Figure 417a

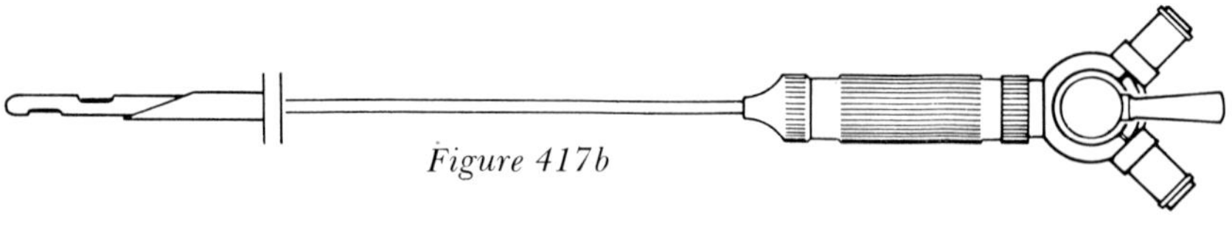

Figure 417b

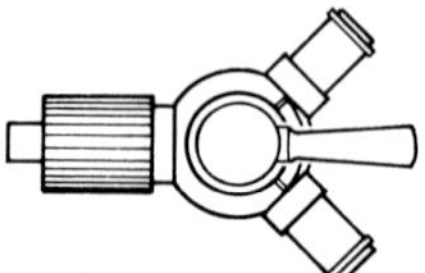

Figure 417c

B

Hysteroscopy

I
Introduction

The revolutionary improvements in optics and lighting and the renewed interest, starting with Lindemann (1971), in carbon dioxide gas insufflation for improved hysteroscopic visualization led to the development of "CO_2-hysteroscopy." It offers for the first time a reproducible procedure that provides photographic and cinematographic documentation of satisfactory quality from the uterine cavity.

CO_2 hysteroscopy initially was used only in the sense of macroscopy, i.e., magnifying glass hysteroscopy. Microhysteroscopy, further developed especially by Marleschki (1966), in which 10× to 20× magnification was made available, offers a considerably different picture of the findings as compared to macrohysteroscopy. CO_2 hysteroscopy for the first time makes it possible to observe the entire uterine cavity visually in its macroscopic structure and to capture it in still and motion pictures (full-format 16 mm film, Rimkus and Semm, 1972). Microhysteroscopy permits the study of changes in the blood vessels, and other structures in the endometrium. At present, scientific research is exploring the question whether, with the aid of this in vivo study of the endometrial structure, clinically valuable diagnoses can be reached with regard to function and changes in the endometrium.

Parallel to these instrumental and technologic improvements there were attempts to expand the uterine cavity with various transparent media (Fig. 418).

Aqueous solutions had the disadvantage of quickly becoming clouded by secretions and blood. Highly viscous solutions such as lumiscol, silicone oils, and

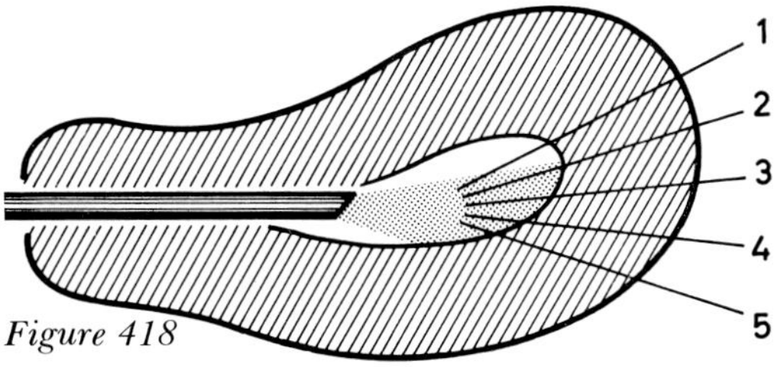

Figure 418

(1) NaCl (physiologic)
(2) Polyvinylpyrrolidone
(3) Dextran
(4) Silicone oils
(5) CO_2 gas

dextran do not afford consistently good visibility, and there are many problems connected with their use. A gaseous medium has all the advantages of clear visibility, but shows a tendency to pass through the tubes into the abdomen, creating a risk of emboli.

Only after the development of sophisticated mechanisms was it possible to develop an apparatus utilizing carbon dioxide that was free from the above disadvantages of gas insufflation. Figure 419 shows the Semm hysteroscopic insufflator.

The following physical considerations influenced the construction of this instrument. The uterine cavity has an average length of about 7 cm, including the cervical canal, and an internal surface of 8 to 16 square cm. On the basis of physical experimentation by Fikentscher and Semm in 1956, the dilation pressure of the cavity was found to be about 50 mm Hg. Figure 420 demonstrates the start of insufflation with carbon dioxide gas. The arrow indicates elevation of the machine-produced pressure of 50 mm Hg to 100 mm Hg, signifying increasing dilatation of the uterine cavity.

On the basis of physical pressure conditions (the ratio of surface area of the

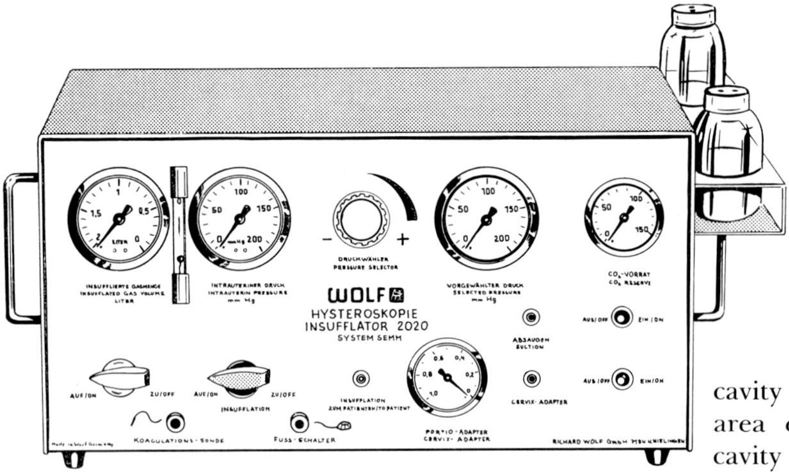

Figure 419

cavity to the cross-section area of the tubal os), the cavity distends before the oviducts open. The total force of dilation on the muscle of the uterus is between 0.6 and 1.6 kg, depending on size. From these properties the formula was derived on which the gas dilation of the uterine cavity must be based for hysteroscopy:

"Constant volume at variable pressure."

The hysteroscopic insufflator constructed on this basis makes it possible to dilate the cavity with carbon dioxide gas and to inspect it without the gas escaping through the oviducts.

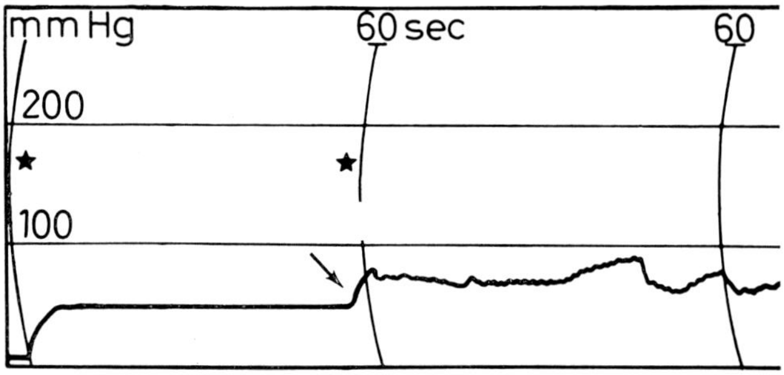

Figure 420

If higher pressures are employed, the physical laws shown in Figure 421 come into play. According to these, the gas volume (1) flowing into the cavity must always be greater than the possible outflow (2) through the two oviducts, in order to maintain the pressure supplied by the apparatus (3) in the uterine cavity (4). But then gas flow volumes in liters would occur, according to the gas flow law of Poiseuille,* and this would be impractical for hysteroscopy, since after about

$$*W = \frac{(P_1 - P_2) \cdot r^4 \cdot t}{l \cdot n}$$

in which W = amount of gas flow, r = radius of the conducting tube, l = length of this tube, $(P_1 - P_2)$ = difference in pressure, n = viscosity (force of cohesion), t = time.

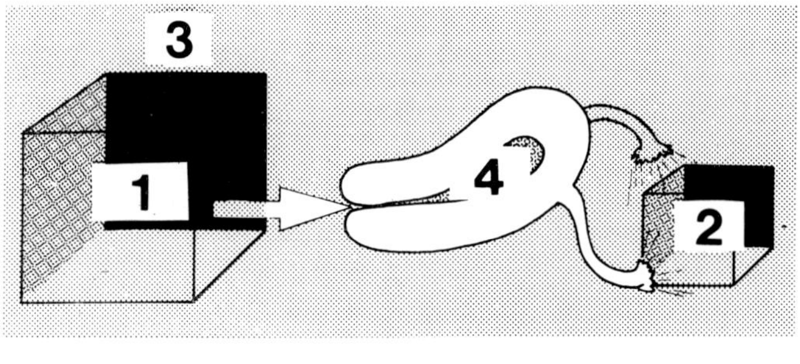

Figure 421

five to ten minutes of hysteroscopy a pneumoperitoneum would be produced equal to that used in laparoscopy.

With such high flow-through volumes, even when employing CO_2 gas, there is

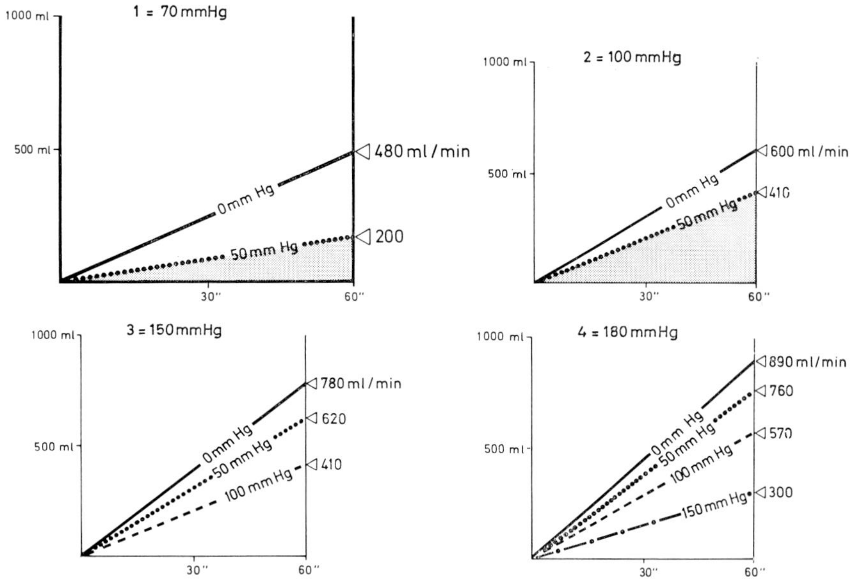

Fig. 422. In 1, 2, 3, and 4 the same uterus-oviduct model was insufflated. The CO_2 gas flows out either against the free atmospheric pressure (0 mm Hg) or against a tubal and intra-abdominal resistance of 0 to 150 mm Hg. Depending on the maximum preselected pressure, ranging from a possible 70 to 180 mm Hg, the flow-through volume per minute increases.

danger to the patient of gas emboli. This makes itself evident in increasing tachycardia upon intravascular intrusion of CO_2 gas, and it can be detected early on the electrocardiogram.

In order completely to eliminate such danger during hysteroscopy, the flow-through of carbon dioxide in the hysteroscopic insufflator is limited to 100 ml/min. Even if all this volume of gas enters the bloodstream, it constitutes no danger to the patient. Human tolerance to carbon dioxide insufflation with intravascular absorption was stated independently by Lindemann and Palmer in 1973 to be 200 ml/min.

The technologically refined hysteroscopic instruments of today, in conjunction with the carbon dioxide gas control unit developed especially for them, afford the opportunity for routine inspection of the uterine cavity. Scientific interest is predominant in this matter. To what extent hysteroscopy will also acquire significance in routine clinical diagnostic procedures cannot yet be predicted in these initial stages.

Especially under discussion at the moment is transuterine tubal sterilization by coagulation of the internal tubal os, extensively attempted and histologically investigated as early as 1916 by Dickinson and in 1929 by Mikulicz-Radecki in an experiment in rabbits with successful optically-monitored extraction of an early pregnancy by suction. Recently Lindemann obtained significant experimental data concerning sealing of the intramural portion of the tubes, not by thermal coagulation, but rather by the necrotizing effect of tissue adhesives such as methyl$_2$–cyano–acrylate.

II

Risks and Dangers in CO_2 Hysteroscopy

The risks and dangers connected with dilation of the cavity by the use of carbon dioxide gas can be stated briefly:

(1) Danger of intravascular insufflation of gas;

(2) Possible intrusion of bacteria;

(3) Possible injury to the uterus through dilation and probing.

Remarks:

On (1): In a normal insufflation of the oviducts for diagnostic purposes, using the Universal Insufflator (Fikentscher and Semm) and the atraumatic flexible cervical adapter (Fig. 423), a vascular lesion is exceptionally rare. Because of the traumatic dilation of the cervical canal prior to a hysteroscopy, however, possible vascular damage can never be ruled out. Tangentially opened blood vessels are especially liable to pick up and pass on gas being insufflated into the cavity (see

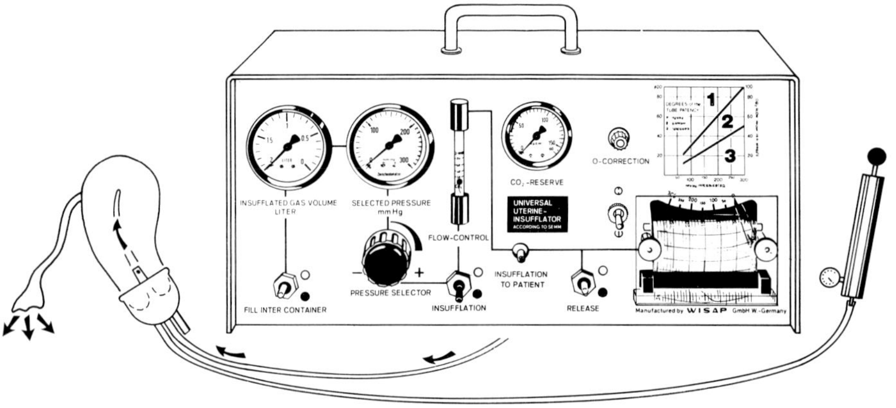

Figure 423

also Fig. 299). A hysteroscopy with CO_2 gas insufflated in an uncontrolled amount and pressure therefore involves a life-threatening risk of emboli for the patient.

On (2): With a transvaginal procedure and dilation of the uterus, it is impossible to keep bacteria from ascending with the dilators and hysteroscope, being carried along into the cavity, and possibly finding their way via the tubes into the cul-de-sac. This danger cannot yet be avoided in the present state of the technique. Hysteroscopy therefore requires the same restrictive precautions that have been obligatory for decades for tubal insufflation:

(1) Control of the vaginal flora by preoperative treatment of the vagina with local sulfonamides or other antibiotics;

(2) Observing the patient for evidence of febrile illness;

(3) Blood work, including sedimentation rate.

In addition, top priority must be given to asepsis of the instruments throughout the procedure itself.

On (3): Unfortunately a dilation of the cervical canal to a size 8 Heger is still necessary for employment of the hysteroscopic instruments presently available. In the course of the probing of the cavity that must precede this procedure, there is the usual danger of trauma to the uterus common to such gynecologic interventions, namely, perforation, laceration of the cervix, etc. The hysterophotograph in Figure 448 shows the traumatizing effect of even simple contact by the dilator against the endometrium in the fundal area.

The danger to the patient mentioned under point 3 is less than the general risk of any gynecologic vaginal operation, and is not a valid reason for special condemnation of this technique if all indicators are strictly observed.

III
Hysteroscopic Instruments

1. THE OPTIC FOR HYSTEROSCOPY

The structural principles for the optic are the same in hysteroscopy as in laparoscopy. They vary slightly in different makes (Storz is the same as the Hopkins optic, (Fig. 424), and Wolf as the Lumina optic, (Fig. 425) and all are fitted with the cold light fiberoptic equipment now regarded as standard. These optics are about 30 cm long and give a direct forward view (0° or 180°) or a 30° or 150° angle (Fig. 40).

The smallness of the cavity is a great handicap, making it all but impossible to avoid contact with the endometrium by the lens, which in consequence is usually smeared. A sort of "windshield-wiper" effect (Fig. 426) in the Lumina model affords some help here. In this, the CO_2 gas escapes in a fine stream through a ring-shaped slit encircling the lens and tends to keep it clean. The lens need be withdrawn for cleaning only in case of heavy smearing.

The sheath surrounding the optic (Fig. 427,1) can also be fitted with a working cannula (Fig. 427,2) for ancillary instruments (p. 271), and in the Wolf model likewise serves for transmission of the CO_2 gas for the "windshield-wiper" effect. In the Hopkins model the gas enters through the adapter shaft (Fig. 428).

In place of the trocar used in laparoscopy, a vacuum cervical adapater is required in order to make the system leak-proof. It is available in various sizes (Fig. 429) to fit different sized cervices. The adapter is placed under suction on the cervix, thus assuring a gas-tight seal to permit inflation of the cavity, which

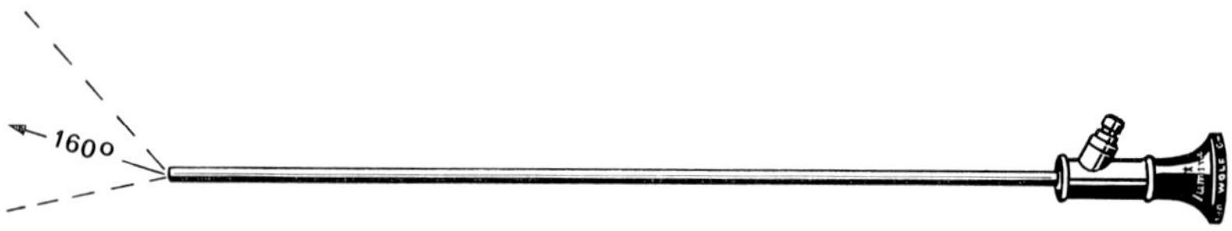

Figure 424

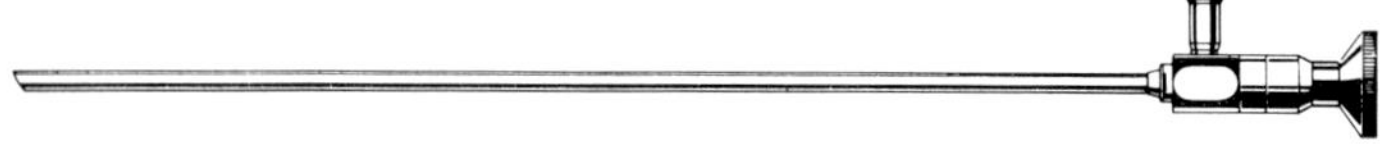

Figure 425

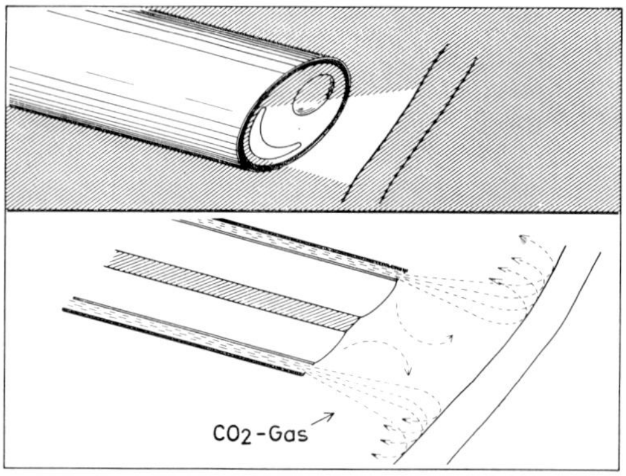

Figure 426

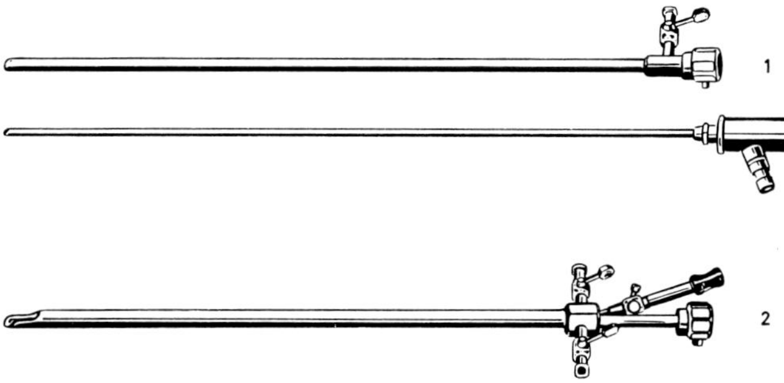

Figure 427

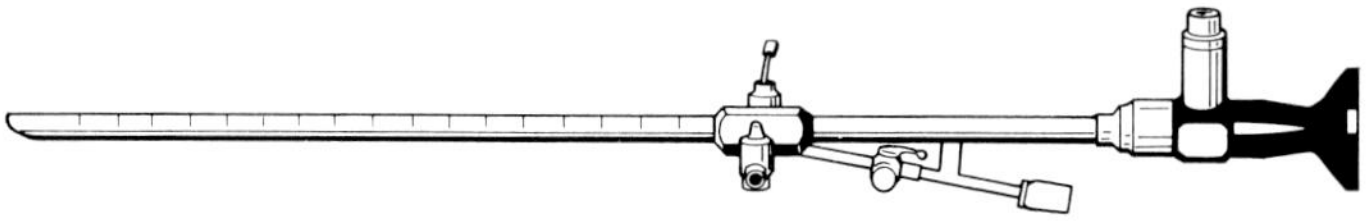

Figure 428

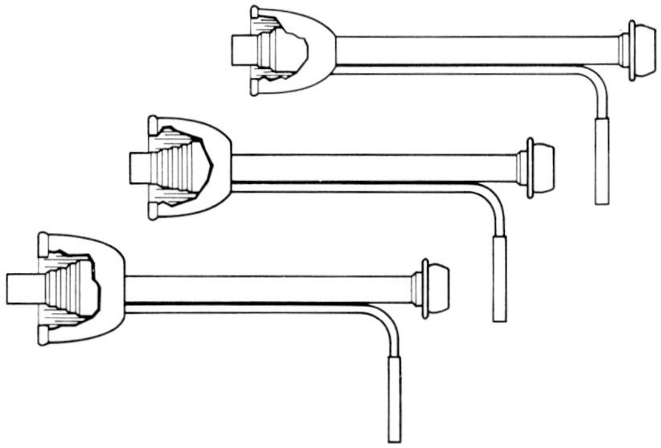

Figure 429

has become routine since the introduction in 1953 of the cervical adapter for insufflation of the oviducts (Fikentscher and Semm).

2. THE HYSTEROSCOPIC LIGHT

The modern technique of hysteroscopy did not become possible until the introduction of fiberoptics in endoscopy. Illumination of the cavity now presents no visual or photographic difficulties (see Chap. 4A, Section 2).

3. THE PNEUMO- OR HYDROMETRA

Because of the fear of transtubal bacterial invasion, expansion of the cavity was carried out for decades exclusively with high viscosity fluids, which to a greater or lesser extent resisted intrusion into the tubes.

All the fluids tried (Fig. 418), however, afforded an optically unsatisfactory image. There is now a real hope of progress in hysteroscopy through the use, not of a fluid but a gas, as is shown here with CO_2 hysteroscopy.

After several years of development a hysteroscopic insufflator is now available (Fig. 430) which permits hysteroscopic inspection of the cavity without at the same time insufflating the tubes. This technique became possible through exploitation of the natural conditions whereby less pressure is needed for expanding the cavity, because of its greater internal surface area, than is needed to dilate the far smaller os and lumen of the tubes.

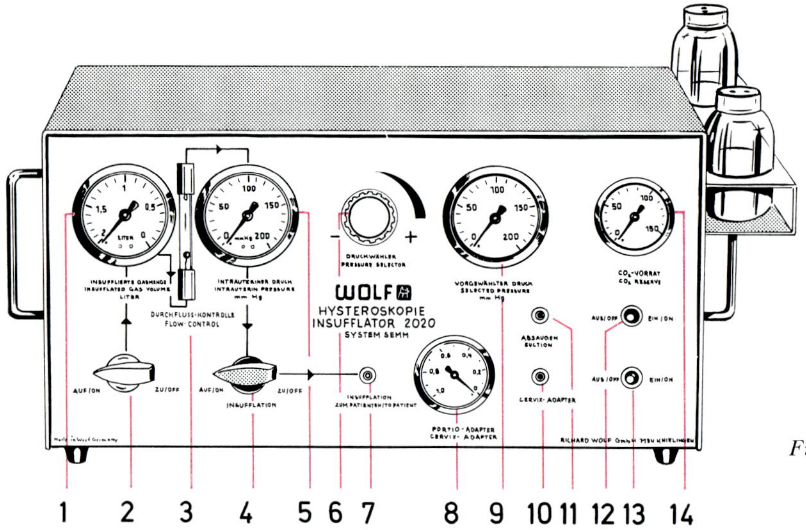

Figure 430

1. Dial showing quantity of gas used (somewhat the same as the intra-abdominal gas bubble).
2. Valve for filling the insufflation container (max. 2 liters for safety).
3. Flow-through indicator, calibrated 0 to 100 ml/min.
4. Valve for liberation of gas into the cavity.
5. Dial for continuous monitoring of intrauterine pressure.
6. Knob for pressure selection (10 to 180 mm Hg) with dial indicating preselected pressure.
7. Hose connection for uterine insufflation.
8. Dial showing negative pressure to indicate proper suction placement of cervical adapter.
9. Dial showing preselection insufflation pressure.
10. Hose connection for cervical adapter.
11. Hose connection for aspirator pump.
12. Switch for aspirator pump (blood, mucus, etc.).
13. Switch for vacuum pump (cervical adapter).
14. Dial for monitoring CO_2 reserve.

The hysteroscopic insufflator works according to the principle of "*constant volume, variable pressure—100 ml/min at 0 to 200 mm Hg.*" This was achieved by the possibility of presetting the hysteroscopic insufflator for any pressure between 10 and 180 mm Hg. Thus, independently of the resistance to gas flow, the maximum volume input is limited to a constant 100 ml/min. In other words, the gas inflow is always stopped automatically when the preselected pressure is attained in the system and the dilation of the uterus is achieved.

Thus, if a blood vessel is injured through dilation of the cervical canal, no more than a maximum of 100 ml of CO_2 gas per minute can possibly escape intravascularly, a quantity that carries with it no danger of emboli in the human body.

Recently, Lindemann (New Orleans, 1973) recommended a new hysteroscopic insufflator that works on exactly the opposite principle, namely, *constant pressure with variable volume.* Here the apparatus is permanently set for a maximum pressure of 200 mm Hg. The flow-through volume can be set for any rate from 0 to 100 ml/min and can be read on an electrovolumeter. Depending on the volume-per-minute setting, and independently of time, according to this principle a pressure is produced in the cavity of up to a maximum of 200 mm Hg, provided the gas flow is not shut off sooner manually. With this method a patent tube is invariably opened, since the operator cannot constantly regulate by hand the necessary gas replenishment in the range of the slight difference between the pressure needed to dilate the cavity and that needed for dilation of the tubes. Manual control is theoretically possible but is not practicable in fact, since the operator's attention would be overburdened and distracted from his main task, the hysteroscopy itself.

An apparatus constructed on the opposite principle of "constant volume with variable pressure," however, automatically turns off the gas when the preselected pressure is reached.

Since, in every hysteroscopy, negative pressure both for the cervical adapter bell and for rinsing the cavity is needed simultaneously, the hysteroscopic insufflator includes separate vacuum pumps for these two functions. The secure placement of the suction adapter bell on the cervix can be monitored on its respective dial. Glass jars safely collect the aspirate from the cavity for subsequent histologic examination.

The liquid media tested for dilation of the uterus during the period of development of hysteroscopy are no longer worthy of consideration. No liquid medium gave endoscopic visibility comparable to that afforded by the pneumometra.

4. AUXILIARY INSTRUMENTS FOR HYSTEROSCOPY

The guide shafts in hysteroscopes permit the introduction of only very slender ancillary instruments such as have been commonly used in gastrointestinal endoscopy. A biopsy forceps for histologic preparation of the tissue successfully visualized (as in colposcopy) is of interest for the study of the endometrium. For endocrine and particularly for immunologic research in the reproductive process, CO_2 hysteroscopy for the first time offers the chance of aspiration of tubal and endometrial secretions during various phases of the menstrual cycle. In the field of research in human reproduction, hysteroscopy can bring to light new knowledge about immunology.

Dickinson as early as 1916 attempted to seal off the tubal lumina by intrauterine cautery, calling his technique in 1929 "sterilization without unsexing."

Lindemann (1972) tested a high-frequency probe for coagulation of the intramural portion of the tube for the purpose of transuterine sterilization. Owing to the limitations of the system, the probe can be only 1 to 1.5 mm in diameter and 1 cm long. It is difficult on a surface this small to create a sufficient electrical

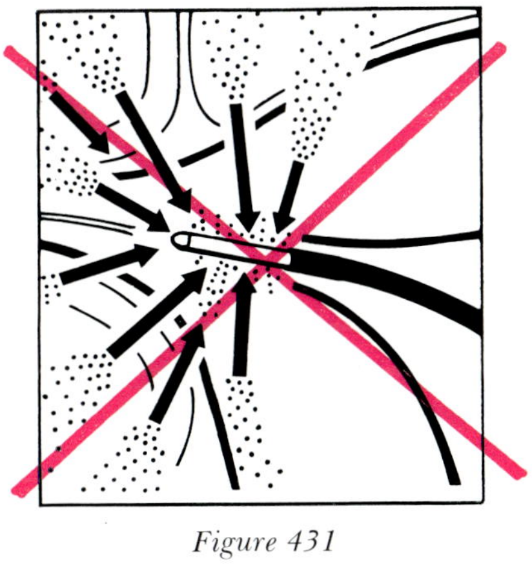

Figure 431

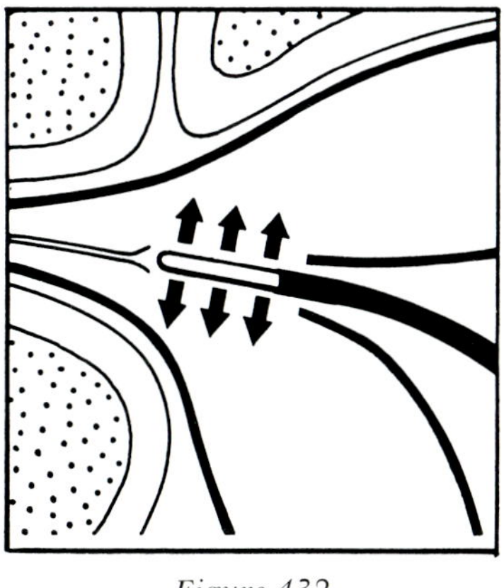

Figure 432

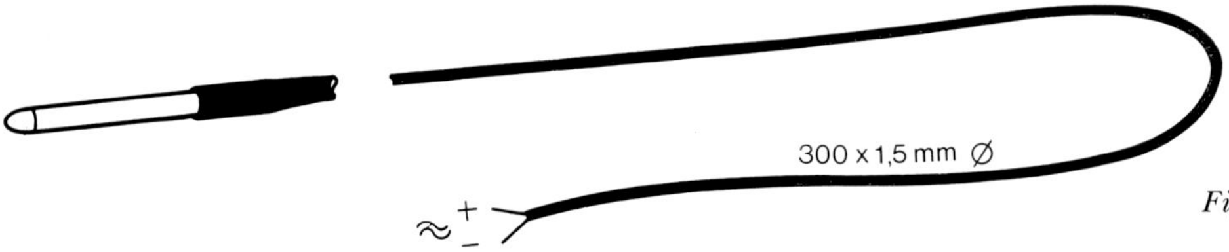

Figure 433

field density to denature by heat an adequate cylinder of tissue without giving rise to exsiccation of the neighboring tissue. Exsiccation leads to simultaneous electrical insulation of the active probe, which thus automatically cuts out the coagulation process. Therefore, a regulated and successful cylinder of coagulation, uniform at all points, cannot be achieved by the use of high-frequency current (see previous discussions on the uncontrollability of high-frequency current).

Moreover, this high-frequency probe involves the calculated risk that the main current may be drawn from the bowel that lies in direct contact with the point of tubal attachment to the uterus (Fig. 431), the intestines being excellent conductors because of their highly electrolytic contents. Field intensifications can build up at the point of transfer from the intestinal contents through the intestinal wall, causing secondary burn necroses (see also Fig. 98). The idea of trying to eliminate the possibility of such intestinal burns by putting a plastic tip on the tubal probe is sheer nonsense from the electrophysical point of view. In addition, the high-frequency coagulation probe has the disadvantage that, after the coagulation of the first tube, it is encrusted with hardened mucus and tissue, so that when it is inserted into the second tubal orifice this encrustation reduces the conductivity and, therefore, the coagulation effect.

On the other hand, the coagulation of a tissue cylinder of uniform length and diameter is possible with the Semm coagulation probe, heated from within and under controlled temperature and duration of burn (Fig. 432). This probe (Fig. 433) is a further development of the Thermoprobe developed by Semm in 1963 for the therapy of endocervicitis (Coagulator for Treatment of Benign Portio-erosion, 1963). After its introduction this probe was developed further by Hegemann in 1968 for the treatment of inoperable carcinoma of the esophagus (Wittrin, 1973). An insulating cap at the tip of this probe has proved its value, since the heat generated in the interior of the probe is prevented by the cap from radiating distally. The heat produced in the interior of the cylindric probe emanates only radially, so that if a probe is introduced a little too close to the peritoneal coating of the uterus (Fig. 471) it has no distal heating effect at its tip.

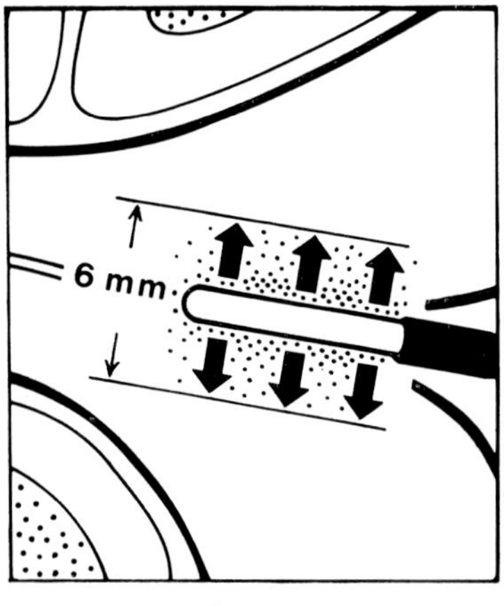

Figure 434

However, the principle should be stressed that transuterine tubal sterilization at hysteroscopy is still in its experimental stage, and cannot be recommended at present as a routine method of sterilization.

In the future it is hoped that a technique will be developed for complete tubal occlusion, but at present there is no experimental series that demonstrates this.

5. HYSTEROSCOPIC COAGULATION CURRENT

In Chapter IVA, Section 8b, we stated that high-frequency current has not stood the test of time for hysteroscopy. This can be ascribed chiefly to the reduced size of the active electrodes. In addition, the field intensification around the electrode is produced irregularly because of the irregular electrolytic content of its immediate environment. For this reason, the surface of the electrode rapidly becomes encrusted with exsiccated tissues. This incrustation produces an insulating effect that is not hysteroscopically controllable. Thus, a successful therapeutic effect, as (for example) the creation of a cylinder of coagulation of equal dimensions in each of the tubes, is not possible with high-frequency current.

The low voltage Endotherm, as described in Chapter IV, Sec. 8c, has proved its value as the source of electric current for hysteroscopy. With a potential below 6 volts and at not over 2 to 5 watts, all coagulation procedures that have become necessary to date for hysteroscopic purposes in the cavity and uterine musculature have been performed without any harm to the patient. The electronic regulator continuously measures the effective temperature of the probe as it lies in the tubal canal. The preset coagulation temperature regulates this heating current. The coagulated cylinder of tissue is consistently reproducible, depending on wattage and duration. Figure 434 shows this in the sketch. Figure 468 documents the size of the coagulation effect of 5 watts and 20 seconds' duration.

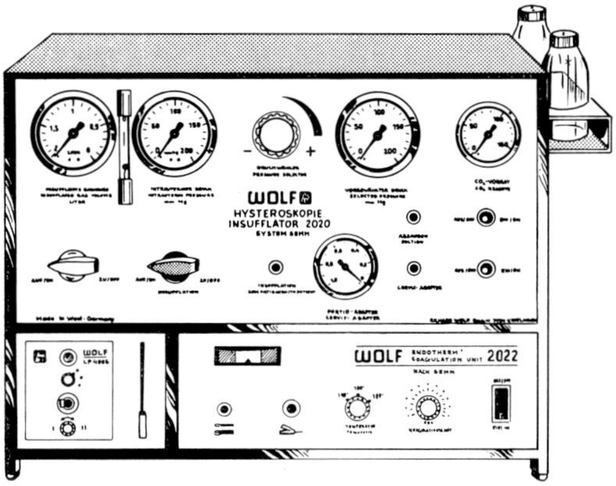

Figure 435

6. CARE OF THE HYSTEROSCOPIC INSTRUMENTARIUM

For the care and sterilization of hysteroscopic instruments see that for laparoscopic instruments in Chapter IV, Sec. 10.

7. COMBINATION HYSTEROSCOPIC APPARATUS

The gradual development of hysteroscopy has led to a proliferation of apparatus: light source for the optic; hysteroscopic insufflator for dilation of the cavity; high-frequency generator or the more recent power sources for tubal sterilization. In acquiring new equipment for hysteroscopy, a combination unit is recommended (Fig. 435) to collect all these power sources in a single housing: CO_2 gas under controlled pressure and volume, coagulation current, light, and vacuum suction. For adaptation to its several applications this combination apparatus can either be mounted on a cart or be wall-mounted (Figs. 107–110).

8. RECORDING HYSTEROSCOPY ON FILM AND TAPE

Photography, cinematography, and television depend chiefly on adequate light, and the very small uterine cavity can be well illuminated with the available fiberoptic sources. Hysteroscopic photography has been satisfactory from the outset. If no demand for a larger optical lens is made on the operating canal in the guide-shaft, color slides with a circular diameter of 24 mm or full-frame 16 mm movies can be obtained readily (Rimkus and Semm, 1971/72). Compare also Chapter V, Secs., 1–3.

IV

The Technique of CO_2 Hysteroscopy

Hysteroscopy, and especially CO_2 hysteroscopy, is still in its infancy. The technique outlined below seems optimal at the moment. However, since both changes in the instruments and their possibilities for technical application are to be anticipated, the following suggested procedures cannot yet be considered as definitive or authoritative.

1. INDICATION AND CONTRAINDICATION FOR HYSTEROSCOPY

The CO_2 hysteroscopic technique is still too new even for a fully developed catalogue of indications and contraindications. The following themes are emerging at present for a diagnostic and therapeutic technique.

(*a*) Optical research into principles of physiologic processes in the uterine cavity, including the gestation processes.

(*b*) Clinical diagnosis of the cavity:

(1) in sterility;

(2) in suspected malformations such as septa, or with pathologic changes such as carcinoma of the endometrium or with benign polyps;

(3) in possible performance and monitoring of sterilization measures in the tubal region;

(4) in optically monitored aspiration of early nidation processes (therapeutic abortion).

(*c*) Procurement of material out of the cavity and tubal lumina:

(1) for histologic purposes;

(2) for immunologic studies;

(3) for nidation research.

Present-day contraindications include:

(1) All diseases of the female genital tract that previously have precluded instrumental invasion of the uterus.

(2) Infections of the genital tract, e.g., vaginitis, cervicitis, endometritis, and adnexitis.

(3) Situations in which the operative risk, either through anesthesia or other circumstances, for an intended procedure would be increased by an additional hysteroscopic examination of the patient.

The individual operator should extend this list of contraindications as much as possible at the outset and feel his way only slowly and with deliberation toward recognizing both the possibilities and the limitations of hysteroscopy.

2. PREPARATION OF THE PATIENT FOR HYSTEROSCOPY

The hysteroscopic procedure is in every way a routine operation. The patient, therefore, should be prepared according to classic precepts, whether it is proposed to use general or local anesthesia.

The patient is placed in a reclining position, her legs positioned as for a classic dilatation and curettage in winch leg-holders (Fig. 436). So far as is known, hysteroscopic procedures require no special patient preparatory measures.

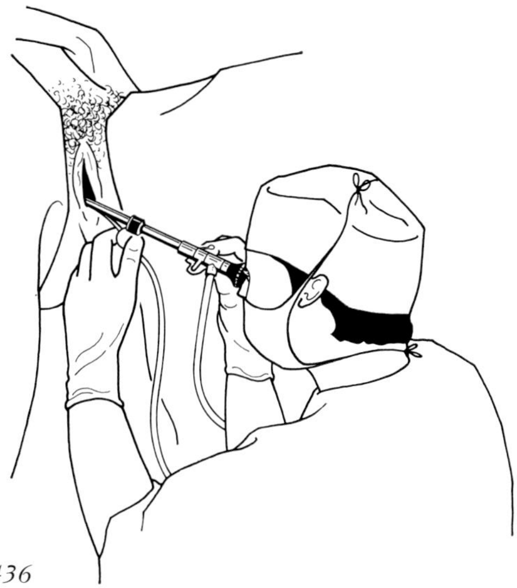

Figure 436

3. ANESTHESIA AND HYSTEROSCOPY

In most cases today, hysteroscopy will be undertaken chiefly for purely scientific reasons ancillary to some classic procedure. For this, the customary anesthetic procedure will be carried out. Hysteroscopy demands no special anesthetic considerations over and above the intended procedure, but it must be discussed in advance with the anesthesiologist.

Hysteroscopy is also possible under local anesthesia, especially when only a specific procedure, for example, tubal sterilization, is planned. It is possible by means of paracervical block to reduce to a minimum the sensation of pain for the patient in hysteroscopic procedures. Here, too, experience must necessarily be gained before any recommendation for a routine clinical technique can be given.

4. PLACEMENT OF THE SUCTION CERVICAL ADAPTER AND INSERTION OF THE HYSTEROSCOPE

After the bimanual examination of the internal genitalia, which precedes any intrauterine procedure (Fig. 131), routine disinfection of the vulva and vagina is performed. After the anterior lip of the cervix is grasped with a tenaculum the uterine cavity is sounded cautiously, because even slight contact by the probe against the fundus injures the endometrium. Then the cervical canal is gently dilated to permit ready entrance of the size 8 Hegar dilator. Here, again, pains

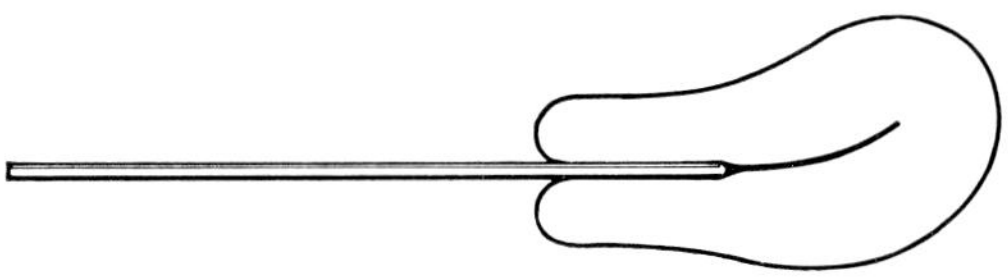

Figure 437

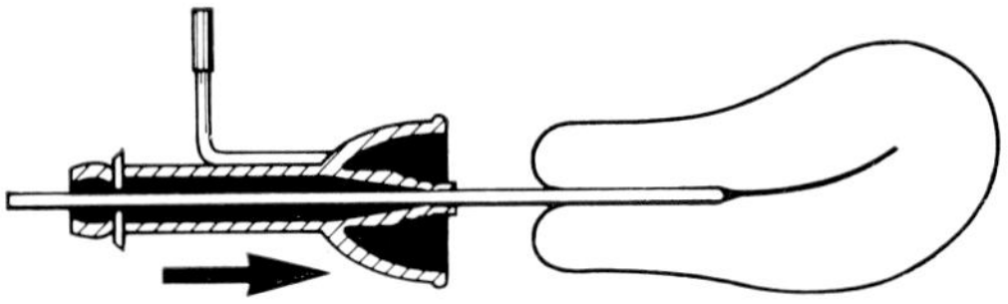

Figure 438

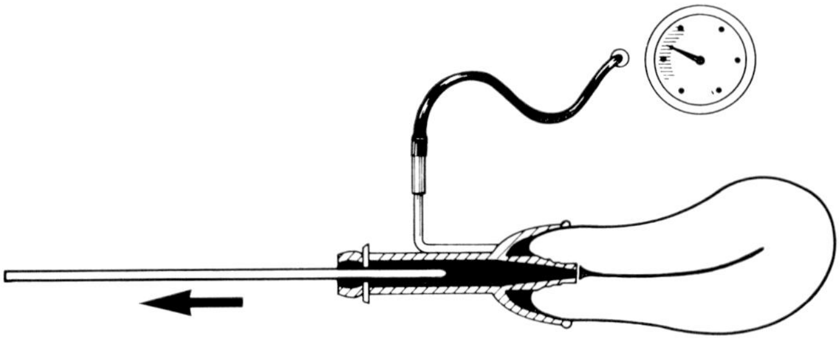

Figure 439

must be taken not to touch the fundus with the dilators, as this leads to trauma of the endometrium with subsequent bleeding.

After a size 8 Hegar dilator has finally been inserted, it is replaced by the straight guiding dilator with uniform external diameter (Fig. 437). Over this straight guiding dilator the cervical adapter is slipped slowly into the cervical canal and placed under negative pressure to the cervix (Fig. 438). The hystero-

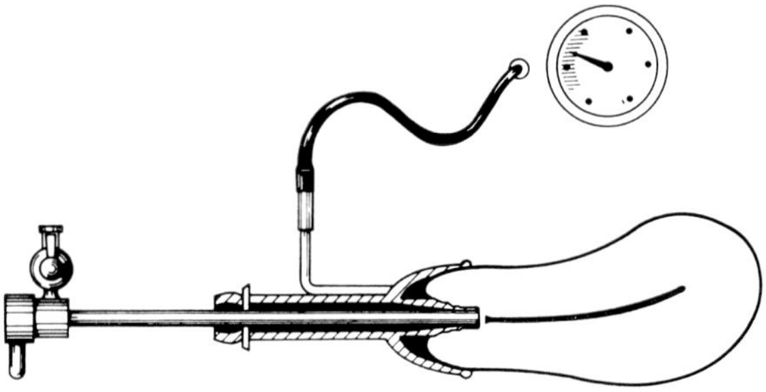

Figure 440

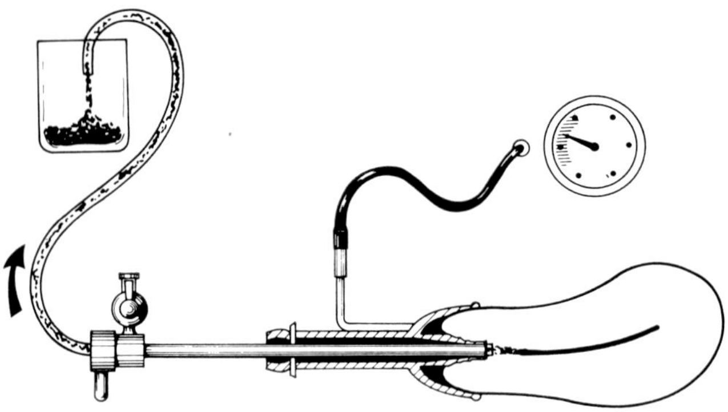

Figure 441

scopic insufflator or hysteroscopic unit (Fig. 435) furnishes the suction. Then the operator removes the straight guiding dilator (Fig. 439) which has assured the correctly angled suction placement of the adapter, a matter of great importance for the subsequent inspection of the cavity.

After the insertion of the guide shaft (Fig. 440) maximally to the end of the adapter shaft, it is wise to activate the vacuum mechanism after instillation, if

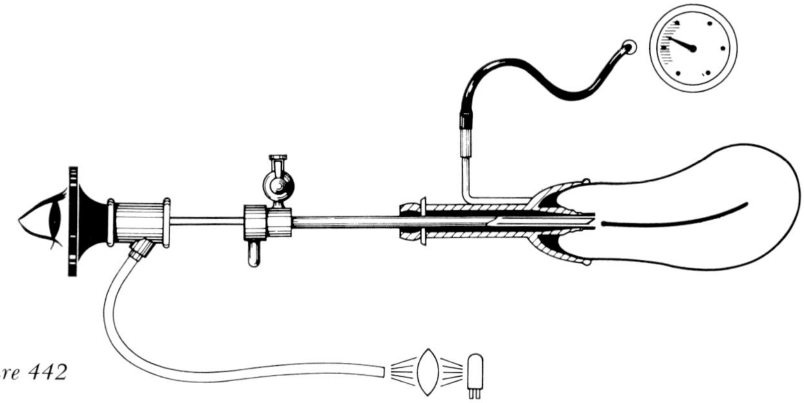

Figure 442

desired, of a few milliliters of physiologic saline solution (Fig. 441). This prevents any blood, drawn into the guide shaft as a result of traumatizing dilation, from lying directly in front of the sheath, blocking the view when the lens is inserted.

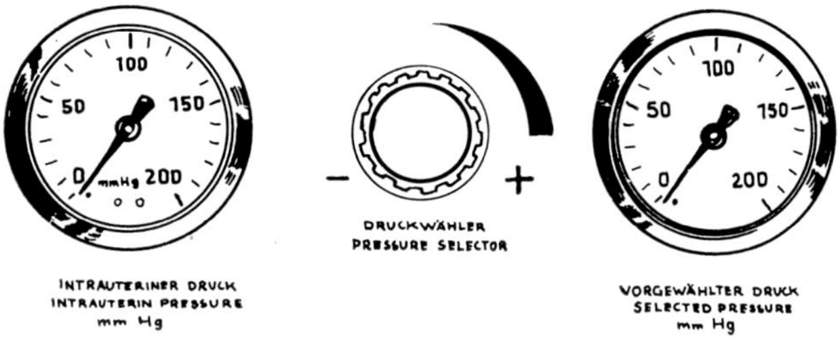

Figure 443

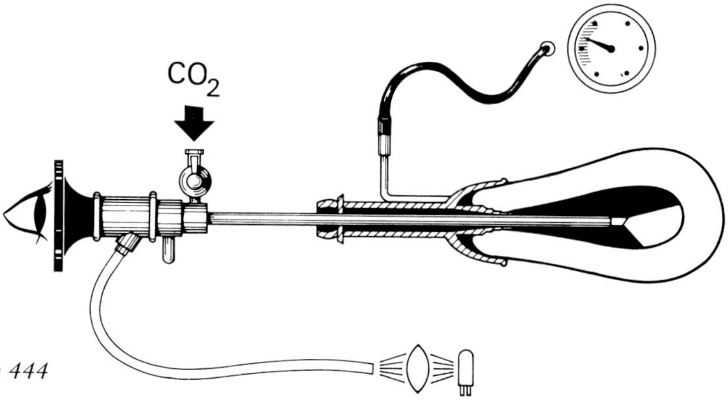

Figure 444

After the opening of the cervical canal and of the uterine cavity as described below, a repetition of this procedure is recommended as conditions require.

Once the guide shaft is clean, the lens is inserted and rendered gas-tight (Fig. 442). After this, the lens is advanced into the guide shaft until the light-colored endothelium of the collapsed cervix is seen. Now the operator increases the insufflation pressure with simultaneous endoscopic monitoring by continuous steady turning of the knob on the hysteroscopic insufflator (Fig. 443), starting at 10 mm Hg. Beyond 40 mm Hg it is turned only a little at a time. With this gradual increase of pressure the operator suddenly becomes aware of a fluttering of the cervical canal in the range of about 50 mm Hg ± 20 mm Hg, followed by the springing open of the whole uterine cavity (Fig. 444). Now the pressure can be reduced again by 3 to 5 mm Hg and the lens can be pushed into the cavity as required.

By means of this step-by-step expansion of the cervical canal and the uterine cavity, the internal ora of the oviducts in almost all cases remain closed within this pressure range, according to the principle of "constant volume with variable pressure." The endoscopic inspection of the cavity can then be carried out without tubal insufflation on either side. It is important to achieve this border state. If the tubes open, gas immediately escapes. In consequence of the machine-controlled cut-off at 100 ml of CO_2 gas per minute, it can easily happen in the case of highly patent, wide-diameter, rigid tubes that this gas volume per minute is no longer able to maintain sufficient dilation of the cavity. However, an increase of the rate of volume-per-minute is perilous, as already established in Figure 422, because of the danger of gas emboli.

5. OBTAINING SPECIMENS AND BIOPSY

It is possible during hysteroscopic observation to introduce various instruments through the working tube, such as biopsy forceps, suction cannula and the coagulation probe. Through appropriate tilting of the guide shaft and the vacuum adapter shaft, the lens, and thus the biopsy instrument, can be brought into the region of the left or right tubal os (Fig. 453). Difficulties arise only if visibility is reduced and freedom of movement is limited by intramural myomas, polyps, and the like.

6. CONCLUSION OF THE CO_2 HYSTEROSCOPY

After finishing the visual observation of the cavity and any further planned diagnostic (e.g., biopsy, aspiration of secretions) and therapeutic measures (such as sterilization), the CO_2 gas flow is first turned off, the lens is withdrawn from the cavity, and following release of the negative pressure the cervical cap is removed. Any hematoma that may have been produced on the cervix in the area of the cervical adapter by the negative pressure is of no consequence.

7. POSTOPERATIVE CARE AFTER HYSTEROSCOPY

Postoperative care after the performance of a CO_2 hysteroscopy depends primarily on the nature of the anesthesia used. Otherwise, the usual precautions are taken in accordance with prevailing custom for any intrauterine procedure performed.

Since, in surgical gynecology, the discussion has not yet been finalized as to whether a uterine curettage or tubal insufflation should be performed on an ambulatory basis, the same considerations apply to hysteroscopy. At the present stage of this new discipline it might be well to mention again that exceptional caution is of more importance than minimizing the risks involved. It is to be hoped that hysteroscopy may enjoy a happier fate than laparoscopy, in which there was a failure to realize dangers initially.

A pneumoperitoneum produced with CO_2 gas, such as on occasion may occur in the course of a hysteroscopy, is of no consequence. A maximum of 100 ml/min is insufflated, and a hysteroscopy, even with ancillary operative procedures, does not exceed five to ten minutes. The resorption rate for CO_2 gas via the peritoneum is about 100 ml/min (Semm, 1969; Kastendieck and Kühnel, 1973).

V

Hysteroscopic Atlas

(Some classic hysteroscopic macrophotographs are reproduced below.)

1. DILATION OF THE UTERINE CAVITY

Fig. 445. First the hysteroscope is inserted at the end of the cervical shaft, and the insufflation pressure is increased until the cervical canal pops open. This moment is shown in this picture.

Through suction placement at the proper axis (Fig. 438), the cervical canal presents as a straight line to the entering lens. Usually no bleeding occurs in a dilation performed during the proliferative phase of the menstrual cycle.

Fig. 446. In the second phase of the cycle, or if metrorrhagia exists, the dilation of the cervical canal is usually bloody. The blood is aspirated *before* the lens is inserted and the gas flow is turned on. The cervical canal in this picture shows the situation prior to a curettage that was indicated because of metrorrhagia.

Fig. 447. In the early proliferative phase, the cavity is lined with a thin, pinkish layer of endometrium. There is hardly any danger of bleeding. The right tubal os can be seen clearly.

Fig. 448. In the early secretory phase the uterine lining appears more reddish, corresponding to the more thickly-layered endometrium. The red areas in the central region of the fundus have been caused by trauma in the course of dilation of the cervix. The dilators have intruded all the way to the fundus and have impinged on it, causing dark red discoloration.

In addition, the mechanical cavity dilator (Rimkus), which is to replace the CO_2 gas flow during the endoscopic examination, is just being introduced.

Fig. 449. The dilator already mentioned in the legend for Figure 448 is here passing through the cervical canal, which is already dilated by the CO_2 gas pressure.

Fig. 450. The CO_2 gas pressure has been released. The cavity is held open solely by the mechanical cavity dilator. The left tubal ostium is clearly visible.

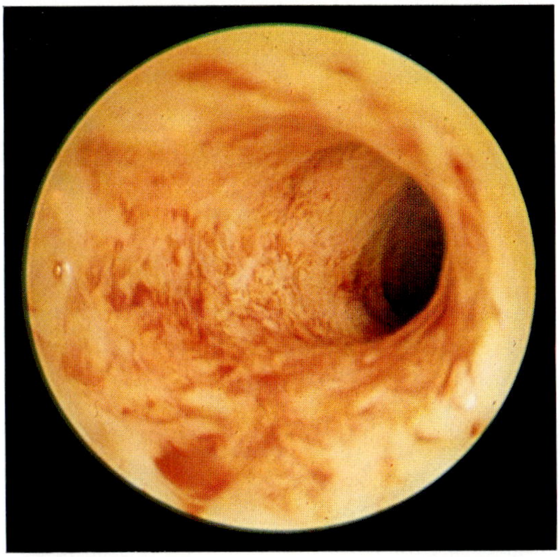
445

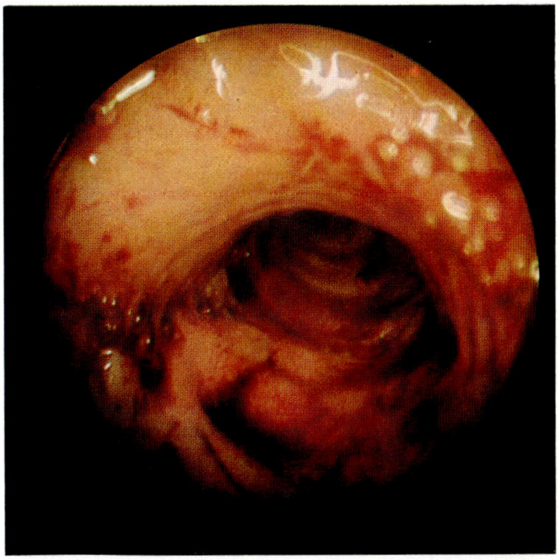
446

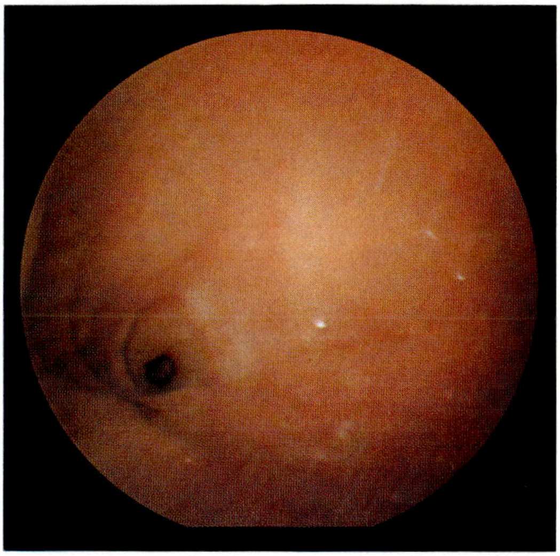
447

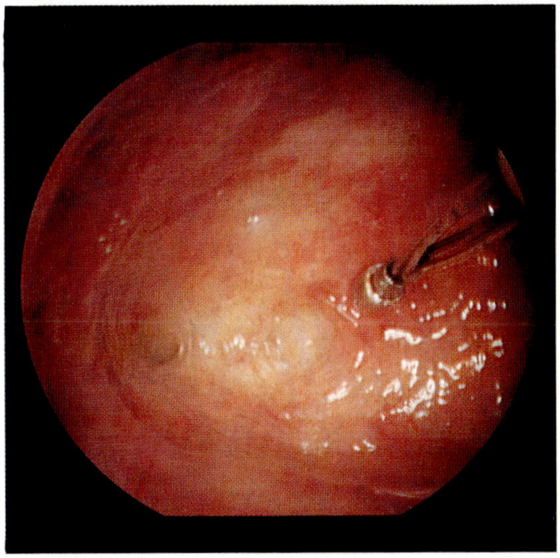
448

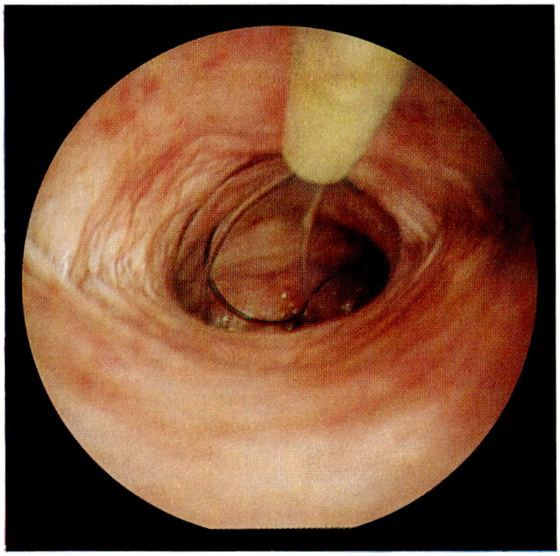
449

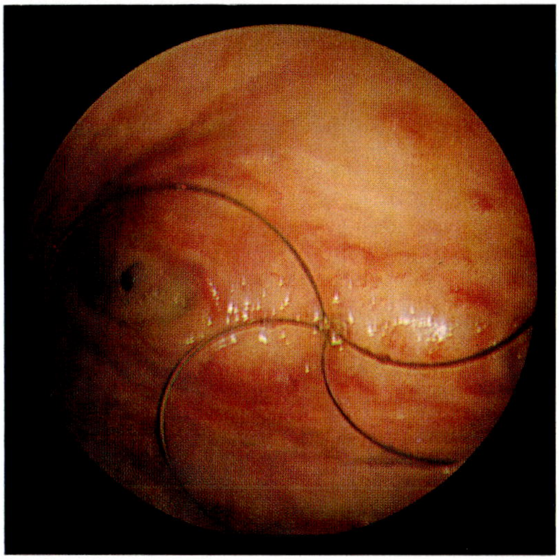
450

2. PHYSIOLOGY AND PATHOLOGY OF THE CAVITY

Fig. 451. A total view of the uterine cavity in the secretory phase. In the foreground at the transition from cervix to cavity two submucous leiomyomata can be seen. Both tubal angles show normal configuration. A mucous membrane polyp is present in the vicinity of the left tubal os.

Fig. 452. Under greater magnification, the mucous membrane polyp already seen in Figure 451 in the vicinity of the left tubal os. The polyp is somewhat bizarrely deformed and although normally dark red, it here appears yellowish because of over-illumination. The polypoid swelling of the mucous membrane in the vicinity of the left tubal os, mechanically displacing it, is worthy of note. This observation is interesting for the evaluation of incorrectly *negative* results of tubal patency by tubal gas insufflation, hysterosalpingography, or tubal dye insufflation.

Fig. 453. In this case of polyps of the endometrium, a biopsy is being performed. Polyps fill the cavity, especially in the region of the fundus. Both tubal ora are visible, the left one being surrounded by a polypoid wall.

Fig. 454. View into the cavity in the direction of the left tubal ostium at the start of the menstrual phase. The mucous membrane is detaching itself from the basal endometrium in large and small patches.

Fig. 455. The view into this cavity is narrowed by endometrial mucous membrane swollen by numerous myomata, some of them polypoid. A further dilation of the cavity in order to enlarge the field of vision is not possible in this case.

Fig. 456. At the start of the proliferative phase the cervix here was dilated in the normal way, in the course of which the endometrium in the vicinity of the fundus was traumatized by the dilator. Intense fresh bleeding is seen in the inspection of such a cavity.

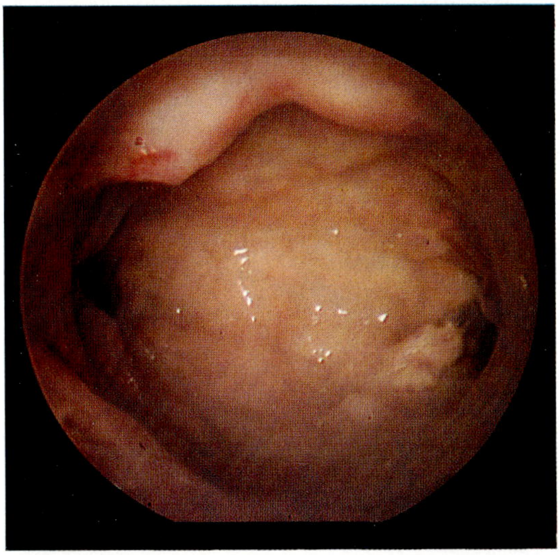
451

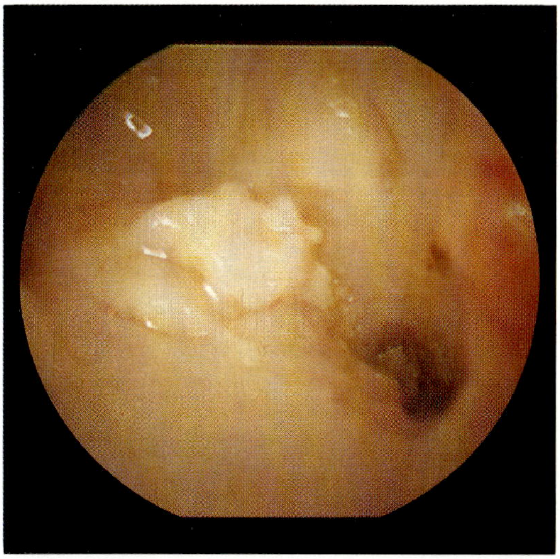
452

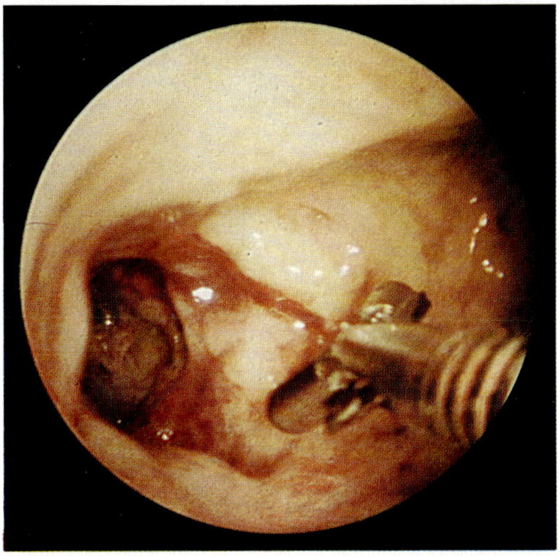
453

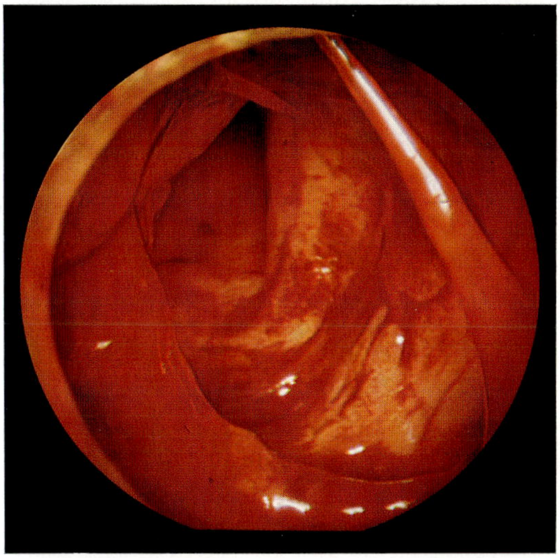
454

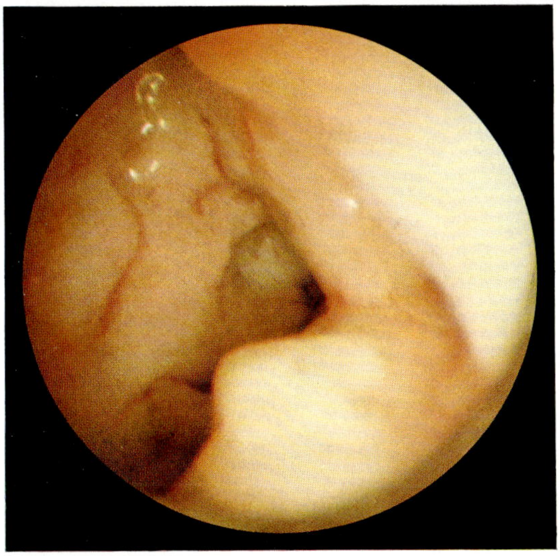
455

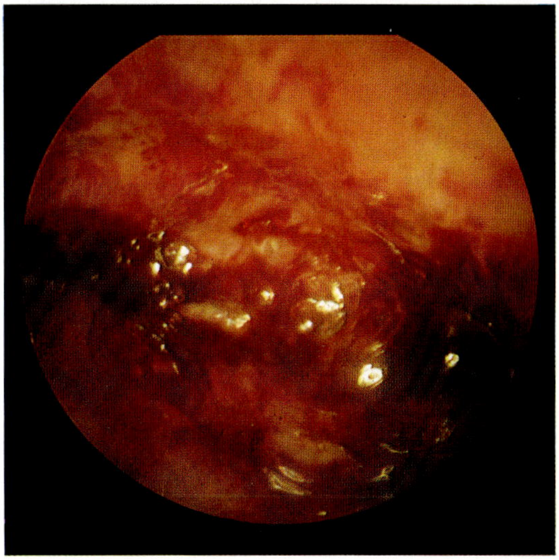
456

Fig. 457. The endometrium, in which bleeding is ceasing in an irregular pattern, shows some thick and some thin layering, together with both fresh and old blood with fibrin structurings.

Fig. 458. The right tubal ostium is rimmed with mostly polypoid uterine mucous membrane, some of it with pronounced vascularization.

Fig. 459. In this case of menstrual bleeding, the endometrium for the most part is being shed in flat chunks. The thick-layered functional layer is detaching itself in large patches from its basal layer.

Fig. 460. Two rather large submucous myomata grown into the uterine lumen and covered with normal endometrium can be seen through the cervical canal.

Fig. 461. In the matrix of these multiple mucous membrane polyps growing in the fundus, a histologically proved carcinosarcoma is visually detectable.

Fig. 462. The irregularly bleeding endometrium seen here with smooth areas and papillary projections proved histologically to be adenocarcinoma.

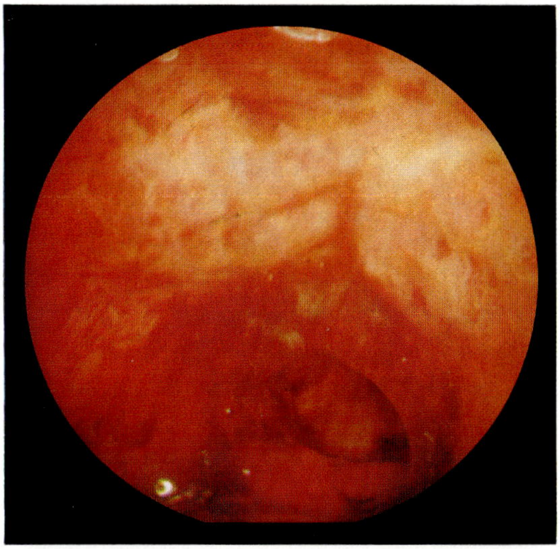

457

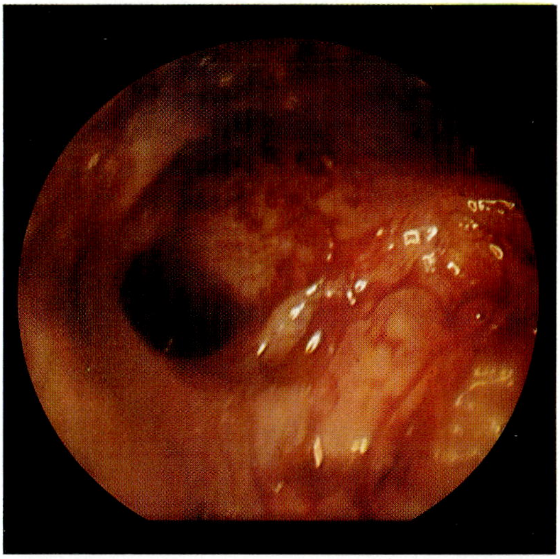

458

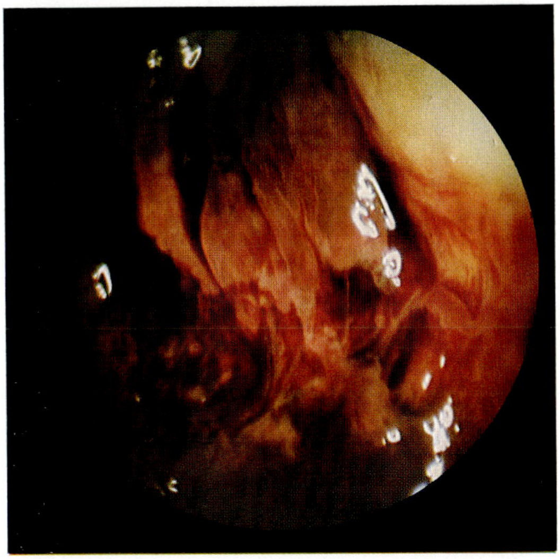

459

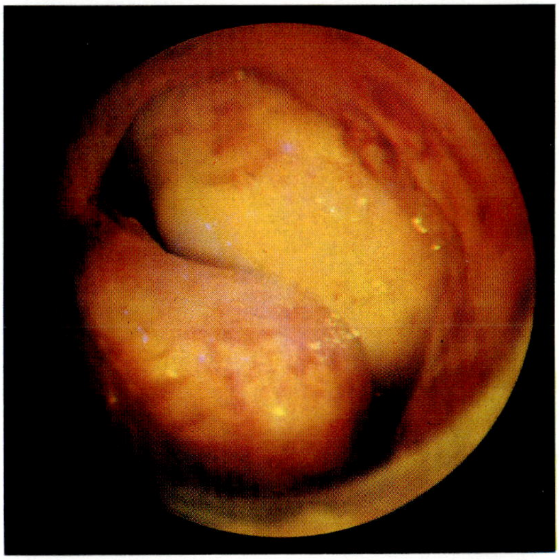

460

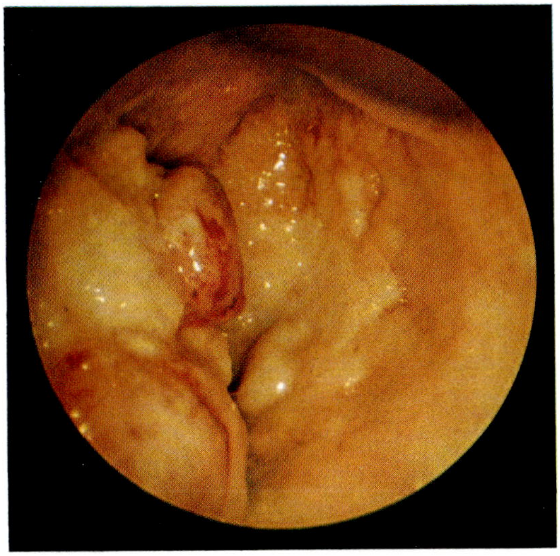

461

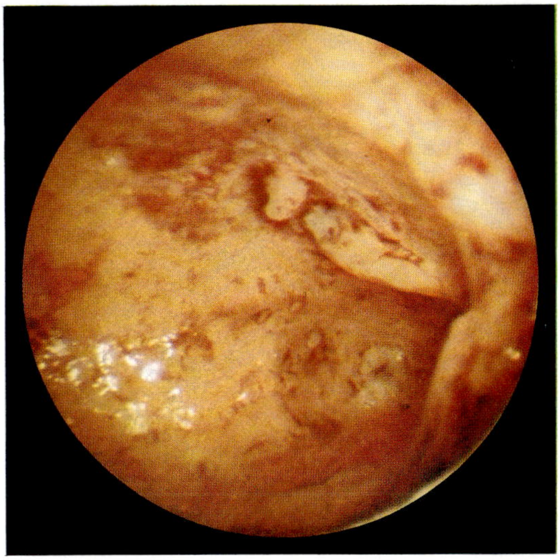

462

3. TRANSUTERINE TUBAL COAGULATION

Fig. 463. Since the inauguration of CO_2 hysteroscopy, the possibility has been discussed of effecting sterilization by sealing the tubes at hysteroscopy through coagulation of the tubal ostia. Here the entry of the coagulation probe into the cervical canal can be seen. The fundus of the uterus is also clearly visible.

Fig. 464. The hysteroscope is aimed at the right tubal ostium which the high-frequency coagulation probe is approaching.

Fig. 465. The coagulation probe (in this case a thermocoagulation model) is in the right tubal ostium. The formation of bubbles indicates the progress of the coagulation of the tubal lumen for about 1 cm of its length.

Fig. 466. After withdrawal of the coagulation probe from the tubal ostium (Fig. 465), we see the intramural course of the tube coagulated cylindrically about 3 mm deep and for a distance of 1 cm.

Fig. 467. If too much gas pressure is applied to dilate the cavity for CO_2 hysteroscopy, the tubes also dilate and a normal tubal insufflation takes place.

This picture demonstrates CO_2 insufflation during such a hysteroscopy. The bubbles are normal for a tubal insufflation for diagnostic purposes with the pertubation apparatus. One must bear in mind that, even with a flow limited to 100 ml/min, 1 liter of pneumoperitoneum has been blown in after about ten minutes.

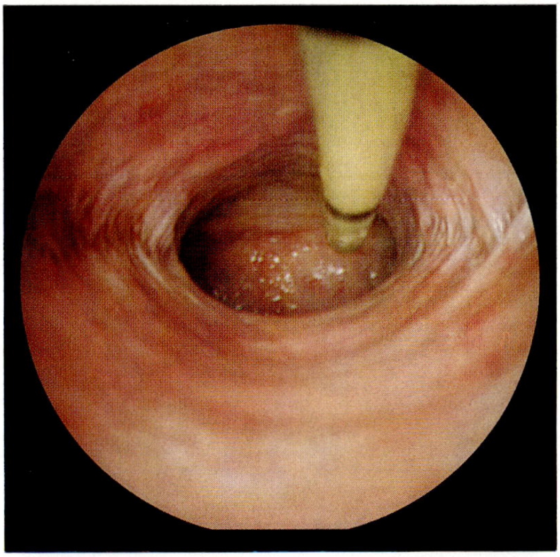

463

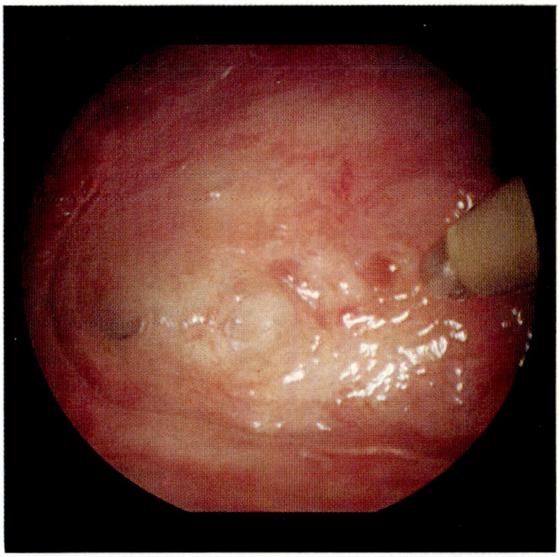

464

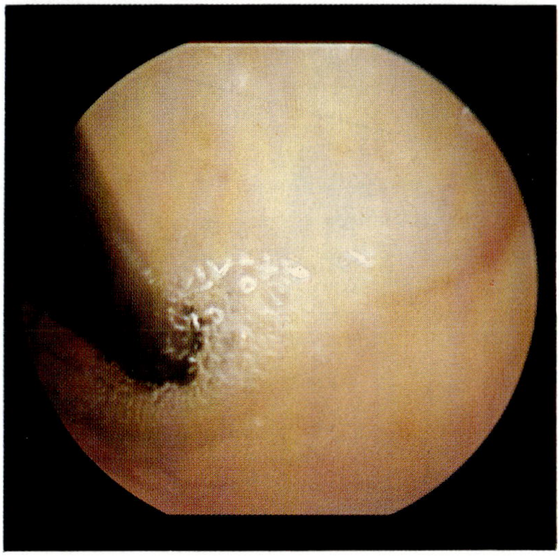

465

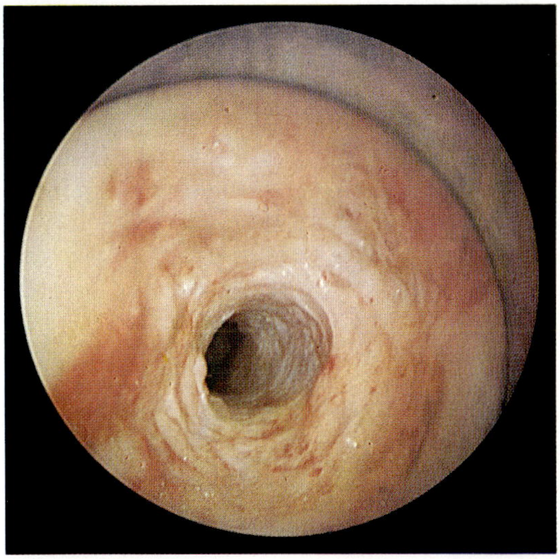

466

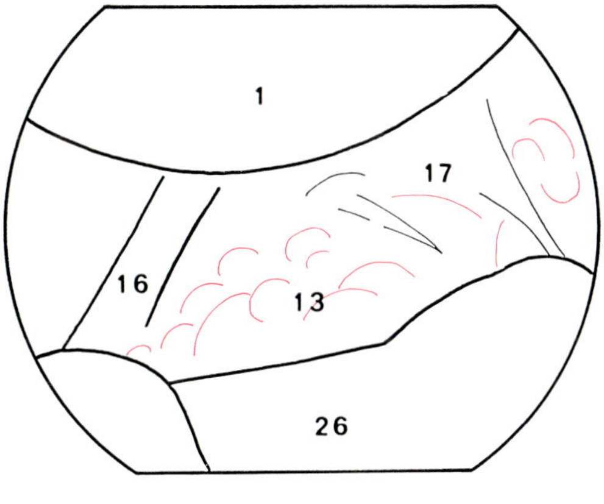

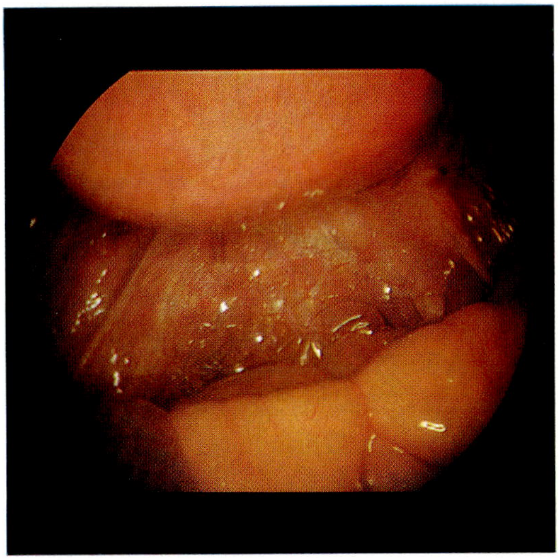

467

Fig. 468. The histochemical specimen dyed with succinate dehydrogenase demonstrates the cylindric biologic denaturalization of the tubal endothelium and the uterine musculature surrounding it. The zone capable of active fermentation, and therefore bluish-colored, contrasts distinctly with the pinkish biologically inactive zones. Coagulation time was 20 seconds at 5 watts.

Fig. 469. This picture shows a coagulation probe introduced into the right tubal ostium.

4. DANGERS OF TRANSUTERINE TUBAL PROBING

Fig. 470. In tubal probing at hysteroscopy, as in any blind probing of the uterus, there is always the danger of perforation.

This dangerous hysteroscopic situation is demonstrated by a picture at laparoscopy. The experienced hysteroscopist was confident he was probing the entrance of the lumen because of slight motion. The hope of probing the intramurally occluded tubes in this sterility case by a transuterine approach was doomed to failure.

Fig. 471. This laparoscopic picture was taken in connection with a tubal coagulation at hysteroscopy. We see clearly how the probe has been pushed too far into the uterine musculature and the resultant whitish color of the peritoneum. Without laparoscopic monitoring, the adjacent intestine also would have been coagulated.

Figures 470 and 471 should make evident what potential dangers lurk in probing or coagulating a tube in an area out of the visual range of the hysteroscope.

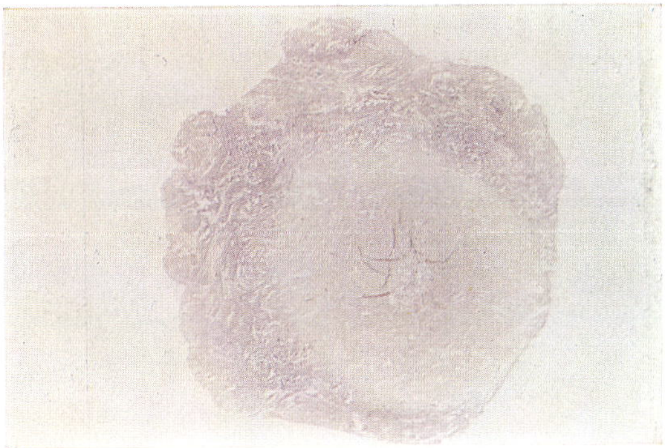

468

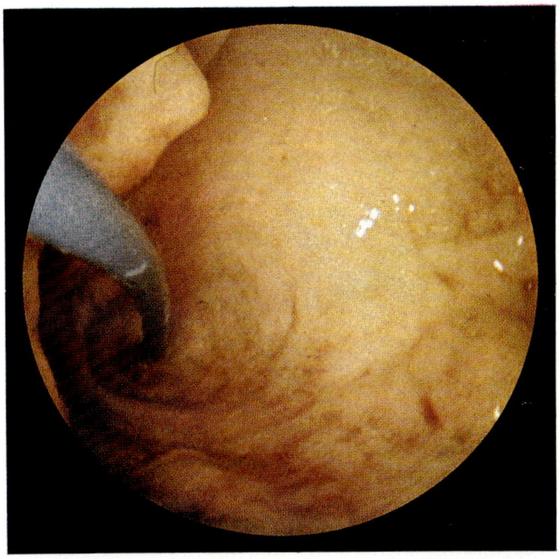

469

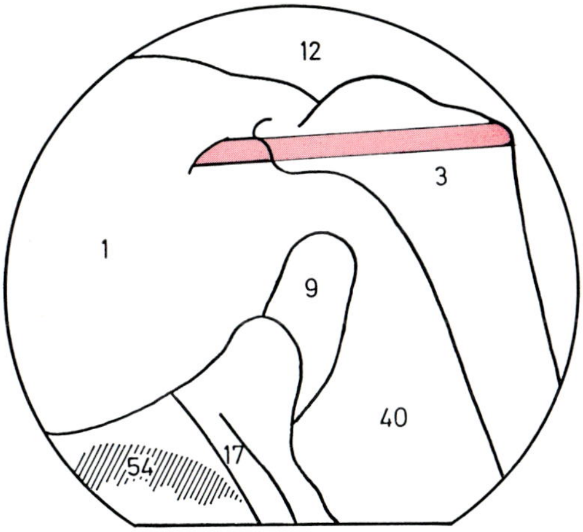

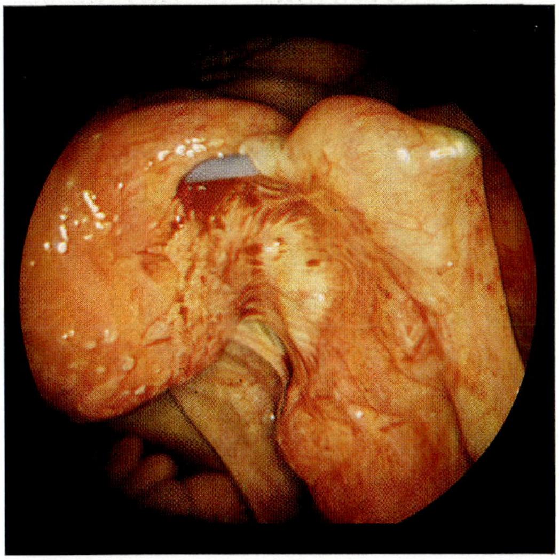

470

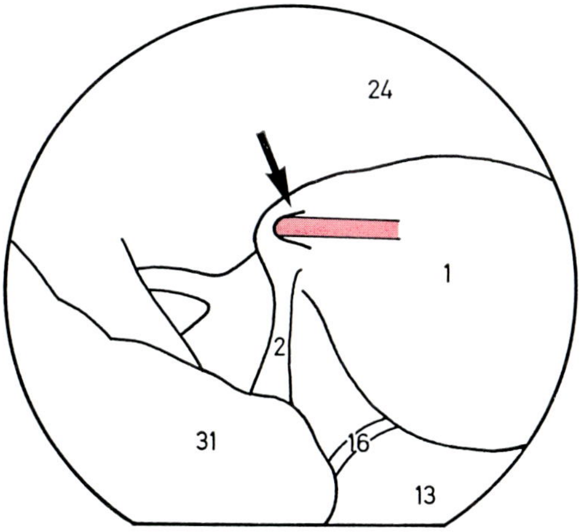

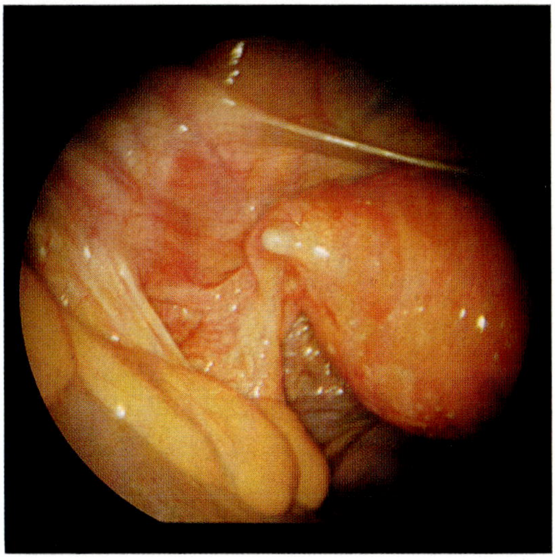

471

REFERENCES

MONOGRAPHS AND TEXTS ON LAPAROSCOPY

Abarbanel, A.: Transvaginal pelviscopy. Further studies in infertility. Proc. Second World Congress on Fertility and Sterility. Vol I, p. 1140. Neapel 1956.

Abstracta I. European Congress of Endoscopy, 12.–16. October, Munich 1970.

Adler, D.: The use of peritoneoscopy for tubal sterilization. Los Angeles 1970.

Albano, V., E. Cittadini: La celioscopia in ginecologia, (monografia). p. I 420. Denaro, Palermo 1962.

Albano, V., E. Cittadini: La celioscopia nella diagnosi della tuberculosi genitale femminile. Proceedings of the First International Symposium of Gynecology, Celios, 1964, p. 305.

Albano, V., E. Cittadini, P. Quartararo: Celioscopic findings after estro-progestational treatments. Proc. 2nd Int. Cong. Horm. Steroids, Milano. Excerpta Medica Foundation, Amsterdam 1966.

Albano, V., E. Cittadini: Intérêt de la coelioscopie dans l'étude des algies pelviennes d'origine endométriosique. Atti Congresso S.M.I.E.R., Marsiglia 1970.

Alfonsin, A. E.: Laparoscopy for the study of sterility. Proceedings of the VIII. World Congress on Fertility and Sterility, 2.–9. November, Buenos Aires 1974.

Armas, O. R.: Laparoscopy and sterility. Proc. VII. World Congress on Fertility and Sterility. p. 795–796. Excerpta Medica, Amsterdam 1973.

Bailey, H.: Emergency surgery. Ed. 8. McNair (ed.). Williams & Wilkins, Baltimore, 1967.

Banyai, A. L.: Pneumoperitoneum treatment. Mosby, St. Louis 1946.

Beck, K.: Atlas der Laparoskopie. Schattauer, Stuttgart 1968.

Benedict, E. B.: Endoscopy. Williams & Wilkins, Baltimore, 1951.

Bismuth, E.: La coelioscopie gynécologique—Son application à l'étude de la stérilité. Foulon, Paris 1945.

Botella-Llusia, J., S. Dexeus Jr.: La coelioscopia nella diagnostica ormonale ginecologica. Proc. I. Intern. Symp. On Gynec. Celioscopy. I.R.E.S., Palermo 1964, p. 209.

Bruneau, Y., et al.: Traité pratique de photographie et de cinématographie médicales. Vol. I. Montel, Paris 1960.

Burgio, G. R., G. Arcara: La celioscopia nello studio della patalogia del sesso nell'età infantile e prepuberale. Proc. I. Intern. Symp. on Gynec. Celioscopy. I.R.E.S., Palermo 1964, p. 285.

Cittadini, E.: La celioscopia nel bilancio della sterilità coniugale. Fertilità e sterilità. Piccin, Padova 1971.

Cittadini, E., T. Rossi: L'interesse della celioscopia nella diagnosi delle malformazioni genitali. Proc. Ist. Intern. Symp. on Ginec. End. I.R.E.S., Palermo 1964.

Cittadini, E., T. Rossi: Celioscopia e techniche ausiliarie. Piccin, Padova 1973.

Clauss, J.: Lokalisation von Tubenverschlüssen durch Foto-Douglasskopie. Proceedings of the Second World Congress on Fertility and Sterility. Vol I., p. 1188. Neapel 1956.

Clyman, M.: Operative culdoscopy in female sterilization. Female sterilization: Prognosis for simplified outpatient procedures. G. W. Duncan, R. D. Falb, J. J. Speidel (eds.). Academic Press, New York 1972.

Clyman, M. J.: Tubal sterilization by operative culdoscopy. In: Female sterilization: Prognosis for simplified outpatient procedures. G. W. Duncan, R. D. Falb, J. J. Speidel (eds.). Academic Press, New York, London 1972.

Clyman, M. J.: Tubal sterilization by operative culdoscopy. Human sterilization. R. Richart, D. J. Prager (eds.). Thomas, Springfield, Ill., 1972.

Cocchi, V.: Retropneumoperitoneum und Pneumomediastinum. Thieme, Stuttgart 1957.

Cohen, M. R.: Laparoscopy, culdoscopy and ginecography: Technique and atlas. Saunders, Philadelphia 1970.

Corson, S. L.: Bipolar laparoscopic instrument suitable for sterilization and biopsy procedures. Proceedings of the VIII. World Congress on Fertility and Sterility, 3.–9. November, Buenos Aires 1974.

David, Ch.: L'endoscopie utérine, applications au diagnostic et au traitement des affections intrautérines. Jacques, Paris 1908.

Dawn, C. S.: Culdoscopic tubal ligation in India. Advances in voluntary sterilization. Proceedings of the Second International Conference. p. 50–54. Excerpta Medica American Elsevier Publ. Co. Inc., New York 1974.

Decker, A.: Pelvic culdoscopy. In: J. V. Meigs, S. H. Sturgis: Progress in gynecology. p. 95. Grune & Stratton, New York 1946.

Decker, A.: Culdoscopy. Saunders, New York 1952.

Decker, A.: Proceedings of the First International Symposium on Gynecological Celioscopy. I.R.E.S., Palermo 1964.

Decker, A.: Culdoscopy. Davis, Philadelphia 1967.

De Brux, J., J. Dupre-Fromet, J. Cohen, M. Mintz, R. Palmer: Proceedings of the First International Symposium on Gynecological Celioscopy, I.R.E.S., Palermo 1964.

De Brux, J., H. Wenner-Mangen: Résultats et intérêt de l'examen histologique systématique des biopsies tubaires per-opératoires et sous coelioscopie. In: La fonction tubaire et ses troubles. Société nationale pour l'étude de la stérilité et de la fécondite, Paris, 2–3 juillet 1955, p. 218–234. Masson, Paris 1955.

Deichman, J. L.: Imaging techniques for female reproductive system. In: Female sterilization: Prognosis for simplified outpatient procedures. G. W. Duncan, R. D. Falb, J. J. Speidel (eds.). Academic Press, New York 1972.

Dellepiane, G., C. Durando: Proceedings of the First International Symposium on Gynecological Celioscopy, I.R.E.S., Palermo 1964.

Désormeaux: Sitzungsber. der Société de Chir. in Paris. Gazette des Hôp. 1865.

Dexeus, J. S., F. J. Fontaine: La celioscopia en ginecologia. S. A. Sandoz, Barcelona 1965.

De Watteville, P. H.: Proceedings of the First International Symposium on Gynecological Celioscopy, I.R.E.S., Palermo, 1964.

Diepgen, P.: Geschichte der Medizin II. Bd., I. Hälfte. de Gruyter, Berlin 1951.

Diepgen, P.: Geschichte der Medizin. II. Bd., 2. Hälfte. de Gruyter, Berlin 1955.

Dittel: Referat über das Endoskop. Med. Jahrb. *XIX*, II:73.

Duffieux, P.: L'intégral de Fourier et ses applications a l'optique. Rennes 1946.

Duncan, G. W., R. D. Falb, J. J. Speidel (eds.). Female sterilization. Workshop on Female sterilization held at Airlie House, Airlie, Virginia, December 2–3, 1971. Academic Press, New York 1972.

Duncan, R. D., J. J. Speidel: Female sterilization: Prognosis for simplified outpatient procedures. Academic Press, New York 1972.

Espagno, G.: Proceedings of the First International Symposium on Gynecological Celioscopy, I.R.E.S., Palermo, 1964, p. 367.

Eulenburg, A.: Real-Encyclopädie der gesamten Heilkunde. S. 265–293. Urban & Schwarzenberg, Wien, Leipzig 1886.

Fikentscher, R., K. Semm: Fortschritte in der utero-tubaren Persufflation. Proceedings of the III. World Congress on Fertility and Sterility, Amsterdam, 1961, p. 635–637.

Frangenheim, H.: Coelioskopie und Douglaspunktion. In O. Käser, V. Riedberg, K. G. Ober, K. Thomsen, J. Zander (Hsgb.): Gynäkologie und Geburtshilfe. Bd. I, S. 875. Thieme, Stuttgart 1964.

Frangenheim, H.: Die Laparoskopie und die Kuldoskopie in der Gynäkologie. Thieme, Stuttgart, Aufl. I. 1959, 2., erw. Aufl. 1970.

Frangenheim, H.: Die Coelioskopie bei der Sterilitätsdiagnostik. Proc. I. Intern. Symp. on Gynec. Celioscopy, I.R.E.S., Palermo, 1964, p. 195.

Frangenheim, H.: Indikationen für die Coelioskopie in der Gynäkologie. In L. Demling, R. Ottenjann: Endoskopie—Methoden, Ergebnisse. S. 180–185. Banaschewski, München 1967.

Frangenheim, H.: Resultate der selektiven Eileiterchirurgie (1956–1965) sowie Vorschlag zur Einteilung der Tubenerkrankungen bei Sterilität. Atti I°-Congresso Europeo Sulla Sterilità, Venezia. S.A.G.A., Genova 1967, p. 440.

Frangenheim, H.: Laparoscopy in the diagnosis of sterility. In P. C. Steptoe: Laparoscopy in gynaecology. Livingstone, Edinburgh 1967.

Frangenheim, H.: Zur Differentialdiagnose der Genitaltuberkulose unter Sicht mit dem Laparoskop. Proc. VI. World Congr. on Fertil. and Steril. 1968.

Frangenheim, H.: Möglichkeiten und Grenzen cölioskopischer Untersuchung in der Gynäkologie. In L. Demling, R. Ottenjann: Endoskopie—Methoden, Ergebnisse. Banaschewski, München 1969.

Frangenheim, H.: Möglichkeiten und Grenzen der laparoskopischen Diagnostik der Ovarialerkrankungen und der Funktionsstörungen der Ovarien. Bücherei des Frauenarztes Nr. 4. Enke, Stuttgart 1971.

Frangenheim, H.: Die Laparoskopie und Kuldoskopie in der Gynäkologie. 2. Aufl. Thieme, Stuttgart 1971.

Frangenheim, H.: Über die Notfall-Laparoskopie bei akuten Unterbaucherkrankungen in der Gynäkologie und in der Chirurgie. In R. Ottenjann: Fortschritte der Endoskopie. Bd. 3, S. 151–153. Schattauer, Stuttgart 1972.

Frangenheim, H.: Einfluß der Laparoskopie auf die Indikation für Sterilitätsoperationen. In R. Ottenjann: Fortschritte der Endoskopie, S. 189. Schattauer, Stuttgart 1973.

Frangenheim, H.: Laparoscopy, including tubal sterilization. Proceedings of the VIII. World Congress on Fertility and Sterility, 3.–9. November, Buenos Aires 1974.

Franke, G.: Fotografische Optik. Akad. Verlagsanstalt, Frankfurt 1964.

Gares, R.: Étude per-coelioscopique des ganglions pelviens. Proc. I. Intern. Symp. on Gynec. Celioscopy, I.R.E.S., Palermo 1964, p. 163.

Giri, K.: Experience of outpatient laparoscopic sterilization in Naples. Advances in voluntary steriliza-

tion. Proc. Second International Conference, p. 36–41. Excerpta med. American Elsevier Publ. Comp. Inc., New York 1974.
Goes, J. S. Jr., F. Chammas: Evaluation of videoscopy and 70 mm intensified fluorography in the diagnosis and treatment of infertility (Abstract). Proc. VII. World Congress on Fertility and Sterility, p. 807. Excerpta Medica Foundation, Amsterdam 1973.
Goldsman, T., et al.: Valor de la celioscopia en esterilidad. Abstr. World Congress on Fertility and Sterility, Israel 1968, p. 174.
Goldsman, T.: Celioscopia en el estudio de esterilidad. Actas del I. Congreso Argentino de Esterilidad, Rosario, 1968, p. 780–782.
Goldsman, T.: Diagnostico de las malformaciones uterinas – Correlacion anatomo clinica – radiologica celioscopica y de anatomia comparada. Cordoba, Argentina 1972.
Gordji, M., F. Javadi: A palpator needle for use in laparoscopy. Proc. VII. World Congress on Fertility and Sterility. p. 805. Excerpta Medica Foundation, Amsterdam 1973.
Gorga, R. S.: La endoscopia abdomino pelviana. Ortiz, Sao Paulo 1955.
Grant, J, G. Mackey: Conference of Sterility and Infertility, USA, 1947.
Grünfeld: Über Vergrößerung resp. scheinbare Annäherung endoskopischer Sehobjekte. Sitzungsber. d. Ges. d. Ärzte in Wien vom 9. April. Anzeiger Nr. 23. 1875.
Grünfeld, J.: Zur Geschichte der Endoskopie. Med. Jahrbuch, Wien 1879.
Gutierrez, A.: Culdoscopy as an aid in family planning. In: Female sterilization: Prognosis for simplified outpatient procedures. G. W. Duncan, R. D. Falb, J. J. Speidel (eds.). Academic Press, New York, London 1972.
Haase, E.: Der Verwendungsbereich für Farbfilm in der Endoskopie. In L. Demling, R. Ottenjann: Endoskopie – Methoden, Ergebnisse. S. 9–11. Banaschewski, München 1967.
Hayashi, M.: Tubal sterilization by coronal coagulation under hysteroscopy. In: Human sterilization. Chapter 28. R. M. Richart, D. J. Prager (eds.), 402 pp. Thomas, Springfield, Ill., 1972.
Hayashi, M., N. Nishio: The application of tubal staples under culdoscopy. Proc. 7th Int. Conf. of the IPPF, Singapore, February, 1963. G. W. Cadbury, H. D. Connolly, K. V. Earle, A. S. Parkes (eds.), p. 623. Excerpta Medica Foundation, Amsterdam.
Hayashi, M., F. Ishikawa: The improvement of uterine cornual coagulation techniques. Proc. III. European Congress on Fertility and Sterility. Athen 1974.
Heinkel, K.: Beleuchtungsmöglichkeiten in der Endophotographie. In Demling, L., R. Ottenjann: Endoskopie – Methoden, Ergebnisse. S. 11–17. Banaschewski, München-Gräfelfing 1969.
Heymans, M., R. Palmer: La coelioscopie dans l-indication opératoire pour stérilité tubaire. Proc. I. Intern. Symp. on Gynec. Celioscopy, I.R.E.S., Palermo 1964, p. 205.
Hoffbauer, H.: Das kolpophotographische Bild des unteren Eipols. In Demling, L., R. Ottenjann: Endoskopie – Methoden, Ergebnisse, S. 193–194. Banaschewski, München-Gräfelfing 1969.
Hopkins, H. H.: Neue Fortschritte in der medizinischen Endoskopie. 70. Tagung der Deutschen Ges. f. angew. Optik, Lübeck 1969.
Hulka, J. F.: Anatomy, biochemistry, physiology and bioengineering of the oviduct and the uterus as they pertain to sterilization techniques. In: Female sterilization: Prognosis for simplified outpatient procedures. G. W. Duncan, R. D. Falb, J. J. Speidel (eds.). Academic Press, New York, London 1972.
Hulka, J. F., K. F. Omran: Cauterization for tubal sterilization. In: Human sterilization. Chapter 27. R. M. Richart, D. J. Prager (eds.). Thomas, Springfield, Ill., 1972.
Hulka, J. F., K. F. Omran: New methods of female sterilization. In: New concepts in contraception. M. Potts, C. Wood (eds.), p. 57. University Park Press, Baltimore, Md., 1972.
Ihavery, C. L., K. Sankari, S. C. Patel: Gynaecological endoscopy-laparoscopy. Proc. XVIth All India Obstetrics and Gynecological Congress, New Delhi, 10–12 March, 1972, p. 86. Dr. C. L. Ihaveri at the Popular Press (Bomb.). Private Ltd., Bombay 1972.
Kalk, H.: Cirrhose und Narbenleber. Enke, Stuttgart 1957.
Kalk, H., W. Brühl: Leitfaden der Laparoskopie und Gastroskopie. Thieme, Stuttgart 1951.
Kalk, H., E. Wildhirt: Lehrbuch und Atlas der Laparoskopie und Leberpunktion. Thieme, Stuttgart 1962.
Klaften, E.: Lichtdiagnostik gynäkologischer Erkrankungen. In Seitz-Amreich: Biologie und Pathologie des Weibes. Bd. II, S. 923–933. Urban & Schwarzenberg, München 1952.
Korbsch, R.: Lehrbuch und Atlas der Laparoskopie und Thorakoskopie. Lehmann, München 1927.
Kratochwil, A.: Laparoskopie bei unklaren gynäkologischen Befunden. Proc. I. Intern. Symp. on Gynec. Celioscopy, I.R.E.S., Palermo 1964, p. 87.
Kröhl, R.: Vergleichende Füllung des Pneumoperitoneums mit CO_2 und N_2O. In R. Ottenjann: Fortschritte der Endoskopie. Verh.-Bericht Bd. 2, S. 247–250. Schattauer, Stuttgart, New York 1970.
Lahiri, B. C.: Value of culdoscopy in infertility problems. Proc. XVIth All India Obstetrics and Gynaecological Congress, New Delhi, 10–12 March 1972. p. 84. Dr. C. L. Ihaveri at the Popular Press (Bomb.) Private Ltd., Bombay 1972.
Laufe, L. E., S. Summerson: Interval vaginal tubal ligation. Female sterilization: Prognosis for simplified outpatient procedures. G. W. Duncan, R. D. Falb, J. J. Speidel (eds.). Academic Press, New York 1972.
Laufe, L.: Current methods of female sterilization, an overview. In: Advances in voluntary steriliza-

tion. Proc. of the second International Conference. Excerpta Medica American Elsevier Publishing Co. Inc., New York 1974.
Leiter, J.: Elektro-endoskopische Instrumente mit 82 Holzschnitten. Wien 1880.
Lenzi, G., C. B. Cavassini, E. Lenzi: La laparoscopie. Masson, Paris 1960.
Lenzi, G., C. B. Cavassini, E. Lenzi: La laparoscopia. Capelli, Bologna 1960.
Levinson, J.: Manual de laparoscopia. Diagnóstico y consideraciones terapéuticas preparadas bajo los auspicios de: La Asociacion Americana de Laparoscopistas Ginecólogos. Departamento de Educación Professional de los Laboratorios Searle, Parte de G. D. Searle & Compania, Downey, Calif., 1974.
Liess, J.: Die Endoskopie beim Rinde. Scharper, Hannover 1936.
Little, W.: Culdoscopic outpatient sterilization procedures. Female sterilization: Prognosis for simplified outpatient procedures. G. W. Duncan, R. D. Falb, J. J. Speidel (eds.). Academic Press, New York 1972.
Loginov, A. C.: Laparoszkopija. Medicina, Leningrad 1964.
Lübke, F.: Prognostic value of tubal diagnosis using laparoscopy. Proc. VII. World Congress on Fertility and Sterility, p. 797–798. Excerpta Medica Foundation, Amsterdam 1973.
Lübke, F.: Vergleich diagnostischer Ergebnisse der Hysterosalpingographie und der gynäkologischen Laparoskopie. In R. Ottenjann: Fortschritte der Endoskopie. S. 191. Schattauer, Stuttgart 1973.
Manual for the safe use of high frequency electronic equipment in hospitals. National Fire Protection Association, Boston 1970.
Marchesi, F., V. Albano, E. Cittadini: L'intérêt de la coelioscopie dans l'étude des hypoplasies et malformations de l'appareil génital féminin interne. C. R. Soc. franç. Gynéc. Colloque sur la Contraception, 1964.
Marchesi, F.: Il ruolo della celioscopia nella diagnostica ginecologica. Proc. I. Intern. Symp. on Gynec. Celioscopy, I.R.E.S., Palermo 1964, p. 7.
Marchesi, F., V. Albano, E. Cittadini: La nostra esperienza in tema di celioscopia nella diagnosi della sterilità femminile. In: Studi sulla sterilità. Minerva med. 1965.
Marchesi, F., V. Albano, E. Cittadini: Possibilità e limiti dell'indagine laparoscopica in ginecologia. Atti Soc. Ital. Gastroenterolaparoscopia, 1968.
Marchesi, F., V. Albano, E. Cittadini: La sterilità coniugale (monografia). Minerva med., Torino 1968.
Menken, F.: Photokolposkopie und Photodouglasskopie—Indikation und Technik. Girardet, Wuppertal 1955.
Menken, F.: Neue Erkenntnisse zur gynäkologischen Sterilitätsdiagnose durch Photokolposkopie und Photodouglasskopie. Proc. of the Second World Congress on Fertility and Sterility. Neapel 1956. p. 1179.
Menken, F.: Endoscopie en gynécologie. Rev. Méd. intern. de Photo-Cinéma-Television 1959.
Menken, F. C.: Photographische Dokumentation kolposkopischer Befunde. In L. Demling, R. Ottenjann: Endoskopie—Methoden, Ergebnisse. S. 186–193. Banaschewski, München-Gräfelfing 1969.
Menken, F.: Fortschritte der gynäkologischen Endoskopie. In L. Demling, R. Ottenjann: Fortschritte der Endoskopie. Schattauer, Stuttgart 1969. S. 203.
Menken, F. C.: Glasfiberendoskopie in der Gynäkologie. In R. Ottenjann: Fortschritte der Endoskopie. S. 176. Schattauer, Stuttgart 1973.
Mestwerdt, G., H.-J. Wespi: Atlas der Kolposkopie. 4. Aufl. Thieme, Stuttgart 1974.
Milliot: Die Methode der Durchleuchtung eines Theiles der Unterleibshöhle durch helles Glühlicht mit dem Mitteldorpf'schen Apparate. Schmid's Jahrbücher *136*:143 (1864).
Mintz, H., H. Elmach, J. De Brux: Cancer de l'ovaire décelé par ponction d'un kyste sous coelioscopie. XXe Congrès des Fed. de Gyn. et Obst. de Langue Française, Lille 1963. Masson, Paris 1964.
Mintz, M.: Per-celioscopic biopsy of the ovary and disorders of ovulation (Abstract). Proc. VII. World Congress on Fertility and Sterility, p. 806. Excerpta Medica Amsterdam, American Elsevier Publ. Co. Inc., New York 1973.
Mohri, T.: Demonstration of the Machida histeroscope. In: Proc. of the Seventh World Congress on Fertility and Sterility, Tokyo and Kyoto, October, 1971.
Mohri, T.: Research of Tubaloscopy. In R. Ottenjann: Fortschritte der Endoskopie. S. 176. Schattauer, Stuttgart 1973.
Morócz, K.: Az endoskopia jelentösége a nögyógyászatban. Elöadás; Nögyógyász szakcsoport 1961. II., 17.
Morócz, K., K. Varga: A laparoszkopia jelentösége a méhenkivüli terhesség diagnosztikájában. Elöadás; Nögyógyász szakcsoport 1961. II. 17.
Mueller, P.: Atlas d'endoscopie. II–III. Gynécologie et obstétrique. Laboratoires Roussel, Paris 1972.
Mueller, P.: Atlas d'endoscopie. Laboratoires Roussel, Paris 1973.
Narula, R. K., P. K. Maikani, S. Vhargava, V. Goyie, J. Rairana, S. Sidh: Comparative value of transabdominal and transuterine gynaecography. Proc. XVIth All India Obstetrics and Gynaecological Congress, New Delhi, 10–12 March 1972, p. 90. Dr. C. L. Ihaveri at the Popular Press (Bomb.). Private Ltd., Bombay 1972.
Neuwirth, R. S.: Nonpuerperal sterilization by laparoscopy. In R. Richart, D. J. Prager (eds.). p. 101–105. Human sterilization. Thomas, Springfield, Ill., 1972.
Neuwirth, R. S.: Nonpuerperal sterilization by laparoscopy. In: Human sterilization. Chapter 11.: R. M. Richart, D. J. Prager (eds.). Thomas, Springfield, Ill., 1972.

Ottenjann, R.: Fortschritte der Endoskopie. Kongreßbericht der Deutschen Gesellschaft für Endoskopie e. V., 1969. Bd. I. Schattauer, Stuttgart 1970.
Ottenjann, R.: Fortschritte der Endoskopie. Kongreßbericht der Deutschen Gesellschaft für Endoskopie e. V., 1970. Bd. 2. Schattauer, Stuttgart 1971.
Ottenjann, R.: Fortschritte der Endoskopie. Kongreßbericht der Deutschen Gesellschaft für Endoskopie e. V., 1972. Bd. 3. Schattauer, Stuttgart 1973.
Owen, R.: On the anatomy of vertebrates. Longinans, Green & Co, London 1868.
Pacheco-Mena, M.: Female sterilization by culdoscopy: an effective, simple, and inexpensive method. In: Advances in voluntary sterilization. Proc. of the Second International Conference, p. 55–61. Excerpta Medica Elsevier Publ. Co. Inc., New York 1974.
Palmer, R.: Abdominal coelioscopy in the diagnosis and treatment of sterility. Int. Congress of Obstetrics and Gynecology, Dublin 1947. p. 214.
Palmer, R.: La stérilité involontaire. Masson, Paris 1950.
Palmer, R., E. Palmer: Coelioscopie et tests d'ovulation. In: Anais do I. Convenio da Sociedade Brasileira de Esterilidade. p. 711–714. Rio de Janeiro 1951.
Palmer, R.: Discussion du rapport de M. Decker sur coelioscopie et troubles de l'ovulation. 1er Congrés mondial de Fertilité et Stérilité. New York, 26 Mai 1953. In: Proceedings *1*:pp. 378–379.
Palmer, R.: Indications et résultats de la coelioscopie dans la stérilité tubaire. Rapport au Colloque sur la fonction tubaire, Paris, 3 juill. 1955. In: La fonction tubaire. 1. vol. pp. 204–217. Masson, Paris 1955.
Palmer, R.: Possibilités actuelles de la coelioscopie et de la photocinématographie coelioscopique. Proc. 2nd World Congress on Fertility and Sterility, p. 1134, Neapel 1956.
Palmer, R.: La place de la coelioscopie dans le diagnostic des tumeurs de l'ovaire. Congrés chilien de Gynécologie et d'Obstétrique. Santiago du Chili, 2 déc. 1957.
Palmer, R.: Ce que l'on peut attendre actuellement de la coelioscopie en gynécologie. Journées gynécologiques et obstétricales de Lisbonne, 19 sept. 1959. Sopima, Porto 1959.
Palmer, R.: Photo et cinéma coelioscopiques. In J. Bruneau, D. de Montreynaud: Traité pratique de photographie et de cinématographie médicales. p. 222–223. Montel, Paris 1960.
Palmer, R.: Les explorations fonctionnelles gynécologiques. Masson, Paris 1963.
Palmer, R., J. Cohen: Biopsie percoelioscopique. Proceedings of the First International Symposium of Gynecology, Celios, 1964, p. 133.
Palmer, R.: Les techniques chirurgicales et coelioscopiques de stérilisation tubaire et leurs résultats. Paper presented at the May, meeting of the Association Nationale pour L'Etude de L'Avortement, Paris, International Conference on Contraception, Sterilization and Abortion.
Palmer, R., J. Cohen: Biopsias coelioscopiques. Proc. I. Internat. Symposium on gynecological celioscopy, Palermo 1964.
Palmer, R., E. Palmer: Les explorations fonctionnelles gynécologiques. p. 345. Masson, Paris 1963.
Pedrosa, F., J. Bernat, C. Stadnick: Laparoscopy, indication and technique. Proc. of the VIIIth World Congress on Fertility, 3.–9. November, Buenos Aires 1974.
Phillips, J. M., L. Keith: Gynecological laparoscopy: Principles and techniques. Symposia Specialists, Miami, Florida, 1975.
Phillips, J. M.: Laparoscopy—1970–1972. Off-line bibliographic citation list generated by NLM/Hedline, National Library of Medicine's Remote-Access Retrieval Service, Downey 1974.
Pous-Ivern, L. C., J. Massanas Rosado, M. A. Canosalazar, J. Esteban-Altirriba: Laparoscopy in gynecology. Proc. of the VIIIth World Congress on Fertility and Sterility, 3.–9. November, Buenos Aires 1974.
Proceedings of the First International Symposium on Gynecological Celioscopy, I.R.E.S., Palermo, 1964.
Pye, A.: Absence congénitale d'utérus et aplasie vaginale. Aspects endoscopiques. Proc. I. Intern. Symp. on Gynec. Celioscopy, I.R.E.S., Palermo 1964, p. 277.
Rao, A. P., K. M. C. Manipal, S. Kanara: Value of laparoscopy in the investigation of infertility. Proc. XVIth All India Obstetrics and Gynecological Congress, New Delhi, 10–12 March 1972, p. 94. Dr. C. L. Jhaveri at the Popular Press (Bomb.) Private Ltd., Bombay 1972.
Revelli, E., G. Durando: La necessità della indagine celioscopic sistematica nella diagnose della tuberculosi femminila genitopelvica. Proc. of the International Symposium on Gynecology and Celioscopy, I.R.E.S., Palermo, 1964. p. 355.
Richardt, R., D. J. Prager: Human sterilization. Thomas, Springfield, Ill., 1972.
Ringleb, O.: Das Kystoskop. Leipzig 1910.
Robert, H. G.: Técnicas de exploración y de tratamiento en ginecologia. Toray, Barcelona 1961.
Roland, M.: Management of the infertile couple. Thomas, Springfield, New York 1968.
Rosenfeld, A. G., D. Muangman: Sterilization procedures—their role in national family planning programs. In: Advances in voluntary sterilization. Proc. of the Second International Conference. Excerpta Medica American Elsevier Publ. Co., Inc., New York 1974.
Rossi, T., A. Scio: Interesse terapeutico delle biopsie-exeresi multiple percelioscopiche dell'ovaio con lo strumento di Palmer-Drapier. In: Atti del 52° Congr. Soc. Ital. Ost. e Ginec., Roma 1966.
Rubin, I. C.: Uterotubal insufflation. Mosby, St. Louis 1947.
Schima, M. E., I. Lubell, J. E. Davis, E. Connell: Advances in voluntary sterilization. Proc. of the Second International Conference. Excerpta Medica American Elsevier Publishing Co., Inc., New York 1974.

Schmidt, K. E. A.: Laparoskopische Tafeln. Deutsche Hoffmann-LaRoche AG, Baden. Neuauflage 1951, 1952.
Schmidt-Gollwitzer, M., E. Lorenz: Zur endoskopischen Diagnostik der Tubargravidität. In R. Ottenjann: Fortschritte der Endoskopie. S. 205. Schattauer, Stuttgart 1973.
Schwalm, H.: Die Laparoskopie in der gynäkologischen Diagnostik. In: Klinik der Frauenheilkunde und Geburtshilfe. I. S. 315. Urban & Schwarzenberg, München 1964.
Sciarra, J. J.: Research and developments programs to achieve practical outpatient sterilization. In: W. G. Duncan, D. R. Falb, J. J. Speidel (eds.). Female sterilization, Academic Press, New York and London 1972.
Sciarry, J. J.: Sterilization of women: a review of new and potentially reversible techniques. In: Advances in voluntary sterilization. Proc. of the Second International Conference. Excerpta Medica Elsevier American Elsevier Publ. Co. Inc., New York 1974.
Segalas, P. S.: Traité des rétentions d'urine etc. Paris 1828.
Semm, K.: A portio-adapter for cervical collection of menstrual blood. In: Latent female genital tuberculosis, p. 154. Karger, Basel, New York 1966.
Semm, K.: Tratamiento de las lesiones benignas de cuello. In: Temas selectos de gineco-obstetricia; Libro homenaje ofrecido al Prof. Dr. Alfonso Alvarez Bravo. S. 89. Division Lederle de Cyanamid de Mexico, S. A., Mexico 1967.
Semm, K.: Das Pneumoperitoneum mit co_2. In L. Demling, R. Ottenjann: Endoskopie-Methoden, Ergebnisse. S. 167–169. Banaschewski, München 1967.
Semm, K.: Newer methods. In S. J. Behrman, R. W. Kistner: Progress in infertility, p. 869–893. Little, Brown & Co., Boston 1968.
Semm, K.: Zur Technik der Tubenkatheterisierung bei Sterilitätsoperationen. In Proc. of the I. European Congress on Sterility, Venedig 6.–7. Mai 1967, p. 607–609. Genua 1968.
Semm, K.: Prüfung der Tubendurchgängigkeit. In O. Käser, V. Friedber, K. G. Ober, K. Thomsen, J. Zander: Gynäkologie und Geburtshilfe. Bd. 2, S. 857. Thieme, Stuttgart 1969.
Semm, K.: Weitere Entwicklungen in der gynäkologischen Laparoskopie—Gynäkologische Pelviskopie. In H. Schwalm, G. Döderlein: Klinik der Frauenheilkunde und Geburtshilfe, Bd. 1 Erg. 5, S. 326/1–326/39. Urban & Schwarzenberg, München, Berlin, Wien 1970.
Semm, K.: Die gynäkologische Pelviskopie. In: Probleme der Sterilität in Klinik und Praxis. S. 15. München 1971.
Semm, K.: Pelviskopische, kolposkopische und amnioskopische Befunde. In H. Orbach: Medizinische Fotografie und Kinematografie. S. 146–154. Thieme, Stuttgart 1971.
Semm, K.: Gynecological pelviscopy in female sterility. Proc. VII. World Congress on Fertility and Sterility. p. 34–37. Excerpta Medica, American Elsevier Publ. Co. Inc., New York 1973.
Semm, K.: The technique of gynecological pelviscopy in human reproduction. In A. Campos Da Paz, T. Hasegawa, M. P. Notake, M. Hayashi: Human reproduction, p. 101–112. Igaku Shoin, Kyoto 1974.
Semm, K.: Tubal sterilization finally with cauterization or temporary with ligation via pelviscopy. In J. M. Phillips, L. Keith: Gynecological laparoscopy—principles and techniques. p. 337–359. Symposia Specialists, Miami, Florida, 1975.
Semm, K.: Elektronisch gesteuerter Schwachstrom als Ersatz des Hochfrequenzstromes in der Endoskopie. In: R. Ottenjann: Fortschritte der Endoskopie, Bd. 6, S. 17–21. Schattauer, Stuttgart 1975.
Siede, W., H. Schneider: Leitfaden und Atlas der Laparoskopie. Lehmann, München 1962.
Siegler, A.: Laparoscopy and hysteroscopy. Proc. of the VIIIth World Congress on Fertility and Sterility, 3.–9. November, Buenos Aires 1974.
Šimić, S.: Proc. of the First International Symposium on Gynecological Celioscopy, I.R.E.S., Palermo, 1964.
Šimić, S.: Coelioskopija u ginekologiji Svjetlost, Izdavačko Preduzeće, Sarajevo 1969.
Sjövall, A.: The possibility of an extended postcoital test by laparoscopy in cases of sterility. Proc. I. Intern. Symp. on Gynec. Celioscopy, I.R.E.S., Palermo 1964, p. 227.
Sjövall, A.: Laparoscopy in the diagnosis of acute salpingitis. Proc. I. Intern. Symp. on Gynec. Celioscopy, I.R.E.S., Palermo 1964, p. 329.
Speidel, J. J.: The role of female sterilization in family planning programs. In: Female sterilization: Prognosis for simplified outpatient procedures. W. G. Duncan, R. D. Falb, J. J. Speidel (eds.). Academic Press, New York, London 1972.
Speidel, J. J., M. I. Perry, G. W. Duncan: Research approaches to new sterilization. Proc. of the Second International Conference. Excerpta Medica American Elsevier Publ. Co. Inc., New York 1974.
Speidel, J. J., M. I. Perry, G. W. Duncan: An overview of research on new sterilization technology. In: Advances in voluntary sterilization. Proc. of the Second International Conference. p. 194–199. Excerpta Medica American Elsevier Publ. Co., New York 1974.
Stein, A., W. H. Stewart: Pneumoperitoneal roentgen-ray diagnosis. Southworth Co., Troy, New York 1919.
Stein, S.: The endoscope as an aid in the diagnosis and treatment of granular urethritis and stricture. East River Med. Association 1. Oct b. The Med. Record New York 1868, vol 2, pag. 416.
Stephan, J., E. H. Kellogg: The world's laws on voluntary sterilization for family planning purposes. Law and Population Monograph Series No. 8. Law and Population Program. The Fletcher School of Law and Diplomacy, Medford, Mass., 1973.

Steptoe, P. C.: Proc. of the First International Symposium on Gynecological Celioscopy, I.R.E.S., Palermo 1964.
Steptoe, P. C.: Laparoscopy in gynecology, p. 75. Livingstone, Edinburgh 1964.
Steptoe, P. C.: Laparoscopy in the study of pelvic flogosis excluding tuberculosis. Proc. I. Intern. Symp. on Gynec. Celioscopy, I.R.E.S., Palermo 1964, p. 321.
Steptoe, P. C.: Laparoscopy in gynaecology. Livingstone, Edinburgh, London 1967.
Steptoe, P. C., A. J. Smith: Contraception today. London Family Planning Assoc. p. 108–112. London 1971.
Symposium Laparoscopic Sterilization. In: Contemporary Obstetrics and Gynecology *11*:71 (1973).
Thews, G.: Nomogramme zum Säure-Basen-Status des Blutes und zum Atemgastransport. Springer, Berlin, Heidelberg, New York 1971.
Thompson, H. E., T. Moulding, C. Dafoe, D. L. Osterling: Transvaginal delivery of sterilizing chemicals. In Richart, R. M., D. J. Prager: Human sterilization. Chapter 30. Thomas, Springfield, Ill., 1972.
Thoyer-Rozat, J.: La coelioscopie. Technique—Indications. Masson, Paris 1962.
Thoyer-Rozat, J.: La coelioscopie dans les grossesses extrautérines et la pathologie gravidique. Proc. I. Intern. Symp. on Gynec. Celioscopy, I.R.E.S., Palermo 1964, p. 297.
Un Manual de Laparoscopia. Departamento de Educación Professional de los Laboratorios, Seccion I. Introducucción. Searle, Parte de G. D., Searle & Compania.
Unverricht: Technik und Methoden der Thorakoskopie. Leipzig 1925.
Wheeless, C. R., Jr.: Outpatient sterilization by laparoscopy under local anesthesia in less developed countries. In: Female sterilization: Prognosis for simplified outpatient procedures. G. W. Duncan, R. D. Falb, J. J. Speidel (eds.). pp. 125–129. Academic Press, New York, London 1972.
Wheeless, C.: Techniques for female sterilization by laparoscopy with local anesthesia under field conditions. In: Female sterilization: Prognosis for simplified outpatient procedures. G. W. Duncan, R. D. Falb, J. J. Speidel (eds.). Academic Press, New York 1972.
Whitelaw, M. J., V. F. Nola: Removal of fimbrial protheses by laparoscopy. Proc. VII. World Congress on Fertility and Sterility, p. 802–804. Excerpta Medica Foundation, Amsterdam 1973.
Williams, W. W.: Sterility: The diagnostic survey of the infertile couple. Williams, Springfield, Mass., 1953.
Wintz-Dyroff: Das Pneumoperitoneum in der Gynäkologie. Thieme, Stuttgart 1924.
Wittmann, I.: A laparoskopia atlasza. Medicina Könyvkiadó, Budapest 1965.
Wittman, I.: Peritoneoscopy. Publishing House of the Hungarian Academy of Sciences, Budapest 1966.
Wortman, J., P. T. Piotrow: Laparoscopic sterilization, a new technique. Sterilization, Pop. Rep., Series C, No. 1, 1973.
Wortman, J., P. T. Piotrow: Laparoscopic sterilization. II. What are the problems? Pop. Rep. Series C, No. 2, 1973.
Wrage, D., H. J. Lindemann: Pelviskopische Nachuntersuchungen an durch Elektrokoagulation sterilisierten Tuben. In R. Ottenjann: Fortschritte der Endoskopie. S. 201. Schattauer, Stuttgart 1973.
Zipper, J., M. Medel, E. Stachetti, L. Pastene, M. Rivera, R. Prager: Chemical agents for transvaginal sterilization. In R. M. Richart, D. J. Prager: Human sterilization. Chapter 29. Thomas, Springfield, Ill., 1972.

CLASSIC WORKS ON LAPAROSCOPY

Abarbanel, A.: "Unexplained" infertility and culdoscopy; observations in fifty consecutive cases. Urol. Rev. *55*:339 (1951).
Abarbanel, A. R.: Transvaginal pelviscopy (peritoneoscopy); simplified and safe technic as office procedure. Amer. J. Surg. *90*:122–128 (1955).
Abay, H.: Über Endoskopie. Pester med. chir. Presse 1882.
Albano, V., E. Cittadini: La laparoscopia in ginecologia. Riv. Ost. Ginec. *17*:201 (1962).
Albano, V., E. Cittadini, P. Quartararo: L'interesse della laparoscopia nello studio delle sindromi da corpo luteo permanente. Atti V. Congr. Intern. Ripr. Anim. e Fecond. artif. *5*:208 (1964).
Albano, V., E. Carollo, E. Cittadini: Il ruolo della laparoscopia nella diagnosi delle disgenesie gonadiche. Min. pediat. *10*:603 (1965).
Alexander, G. D., E. M. Brown: Physiologic alterations during pelvic laparoscopy. Amer. J. Obstet. Gynec. *105*:1078–1081 (1969).
Alexander, G. D., F. E. Noe, E. M. Brown: Anesthesia for pelvic laparoscopy. Anesth. Analg. *48*:14–18 (1969).
Alfonsin, A. E.: Stérilisation tubaire par section—Electrocoagulation per célioscopique des isthmes tubaires. C. R. Soc. franç. Gynéc. *37*:147 (1967).
Alfonsin, A. E., A. Chaulet, J. Bottaro: Morbididad en laparoscopia. Obstet. Ginec. Lat. Amer. *32*:102 (1974).
Allodi, A., M. Banche, F. Muratori: L'indagine endoscopie della cavita abdominale. (Nostre prime esperienze.) Minerva med. *43*, 2:11–15 (1952).

Amin, H. K., R. S. Neuwirth: Further experience with laparoscopic sterilization concomitant with vacuum curettage for abortion. Fertil. and Steril. *24*:592–594 (1973).
Aminev, A. M.: Vozrodit peritoneoszkopiju. Vracs. delo *6*:(1939).
Aminev, A. M.: Peritoneoscopy. Vesztny. Hir. *58*:334–337 (1939).
Aminev, A. M.: Peritoneoscopy, pneumoperitoneum and problems of intra-abdominal pressure. Vesztny. Hir. *3*:44–50 (1949).
Anderson, E. T.: Peritoneoscopy. Amer. J. Surg. *35*:36 (1937).
Anita, F. P.: Peritoneoscopy. J. int. Coll. Surg. *17*:679 (1952).
Anonymous: Sterilization for both sexes. Time *95*:38 (1970).
Anonymous: Laparoscopy. Short cut to sterilization. Med. World News *11*:20 (1970).
Anonymous: Control of fertility by sterilization. Canad. med. Ass. J. *104*:527–528 (1972).
Anonymous: Sterilization—Simpler methods boast public acceptance. Family Planning Digest *1*:4–7 (1972).
Anonymous: Low cost sterilization. Bulitin Keluarga (Malaysia) *51*:7 (1972).
Ansari, A. H.: The cul-de-sac approach to induction of pneumoperitoneum for pelvic laparoscopy and pneumography. Fertil. and Steril. *21*:599–605 (1970).
Antonovitsch, E.: Zölioskopie, insbesondere Douglasskopie. Zbl. Gynäk. *9*:896–897 (1949).
Antonovitsch, E.: Die Endoskopie des Douglasraumes (Die Douglasskopie). Zbl. Gynäk. *74*:1387 (1952).
Aramaki, N.: Peritoneoscopy and surgery (Jap.) Shujutsu *23*:771–779 (1969).
Ardizzone, G.: La coelioscopia gynecologica. Minerva med. *50*:2423–2424 (1959).
Aresin: Über Douglasskopie. Zbl. Gynäk. *74*:401–410 (1952).
Aronson, A. R., G. W. Parker: Peritoneoscopy: its value as a diagnostic aid. Amer. J. digest. Diseases *5*:931 (1960).
Arronet, G. H., S. Y. Eduljee, J. R. O'Brien: A nine-year survey of fallopian tube dysfunction in human infertility. Diagnosis and therapy. Fertil. and Steril. *20*:903–918 (1969).
Aubinais: Un Med. Provence. (Marseille) *24*:591 (1864).
Bachmann: Intraperitoneale Blutung aus einem Corpus luteum. Zbl. Gynäk. *49*:1915–1918 (1955).
Bailer, P.: Laparoskopische Tubensterilisation—Kontrazeptivum auf Dauer. Mediz. Mschr. *26*:49–50 (1972).
Balin, H., L. S. Wan, L. S. Israel: Recent advances in pelvic endoscopy. Obstet. and Gynec. *21*:343 (1963).
Balin, H., L. S. Wan, L. S. Israel: Recent advances in pelvic endoscopy. Obstet. and Gynec. *27*:30 (1966).
Balin, H., L. S. Wan, R. Rajan, A. Kaiser, R. H. Macmann: Experimental applications of endoscopy. Clin. Obstet. Gynec. *12*:534–552 (1969).
Baratz, R. A., H. Karis: Blood gas studies during laparoscopy under general anesthesia. Anesthesiology *30*:463–464 (1969).
Battig, C. G.: Electrosurgical burn injuries and their prevention. Amer. med. Ass. *204*:1025–1029 (1968).
Belbenoit, S. F. Louison: Accidents et complications du pneumopéritonie. Presse méd. *62*:22 (1954).
Beling, C. A.: Experiences in diagnosis with the peritoneoscopy: Indications for it. J. med. Soc. N. J. *36*:602–605 (1939).
Beling, C. A.: Selection of cases for peritoneoscopy. Arch. Surg. *42*:872–889 (1941).
Benaim Pinto, V., A. Ortega Borjas, A. Diaz-Bruzal: Gynecological coelioscopy. Rev. Obstet. Gynec. *20*:285–296 (1960).
Belbenoit, S., J. F. Louison: Accidents et complications du pneumopéritonie. Presse méd. *62*:22 (1954).
Bernhard, J., K. Semm: Reaktion des Portiogewebes nach mechanischer Traumatisierung. Arch. Gynäk. *204*:63 (1967).
Bishop, H. L., T. F. Halpin: Dehiscence following laparoscopy: Report of an unusual complication. Amer. J. Obstet. Gynec. *116*:585 (1973).
Bismuth, E.: La coelioscopie gynécologique, son application à l'étude de la stérilité. Thèse, Paris 45, 1945.
Black, W. P.: Sterilisation by laparoscopic tubal electrocoagulation: an assessment. Amer. J. Obstet. Gynec. *111*:979–983 (1971).
Black, W. P., A. D. T. Govan: Laparoscopy and ovarian biopsy for the assessment of secondary amenorrhea. Amer. J. Obstet. Gynec. *114*:739–747 (1972).
Bleier, W.: Eine neue Methode der Tubensterilisation mit Polyacetal-Clip. Vortrag auf dem Oberrheinisch-Schweizerischen Gynäkologenkongreß. Freiburg 1973.
Bleier, W.: Transvaginaler Tubenverschluß mit Kunststoff-Clips. Vortrag auf dem Nordwestdeutschen Gynäkologen-Kongreß. Hamburg, April 1975.
Bleier, W.: Tuben-Sterilisation mit einem Polyacetal-Clip. Hug, D-7801 Umkirch.
Bombalgini: Arch. Générales, Jan. 1827.
Bonte, M., R. Palmer: Résultats de la coelioscopie dans l'etude des échecs de la chirurgie tubaire. C. R. Soc. franç. Gynéc. *31*:83–89 (1961).
Bosworth, B. M.: Peritoneoscopy versus exploratory laparotomy. Comparison of morbidity and mortality. Amer. J. Surg. *54*:502–504 (1941).

Botella-Llusia, J., J. M. Bedoya, Y. F. La Fuente: La coelioscopie transvaginale. Acta ginec. (Madr.) *3*:481 (1952).
Bozorgi, N., R. C. Steptoe, H. Havdala, M. Prenzlau, B. Salvo: The use of Ketamine anesthesia for Laparoscopy. Obstet. and Gynec. *39*:639 (1972).
Bradfield, G. F.: Laparoscopic sterilization. First international Planned Parenthood Federation Publication, Regional Medical and Scientific Congress, South-East Asia and Oceania, 1972, pp. 46–47.
Branco, J. M. C., S. R. Barbosa: Peritoneoscopia. Clin. Physiol. *6*:451–457 (1951).
Brooks, M. J.: Sterilization short cut. Med. World News *11*:12 (1970).
Brown, A. B., K. M. Croker: Culdoscopy. Amer. J. Obstet. Gynec. *80*:25–29 (1960).
Brubaker, J. H., Brubaker, J. D., and P. H. Hollinger: Recent progress in open-tube endoscopic and cavity still and motion picture photography. J. Biol. Photographic A., 1957.
Brühl, W.: Zur Technik der Laparoskopie – Komplikationsmöglichkeiten bei der Einführung des Laparoskopschaftes und ihre Verhütung. Gastroenterologie *9*:525–529 (1971).
Budge, B. C.: Office culdoscopy. Northw. Med. (Seattle) *53*:132 (1954).
Bunch, C.: Peritoneoscopy. J. S. C. med. Ass. *45*:74–75 (1949).
Burch, L. E., J. Seitchik: Ectopic gestation. The diagnostic value of cul-de-sac aspiration. Amer. J. Obstet. Gynec. *50*:765 (1945).
Buxton, C. L.: (Felszólalás cim Nélkül). Amer. J. Obstet. Gynec. *63*:675 (1952).
Buxton, C. L., W. Hermann: An analysis of one hundred culdoscopies. Amer. J. Obstet. Gynec. *68*:786 (1954).
Buxton, C. L., et al.: Culdoscopy, colpotomy, or culdocentesis as diagnostic procedures: Which one? Trans. New Engl. obst. gynec. Soc. *14*:47 (1960).
Buytaert P. M. H. G., E. V. van Hall: Hundert gynäkologische Laparoskopien. Ned. T. Geneesk. *113*:553–555 (1969).
Calamé, A.: Laparoscopie, cholangiographie et photographie laparoscopique. Gastroenterologia (Basel) *82*:88 (1954).
Calamé, A.: La photographie laparoscopique. Presse méd. *63*:1848 (1955).
Calamé, A.: Laparoscopic photography. Med. Biol. Ill. *6*:148 (1956).
Carmichael, D. E.: Laparoscopy in gynecology. J. med. Ass. Ala. *39*:241–242 (1969).
Carmichael, D. E.: Laparoscopy – Cardiac considerations. Fertil. and Steril. *22*:69–70 (1971).
Caroli, J., A. Fourés: La laparophotographie. Sem. Hôp. Paris *33*:2389–2392 (1957).
Caspi, E., H. Hirsch: Laparoscopy in gynecology. Report on 150 Laparoscopies. Harefuah *75*:460–463 (1968).
Castleton, K. B.: Peritoneoscopy. Rocky Mtn. med. J. *41*:247–251 (1944).
Catarivas de Ansaldo, V.: Celioscopia transparietal en ginecologia. Tesis de doctorado. Univ. Nac. Córdoba 1971.
Caviglia: Sobre laparoscopia. Bol. Soc. Cirug. B. Aires *8*:913 (1924).
Cekanski, A.: Culdoscopy. (Pol.) Wiad lek. *21*:461–467 (1968).
Chaffe, J. S.: Postmortem peritoneoscopy; Means of learning peritoneoscopy. Ann. Surg. *116*:843–850 (1942).
Chaturachinda, K.: Laparoscopy: a technique for a tropical setting. Amer. J. Obstet. Gynec. *112*:941 (1972).
Chaturachinda, K.: Interval sterilization by peritoneoscope. J. med. Ass. Thailand *55*:395–399 (1972).
Cherigié, E.: La télévision médicale. Ann. Chir. *3*:26–28 (1957).
Chun, D., H. K. Ma, J. K. Yip, P. K. Chan: Laparoscopic tubal sterilization. International Planned Parenthood Federation (IPPF) Medical Bulletin *4*:1–3 (1970).
Cismeres: Considerations sobre laparoscopia. Bol. Soc. Cirug. B. Aires *8*:893–909 (1924).
Cittadini, E., P. Quartararo: L'apporto della laparoscopia alla diagnosi dell'endometriosi esterna. Aggiorn. Ostet. e Ginec. (Palermo) *3*:221 (1961).
Cittadini, E.: Interesse della celioscopia nella diagnosi della gravidanza ectopica extracoriale – Descrizione di due casi di aborto tubo addominale. Sicilia sanit. *15*:671 (1962).
Cittadini, E., D. Funaro, F. Romano: L'aspirazione percelioscopica del sangue refluo dalle tube nella verifica della teoria di Sampson. Clin. ginec. *9*:533 (1967).
Cittadini, E., T. Rossi: L'impiego della camera Polaroid-Land nella celiofotografia. Clin. ginec. *12*:115 (1970).
Clarce, B.: Female sterilization using the laparoscope. Med. J. Aust. *1*:493 (1972).
Clarce, H.: Laparoscopy – New instruments for suturing and ligation. Fertil. and Steril. *23*:274–277 (1972).
Clauss, J.: Douglasskopie und Sterilität. Dtsch. med. Wschr. *22*:886–888 (1954).
Clauss, J.: Ein neuer Douglasskopiestuhl. Zbl. Gynäk. *78*:707–711 (1956).
Clyman, M. J.: A new panculdoscope – Diagnostic, photographic and operative aspects. Obstet. and Gynec. *21*:343 (1963).
Clyman, M. J.: Importance of culdoscopy in sterility studies. N. Y. med. J. *66*:1867 (1966).
Clyman, M. J.: A new approach to the study of tubal physiology in situ. Pacif. med. Surg. *74*:119 (1966).
Clyman, M. J.: Operative culdoscopy. Obstet. and Gynec. *32*:840 (1968).
Clyman, M. J.: Fiber optic cannula for the panculdoscope. Amer. J. Obstet. Gynec. 105281–15. Sept. 1969.
Cognat, M., R. Lyonnet, J. Saint-Arrowman: Stérilisation tubaire per-coelioscopique: Technique et avantages. Lyon méd. *222*:803–806 (1969).

Cohen, M. R.: The role of culdoscopy in infertility. Amer. J. Obstet. Gynec. *78*:266 (1959).
Cohen, M. R.: Culdoscopy vs. peritoneoscopy. Obstet. and Gynec. *31*:310–321 (1968).
Cohen, M. R., et al.: Interval tubal sterilization via laparoscopy. Amer. J. Obstet. Gynec. *108*:458–461 (1970).
Cohen, M.: Hazards of laparoscopy. Arizona Medicine *28*:830 (1971).
Cohen, M., R. M. B. Taylor, M. B. Kass: Internal tubal sterilization via laparoscopy. Amer. J. Obstet. Gynec. *109*:794–809 (1971).
Coltart, T. M.: Laparoscopy in the diagnosis of tubal patency. J. Obstet. Gynaec. Brit. Cwlth. 77:69–71 (1970).
Copenhaver, E. H.: A critical assessment of culdoscopy. (End.) Surg. Clin. N. Amer. *50*:713–717 (1970).
Cordua: (Felszólalás cím nélkül). Zbl. Gynäk. *35*:1389 (1952).
Corson, S. L., R. Bolognese J.: Laparoscopy: An overview and results of a large series. J. repr. Med. *9*:148–157 (1972).
Corson, S. L., R. J. Bolognese: Laparoscopic nuances. Fertil. and Steril. *22*:684–689 (1971).
Corson, S. L., H. P. Th. Hamilton, R. J. Bolognese: Electrical considerations of laparoscopic sterilization. J. repr. Med. *11*:4 (1973).
Cortesi, N., A. Bertaglia, A. Manenti, M. Speranza: A case of symmetric bilateral agenesis of the uterus. (Rokitansky-Kuster's syndrome) diagnosed by peritoneoscopy. Endoscopy *4*:43–45 (1972).
Cortesi, N., B. Cuoghi, F. Boschini: Indagine laparoscopia e gravidanze extrauterina. Riv. Ostet. Ginec. prat *52*:37–49 (1970).
Craft, I., P. Diggory: Problems in male and female sterilization. Lancet *7758*:1011 (1972).
Craft, I., P. Bowen-Simpkins: Puerperal laparoscopic sterilization. Fertil. and Steril. *24*:426–428 (1973).
DaBroi, G. L.: Abdominal endoscopy as a method of clinical examination. Rass. Clin. Ter. *59*:241–253 (1960).
Daley, J., H. Kotz, R. Hausknecht, L. Mastroianni, D. C. Davis, I. Friedmann: Culdoscopy, colpostomy, or culdocentesis as diagnostic procedures. Which one? Trans. New Engl. obstet. gynec. Soc. *14*:47–68 (1960).
Dargent, D., H. Fayette: La stérilisation chirurgicale féminine. Thérapeutique *48*:711–716 (1972); Sem. Hôp. Paris *48Z* 2119–2123 (1972).
Dargent, D., P. H. Fargier, P. Schuster: Le coup d'oeil coelioscopique pré-opératoire dans certaines indications de l'hystérectomie vaginale. C. R. Soc. franç Gynéc. *42*:549–556 (1972).
Dasher, W. A., J. P. M. Black, W. Weiss, E. Bogen: Air embolism complicating pneumoperitoneum: A review. Amer. Rev. Tuberc. *69*:369 (1954).
Daves, M. L., W. C. Diner, G. H. Brenner: Pelvic pneumography. Amer. J. Roentgenol. *92*:390 (1964).
David, A., C. R. Garcia, B. Czernobilsky: Human hydrosalpinx. Histologic study and chemical composition of fluid. Amer. J. Obstet. Gynec. *105*:400–411 (1969).
Davidson, A. C., I. Donald: Female sterilization. Scot. med. J. *17*:210–213 (1972).
de Boer, C. H., G. Dunster: Tubal electrocoagulation under laparoscopic control. Lancet *7654/I*997 (1970).
Debray, C., J. Paolaggi, R. Laumonier, E. Martin: Biopsie à la pince sous controle laparoscopique. Arch. Mal. Appar. dig. *50*:344–349 (1961).
Debray, C., J. Paolaggi, R. Laumonier, E. Martin: La biopsie à la pince sous péritonéoscopie. Sem. Hôp. Paris *37*:1908–1916 (1961).
de Brux, J. A., J. Dupré-Froment, M. Mintz: Cytology of the peritoneal fluids sampled by coelioscopy or by cul-de-sac puncture; its value in gynecology. Acta cytol. (Philad.) *12*:395 (1968).
de Brux, J., R. Palmer, M. Mintz: Cytology of para-uterine tumors punctured under coelioscopy. J. int. Fed. Gynaec. Obstet. *5*:247–254 (1967).
Decker, A.: Culdoscopy: its diagnostic value in pelvic disease. J. Amer. med. Ass. *140*:378 (1949).
Decker, A.: The mechanical treatment of tubal occlusion by culdoscopy and insufflation. Fertil. and Steril. *2*:487 (1951).
Decker, A.: Culdoscopy. Amer. J. Obstet. Gynec. *63*:654–659 (1952).
Dellepiane, G., C. Durando, E. Revelli: Il problema clinico della tubercolosi genitale femminile. Arch. Chir. Orthop. *3*:5 (1957).
Denicker, M.: La ≫coelioscopy≪ en gynécologie. Rev. méd. (Paris) *29*:23–24 (1948).
Derjabina, E. J.: Metod peritoneoszkopii i ginekologii. Zsurn. akus. i ginekol. *5* (1957).
de Senarclens, F.: Celioscopy as method of investigation of general sterility. Praxis *35*:739 (1946).
de Senarclens, F.: Coelioscopie et cycle ovarien. Gynecologia (Basel) *123*:220–237 (1947).
Desneux, J. J., et al.: La laparoscopie au point de vue du médecin. Acta chir. belg. *62*, *5*:564–566 (1963).
Dick, H.: Remarks on the use of the endoscope. Lancet (1866).
Dierschke, D. J., J. L. Hyatt: Peritoneoscopy via a chronically implanted cannula to observe ovarian activity in ewes. J. Anim. Sci. *28*:645–649 (1969).
Dignam, W. J.: The usefulness of culdoscopy in gynecologic diagnosis. Ariz. Med. *8*:132–135 (1961).
Dillon, T. F., B. D. Smith: Culdoscopy. Fertil. and Steril. *21*:104–109 (1970).
Dineen, P.: The ≫sterilization≪ of endoscopic instruments. J. Amer. med. Ass. *176*:772–775 (1961).
Dionisi, H., T. Goldsman: Celioscopia y celiofotografia en ginecologia. Rev. Soc. Obstet. Ginec. B. Aires *47*:406–412 (1968).

Dlhos, E.: Importance of culdoscopy in the diagnosis of sterility. Zbl. Gynäk. *90*:1394–1397 (1968).
Dlhos, E.: Narrowing down the indication for exploratory laparotomy using gynecoscopy. Bratisl. Lek. Listy *53*:230–232 (1970).
Dogu, T. S., D. R. Cook: Extradural analgesia for culdoscopy. Anesth. Annals (Cleveland) *48*:237–241 (1969).
Donaldson, J. K., J. H. Sanderlin, W. B. Harrel jun: Method of suspending uterus without open abdominal incision; Use of peritoneoscope and special needle. Amer. J. Surg. *55*:537–543 (1942).
Dorangeon, P., R. Palmer: La coelioscopie en cancérologie gynécologique. Gynéc. prat. *12*:335–344 (1961).
Dorofeev, N. M.: A simple modification of endoscopy of the cavity of the true pelvis in women. Zsurn. akus. i ginekol. *37*:79–83 (1961).
Doyle, J. B.: Exploratory culdotomy for observation of tuboovarian physiology at ovulation time. Fertil. and Steril. *2*:477 (1951).
Doyle, J. B.: Use of the pelvioscope in culdotomy. Aid to early diagnosis and relief of pelvic disorders. J. Amer. med. Ass. *151*:605 (1953).
Doyle, J. B.: Ovulation and effect of selective uterotubal denervation; Direct observation by culdotomy. Fertil. and Steril. *5*:105–130 (1954).
Drury, W. L., D. A. LaVallee, C. J. Vacanti: Effects of laparoscopic tubal ligation on arterial blood gases. Anesth. Analg. Curr. Res. *1971*:349–351.
Dubois de Montreynaud, J. M., S. Segal: Simplification and standardization in the taking of objective pictures in endoscopy. Ann. Oto-laryng. *77*:227–229 (1960).
Dumont, M.: Criteria of safety during gynecologic celioscopy. Lyon méd. *223*:677–670 (1970).
Durando, C., M. Faccini: L'associazione celioscopia e pneumoginecografia nella diagnostica ginecologica. Minerva ginec. *10*:187–203 (1958).
Durando, C.: Laparoscopy. Minerva med. *51*:1729–1733 (1960).
Durando, C.: Laparoscopy. Minerva ginec. *12*:113–117 (1960).
Edwards, R. L.: Culdoscopia técnica modificado usando dióxido de carbono. Sinops. obstét.-ginec. *14*:76–79 (1967).
Ehrler, P.: Die intramurale Tubenanastomose. Zbl. Gynäk. *85*:393–400 (1963).
Ehrler, P.: Tubeninstrumentarium nach Dr. P. Ehrler. Kurzinformation Dr. Ing. R. Straumann AG, CH-4437 Waldenburg.
Eisenburg, J.: Über eine Apparatur zur schonenden und kontrollierbaren Gasfüllung der Bauchhöhle für die Laparoskopie. Klin. Wschr. *44*:593–594 (1966).
Elizarovszkij, Sz. I.: Szlucsaj szarkomi zseludka, diagnosztirovannij do operacii metodom peritoneoszkopii. Hirurgija *12* (1946).
Elert, R.: Der Mechanismus der Eiabnahme im Laparoskop. Zbl. Gynäk. *1*:38–43 (1947).
Elstein, M.: Sterilization and family planning. Practitioner *205*:30–37 (1970).
Endicott, E. T.: Peritoneoscopy. J. Amer. Women's Ass. *3*:192–194 (1948).
Epple, H., F. Funk: Die Laparoskopie in der gynäkologischen Ambulanz. Dtsch. Ärztebl. 1982–1984 (1973).
Epstein, M.: Right sided spontaneous pneumothorax and peritoneal effusion complicating therapeutic pneumoperitoneum. Amer. Rev. Tuberc. *66*:90 (1952).
Espagno, G.: Trois ans de pratique de coelioscopie. Réflexions à propos de 160 observations. Bull. Féd. Soc. Gynéc. Obstét. franç. *12*:638–639 (1960).
Espagno, G.: Study of 250 cases of celioscopy in gynecology. Toulouse med. *63*:1086 (1962).
Esposito, J. M.: A method for preventing abdominal burns caused by electrocautery during laparoscopy. Amer. J. Obstet. Gynec. *114*:1105–1106 (1972).
Esposito, J. M.: Electrical burn of the abdominal wall as a complication of fallopian tube cautery. Fertil. and Steril. *24*:158–160 (1973).
Evans, T. N.: Simplified method for sterilization of the female. Amer. J. Obstet. Gynecol. *66*:393–395 (1953).
Fahrländer, H.: Laparoskopie bei abdominellen Notfällen. Helv. chir. Acta *32*:54 (1965).
Fahrländer, H.: Die Laparoskopie bei abdominellen Notfällen. Dtsch. med. Wschr. *94*:890 (1969).
Fahrländer, H., G. Engelhardt, Ch. Baerlocher: Emergency peritoneoscopy. Report on 160 cases. Endoscopy *2*:120–122 (1970).
Fairbrother, P. F., M. C. Anderson: Pregnancy after laparoscopic sterilization. Lancet 1011–1012 (1972).
Fathalla, M. F.: Laparoscopic sterilization in the family planning program in developing communities. Contraception *6*:295–303 (1972).
Fear, R. E.: Laparoscopy: a valuable aid in gynecologic diagnosis. Obstet. and Gynec. *31Z* 297–309 (1968).
Fegerle, H., K. Narik: Die Varicocele pelvina muliebrum als selbständiges Krankheitsbild. Zbl. Gynäk. *10*:392–396 (1954).
Feldman, J. P., C. Sureau: Utilisation de la voie transpariétale suspubienne en coelioscopie gynécologique. Gynéc. et Obstét. (Paris) *69*:55–64 (1970).
Fenger, Chr., Hinde: The endoskope etc. Chicago med. Rev. 1880.
Fervers, C.: Die Laparoskopie mit dem Cystoskop. Ein Beitrag zur Vereinfachung der Technik und zur endoskopischen Strangdurchtrennung in der Bauchhöhle. Med. Klin. *29*:1042–1045 (1933).

Fervers, C.: Die Laparoskopie mit dem Cystoskop. Ein Beitrag zur Vereinfachung der Technik und zur endoskopischen Strangdurchtrennung in der Bauchhöle. Med. Klin. Chir. *118*:288 (1933).

Fikentscher, R.: Die Erfassung der männlichen und weiblichen Faktoren als Sterilitätsursachen und ihre Auswertung für die Prognose und Therapie. Münch. med. Wschr. *112*:1671–1681 (1970).

Fikentscher, R., K. Semm: Beitrag zur Methodik der utero-tubaren Pertubation. Geburtsh. u. Frauenheilk. *15*:313 (1955).

Fikentscher, R., K. Semm: Beitrag zur Deutung der bei der utero-tubaren Persufflation erhaltenen Oscillationen. Arch. Gynäk. *188*:192–200 (1956).

Fikentscher, R., K. Semm: Physikalische Grundlagen zur utero-tubaren Persufflation. Arch. Gynäk. *188*:184–191 (1956).

Fikentscher, R., K. Semm: Weitere Untersuchungen zur Methodik der Pertubation und der Deutung der Pertubationsdiagramme. Geburtsh. u. Frauenheilk. *18*:161–172 (1958).

Fikentscher, R., K. Semm: Ein Portio-Adapter für Persufflation und Hysterosalpingographie. Geburtsh. u. Frauenheilk. *19*:868–870 (1959).

Fikentscher, R., K. Semm: Eine Ballonklemme zur deszendierenden Eileiterdurchblasung. Geburtsh. u. Frauenheilk. *23*:445–449 (1963).

Fikentscher, R., K. Semm: New instruments for insufflation. Int. J. Fertil. *IX*:315–320 (1963).

Fikentscher, R., K. Semm: New instruments and apparatus for ascending and descending insufflation. Int. J. Fertil. *9*:315–320 (1964).

Fikentscher, R., K. Semm: Die apparativ gesteuerte Eileiterdurchblasung. Geburtsh. u. Frauenheilk. *24*:541–551 (1964).

Fikentscher, R., K. Semm: Diagnostik und Therapie der weiblichen Sterilität—Technische Neuerungen. Fortschr. Med. *88*:1052–1056 (1970).

Fort, A. T., et al.: Vaginal Pomeroy sterilization. A description of technique and a review of 100 cases. Obstet. and Gynec. *28*:421 (1966).

Fortier, Q. E.: Retroperitoneal, mediastinal and cervical emphysema following culdoscopy. Fertil. and Steril. *5*:173–181 (1954).

Fowle, A. S. E., E. J. M. Campbell: The immediate carbon dioxide storage capacity of man. Clin. Sci. *27*:41 (1964).

Fourès, A. P., J. Ricordeau, Caroli: La laparophotographie. Sem. méd. (Paris) Suppl. Sem. Hôp. *46*:37 (1956).

Fourestier, M.: La péritonéoscopie. Presse méd. *5*:46 (1943).

Frangenheim, H.: Die Bedeutung der Laparoskopie für die gynäkologische Diagnostik. Fortschr. Med. *76*:451 (1958).

Frangenheim, H.: Die Stellung der Laparoskopie und der Culdoskopie in der Gynäkologie. Medizinischer Bilddienst. Hoffmann-La Roche. Nr. *6*:12 (1959).

Frangenheim, H.: Tubal sterilization under visualization with the laparoscope. Geburtsh. u. Frauenheilk. *24*:470 (1964).

Frangenheim, H.: Tubal sterilization by laparoscopy. Improved technique. Geburtsh. u. Frauenheilk. *31*:622 (1971).

Frangenheim, H.: Erfahrungen mit der Laparoskopie und der Culdoskopie in der Gynäkologie. Med. Welt (Stgt.) *41*:2152–2154 (1960).

Frangenheim, H.: Indikationen, Technik und Komplikationen der Laparoskopie und Kuldoscopie in der Gynäkologie. Geburtsh. u. Frauenheilk. *7*:597 (1962).

Frangenheim, H.: Ein neues Insufflationsgerät zur Anlage des Pneumoperitoneums bei der Zölioskopie. Geburtsh. u. Frauenheilk. *11*:950 (1964).

Frangenheim, H., I. Turanli: Die Vorteile der Kuldoskopie und der Laparoskopie bei der Diagnose der Extrauteringravidität. Geburtsh. u. Frauenheilk. *24*:474–478 (1964).

Frangenheim, H.: Tubal division under endoscopic control. Germ. med. Mthl. *10*:421 (1964).

Frangenheim, H.: Die Tubensterilisation unter Sicht mit dem Laparoskop. Geburtsh. u. Frauenheilk. *24*:470 (1964).

Frangenheim, H.: Technical errors in peritoneoscopy. Germ. med. Mth. *10*:405 (1965).

Frangenheim, H.: Technische Ratschläge für die Foto- und Film-Laparoskopie mit Kaltlicht-Laparoskopen. Acta medicotechnica *8*:377 (1965).

Frangenheim, H.: Erros de técnica durante la celioscopia. Sinops. obstét.-ginec. *12*:280–287 (1965).

Frangenheim, H.: Die Coelioskopie in der Unterbauchchirurgie. Dtsch. med. Wschr. *43*:109 (1965).

Frangenheim, H.: Operative Eingriffe bei der Coelioskopie. Geburtsh. u. Frauenheilk. *25*:1124 (1965).

Frangenheim, H.: Technische Fehler bei der Coelioskopie. Geburtsh. u. Frauenheilk. *25*:22 (1965).

Frangenheim, H.: Vergleichende Untersuchungen zwischen dem Wert der Hysterosalpingographie und der Coelioskopie bei der Sterilitätsdiagnostik. Arch. Gynäk. *204*:2 (1966).

Frangenheim, H.: Vergleichende Untersuchungen zwischen dem Wert der Pertubation und der Hydrotubation unter Sicht mit dem Coelioskop. Beiträge zur Fertilität u. Sterilität. 5. Folge. Beilageheft zu Z. Geburtsh. Gynäk. *168*:189 (1966).

Frangenheim, H.: Welche Möglichkeiten gibt es für die endoskopischen Untersuchungen in der Gynäkologie? Endoscopy *1*:9–14 (1969).

Frangenheim, H.: Was muß der Internist von der gynäkologischen Laparoskopie wissen? Z. Gastroent. *2*:92 (1969).

Frangenheim, H.: Valeur de la coelioscopie dans le diagnostic des algies pelviennes. Rev. méd. normandes *11*:549 (1969).

Frangenheim, H.: Die heutige Stellung der Laparoskopie in der Gynäkologie. Arch. Gynäk. *207*:240–250 (1969).
Frangenheim, H.: Welches ist die beste Einstichstelle für den Trokar zur Anlage des Pneumoperitoneums und des Laparoskops? Z. Gastroent. *1*: (1970).
Frangenheim, H.: Sicherheitsmaßnahmen zur Verhütung von Komplikationen bei der Laparoskopie. Endoscopy *3*:10–20 (1971).
Frangenheim, H.: Die Laparoskopie bei der Diagnostik des »akuten Bauches«. Endoscopy *3*:121–126 (1971).
Frangenheim, H.: Die Laparoskopie in der Gynäkologie, Technik, Indikationen und operative Eingriffe. Dtsch. Ärztebl. *68*:363–370 (1971).
Frangenheim, H.: Die Tubensterilisation unter Sicht mit dem Laparoskop—Neue Technik und Erfahrungsbericht. Geburtsh. u. Frauenheilk. *31*:622–628 (1971).
Frangenheim, H.: Tubensterilisation unter Sicht mit dem Laparoskop. Neue Techniken und Instrumente zur Tuben-Ligatur und zum Tubenverschluß mittels Tantalum-Clips. Geburtsh. u. Frauenheilk. *33*:967–970 (1973).
Frangenheim, H., H. Stockhammer: Die Laparoskopie bei der Differentialdiagnose unklarer Unterbauchtumoren bei Frauen nach der Menopause. Gynaecologia (Basel) *167*:503–510 (1969).
Franke, G.: Hochbrechende Gläser als Grundlage moderner Objektive. Photo-Technik und Wirtschaft *10*:436–438 (1958).
Franke, G.: Endoskope—Prinzipien und Probleme ihrer Optik. Acta medicotechnica *16*:372–374 (1968).
Franke, G.: Der Aufbau moderner Endoskope. Feinwerktechnik *74*:382 (1970).
Frenkel, A., A. Greena, L. Siegler: Technical improvements in culdoscopic examination. Amer. J. Obstet. *64*:1303–1309 (1952).
Frik: Zur Untersuchungstechnik des Pneumoperitoneum. Fortschr. Röntgenstr. *30*:561 (1922/23).
Funk, O.: Technice endoskopii. Gaz. lek. Warszawa 1881.
Funck-Brentano, P.: Hematosalpinx in pregnancy and celioscopy. Gynecology *152*:144–153 (1961).
Funck-Brentano, P., L. Bouccara: Hematosalpinx of pregnancy and celioscopy. A propos of 200 cases of extrauterine pregnancy treated in 10 years at the Broca Hospital. Ann. Chir. *14*:755–761 (1960).
Fürstenheim: Notizen über das Endoskop und seine Verwendbarkeit besonders in Krankheiten der Harnwege. Dtsch. Klinik *32*: (1863).
Garrey, W. E.: Evaluation of peritoneoscopy, with particular reference to diagnosis of abdominal tumors. New Engl. J. Med. *225*:180–184 (1941).
Gaster, J. L.: Peritoneoscopy with color photographs of intraperitoneal organs. Med. Rec. (N. Y.) *154*:368–372 (1941).
Gaujoux, J.: Value of peritoneoscopy in the diagnosis of non-interrupted extrauterine pregnancy. Marseille Chir. *13*:242–246 (1961).
Gear, E. J.: Unusual complications of culdoscopy. Amer. J. Obstet. Gynec. *72*:667 (1956).
Gerber, L.: Peritoneoscopy. Med. Ann. D. C. *12*:348–351 (1943).
Giggleberg, H.: Komplikationen bei der Laparoskopie. Gastroenterologia *91*:375–388 (1959).
Girard, Y., P. Vigeant: Culdoscopy—Necessary or useless method of gynecologic investigation. Un. méd. Can. *99*:1308–1310 (1970).
Girard, Y., S. Bielinski, P. Fugère: Stérilisation tubaire perlaparoscopique par électro-coagulation. Un. méd. Can. *101*:874–876 (1972).
Gleichmann, U., D. W. Lübbers: Die Messungen des Kohlensäuredruckes in Gasen und Flüssigkeiten mit der Pco_2-Elektrode unter besonderer Berücksichtigung der gleichzeitigen Messung von P_2 und pH im Blut. Pflügers Arch. ges. Physiol. *271*:456 (1960).
Goetze, O.: Die Röntgendiagnostik bei gasgefüllter Bauchhöhle; eine neue Methode. Münch. med. Wschr. *65*:1275–1280 (1918).
Golditch, I. M.: Laparoscopy: Advances and advantages. Fertil. and Steril. *22*:306–310 (1971).
Golubev, V. A.: Use of culdoscopy and laparoscopy in gynecological practice. Akush. Ginec. *37*:71–74 (1961).
Gonzalez Lobo, R.: Culdoscopy; Presentation of 80 cases. Gynec. Obstet. mex. *15*:409–412 (1960).
Gordji, M., R. Palmer: Étude critique des ponctions per coelioscopiques des kystes pelviens. C R Soc. franç. Gynéc. *36*:203 (1966).
Gordji, M., F. Djavadi: Codonolyse per coelioscopique. Nouvelle technique (zur Klärung von Sterilitätsursachen). Bull. Féd. Soc. Gynéc. Obstét. Langue franç. *23*:15–16 (1971).
Graber, E. A.: Early diagnosis of ovarian cancer. Clin. Obstet. Gynec. *12*:958–961 (1969).
Graham, J. B., R. Graham: Cul-de-sac puncture in the diagnosis of early ovarian carcinoma. J. Obstet. Gynaec. Brit. Cwlth. *74*:371 (1967).
Grant, A.: Additional sterility factors in endometriosis. Fertil. and Steril. *17*:514 (1966).
Greenhalf, J. O., H. R. Roberts: Laparoscopic sterilization through Cusco's speculum. Brit. med. J. *31*:304 (1971).
Greggersen, D., K. Semm: Kolposkopische und histologische Verlaufskontrollen der thermokoagulierten gutartigen Portioveränderungen. Geburtsh. u. Frauenheilk. *32*:661–667 (1972).
Griaznova, I. M.: Culdoscopy in the diagnosis of gynecological diseases. Akush. Ginec. *37*:66–71 (1961).
Grillo, D., R. H. Stienmeir, D. M. Lowell: Early diagnosis of ovarian carcinoma by culdocentesis. Obstet. and Gynec. *28*:346 (1966).

Grimwade, J., P. Paterson: Female sterilization using the laparoscope. Med. J. Aust. 7:317–19 (1972).
Grünfeld: Die Methoden der künstlichen Beleuchtung im allgemeinen und zu endoskop. Zwecken im besonderen. Wien. med. Ztg. Nr. 25 (1879).
Grünfeld, J.: Eine bequeme Methode zur Demonstration endoskopischer Sehobjekte. Wien. med. Presse 1881.
Grünfeld, J.: Ein Fall von Polypen der Harnblase auf endoskopischem Wege diagnostiziert und operiert. Wien. med. Presse 1885.
Guggisberg, W.: Bericht über 170 Laparoskopien. Gynaecologia (Basel) *142*:290–295 (1956).
Gutierrez-Najar, A., H. Marquez-Monter, J. Ginera-Velazquez, Martinez-Manaut: Presence of corpus luteum as evidence of ovulation in women treated with low doses of chlormadinone acetate. Amer. J. Obstet. Gynec. *102*:1018–1022 (1968).
Gutierrez-Najar, A. J.: Tubal ligation by culdoscopy. To be published (1973).
Haag, B., H. A. Hirsch: Die laparoskopische Tubensterilisation allein und als zusätzlicher Eingriff. Geburtsh. u. Frauenheilk. *34*:350 (1974).
Haag, B., H. P. Mäder: Ergebnisse bei 1000 Laparoskopien an der Universitäts-Frauenklinik Basel. Schweiz. Ges. f. Gynäk. Jahresversammlung, Luzern 1974.
Habermann, G.: Abdominal inner pressure changes dependent on respiration. Pneumographic determination in laparoscopy. Folia Phoniat. (Basel) *12*:60–74 (1960).
Hahn, J.: Elektrokoagulation beider Tuben per laparoscopiam zur Unfruchtbarmachung und histologischen Untersuchung der Tuben. Vortrag vor der Deutschen Gesellschaft für Gynäkologie, 38. Tagung 1970.
Hahn, J.: Schwangerschaft nach Elektrokoagulation der Tuben per laparoscopiam. Arch. Gynäk. *211*:405 (1971).
Hall, E. V. van, P. M. H. G. Buytaert: Laparoskopie in de gynaecologie. Ned. T. Geneesk. *113*:561–565 (1969).
Hall, E. V. van, P. M. H. G. Buytaert: The neonatal laparoscopist. Ned. T. Verlosk, *70*:269–272 (1970).
Hall, H.: Culdoscopy in infertility investigation. Fertil. and Steril. *18*:4 (1967).
Hall, R. E.: Culdoscopy in infertility investigation. Fertil. and Steril. *18*:486 (1967).
Hall, R. E., W. D. Todd: The suspected ectopic pregnancy. Amer. J. Obstet. Gynec. *81*:1220 (1961).
Handley, R. S., A. W. Nurick: Peritoneoscopy; evaluation and report of 136 cases. Brit. med. J. *2*:1211–1214 (1956).
Hankock, A. F.: Peritoneoscopic photography. J. biol. photogr. Ass. *14*:163 (1946).
Harris, J. W., H. G. McQuarrie, H. S. Ellsworth, R. A. Stone, A. E. Anderson: The yield from pelvic endoscopy. Comparison of culdoscopy and laparoscopy. J. Amer. med. Ass. *215*:1117–1121 (1971).
Hartlieb, J.: Luftembolie bei der Laparoskopie. Dtsch. med. Wschr. *80*:1532–1533 (1955).
Haskins, A. L.: Oviductal sterilization with tantalum clips. Amer. J. Obstet. Gynec. *114*:370–377 (1972).
Hasson, H. M.: A modified instrument and method for laparoscopy. Amer. J. Obstet. Gynec. *110*:886–887 (1971).
Havlicek, S.: Neuer Gewindetrokar für die operative Laparoskopie. Endoscopy *4*:153–154 (1972).
Hayashi, M., et al.: Round table conference. Pointers for tubal sterilization per vaginam. Sanfujin Jissai *15*:59 (1966).
Hayden, T.: Exploration of the uterus with the endoscope. The Dublin Quarterly J. of med. Science *XL*:497 (1865).
Hays, I.: Instrumente zur Illumination dunkler Räume. Philad. J. phys. med. Sci. 1827, XIV.
Heath, Chr.: On the endoscopic appearances of the urethra. Lancet 3. Nov. 1866.
Heinkel, K.: Die Möglichkeiten der laparoskopischen Farbphotographie. Verh. dtsch. Ges. Verdau.- u. Stoffwechselkr. 1959.
Heinkel, K.: Die Farbphotographie der Bauchorgane während der Laparoskopie. Med. Bild-Dienst Roche. *21*:353–357 (1957).
Heinkel, K., H. Frotz, H. Hiltner: Die Hopkins Panorama-Optik: Ihre Anwendung in der Laparoskopie. 1. Kongreß der Deutschen Gesellschaft für gastroenterologische Endoskopie, Hamburg 1967.
Heinrichs, O., W. Windemuth: Zur Farbphotographie in der Harnblase der Frau. Med. Bild-Dienst Roche *22*:8–11 (1958).
Herman, L., J. dePietro: Broad-ligament hematoma and emphysema following culdoscopy (Report of a case). Obstet. and Gynec. *5*:211 (1955).
Herrera-Llerandi, R.: Peritoneoscopy. Endoscopic refinement par excellence. Brit. med. J. *5253*:661–665 (1961).
Herstein, A.: Culdoscopy an adjunct in gynecological diagnosis. Amer. J. Obstet. Gynec. *69*:240–243 (1955).
Heynemann, T.: Weibliche Sterilität. Geburtsch. u. Frauenheilk. *3*:467 (1941).
Hibbard, B. M., H. K. Basu: Laparoscopy in gynaecological practice J. Indian med. Ass. *53*:1–6 (1969).
Hinselmann, H.: Die Blauprobe zur Prüfung der Tubendurchgängigkeit. Zbl. Gynäk *53*:1394 (1942).
Hirsch, H. A.: Laparoskopie und Sterilisation. Gynäkologe 7:157–165 (1974).
Hirsch, H. A.: Verbrennungen bei der laparoskopischen Tubensterilisation und Möglichkeiten ihrer Vermeidung. Geburtsh. u. Frauenheilk. *34*:345 (1974).

Hirsch, H. A., E. Roos: Laparoskopische Tubensterilisation mit einer neuen Bikoagulationszange. Geburtsh. u. Frauenheilk. *34*:340 (1974).
Hodez, J. P.: Importance of celioscopy in nonacute pelvic pain. Sci. méd. Lille *79*:176–182 (1961).
Hodgson, C., R. M. A. McClelland, J. R. Newton: Some effects of the peritoneal insufflation of carbon dioxide at laparoscopy. Anaesthesia *25*:382–390 (1970).
Hörmann, J.: Mediastinal-Emphysem bei der Laparoskopie. Münch. med. Wschr. *97*:541–542 (1955).
Hollis, W. J., W. H. Brown: Peritoneoscopy; analysis of its use in 69 cases. New Orleans med. surg. J. *100*:497–504 (1948).
Hope, R. B.: The differential diagnosis of ectopic gestation by peritoneoscopy. Surg. Gynec. Obstet. *64*:229–234 (1937).
Hope, R. B.: Peritoneoscopy as diagnostic adjunct in gastroenterology. Amer. J. Gastroent. *22*:221–230 (1954).
Hope, R. B.: Modified biopsy forceps for peritoneoscopy. Amer. J. Surg. *88*:677–679 (1454).
Hope, R. B.: Endothoracale Photographie. Tuberk.-Arzt *12*:733–736 (1955).
Hope, R. B.: Sterilization short cut. Med. World News *11*:12 (1970).
Hopkins, H. H.: On the diffraction theory of optical images. Proc. roy. Soc. A *217*:408 (1953).
Hopkins, H. H.: The frequency response of a defocussed optical system. Proc. roy. Soc. A *231*:91 (1955).
Hopkins, H. H.: The numerical evaluation of the frequency response of optical systems. Proc. physiol. Soc. B *70*:1002 (1957).
Horan, T. N., C. G. Eddy, E. C. Graham: Intra-abdominal photography in color. Surg. Gynec. Obstet. *73*:273–276 (1941).
Horwitz, S. Th.: Laparoscopy in gynecology. Obstet. gynec. Surv. *27*:1–13 (1972).
Houel, E., R. Gares: La place de la coelioscopie dans l'examen d'une aménorrhée. Rev. franç. Gynéc. Obstét. *12*:765 (1960).
Houel, E., H. Gares: The place of celioscopy in the examination of amenorrhea. Rev. franç. Gynéc. Obstét. *55*:755–771 (1960).
Hulka, J. F.: Controlling tenaculum: Instrument for uterine mobilization during tubal sterilization. Amer. J. Obstet. Gynec. *112*:865–866 (1972).
Hulka, J. F., J. I. Fishburne, J. P. Mercer, K. F. Omran: Laparoscopic sterilization with a spring clip: A report of the first fifty cases. Amer. J. Obstet. Gynec. *116*, 751 (1973).
Hulka, J. F., K. F. Omran: Tubal occlusion: A comparative study. Amer. J. Fertil. *15*:226 (1970).
Hulka, J. F., K. F. Omram: Comparative tubal occlusion: Rigid and spring-loaded clips. Fertil. and Steril. *23*:633–639 (1972).
Hulka, J. F.: Laparoscopic sterilization with spring clips. Chapel Hill, North Carolina, Carolina Population Center, Inter. Fertil. Res. Progr. 1973, p. 60.
Hulka, J. F., B. S. Delhi-Thweatt, L. C. Ulberg: Contained cautery: Studies toward safer laparoscopic sterilization technics. Fertil. and Steril. *24*:912–920 (1973).
Hulka, J. F., R. M. Soderstrom, W. L. Corson, P. G. Brooks: Complications committee of the American Association of Gynecological Laparoscopists. First annual report. J. reprod. Med. *10*:301–306 (1973).
Humke, W.: Kuldoskopie mit einer Nahsichtoptik. Arch. Gynäk. *211*:405 (1971).
Imenitoff, R. Palmer: La coelioscopie dans le diagnostic des grossesses extra-utérines. C. R. Soc. franç. Gynéc. *17*:226–228 (1947).
Jacobaeus, H. C.: Über die Möglichkeit, die Zystoskopie bei Untersuchung seröser Höhlungen anzuwenden. Münch. med. Wschr. *57*:2090–2092 (1910).
Jacobaeus, H. C.: Kurze Übersicht über meine Erfahrungen mit der Laparo-thorakoskopie. Münch. med. Wschr. *58*:2017–2019 (1911).
Jacobaeus, H. C.: Laparo-thorakoskopie. Hygiea (Stockh.) *74*:1070–1091 (1912).
Jacobaeus, H. C.: Über Laparo- und Thorakoskopie. Beitr. Klin. Tuberk. *25*:183–254 (1912).
Jacobaeus, H. C.: Können durch die Laparoskopie Indikationen zu chirurgischen Eingriffen gewonnen werden? Nord. med. Ark. *14*:1 (1914).
Jacobson, L.: Laparoscopy in the diagnosis of acute salpingitis. Acta obstet. gynec. scand. *43*:160 (1964).
Jacobson, L., L. Westrom: Objectivized diagnosis of acute pelvic inflammatory disease. Diagnostic and prognostic value of routine laparoscopy. Amer. J. Obstet. Gynec. *105*:1088–1098 (1969).
Jacobson, L.: The value of visual diagnosis in acute pelvic inflammatory disease. Ned. T. Verlosk. *70*:272–285 (1970).
Jaeger, J., W. Drüner: Die Laparoskopie in der Gynäkologie. Diagnostik *2*:315–318 (1969).
Jäämeri, K. E. U.: Gynecologic laparoscopy. Nord. med. Ark. *34*:919–920 (1947).
Jakobszon, V. L.: Oszvescsenyije brujsnoj golosti po szposzobu prof. D. Otta ventroszkipija. Zsurn. ≫Novoje v medicine≪ 23–24 (1967).
Jamain, B., A. Letessier, J. Bonhomme: Tubal pregnancy celioscopy. Rev. franç. Gynéc. Obstét. *55*:663–668 (1960).
Jamain, B., A. Letessier, J. Baillif: La coelioscopie dans le diagnostic des grossesses extrautérines. Bull. Féd. Soc. Gynéc. franç. *12*:140–143 (1960).
Jamain, B., A. Letessier, J. Bonhomme: Grossesse tubaire et coelioscopie. Rev. franç. Gynéc. *55*:663 (1960).
Jamain, B., A. Letessier, J. Bonhomme: Grossesse tubaire et coelioscopie. Sem. Hôp. Paris *37*:1821–1823 (1961).

Jamain, B., A. Letessier: Intérêt de la coelioscopie en gynécologie; expérience personnelle pour le diagnostic de la grossesse tubaire. Sem. Hôp. Paris *37*:2070–2072 (1961).
Jamain, B., A. Letessier: The problem of ligation of the tubes during cesareans at the Hospital Tenon during a continuous 9-year period (12,000 births). Bull. Féd. Soc. Gynéc. Obstét. franç. *14*:310 (1962).
Jeffcoate, T. N.: Culdoscopy. J. Obstet. Gynec. brit. Emp. *67*:529–538 (1960).
Jernstrom, P.: Air embolism during peritoneoscopy. Amer. J. clin. Path. *21*:573–575 (1951).
Johnson, Diana Schneider: Female sterilization: Prognosis for simplified outpatient procedures. Contraception *5*:155–163 (1972). Summary of Conference held in Virginia, December 2–3, 1971 (P. 158 report by Dr. Clifford Wheeless).
Jones, H. A.: Pneumoperitoneoscopy, cauterisation of adhesions between liver and diaphragm. Amer. Rev. Tuberc. *42*:805–806 (1940).
Jordan, J. A., R. L. Edwards, J. Pearson, P. J. K. Maskery: Laparoscopic sterilization and follow-up hysterosalpingogram. J. Obstet. Gynaec. Brit. Cwlth. *78*:440–466 (1971).
Kai, I.: Key points of our method of transvaginal tubal sterilization. Sanfujin Jissai *19*:408 (1970).
Kalk, H.: Erfahrungen mit der Laparoskopie (zugleich mit Beschreibung eines neuen Instrumentes). Z. klin. Med. *111*:303–348 (1929).
Kalk, H.: Über Laparoskopie. Med. Klin. *28*:995–997 (1932).
Kalk, H.: Über Laparoskopie (Reply to Kelling). Med. Klin. *28*:1747 (1932).
Kalk, H.: Über einen laparoskopisch diagnostizierten, geheilten Fall von Bauchfelltuberculose. Dtsch. med. Wschr. *61*:4–5 (1935).
Kalk, H.: Laparoskopie. (Die Besichtigung der Bauchhöhle am lebenden Menschen.) Ges. Krankenh. *5*:97–99 (1935).
Kalk, H.: Wann sollte man von der Laparoskopie Gebrauch machen? Z. ärztl. Fortbild. *39*:36 (1942).
Kalk, H.: Fortschritte der Laparoskopie. Dtsch. med. Wschr. *68*:677–681 (1942).
Kalk, H., E. Wildhirt: Dir Bedeutung der Leberfunktionsprobleme im Vergleich zum bioptischen Befund der Leber. Med. Klin. *46*:585–591 (1951).
Kalk, H., E. Wildhirt: Beitrag zum Krankheitsbild der Periarteriitis nodosa. Dtsch. med. Wschr. *79*:803–805 (1954).
Kalk, H., E. Wildhirt: Cholangitis-Choledochusstein. Dtsch. med. Wschr. *81*:1235–1257 (1956).
Kapandji, M.: L'hysterio-ligamentopexie laparoscopique des prolapsus du troisième degré (premiers cas). Apport à la chirurgie laparoscopique. Gynéc. et Obstét. *69*:551–560 (1970).
Kastendieck, E.: Zur Anlage des Pneumoperitoneums bei der gynäkologischen Laparoskopie. Geburtsh. u. Frauenheilk. *33*:376–378 (1973).
Kastendieck, E., W. Mestwerdt: Tierexperimentelle und klinische Aspekte zur Technik der laparoskopischen Tubensterilisation. Geburtsh. u. Frauenheilk. *33*:971–978 (1973).
Kayser, H. W.: Unsere Erfahrungen mit der Douglasscopie. Zbl. Gynäk. *74*:1938–1943 (1952).
Keith, L.: Laparoscopic puerperal tubal sterilization (in: Letters to the Editor; response to correspondence from D. Satlop and J. Esposito). J. reprod. Med. 7:77 (1971).
Keith, L.: Sterilisation durch das Laparoskop. Zbl. Gynäk. *14*:1406 (1972).
Keith, L., K. Houser, A. Webster, A. Lash: Puerperal tubal sterilization using laparoscopic technique: A preliminary report. J. reprod. Med. *6*:69–72 (1971).
Keith, L., A. Webster, A. F. Lash: Postpartum laparoscopy for sterilization. Int. J. Gynaec. Obstet. *8*:145 (1970).
Keith, L., A. Webster, A. Lash: A comparison between puerperal and nonpuerperal laparoscopic sterilization. International Surgery *56*:325–330 (1971).
Keith, L., A. Webster, K. Houser, L. Procknicki, A. Lash, J. Barton: Laparoscopy for puerperal sterilization. Obstet. and Gynec: *39*:616–621 (1972).
Keirse, M., R. Vandervellen: Laparoscopy in chronic pelvic pain. Endoscopy *5*:27–30 (1973).
Kelling, G.: Über Oesophagoskopie, Gastroskopie und Cölioskopie. Münch. med. Wschr. *49*:21–24 (1902).
Kelling, G.: Über die Möglichkeit, die Zystoskopie bei Untersuchungen seröser Höhlungen anzuwenden. Bemerkungen zu dem Artikel von Jacobaeus. Münch. med. Wschr. *57*:2358 (1910).
Kelling, G.: Zur Cölioskopie und Gastroskopie. Arch. klin. Chir. *126*:226 (1923).
Kelling, G.: Zu dem Artikel von Kalk über Laparoskopie. Med. Klin. *28*:1747 (1932).
Kelly, J. C., J. Rock: Culdoscopy for diagnosis in infertility. A report of 492 cases. Amer. J. Obstet. Gynec. *72*:523 (1956).
Kelman, G. R., G. H. Swapp, I. Smith, R. J. Benzie, N. L. M. Gordon: Herzminutenvolumen und arterielle Blutgasdrucke während der Laparoskopie. (Cardiac output and arterial bloodgas tension during laparoscopy.) Brit. J. Anaesth. *44*:1155 (1972); Geburtsh. u. Frauenheilk. *33*:418 (1973).
Keyes, E. L.: On urethral chancre observed by Désormeaux's endoscope. Amer. J. Syphil. Dermat. New York, Januar 1870.
Khalife, F.: Personal examples of the diagnostic possibilities of coelioscopy. Rev. méd. Moy. Or. *17*:184–186 (1960).
Kiessling, J.: Laparoskopie: Indikation, Kontraindikation und Zwischenfälle. Z. ärztl. Fortbild. *57*:399–402 (1963).
Klaften, E.: Die Kolpolaparoskopie; eine Methode zur direkten Betrachtung der Organe der Becken-Bauchhöhle vom hinteren Scheidengewölbe. Wien. klin. Wschr. *59*:829–831 (1947).

Klaften, E.: Kolpolaparoskopie; ein weiterer Beitrag zur gynäkologischen Endoskopie. Wien. med. Wschr. *106*:295–297 (1956).
Korbsch, R.: Die Laparoskopie nach Jacobaeus. Berl. klin. Wschr. *58*:696 (1921).
Korbsch, R.: Technik und Grenzen der Laparoskopie. Münch. med. Wschr. *69*:426 (1922).
Kramarenko, J. J.: Voproszi o novoj tyechnyike nalozsenyija pnevmoperitoneuma. Russzk. klin. *14*:3 (1925).
Kratochwil, A.: Die Bedeutung der Laparoskopie in der Sterilitätsdiagnostik. Wien. klin. Wschr. *80*:581–583 (1968).
Kraûse, N. I.: Vnutribrjusnoe davlenyie v predelah poddiafragmalnogo prosztransztva i nadcsrevja i jevo znacsenyije v hirurgiji pecsenyi i zseludka. Nov. khir. Arkh. *3*:5 (1924).
Krautwald, A., F. Regner: Röntgenologische Darstellung der Bauchorgane nach Pneumoperitoneumanlage als Voruntersuchung zur Laparoskopie. Dtsch. Gesundh.-Wes. *27*:850–941 (1952).
Kreel, L., J. Gensburg, M. F. Green: Gynecography in premature ovarian failure and ovarian dysgenesis. Brit. med. J. *1*:682 (1969).
Kress, D., F. W. Dittmar: Indikationen zur gynäkologischen Pelviskopie. Arch. Gynäk. *211*:406–407 (1971).
Kress, D., F. W. Dittmar, K. Semm: Statistische Auswertung von 600 gynäkologischen Pelviskopien. Arch. Gynäk. *211*:406–407 (1971).
Kunstadte, R. H., A. Tulsky: Diagnostic transabdominal pneumoperitoneum in children. Amer. J. Obstet. Gynec. *68*:819 (1954).
Kunz, J.: Letale Komplikationen bei der Laparoskopie und Leberpunktion. Z. ges. inn. Med. *18*:337–342 (1963).
Künzel, W., E. Kastendieck, G. Ferneding: Der Säure-Basen-Status und die Ventilation während gynäkologischer Laparoskopien. Anaesthesist *21*:249–298 (1972).
Kush, N. L., A. D. Timchenko, V. P. Sleptsov, M. L. Shparkovskaya: Diagnostic value of laparoscopy in sex determination. Probl. Endokr. (Mosk.) *16*:41–43 (1970).
Kuthan, S.: Clinical significance of laparoscopy. Čas. Lék. čes. *78*:46–48 (1939).
Labbé: Gaz. hebd. 21. Juillet, p. 464 (1865).
Lamb, E. J., A. M. Guderian, A. L. Cruz: Culdoscopy in infertility. Obstet. Gynec. *33*:822–826 (1969).
Lane, E., G. A. Souza: Culdoscopy. Matern. Infanc. (S. Paulo) *29*:65–70 (1970).
Lang, W. R., B. L. Wellenbach: Colpocentesis, colpotomy. Culdoscopy and colposcopy: their applications in vaginal surgery. Clin. Obstet. Gynec. *4*:149–159 (1961).
Larson, S. L.: Laparoscopic sterilization. Minn. Med. *55*:369–371 (1972).
Laubie, B., J. L. Latapie, F. Moreau: Bilan de 80 coelioscopies dans les affections génitales féminines chez le sujet jeune. France méd. *29*:395 (1966).
Lazarewitsch: Separatabdruck der Beilage zu den Sitzungsprotokollen des Universitäts-Senates in Charkow 1868. Diaphanoskopie – Untersuchung des weiblichen Beckens.
Leising, K., K.-J. Rosenbruch: Möglichkeiten für die Ermittlung meßbarer und vergleichbarer Kennzahlen für Endoskopoptiken. Endoscopy *3*:94–102 (1971).
Lent, H.: Technik und diagnostische Möglichkeiten der Photolaparoskopie. Medizinischer Bild-Dienst *18*:300–302 (1957).
Lent, H.: Das Photolaparoskop, seine Technik und Handhabung. Medizinalmarkt *6*:14 (1958).
Lent, H., H. H. Jansen: Die Beobachtung der Leberoberfläche mit dem Photolaparoskop und Bedeutung für die klinische Praxis. Dtsch. med. Wschr. *83*:24 (1958).
Lent, H.: Photolaparoskopie mit neuen Beleuchtungseinrichtungen. Tg. Med. Photographie u. Kinematographie. Köln 1958.
Lent, H.: Ein neues Film – und Photolaparoskop. Medizinalmarkt 7:27 (1959).
Lent, H.: Die Entwicklung der Photolaparoskopie mit dem Elektronenblitz. Acta hepato-splenol. (Stuttg.) *9*:195–202 (1962).
Le Lorier, G.: La coelioscopie gynécologique. Sem. Hôp. Paris *5*:215–219 (1951).
Leonard, P.: The indications for laparoscopy. Its possibilities and limitations. Scalpel *113*:821–832 (1960).
Le Perre, F.: La laparoscopia. Acta chir. belg. *55*:777 (1956).
Leppert u. Gasenius: Laparoskopie in der Tierheilkunde. Berl. tierärztl. Wschr. *51*:180 (1931).
Leroux, P.: La coelioscopie et la culdoscopie en gynécologie et en obstétrique. A propos de 30 cas. Bull. Féd. Soc. Gynéc. Obstét. franç. *12*:212–217 (1960).
Levinson, C. J., S. F. Schwartz, E. C. Salzstein: Complication of laparoscopic tubal cauterization. Small bowel perforation. Obstet. and Gynec. *41*:253–256 (1973).
Liehr, H.: Die Polaroid-Kamera zur Dokumentation laparoskopischer Befunde. Materia Medica, Nordmark (1968).
Lindemann, H. J., B. Karacz: Die erweiterte Laparoskopie in der Gynäkologie. Hamb. Ärztebl. *25*:11 (1971).
Lindemann, H. J.: Second-look-Pelviskopie nach Tubensterilisierung durch Elektrokoagulation. Zbl. Gynäk. *95*:578 (1973).
Lindenschmidt, T. O., F. W. Unger-Sternberg: Probelaparotomie oder ≫chirurgische Laparoskopie≪. Med. Welt. (Stuttg.) *36*:1789–1793 (1963).
Lingemann, O.: Kasuistischer Beitrag zum Pneumoperitoneum. Med. Klin. *44*:20 (1949).
Liston, W. A., J. Downie, W. Bradford, M. G. Kerr: Female sterilisation by tubal electro-coagulation under laparoscopic control. Lancet *1*:382–383 (1970).

Liu, D. T. Y., H. A. H. Melville, B. Measday: Suggested technique for laparoscopic sterilization (letter). Lancet *1*:1230 (1972).
Lode, H., U. Hüttemann, Ch. v. Wolff: Einfluß endoskopischer abdomineller Untersuchungen auf die Atmung. 77. Tagung der Dtsch. Ges. f. Inn. Med., Wiesbaden April 1971.
Loginov, A. SZ.: O fotolaparoszkopii. Ter. Arch. *35*:34–37 (1963).
Loginov, A. SZ.: Diagnoszticseszkije vozmozsnosztyi laparoszkopii pri zabolevanijah pecsenyi i zselecsnüh putyej. Vestn. Khir. *93*:9–13 (1964).
Lorey, A.: Hydropneumoperitoneum. Verh. dtsch. Röntg.-Ges. 46–52 (1912).
Lorey, A.: Über einen eigenartigen Zwischenfall bei der Anlegung eines Pneumoperitoneums. Münch. med. Wschr. *69*:86–87 (1922).
Lübke, F.: Die Bedeutung der Laparoskopie für die Diagnostik der Tubensterilität. Beiträge zur Fertilität und Sterilität, 4. Folge. Beilageheft zu Z. Geburtsh. Gynäk. *62*:58 (1964).
Lübke, F.: Die Laparoskopie als diagnostisches Hilfsmittel in der Gynaekologie. Zbl. Gynäk. *86*:260 (1964).
Lübke, F.: Hilfsinstrumente für die zölioskopische Tubendiagnostik. Geburtsh. u. Frauenheilk. *12*:1172 (1965).
Lübke, F.: Diagnostische Aspekte des Sterilitätsproblems. Dtsch. Ärztebl. 2143 (1970).
Lübke, F.: Zur diagnostischen Aussagefähigkeit und zum Risiko der gynäkologischen Laparoskopie. Arch. Gynäk. *211*:401 (1971).
Lund, E.: On the detection and treatment of foreign bodies in the bladder with remarks on the use of the endoscope. Brit. med. J. 31. July.—Canst. Jahresb. II. p. 168, 1869.
Maathuis, J. B., J. H. M. Horbach, E. V. van Hall: A comparison of the results of hysterosalpingography and laparoscopy in the diagnosis of fallopian tube dysfunction. Fertil. and Steril. *23*:428–431 (1972).
MacFayden, B. V., W. A. Reichstein, A. R. Kannapel: Endoscopy in gynecology. Amer. J. Obstet. Gynec. *64*:319–325 (1952).
Mackey, R.: Management of the sterile but normal couple. Int. J. Fertil. *8*:419 (1963).
Mäder, H. P.: Abklärung gynäkologischer Schmerzzustände durch die Laparoskopie. Arch. Gynäk. *211*:401 (1971).
Magendie, J., J. P. Secousse, M. Regnier: Sur l'intérêt de la coelioscopie en gynécologie (à propos de 45 laparoscopies effectuées dans service de clinique gynécologique). J. Méd. Bordeaux *133*:265–268 (1956).
Magendie, J., J. P. Secousse, G. Lassalle, P. Daraignez: Importance of coelioscopy in the early diagnosis of extrauterine pregnancy. Bordeaux chir. *4*:161–163 (1959).
Majewski, A.: Die Douglasskopie. Arch. Gynäk. *207*:250 (1969).
Mallik, M. K. B.: Value of pelvic pneumography as a diagnostic aid in amenorrhea. Int. Surg. *47*:57 (1967).
Manszurov, H. H., D. G. Rudoj: Analiz 625 szlucsejev iglovoj biopszii pecsenyi. Ter. Arch. *34*:72–78 (1962).
Marchesi, F., E. Cittadini: Quadri celioscopici ovarici nella menopausa precoce. Atti Soc. ital. Ostet. Ginec. *51*:25 (1965).
Mark, P. M., G. A. Webb: A disappearing incision for postpartum tubal ligation. Obstet. and Gynec. *32*:174 (1968).
Marquez-Monter, H., A. Gutierrez-Najar, J. Casasola: Anatomical findings in fallopian tubes under fertility control by culdoscopic clipping. Fertil. and Steril. *23*:823 (1972).
Marshall, J. R., Ch. B. Hammond: Biopsia de ovario por culdosopia. Obstet. y Ginec. *27*:733–737 (1966).
Marshall, J. R.: Recent advances in culdoscopy. Clin. Obstet. Gynec. *12*:504–513 (1969).
Mathié, C.: Indications et limites de la coelioscopie. Faculté de Médicine, Thèse (Paris) *350*:37 (1950).
Mayer, H. G. K. von: Die operativen Methoden der Sterilisation der Frau. Dtsch. med. J. *22*:633–634 (1971).
Mäder, H., O. Käser, B. Haag: Die Bedeutung der Laparoskopie bei unklarem Unterbauchsschmerz. Gynäkologe *6*:126–128 (1973).
McDonough, P. G., O. E. Taledo, R. G. Owen: Pelvic laparoscopy: an instrument (modified) to provide uterine elevation. Amer. J. Obstet. Gynec. *110*:1017–1018 (1971).
McQuaide, J. R. F. C. S.: Air embolism during peritoneoscopy. S. Afr. Med. J. *46*:422 (1972).
Medgyes, A.: A laparoszkopia szerepe a peritonaeum elváltozásainak diagnosztikájában. Orv. Hetil. *103*:1802–1806 (1962).
Medgyes, A.: Laparoskopia szerepe a hasüregi szervek daganatainak diagnosztikájában. 25 év a rákellenes küzdelem szolgálatában. Bp. 293–301 (1963).
Medgyes, A.: Laparoskopia szerepe a retroperitonaealis és a retroperitonaealis szervekböl künduló daganatok diagnosztikájában. Orv. Hetil. *104*:727–731 (1963).
Medgyes, A.: Über laparoskopische Untersuchungen nach abdominalen Operationen. Dtsch. Z. Verdau.- u. Stoffwechselkr. *23*:1–6 (1963).
Medgyes, A., F. Hartai: Laparoskopos vizsgálat után jelentkezett pitvarfiblillation. Orv. Hetil. *104*:1801–1802 (1963).
Meirelles, E. A.: Laparoscopia. Tribuna méd. (Rio de Jan.) 199 (1913).
Menken, F. C.: Genitaltuberkulose im photo-kolposkopischen und photo-douglasskopischen Farbbild. Arch. Gynäk. *186*:303–309 (1959).

Menken, F. C.: Endoscopic observations of endocrine processes and hormonal changes. Simposio Esteroides Sexuales, Bogotá, Columbia 1968. *92*:13 (1970).
Mercer, J. P., H. J. Lefler, J. F. Hulka, J. I. Fishburne: Development of an outpatient program for laparoscopic sterilization. Obstet. and Gynec. *44*:444–449 (1974).
Michaud, J. T.: Utilité et limitations de la péritonéoscopie. Laval méd. *16*:427–432 (1951).
Michelon, B.: Qu'apporte la coelioscopie dans les douleurs pelviennes chez la femme? A propos de 62 cas. Rev. franç. Gynéc. *66*:437–442 (1971).
Mikulicz-Radecki, F. von: Experimentelle Untersuchungen über Tubenbewegungen. Arch. Gynäk. *128*:318 (1926).
Mikulicz-Radecki, F. von: Experimentelle Untersuchungen über Tubensterilisation durch Elektrokoagulation. Z. Geburtsh. Gynäk. *94*:318 (1929).
Mintz, M.: La coelioscopie dans le syndrome de Stein-Leventhal. Gynéc. prat. *18*:96–101 (1967).
Mintz, M., J. Dupre-Froment, J. de Brux: Ponctions de 94 kystes parautérins sous coelioscopie et étude cystologique des liquides. Gynaecologia *163*:61 (1967).
Moggi, G., G. Santoli: Sulla biopsia ovárica per celioscópia. Minerva ginec. *20*:2 (1968).
Mohri, T., C. Mohri, F. Yamadori: Tuboloscope. Endoscopy *2*:227 (1970).
Motschmann, H.: Pneumothorax, als Zwischenfall bei der Laparoskopie. Med. Klin. *49*:401–403 (1954).
Müller, Fr. Die elektrische Beleuchtung der natürlichen Körperhöhlen. Oester. ärztl. Vereinsztg. 1879, Nr. 13, 15, 22.
Müller, H. O., E. Gundel, H. Kollmeier: Laparoskopie mit Kohlensäuregas. Mögliche Fehldeutung eines endoskopischen Gefäßbefundes. Endoscopy *2*:58–61 (1970).
Müller, K.: Zur Frage der sedativen Prämedikation in der Kaparoskopie. Med. Klin. *59*:1472–1474 (1964).
Mur Linares, J.: Laparofotografia en color. Med. esp. *38*:470–481 (1957).
Nadeau, O. E., O. F. Kampmeier: Endoscopy of the abdomen; Abdominoscopy; a preliminary study, including a summary of the literature and a description of the technique. Surg. Gynec. Obstet. *41*:259–271 (1925).
Neely, M. R., A. A. Elkady: Modified technique of puerperal laparoscopic sterilization. J. Obstet. Gynaec. Brit. Cwlth. *79*:1025–1027 (1972).
Neill, J. G.: A follow-up study of one hundred cases of sterilization by tubal ligation. Ulster med. J. *38*:119–122 (1969).
Neumann, H. H., H. C. Frick: Occlusion of the Fallopian tubes with tantalium clips. Amer. J. Obstet. Gynec. *81*:803 (1961).
Neuwirth, R. S.: Laparoscopy. Clin. Obstet. Gynec. *12*:514 (1969).
Neuwirth, R. S.: Recent experience with diagnostic and surgical laparoscopy. Amer. J. Obstet. Gynec. *106*:119–121 (1970).
Neuwirth, R. S.: A method of bilateral ovarian biopsy at laparoscopy in infertility and chronic anovulation. Fertil. and Steril. *23*:361–366 (1972).
Neuwirth, R. S., M. Cejas: Sterilization by tubal cauterization and transection at laparoscopy. Amer. J. Obstet. Gynec. *105*:632–633 (1969).
Nitze, M.: Über eine neue Beleuchtungsmethode der Höhlen des menschlichen Körpers. Wien. med. Presse 1879, Nr. 26.
Noble, A., Contreras, L.: Pelvic endoscopy in sterility. Ginec. Obstet. Méx. *24*:153–159 (1968).
Nordentoeft, S.: Über Endoskopie geschlossener Cavitaeten mittels meines Trokart-Endoskops. Verh. dtsch. Ges. Chir. *41*:78–81 (1912).
Nordvall, S.: An instrument to aid laparoscopic diagnosis. Acta obstet. gynec. scand. *49*:111–112 (1970).
Oaks, W. W.: Evaluation of peritoneoscopy in abdominal disease. Clinics *4*:841–849 (1945).
Olim, C. B.: Peritoneoscopy: Analysis of 150 cases. Surgery *10*:391–404 (1949).
Oliveira, H. M.: Les renseignements fournis par l'utilization conjuguées du bleu et de l'insufflation dans les coelioscopies pour stérilité. C. R. Soc. franç. Gynéc. *31*:79 (1961).
Oliveira, E. M., R. Palmer: A propos des biopsies tubaires percoelioscopiques. C. R. Soc. franç. Gynéc. *32*:625 (1962).
Orlov, G. A.: O tyehnyike peritoneoszkopii. Hirurgija *12* (1947).
Orlovszkij, A. SZ.: Differencialnaja diagnosztyika i hirurgija neparazitannih kiszt pecsenyi. Hir. Arch. *1*:41 (1938).
Orlovszkij, A. SZ.: O primenyejii metoda Kelling-Jakobeusza dlja diagnosztyiki tuberkuleznih peritonitov. Probl. tuberk. *1*: (1938).
Orndoff, B. H.: The peritoneoscope in diagnosis of diseases of the abdomen. J. Radiol. *1*:307–325 (1920).
Ott, D. von: Ventroscopic illumination of the abdominal cavity in pregnancy. Zh. Akus. i. Zsensk. bolez. *15*:7 (1901).
Ott, D. von: Die Beleuchtung der Bauchhöhle (Ventroskopie) als Methode bei vaginaler Cöliotomie. Zbl. Gynäk. *26*:817 (1902).
Ott, D. von: Nyeposzredsztvennom oszvescsenyii brjusnoj polosztyi, pzirja, tolsztoj kiski i mazkidlja celej diagnosztisceszkih i operatyivnih. Zh. Akus. i Zsenszk. bolez. *XVII*:7–8 (1903).
Ott, D. von: Die unmittelbare Beleuchtung der Bauchhöhle, der Harnblase, des Rektum und der Gebärmutterhöhle zu diagnostischen und operativen Zwecken. Zh. Akus. i Zsenszk bolez. Nr. 7 (1903).

Ott, D. von: Die direkte Beleuchtung der Bauchhöhle, der Harnblase, des Dickdarms und des Uterus zu diagnostischen Zwecken. Rev. med. tchèque, Prague *2*:27 (1909).
Ottenjann, R.: Die Entwicklung der medizinischen Endoskopie. Med. Technik *92*:273–276 (1972).
Otturi, J. E.: Culdoscopy. Sem. méd. (B. Aires) *118*:819–822 (1961).
Overstreet, E. W.: Techniques of sterilization. Clin. Obstet. Gynec. 7:109 (1964).
Palliez, R., M. Delecour, J. C. Monnier, P. Y. Leroy, M. Declerco, P. Branle: La sterilisation tubaire percoelioscopique par électro-coagulation isthmique. Bull. Féd. Soc. Gynéc. Obstét. franç. *22*:449–451 (1970).
Palla: Die Laparoskopie beim Hunde. Wien. tierärztl. Mschr. *6*:865 (1929).
Palmer, R.: La coelioscopie gynécologique. Rapport du Professeur Mocquot. Acad. de Chir. *72*:363–368 (1946).
Palmer, R.: Abdominal coelioscopy in the diagnosis and treatment of sterility. Int. Congr. of Obst. and Gyn., Dublin, 10 juill. 1947, p. 214.
Palmer, R.: Instrumentation et technique de la couldoscopie gynécologique. Gynéc. et Obstét. *46*:422 (1947).
Palmer, R.: Technique et instrumentation de la coelioscopie transpariétale. Gynéc. et Obstét. *46*:420 (1947).
Palmer, R.: La coelioscopie dans le diagnostic des grossesses extra-utérines. C. R. Soc. franç. Gynéc. *17*:226 (1947).
Palmer, R.: La coelioscopie. Brux.-méd. 305–312 (1948).
Palmer, R.: La coelioscopie transvaginal. Gynéc. et Obstét. *48*:206–213 (1949).
Palmer, R.: La coelioscopia ginecologia. Ginec. Obstet. Méx. *8*:301–316 (1953).
Palmer, R.: La coelioscopie gynécologique; ses possibilités et ses indications actuelles. Sem. Hôp. Paris. *30*:4040–4043 (1954).
Palmer, R.: Gynecological coelioscopy as applied to problems in sterility. Soc. anglaise de stérilité, Londres, 19 juill. 1954. In: Studies on Sterility *6*:95–115 (1954).
Palmer, R.: Les enseignements de la coelioscopie dans les tuberculoses génitales latentes chez la femme. Gaz. méd. *62*:1075–1077 (1955).
Palmer, R.: La coelioscopie dans la grossesse extra-tubaire. Gaz. méd. Fr. *63*:1235–1239 (1956).
Palmer, R.: La place actuelle de la coelioscopie dans le diagnostic de la tuberculose génitale féminine. Gynéc. prat. *7*:211–214 (1956).
Palmer, R.: La coelioscopie gynécologique. Encyclopédie médico-chirurgicale *76–C1*°:1–10 (1956).
Palmer, R.: Zölioskopie und Tubenbiopsie bei Eileiter–Tuberkulose. Österreichische Gesellschaft zum Studium der Sterilität und Fertilität 23. Mai 1957; in: Klin. Med. *12*:517 (1957).
Palmer, R.: La celioscope dans les malformations congénitales de l'appareil génital révélées à la puberté. A propos du rapport de MM. Lumbroso, Netter et Mauvais aux XIXe assises françaises de Gynécologie, Annecy, 26 mai 1958. In: C. R. Soc. franç. Gynéc. *29*:261–262 (1958).
Palmer, R.: Discussion de la communication de M. Thoyer-Rozat: Présenation d'un générateur flash pour l'endoscopie gynécologique: projection de clichés. Soc. nat. Gynéc. Obstét. franç. Paris, 2 nov. 1959. In C. R. Soc. franç. Gynéc. *2*:444–445 (1959).
Palmer, R.: La coelioscopie dans le diagnostic des algies pelviennes rebells. Rev. Prat. *9*:2375–2379 (1959).
Palmer, R.: Celioscopy in the diagnosis of refractory pelvic pains. Rev. Prat. *9*:2375–2381 (1959).
Palmer, R.: Celioscopy in amenorrhea. Gaz. méd. Fr. *66*:1153–1156 (1959).
Palmer, R.: What can be expected at the present time from celioscopy in gynecology. Acta gynec. obstet. hisp. lusit. *9*:19–29 (1960).
Palmer, R.: Progrès récents et indications actuelles de la coelioscopie abdominale en gynécologie (avec présenation de film). Mém. Acad. Chir. *86*:659–663 (1960).
Palmer, R.: Ce que l'on peut attendre actuellement de la coelioscopie en gynécologie. Presse therm. climat. Avril-mai 1960, n° 3.
Palmer, R.: Essai de stérilisation tubaire coelioscopique par électrocoagulation isthmique. R. C. Soc. franç. Gynéc. Séance du *5*:3 (1962).
Palmer, E. D.: Peritoneoscopy technic. Gastroint. Endosc. *14*:105 (1967).
Palmer, R.: Laparoscopy in diagnosis and treatment of endometriosis and pelvic adhesions. Ned. T. Verlosk. *70*:293–296 (1970).
Palmer, R.: J. de Brux: La biopsie tubaire coelioscopique dans le diagnostic de la tuberculose tubaire (avec film). Soc. nat. Gynéc. Obstét. Fr., groupe Paris, 8 mai 1961. In: Bull. Féd. Soc. Gynéc. Obstét. franç. *13*:279–283 (1961).
Palmer, R., J. de Brux: Résultats histologiques, biochimiques et thérapeutiques obtenus chez les femmes dont les ovaires avaient été diagnostiqués Stein-Leventhal à la coeliscopie. Bull. Féd. Soc. Gynéc. Obstét. franç. *19*:405 (1967).
Palmer, R., P. Dorangeon: La coelioscopie dans les ovarites. Rapport aux Assises françaises de Gynécologie; Bordeaux, 26 mai 1953, 1: pp. 111–114.
Palmer, R. P. Dorangeon: La coelioscopie dans les dysharmonies sexuelles. J. méd. France, Reims, 27 mai 1960.
Palmer, R., P. Dorangeon: La coelioscopie en cancérologie gynécologique. J. méd. France, Reims, 27 mai 1960. In: Gynéc. prat. (1961).
Palmer, R. M. Imenitoff: La place de la coelioscopie dans le diagnostic et le traitment des stérilités et des grossesses ectopiques. Rev. franç. Gynéc. *42*:113–155 (1947).

Palmer, R., R. Moricard, P. Le Bourg: Un cas de tuberculose tubaire vérifié par biopsies coelioscopiques avant et après traitement antibiotique et ayant abouti à un accouchement normal. Soc. nat. Gynéc. Obstét. France, groupe Paris, 8 mai 1961. In: Bull. Féd. Soc. nat. Gynéc. franç. *13*:276 (1961).
Palmer, R., E. Palmer: Coelioscopie et tests d'ovulation. Anais do I Convenio da Sociedade Brasileira de Esterilidade. Rio de Janeiro, 14 Oct. 1951. p. 711–714.
Palmer, R., J. Vallve: Progrés récents et causes d'échec de la coelioscopie cinématographique. Soc. franç. Gynéc. 21 avril 1958. In: C. R. Soc. franç. Gynéc. *28*:209 (1958).
Palmer, R., J. Vallvé: Deux nouveaux accessoires pour coelioscopie; péritonéostat et aiguille a pnéumopéritoine. Bull. Féd. Soc. Gynéc. Obstét. Fr. *10*:291–294 (1958).
Palmer, R., J. Vallve: Kymographical utero-tubal insufflation in the light of celioscopy and operations for sterility. Acta obstet. gynec. scand *38*:618–630 (1959).
Pantaleoni: On endoscopic examination of the cavity of the womb. Med. Press and Circ. 14. July. – Canst. Jahresb. *III*:582 (1869).
Partsch, F.: Das diagnostische Pneumoperitoneum in der Chirurgie. Forschr. Röntgenstr. *35* (1924).
Patel, J.-Cl.: Stérilisation féminine par électro-coagulation tubaire sous lapraoscopie. Presse méd. *78*: 1114–1117 (1970).
Paterson, J., J. C. Grimwade: Laparoscopic sterilization during the puerperium. Med. J. Aust. *2*:312–313 (1972).
Pent, D.: Laparoscopy: Its role in private practice. Amer. J. Obstet. Gynec. *113*:459 (1971).
Pent, D.: Laparoscopy: Its role in private practice. Amer. J. Obstet. Gynec. *113*:459–468 (1972).
Peretz, A., M. Sharf: Culdoscopy in gynecologic diagnosis. Amer. J. Obstet. Gynec. *82*:582 (1961).
Pérez-Fernandez, E.: Utilidad de la laparoscopia en la clinica; a proposito de 50 exámenes ralisados. Arch. urug. Med. *50*:480–490 (1957).
Pergola, F.: La cinématographie laparoscopique. Sem. Hôp. Paris *33*:2399–2400 (1957).
Peterson, E. P.: Laparoscopy best in infertility study. Obstet. Gynec. News *5*:6 (1970).
Peterson, E. P.: Anesthesia for laparoscopy. Fertil. and Steril. *22*:695–698 (1971).
Peterson, E. P., S. J. Behrman: Laparoscopy of the infertile patient. Obstet. and Gynec. *36*:363–367 (1970).
Peterson, E. P., J. Behrmann: Laparoscopic tubal sterilization. Amer. J. Obstet. Gynec. *110*:24–31 (1971).
Peterson, R.: Pneumoperitoneum and roentgenology as aides to more accurate obstetric and gynecologic diagnosis. Amer. J. Obstet. Gynec. *2*:349 (1921).
Petty, P. G., A. J. Lim, R. Stahl: A solid state pulsed coagulating diathermy instrument: preliminary report. Aust. N.Z.J. Surg. *38*:2 (1968).
Phillipp, E., K. Semm: Die diagnostische Wertstellung der gynäkologischen Pelviskopie. Geburtsh. u. Frauenheilk. *32*:46–50 (1972).
Pirlet, F.: Gynecological celioscopy. Rev. méd. Liège *15*:698–699 (1960).
Playfair, P. L.: Sterilisation with peritoneoscope. S. Afr. med. J. *22*:711–714 (1948).
Pous-Ivern, L. C., M. A. C. Salazar, O. L. Paouli: Tecnica i complicaciones de la laparoscopia en ginecologia. Clin. invest. gin. obst. *2*:32–80 (1975).
Power, F. H., A. C. Barnes: Sterilization by means of peritoneoscopic tubal fulguration. A preliminary report. Amer. J. Obstet. Gynec. *41*:1038–1043 (1941).
Presser, H. B.: Voluntary sterilization: A world view. Reports on Population/Family Planning *5*:36 (1970).
Prem, K. A.: Culdoscopy. Clin. Obstet. Gynec. *12*:484 (1969).
Pretz, A., M. Sharf: Culdoscopy in gynecological diagnosis. A review of 404 cases of endoscopic examinations. Amer. J. Obstet. Gynec. *82*:582–587 (1961).
Pye, A., M. Fourestier: La culdoscopie. (Exploration de la cavité pelvienne chez la femme par voie vaginale.) Presse méd. *72*:679–683 (1964).
Quatrochi, G., R. Alicino: Indicazioni e limiti della celioscopia ginecològica. Minerva ginec. *20*:688–690 (1968).
Rakos, L.: L'utilisation de la coelioscopie en vue de choisir la voie d'abord dans l'hystérectomie totale. Gynéc. prat. *17*:465–470 (1966).
Rautenberg, E.: Röntgenphotographie der Leber, der Milz und des Zwerchfells. Dtsch. med. Wschr. *40*:1205–1208 (1914).
Ravina, A.: La coelioscopie par voie vaginale. Presse méd. *58*:81–82 (1950).
Ravina, A.: Hémorrhagie mortelle consécutaire a une ponction biopsie du foie dans un cas de cancer secondaire de cet organe. Bull. Soc. méd. Hôp. Paris *66*:1216–1217 (1950).
Ravina, J. H.: Stérilisation coelioscopique des trompes. Presse méd. *79*:141 (1971).
Redi, R.: Über ein neues endoskopisches chirurgisches Instrument, das Splanchnoskop. Zbl. Chir. 558 (1935).
Renaer, M.: Experiences with laparoscopy in the investigation of chronic pain syndromes in gynaecological practice. Ned. T. Verlosk. *70*:285–293 (1970).
Rettenmaier, G.: Bewertung und Einschränkung des Risikos bei der Laparoskopie. Endoscopy *1*:115–122 (1969).
Revaz, C.: Problèmes chirurgicaux de la stérilité tubaire. Gynécologia *165*:178 (1968).
Reynaud: Étude sur les rétrécissements de l'urèthre. Thèse de Paris, 1868.
Richart, R. M., A. J. Gutierrez-Najar, R. S. Neuwirth: Transvaginal human sterilization, a preliminary report. Amer. J. Obstet. Gynec. *III*:108 (1971).

Rioux, J. E., A. F. Bastide, S. Lemire: Laparoscopy in gynecology. I. General concepts. Un. méd. Can. *99*:698–706 (1970).
Riva, H. L., R. D. Hatch, J. L. Breen: Culdoscopy for infertility. Amer. J. Obstet. Gynec. *78*:1302 (1959).
Riva, R., P. S. Anderson, J. L. des Rosiers, J. L. Breen: Further experience with culdoscopy. An analysis of 2850 cases. J. Amer. med. Ass. *178*:873 (1961).
Robinson, S.: Instrument for retraction of viscera during peritoneoscopy. Med. Surg. Tributes 417–429 (1942).
Rodgers, J., Q. Female sterilizations book Hopkins. The News American, April 12, 1970, pp. iA and 44.
Roitman, M. J.: Fiber optic culdoscopy. J. Amer. osteopath. Ass. *67*:1241–1247 (1968).
Roland, M.: Endoscopic methods in gynecology and infertility. A comparison of experiences with culdoscopy and laparoscopy. Endoscopy *4*:145–149 (1969).
Roland, M.: Culdoscopy and laparoscopy: competitive or complementary technics? Fertil. and Steril. *21*:361–376 (1970).
Romsing, J.: Sterilization of women by means of puerperal sterilization. Ugeskr. Laeg. *134*:439–440 (1972).
Rosen, A. D.: Diagnostic and operative applications of laparoscopy. Texas Med. *68*:94–101 (1972).
Rosenbruch, K.-J.: Some remarks about the measurement and calculation of optical transfer functions. SPIE Seminar, Proc. *13*:157 (1968).
Rosenbruch, K.-J.: Die Bedeutung der optischen Übertragungsfunktion bei der Konstruktion optischer Systeme. Optik *30*:346 (1970).
Rosenbruch, K.-J., K. Rosenhauer: Ein Verfahren zur Messung der Kontrastübertragungsfunktion photographischer Objektive. Optica Acta *4*:21 (1957).
Rosenbruch, K.-J., K. Rosenhauer: Die Messung der Kontrastübertragungsfunktion aus der Kantenbildanalyse. Z. Instr.-Kde. *67*:179 (1959).
Rossi, T.: L'interesse della celioscopia nella diagnosi della gravidanza ectopica. Aggiorn. Ostet. Ginec. *4*:120 (1963).
Roitman, M. J.: Fiber optic culdoscopy for infertility. J. Amer. osteopath. Ass. *67*:1423–1426 (1968).
Rubin, I. C.: J. Amer. med. Ass. *75*:661 (1920).
Ruddock, J. C.: Peritoneoscopy. West. J. Surg. *42*:392–405 (1934).
Ruddock, J. C.: Peritoneoscopy. Surg. Gynec. Obstet. *65*:623–639 (1937).
Ruddock, J. C.: Peritoneoscopy. Sth. Surg. *8*:113–135 (1939).
Ruddock, J. C.: Application and evaluation of peritoneoscopy. Calif. Med. *71*:110–116 (1949).
Ruddock, J. C.: Peritoneoscopy, a critical clinical review. Surg. Clin. N. Amer. *37*:1249–1260 (1957).
Ruddock, J. C., R. B. Hope: Coccidial peritonitis; diagnosis by peritoneoscopy. J. Amer. med. Ass. *113*:2054–2055 (1939).
Ruhman, W.: Über viscerale Reflexe auf lokale thermische Hautreize. Z. ges. exp. Med. *57*:768 (1927).
Sabagh, R. A., I. A. Coppola: Color laparophotography. Acta cytol. (Philad.) *5*:83–102 (1961).
Sala, S., M. Simonetti, R. Pomares: La importancia de la laparoscopia como medio de diagnostico en el embarazo extrauterion. Bol. Soc. Obstet. Ginec. (B. Aires) *25*:167–185 (1946).
Samuelsson, S.: Coelioskopi som gynekologisk undersökningsmetod. Nord. Med. *63*:270 (1960).
Samuelsson, S.: Needle biopsy from uterus and myoma during peritoneoscopy. Acta obstet. gynec. scand. *44*:153 (1965).
Samuelsson, S., S. Sjöstedt: Transperitoneal liver biopsy under peritoneoscopic control. Acta med. scand. *170*:627 (1961).
Samuelsson, S., A. Sjövall: On the diagnostic value of laparoscopy in ovarian endometriosis. Acta obstet. gynec. scand. *47*:350–360 (1968).
Samuelson, S., A. Sjövall: The value of laparoscopy in the differential diagnosis between uterine fibromyomata and adnexal tumours. Acta obstet. gynec. scand. *49*:175–178 (1970).
Sarto, G. E., M. Crumpacker, W. Kiekhofer, A. E. Schultz: Culdoscopy at university hospitals 1964–1967. Review of 100 consecutive cases. Wis. med. J. *67*:514–518 (1968).
Sawyer, C. D.: Peritoneoscopy. N. Y. St. J. Med. *39*:2022–2025 (1939).
Scott, D. B.: Some effects of peritoneal insufflation of carbon dioxide at laparoscopy. Anaesthesia *25*:590 (1970).
Seed, R. F., T. F. Shakespeare, M. J. Muldoon: Carbon dioxide hemostasis during anesthesia for laparoscopy. Anaesthesia *25*:223 (1970).
Sellheim, H.: Ein einfacher, zuverlässiger und ungefährlicher Tubenschneuzer. Sbl. Gynäk. *30*:1206 (1923).
Semm, K.: Zur Technik der Eileiterdurchblasung. Z. Geburtsh. Gynäk., Beilageheft, *162*:48–53 (1964).
Semm, K.: Die gezielte und dosierbare Wärme-Koagulation der gutartigen Portio-Veränderung. Geburtsh. u. Frauenheilk. *25*:795–802 (1965).
Semm. K.: Ein neuer Apparat zur Behandlung der gutartigen Portioerosion und der chronischen Zervizitis. Geburtsh. u. Frauenheilk. *26*:657–663 (1966) und Monit. ostet. ginec. *36*:367–372 (1966).
Semm, K.: New apparatus for ≫cold-coagulation≪ of the benign cervical lesions. Amer. J. Obstet. Gynec. *95*:963–966 (1966).
Semm, K.: Die Behandlung der gutartigen Portioveränderungen und der Zervizitis in der Sterilitätspraxis. Wien. med. Wschr. *116*:385–387 (1966).

Semm, K.: Die Laparoskopie in der Gynäkologie. Geburtsh. u. Frauenheilk. *27*:1029 (1967).
Semm, K.: Neue Möglichkeiten durch die Vakuum-Intrauterin-Sonde. Endoscopy *1*:33–37 (1969).
Semm, K.: Technique of gynaecological pelviscopy. Med. Gynaec. Sociol. *4*:62 (1969).
Semm, K.: Die Technik des Pneumoperitoneums. Endoscopy *1*:68–70 (1969).
Semm, K.: Die kinderlose Ehe. Landarzt *45*:1268 (1969).
Semm, K.: Gynaecological pelviscopy and its instrumentarium. Acta Europ. Fertil. *1*:81–97 (1969).
Semm, K.: Heute zur Verfügung stehende Laparoskopie. Z. Gastroent. *1*:152–155 (1970).
Semm, K.: La pelviscopie gynécologique. Gynéc. prat. *1*:9–26 (1970).
Semm, K.: Das Instrumentarium der gynäkologischen Pelviskopie. Endoscopy *2*:36–42 (1970).
Semm, K.: Die Pelviskopie bei der sterilen Frau. Gynäkologe *3*:118–125 (1971).
Semm, K.: Aufbau und Herstellung eines gynäkologischen Lehrfilms. Med. Technik *12*:382–400 (1971).
Semm, K.: Gynäkologische Endoskopie. Arch. Gynäk. *211*:396–400 (1971).
Semm, K.: Die fotografische und filmische Dokumentation interessanter Befunde bei der Routinepelviskopie. Endoscopy *4*:150–152 (1972).
Semm, K.: Die moderne Endoskopie in der Frauenheilkunde. Frauenarzt *13*:300–307 (1972).
Semm, K.: Gynecologic pelviscopy. Obstet. Gynec. Digest *14*:21–25 (1972).
Semm, K.: Der technische Stand pelviskopischer Filmaufnahmen. Research Film 7:541–551 (1972).
Semm, K.: Technische Bemerkungen zur Saugkürette. Geburtsh. u. Frauenheilk. *32*:547–550 (1972).
Semm, K.: Modern endoscopy in gynecology and obstetrics. Clin. Excerpts *34*:1094–1103 (1972).
Semm, K.: L'endoscopie moderne en gynécologie et obstétrique. Rev. Progr. Therap. *26*:1118–1127 (1972).
Semm, K.: Die Wertstellung der Endoskopie in Gynäkologie und Geburtshilfe. Urologe B *13*:33–36 (1973).
Semm, K.: Endoskopie in der Frauenheilkunde (Moderatorenbericht). Arch. Gynäk. *214*:235–237 (1973).
Semm, K.: Transabdominale oder transvaginale Eileitersterilisation mit einer neuen Koagulationszange. Endoscopy *6*:40–42 (1974).
Semm, K.: Suction-Palp, a new aid for pelviscopy. Endoscopy 7:85–88 (1975).
Serment, H.: Intérêt de la coelioscopie en pratique gynécologique. Marseille-méd. *90*:509–515 (1953).
Serrano Rebeil, G., F. Balderrama: Valor diagnostico de la peritoneoscopie. Rev. Invest. clin. *9*:111–119 (1957).
Serrano Rebeil, G., H. Jinich, J. L. Gutierrez Sacasa: The utility of peritoneoscopy in clinical practice. Rev. Invest. clin. *12*:329–357 (1960).
Serrano Rebeil, G., H. Jinich, J. L. Gutierrez Sacasa: The use of peritoneoscopy in clinical medicine. Nivar. med. *17*:70–94 (1961).
Shackelford, R. T.: Peritoneoscopy. Surgery *10*:742–746 (1941).
Sharf, M.: Permanent sterilization by electrocoagulation of the Fallopian tubes. Excerpta med. (Amst.) Sect. X *20*:2164 (1967).
Sharf, M., A. Peretz: Diagnosis of tubal pregnancy by culdoscopy as compared with routine methods. Harefuah *59*:105–106 (1960).
Sharf, M., W. Z. Polishuk, A. Peretz: The value of endoscopy in the diagnosis of endocrine disorders. J. Obstet. Gynaec. brit. Cwlth. *5*:834 (1961).
Shell, J. H., R. C. Myers: Small bowel injury after laparoscopic sterilization. Amer. J. Obstet. Gynec. *115*:285 (1973).
Short, A. R.: The use of celioscopy. Brit. med. J. *2*:254 (1925).
Siegler, A. M.: Trends in laparoscopy. Amer. J. Obstet. Gynec. *109*:794–809 (1971).
Siegler, A. M.: Tubal sterilization. Amer. J. Nursing 72:1625–1629 (1972).
Siegler, A. M.: An instrument to aid tubal sterilization by laparoscopy. Fertil. and Steril. *23*:367–368 (1972).
Siegler, A. M.: Removal of ectopic intrauterine contraceptive devices aided by laparoscopy. A report of 3 cases and a review of the literature. Amer. J. Obstet. Gynec. *115*:158–162 (1973).
Siegler, A. M., K. J. Berenyi; Laparoscopy in gynecology. Obstet. and Gynec. *34*:572–577 (1969).
Siegler, A. M., M. Garret: Ancillary technics with laparoscopy. Fertil. and Steril. *21*:763–773 (1970).
Šimić, S., A. Milojković, M. Dzumhur: Ginekologija i opstetricija *3*:173–175 (1963).
Šimić, S., D. Sedlar, P. Konstantinović: Med. arhiv *18*:99–104 (1964).
Sironi, P. G.: Anesthesia in its applications in the endoscopic field. Acta anaesth. (Padova) *11*:393–438 (1960).
Sjövall, A.: Size-measuring at laparoscopy. Acta obstet. gynec. scand. *42*:279 (1963).
Sjövall, A.: Un metodo semplificato di laparoscopia. Minerva ginec. *17*:233 (1965).
Slyke, D. D. van, J. Sendroy jr., S. H. Liu: Manometric analysis of gas mixtures. III. Manometric determination of carbon dioxide tension and pH of blood. J. biol. Chem. *95*:547 (1932).
Smith, I., R. J. Benzie, N. L. M. Gordon, G. R. Kelman, G. H. Swapp: Cardiovascular effects of peritoneal insufflation of carbon dioxide for laparoscopy. Brit. med. J. *3*:410–411 (1971).
Smith, D. C.: Removal of an ectopic IUD through the laparoscope. Amer. J. Obstet. Gynec. *105*:285 (1969).
Smith, V. M.: Clinical peritoneoscopy. Amer. J. Gastroent. *42*:13–22 (1964).
Soderstrom, R. M., M. R. Smith: Instrument and method-Tubal sterilization, a new laparoscopic method. Obstet. and Gynec. *38*:152–154 (1971).

Soonawalla, R.: Vaginal techniques of surgical sterilization. Aust. N. Z. J. Obstet. Gynaec. (in press).
Sousek, O.: Adhesions in the abdominal cavity and laparoscopy. Čas. Lék. čes. *100*:218–220 (1961).
Spellacy, W. N., J. A. Tolien: Gynecography: a neglected adjuvant to culdoscopy. Obstet. and Gynec. *24*:286 (1964).
Svennerud, S. B. Ästedt: Steriliserings-operation via laparoskop. Lakartidningen *65*:3932–3933 (1968).
Svennerud, S., B. Ästedt: Sterilization during laparoscopy. Acta obstet. gynec. scand. *48*:Suppl. *3*:64–65 (1969).
Sweek, W. O.: A new and practical abdominoscope. Surg. Gynec. Obstet. *45*:700–701 (1927).
Swolin, K.: Die Einwirkung von Großen, intraperitonealen Dosen Glukokortikoid auf die Bildung von post-operativen Adhäsionen. Klinische Studien mit Hilfe des Laparoskopes an operierten Extrauteringraviditäten. Acta obstet. gynec. scand. *46*:204 (1967).
Swolin, K.: Spontanheilung nach Querresektion der Tuba Fallopii. Beobachtungen an operierten Eileiter-schwangerschaften. Acta obstet. gynec. scand. *46*:219 (1967).
Swolin, K.: 50 Fertilitätsoperationen. Teil I. Literatur und Methodik. Acta obstet. gynec. scand. *46*:234 (1967).
Swolin, K.: 50 Fertilitätsoperationen. Teil II. Material und Resultate. Acta obstet. gynec. scand. *46*:250 (1967).
Swolin, K., M. Rosencrantz: Laparoscopy vs., hysterosalpingography in sterility investigations. A comparative study. Fertil. and Steril. *23*:270–273 (1972).
Szeprievszkij, Sz. A.: Poszleoperacionnij pnevmoperitoneum i jevo vlijannie na vozniknovenie legocsnih oszlozsneniji. Vesztn. Khir. *2*: (1947).
Schmidt-Matthiesen, H.: Eine neue Methode zur schonenden Laparoskopie. Geburtsh. u. Frauenheilk. *31*:1019–1021 (1971).
Schnitzler: Über Laryngoskopie und Rhinoskopie. Wiener Klinik 1878.
Schramm, J.: Über die diaphanoskopische Untersuchung der weiblichen Beckenorgane. Jahresberichte der Gesellschaft für Nat. und Heilkunde in Dresden, October 1875—Juni 1876, Dtsch. prakt. Med. 1876 Nr. 32.
Schubert, H.: Endoskopische Optik. Medizinalmarkt *5*:135 (1957).
Schubert, H.: Technische Entwicklung und Stand der Endo-Photographie. Medizinalmarkt *5*:269 (1957).
Schustler: Beiträge zur endoskopischen Diagnostik. Wiener med. Wschr. 1886.
Stamm, O.: Indications et résultats de 128 cas de laparoscopie. Bull. Féd. Soc. Gynéc. Obstét. franç. *10*:11 (1958).
Stein, I. F., M. L. Leventhal: Amenorrhoea associated with bilateral polycystic ovaries. Amer. J. Obstet. Gynec. *29*:181–191 (1939).
Stein, I. F.: Why pneumoperitoneum? Radiology *28*:391–398 (1937).
Stein, I. F., M. R. Cohen, R. Elson: Results of bilateral ovarian wedge resection in 47 cases of sterility. Amer. J. Obstet. Gynec. *58*:267 (1949).
Stein, S.: Das Photo-Endoskop. Berl. klin. Wochenschr. H. 3 (1974).
Steinberg, U.: Komplikationen bei der Laparoskopie. I. Beobachtungen bei Anlegung des Pneumoperitoneums. Z. ges. inn. Med. *11*:557–561 (1956).
Steinberg, U.: Komplikationen bei der Laparoskopie. II. Zwischenfälle infolge Leberpunktion. Z. ges. inn. Med. *12*:201–206 (1957).
Steinberg, U.: Zur Technik der gezielten Leberpunktion und anderer Probeentnahmen bei Laparoskopie. Z. ges. inn. Med. *12*:279–282 (1957).
Steiner, O. P.: Abdominoskopie. Schweiz. med. Wschr. *54*:84–87 (1924).
Steptoe, P. C.: Laparoscopy and ovulation. Lancet *II*:913 (1968).
Steptoe, P. C.: Laparoscopic sterilization. In: P. Curzen: Report of scientific meeting, Royal College of Obstetrics and Gynecology. J. Obstet. Gynaec. Brit. Cwlth. *76*:1043 (1969).
Steptoe, P. C.: Laparoscopic studies of the ovaries. Ned. T. Verlosk *70*:296–300 (1970).
Steptoe, P. C.: Recent advances in surgical methods of control of fertility and infertility. Brit. med. Bull. *26*:60–64 (1970).
Steptoe, P. C.: Female sterilization. Nursing Times *67*:1529–1530 (1971).
Steptoe, P. C.: Laparoscopic tubal sterilization—A British viewpoint, IPPF Med. Bull. *5*:4 (1971).
Steptoe, P. C.: Problems of laparoscopic sterilization. Lancet *I*:1115 (1972).
Steptoe, P. C., R. G. Edwards: Laparoscopic recovery of preovulatory human oocytes after priming of ovaries with gonadotrophins. Lancet *I*:683–689 (1970).
Steptoe, P. C., M. Imram: Combined procedure of aspiration termination and laparoscopic sterilization. Brit. med. J. *3*:751–752 (1969).
Stöckli, A.: Laparoskopie mit besonderer Berücksichtigung der Photolaparoskopie. Gyneacologia (Basel) *153*:121–125 (1962).
Stuermer, M. V.: Culdoscopy and the tubal factor. Obstet. and Gynec. *25*:470–474 (1965).
Taylor, M. B.: Flexible arm support for the laparoscopy. Obstet. and Gynec. *37*:918–919 (1971).
Tedesko, F.: Über Endoskopie des Abdomens und des Thorax. Mitt. d. Gesellsch. f. Med. u. Kinderh. in Wien *12*:323 (1912).
Te Linde, R. W., F. N. Rutledge: Culdoscopy; a useful gynecological procedure. Amer. J. Obstet. Gynec. *55*:102 (1948).

Teschendorf, W.: Uber die Verwendung schnell resorbierbarer Gase in der Röntgendiagnostik. Acta radiol. (Stockh.) *36*:297–304 (1961).
Teton, I. B.: Diagnostic culdoscopy. Amer. J. Obstet. Gynec. *60*: 665–670 (1950).
Thom, B.: Die Ektoskopie bei Erkrankungen des Bauches. Münch. med. Wschr. *79*:1909–1912 (1932).
Thompson, B. H., C. R. Jr. Wheeless: Outpatient sterilization by laparoscopy. A report of 666 patients. Obste. and Gynec. *38*:912–915 (1971).
Thompson, B. H., C. R. Wheeless: Gastrointestinal complications of laparoscopy sterilization. Obstet. and Gynec. *41*:669–676 (1973).
Thompson, H.: Remarks on the use of the endoscope. Lancet 1866.
Thompson, R. J., Q. Mojadidi, L. Beadling: Laparoscopy. Sterilization under local anesthesia. Obstet. and Gynec. *39*:635 (1972).
Thomsen, K.: Erfahrungen und Fortschritte bei der Douglasskopie. Geburtsh. u. Frauenheilk. *11*:587 (1951).
Thomsen, K.: Die Stellung der Endoskopie in der Gynäkologie. Geburtsh. u. Frauenheilk. *14*:925 (1954).
Thorsteinsson, V. T., J. H. Pratt: Gynecologic operations for sterilization. Minn. Med. *55*:204–210 (1972).
Thoyer-Rozat, J.: Electronic flash photography in the course of celioscopy. Gynec. Obstet. *59*:71–73 (1960).
Thoyer-Rozat, J.: La photographie laparoscopique en flash electronique. Presse méd. *69*:157–158 (1961).
Thoyer-Rozat, J., M. F. Coudere: Sterilization of the Fallopian tubes by electrocoagulation of the isthmus under celioscopy. Bull. Féd. Soc. Gynéc. Obstét. franç. *22*:11–13 (1970).
Thoyer-Rozat, J., A. Dupay: A propos d'une série de 200 grossesses extrautérines. Sem. Hôp. Paris 632 (1960).
Thoyer-Rozat, J., M. Mintz: Table ronde sur la coelioscopie. Rev. franç. Gynéc. *62*:93 (1967).
Tietze, C.: Stud. Fam. Plan., Nos. 3, 7, 12, 18 (suppl.), 25, 36, published June 1963-May 1918, also 47, 14, November 1969 and Vol. 2, No. 1, January 1971.
Torchinov, A. M.: Significance of endoscopy for the differential diagnosis of myoma of the uterus and ovarian rumors. Akush. i Ginek. *46*:65–67 (1970).
Towbin: Mediastinal emphysema occurring with therapuetie pneumoperitoneum of the cases. Ann. int. Med. *35*:555–592 (1951).
Turner, G., N. Hooper: Sterilization and thrombo-embolism. J. Obstet. Gynaec. Brit. Cwlth. *78*:737–740 (1971).
Unna: Untersuchungsstuhl und Albocarbonlampe zu endoskopischen Zwecken. Mh. prakt. Derm. 1885.
Unverricht, W.: Die Thoracoskopie und Laparoskopie. Berl. klin. Wschr. *2*:502 (1923).
Unverricht: Brauers Beitr. *55*:296 (1923).
Várkonyi, S., T. Zrinyi, E. Tóth: Laparoskópiás tapasztalataink. MÁV. Eü Tud. Közl. *IV*:209–216 (1962).
Vasiliev, R. K.: Complications in peritoneoscopy and their prophylaxis. Gastroent. Abstr. Citations *2*:1156 (1967).
Veress, J.: Neues Instrument zur Ausführung von Brust- oder Bauchpunktionen und Pneumothoraxbehandlung. Dtsch. med. Wschr. *41*:1480 (1938).
Veress, J.: Eine Nadel zur gefahrlosen Anlegung des Pneumoperitoneums. Elöadás a zürichi Gastroenterologiai Kongresszuson, 1960. szeptember 30-án. Gastroenterologia (Basel).
Vieira, V. A.: Peritoneoscopia y culdoscopia en el examen genital. Bol. Soc. chil. Obstet. Ginec. *14*:221–227 (1949).
Vignalou, J., S. Plouin: Amenorrheas of endocrine nature and celioscopy. Rev. méd. franç. *41*:279–282 (1960).
Vojta, M.: Sterilizace na vejcovodech pri laparoskopii. Česk. Gyneck. *35*:602–603 (1970).
Vrobel, T., E. Dlhos, K. Schmidt: Simultaneous culdoscopy and chromosalpingography. Česk. Gynek. *32*:404–407 (1967).
Wadhwa, R., R. McKenzie: Complications of band-aid surgery for sterilization. J. Amer. med. Ass. *222*:1558 (1972).
Walch, E., H. Grünagel: Praktische Erfahrungen mit der Douglasskopie. Zbl. Gynäk. *76*:397 (1954).
Weber, E.: Über die Bedeutung der Einführung von Sauerstoff resp. Luft in die Bauchhöhle für die experimentelle und diagnostische Röntgenologie. Fortschr. Geburtsh. Gynäk. *20*:453–455 (1913).
Weigel, H.: Über Endophotographie, speziell bei der Laparoskopie. Photographie und Wissenschaft *4*:15–18 (1956).
Weill, J. P.: Les indications de la laparoscopie. Strasbourg méd. *9*:522–525 (1958).
Weinberg, J.: Verbesserungen am Metallendoskope. Wien. med. Bl. 1881, Nr. 16.
Weisman, A.: Gynograph, new improved gynoroentgenologic apparatus for use in conjunction with fluoroscopy and radiography of the female genital tract. Radiology *56*:104 (1951).
Wenderoth, H.: Nil nocere!; Mediastinalemphysem bei Laparoskopie. Münch. med. Wschr. *96*:1369–1371 (1954).
Wenderoth, H.: Luftembolie bei Laparoskopie? Dtsch. med. Wschr. *81*:947 (1956).

Wenner, R.: Was kann man in der Gynecologie von der Coelioscopie erwarten? Gynaecologia (Basel) *125*:264–267 (1948).
Werner, H.: Sterilisierung der Frau durch Tubenverkochung. Chirurg 843–845 (1934).
Wheeless, C. R., Jr.: A rapid, inexpensive, and effective method of surgical sterilization by laparoscopy. J. reprod. Med. *3*:65 (1969).
Wheeless, C. R., Jr.: Instrument and method—Elimination of second incision in laparoscopic sterilization. Obstet. and Gynec. *36*:208–211 (1970).
Wheeless, C. R., Jr.: Outpatient tubal sterilization. Obstet. and Gynec. *36*:208–211 (1970).
Wheeless, C. R., Jr.: Anesthesia for diagnostic and operative laparoscopy. Fertil. and Steril. *22*:690–694 (1971).
Wheeless, C. R., Jr.: Outpatient laparoscope sterilization under local anesthesia. Obstet. and Gynec. *39*:767–770 (1972).
Wheeless, C. R., Jr.: International sterilization project (trip report on visit to Nepal and Thailand) submitted to U. S. Agency for International Development, April 1972 (unpublished).
Wheeless, C. R., Jr.: Elimination of second incision in laparoscopic sterilization. Obstet. and Gynec *39*:134 (1972).
Wheeless, C. R., Jr.: The status of outpatient tubal sterilization by laparoscopy: improved technics and review of 1000 cases. Obstet. and Gynec. *39*:635 (1972).
Wheeless, C. R., Jr.: Laparoscopy sterilization; review of 3,600 cases. J. Obstet. Gynec. *42*:751–758 (1973).
Whiteley, P. F.: Laparoscopic sterilization in the puerperium. J. Obstet. Gynaec. Brit. Cwlth. *79*:166–167 (1972).
Wierzbicki, J.: Kliniczne uniti laparoskopie. Pol. Przegl. chir. *35*:137–141 (1963).
Wierzbicki, J.: Kliniczne zastosowanie laparoskopii. Pol. Przegl. chir. *35*:139–141 (1963).
Wildhirt, E.: Mediastinalemphysem bei Laparoskopie und zur Luftembolie bei Laparoskopie. Münch. med. Wschr. *98*:58 (1956).
Willenegger, H.: Klinische und technische Bemerkungen zur temporären Zwerchfellähmung, unterstützt durch das Pneumoperitoneum. Helv. chir. Acta *12*:4–5 (1945).
Williams, P. P., R. P. Bendel: Laparoscopic sterilization. Minn. Med. *54*:887–888 (1971).
Winklemann, P.: Die besonderen Indikationen zur Douglasskopie. Geburtsh. u. Frauenheilk. *14*:934 (1954).
Wittrin, G.: Die palliative Behandlung tumorbedingter inoperabler Oesophagusstenosen mit der Thermosonde. Chirurg *44*:285–287 (1973).
Wood, J.: Sterilization: A working paper, submitted to the U.S. Agency for International Development, April 12, 1972 (unpublished).
Wortman, J., P. T. Piotrow: Laparoscopic sterilization. II. What are the problems? Population Report, Series C, No. 2, 1973.
Yamakawa, K.: Kinelaparography. Med. Biol. *III*:247–251 (1960).
Yupze, A. A., H. H. Allen, J. A. Collins: Tubal sterilization: methodology, postoperative management and follow-up of 2934 cases. Can. med. Ass. J. *107*:115–117 (1972).
Zaufal: Versuche mit dem Nitze Leiter'schen Endoskop. Prager med. Wschr. 11. Februar 1880.
Zhanel, J.: Sterilization by the abdominal route with one suture. Česk. Gynek. *33*:288 (1968).
Zielske, F.: Sterilisation der Frau durch laparoskopische Elektrokoagulation der Tuben. Gynäkologe *5*:175 (1972).
Zollikoffer, R.: Über Laparoskopie. Schweiz. med. Wschr. *104*:264 (1924).
Zuniga, G. A.: Endoscopy in gynecological examination. Rev. med. Honduras *27*:159–162 (1960).

MONOGRAPHS AND BOOKS ON HYSTEROSCOPY

Alvarado, D. A., G. R. Quinones: Histeroscopía. Aparatos, técnica y resultados. In: Asoc. Mex. Ginec. Obstet. (ed.). Actualidades en Ginecología y Obstetricia. p. 362. Méxiko, D. F. 1970.
Anderson, R. K.: Electrical and thermal aspects of high frequency electrosurgical energy as applied to hysteroscopy. In: Hysteroscopic sterilization. p. 19–26. Intercont. Med. Book Corp., New York, London 1974.
Bumm, E.: Verhandlungen der Deutschen Gesellschaft für Gynäkologie. *1895*:524.
Cohen, M. R., W. P. Dmowski: Modern hysteroscopy: Diagnostic and therapeutic potential. Hysteroscopic sterilization. p. 39–49. Intercont. Med. Book Corp., New York, London 1974.
David, Ch.: L'endoscopie utérine, applications au diagnostic et au traitement des affections intrautérines. Jacques, Paris 1908.
Désormeaux, A.-J.: L'endoscope et de ses applications au diagnostic et au traitement des affections de l'urèthre de la vessie, Baillière, Paris 1865.
Duncan, C. W., R. D. Falb, J. J. Speidel (eds.): Female sterilization: prognosis for simplified outpatient procedures. Proc. workshop held at Airlie, Virginia, December 2–3, 1971. p. 125–129. Academic Press, New York 1972.
Edström, K. G.: Intrauterine surgical procedures during hysteroscopy (Abstract). Proc. VII. World Congress on Fertility and Sterility. p. 808. Excerpta Medica Amsterdam, Elsevier Publ. Co. Inc., New York 1973.
Falb, W. R. D., J. J. Speidel (eds.): Female sterilization. p. 131 Academic Press, New York 1972.

Hayashi, M.: Tubal sterilization by coronal coagulation under hysteroscopy. In R. M. Richart and D. J. Prager (eds.): Human sterilization, Chapter 28. Thomas, Springfield, Ill., 1972.
Hayashi, M.: Endoscopy in experimental animals—Photography and cinematography. In: Hysteroscopic sterilization. p. 3–7. Intercont. Med. Book Corp. New York, London 1974.
Hoffbauer, H.: Das kolpophotographische Bild des unteren Eipols. In L. Demling u. R. Ottenjann: Endoskopie—Methoden, Ergebnisse. S. 193–194.
Hulka, J. F., K. F. Omran: In M. Richart (ed.): Cauterization for tubal sterilization. p. 313. Thomas, Springfield, Ill., 1972.
Israngkun, Ch.: The use of hysteroscopic sterilization in less developed countries. In: Hysteroscopic sterilization. p. 145–149. Intercont. Med. Book Corp., New York, London 1974.
Joelsson, I.: Hysteroscopy using dextran with special reference to delineation of the intrauterine extent of corpus carcinoma. In: Hysteroscopic sterilization. p. 35–38. Intercont. Med. Book Corp., New York, London 1974.
Karacz, B., H.-J. Lindemann: Erste Erfahrungen über intramurale Tubensterilisation per Hysteroskop. In R. Ottenjann: Fortschritte der Endoskopie. S. 197. Schattauer, Stuttgart 1973.
Lindemann, H.-J.: Eine neue Methode für die Hysteroskopie. In R. Ottenjann: Fortschritte der Endoskopie. S. 185. Schattauer, Stuttgart 1973.
Lindemann, H.-J.: Hysteroscopy for the diagnosis of intrauterine causes of sterility (Abstract). Proc. VII. World Congress on Fertility and Sterility. p. 807. Excerpta Medica Amsterdam, Elsevier Publ. Co. Inc., New York 1973.
Lindemann, H.-J.: Transuterine tubal sterilization by CO-hysteroscopy. In: Hysteroscopic sterilization. p. 61–73. Intercont. Med. Book Corp., New York, London 1974.
Lübke, F., M. Schmidt-Gollwitzer: Erste Erfahrungen mit der Hysteroskopie. In R. Ottenjann: Fortschritte der Endoskopie. S. 181. Schattauer, Stuttgart 1973.
Marleschki, V.: Moderne Cervicoscopie und Hysteroscopie. In: Abhandlungen der deutschen Akademie der Wissenschafren zu Berlin. S. 421. Akademie Verlag, Berlin. 1966.
Marleschki, B.: Hysteroscopy in gynaecological and obstetric emergencies: Urgent endoscopy of digestive and abdominal diseases. p. 248. Karger, Basel 1972.
Marleschki, V.: The hysteroscopy method of Marleschki. In: Proc. VII. World Congress on Fertility and Sterility. p. 279. Excerpta Medica Amsterdam, Elsevier Publ. Co. Inc., New York 1973.
Marleschki, V.: Hysteroscopy study of uterine circulation in normal labor and in labor involving the use of abdominal decompression. In: Excerpta Medica Amsterdam, Elsevier Publ. Co. Inc., New York 1973.
Marleschki, V.: Hysteroscopie diagnosis of intrauterine synechiae and their treatment (Abstract). In: Proc. VII. World Congress on Fertility and Sterility. p. 806. Excerpta Medica Amsterdam, Elsevier Publ. Co. Inc., New York 1973.
Menken, F. C.: Fortschritte der gynäkologischen Endoskopie. In: L. Demling u. R. Ottenjann: Fortschritte der Endoskopie. Bd. 1 Schattauer, Stuttgart 1969.
Neuwirth, R. S., R. M. Richard, Ch. Israngkun, U. Levine, S. Phaosavsadi: Hysteroscopic sterilization. In: Hysteroscopic sterilization. p. 121–129. Intercont. Med. Book Corp., New York, London 1974.
Newell, J. W.: Comparative study of various hysteroscopes. In: Hysteroscopic sterilization. p. 27–32. Intercont. Med. Book Corp., New York, London 1974.
Porto, R.: Pneumohysteroscopy: Instrumentation and technique. In: Hysteroscopic sterilization. p. 51–58. Intercont. Med. Book Corp., New York, London 1974.
Quiñones, A. A., R. Aznar: Tubal instillation of quinaerine under hysteroscopic control. In: Hysteroscopic sterilization. p. 85–94. Intercont. Med. Book Corp., New York, London 1974.
Quiñones, R., A. Alvarado, R. Aznar: Tubal electrocoagulation under hysteroscopic control. In: Hysteroscopic sterilization. p. 95–106. Intercont. Med. Book Corp., New York, London 1974.
Quint, R.: The rigid hysteroscope. In: Hysteroscopic sterilization. p. 11–18. Intercont. Med. Book Corp., New York, London 1974.
Rimkus, V.: Hysteroskopie—ein neues Gerät zur CO_2-Insufflationstechnik. Kongreßbericht, VI. Kongreß der Deutschen Gesellschaft für Endoskopie. Schattauer, Stuttgart 1974.
Rimkus, V., K. Semm: Hysteroscopic sterilization using carbon-dioxide. In: Selected papers and discussions from the Workshop on Hysteroscopic Sterilization, sponsored by the University of Minnesota, Medical School, Minneapolis, Minnesota. p. 75–84. Intercont. Med. Book Corp., New York, London 1974.
Sciarra, J. J.: Research and developments programs to achieve practical outpatient sterilization. In: W. G. Duncan, D. R. Falb, J. H. Speidel: Female sterilization. Academic Press, New York, London 1972.
Selected papers and discussions from the Workshop on Hysteroscopic Sterilization. Sponsored by the University of Minnesota, Medical School, Minneapolis, Minnesota. Intercont. Med Book Corp., New York 1973.
Semm, K.: Hysteroscopy. In: Proceedings of the VII. World Congress of Obstetrics and Gynaecology. p. 499–512. Excerpta Medica, Amsterdam 1974.
Siegler, A. M.: Learning and teaching hysteroscopic tubal sterilization. In: Hysteroscopic sterilization. p. 133–143. Intercont. Med. Book Corp., New York, London 1974.
Sugimoto, O.: Hysteroscopic sterilization by electrocoagulation. In: Hysteroscopic sterilization. p. 107–120. Intercont. Med. Book Corp., New York, London 1974.

Steptoe, P. C.: Assessment of the potential of hysteroscopic sterilization. In: Hysteroscopic sterilization. Intercont. Med. Book Corp., New York, London 1974.
Williams, W. W., R. A. Grugan: Pneumoperitoneum as an aid in the diagnosis of pelvic pathology. Proc. Sec. World Congress on Fertility and Sterility. Vol. I. p. 1160–1178. Neapel 1956.

CLASSIC WORKS ON HYSTEROSCOPY

Aubiinais: Union Méd. no. 152 (1864).
Aubinais, zit. n. Marleschki, V.: Die moderne Cervikoskopie und Hysteroskopie. Zbl. Gynäk. *88*:637 (1966).
Belvederi, G. D., G. Borghetti: L'isteroscopia: tecnica, indicazioni e limiti. Minerva ginec. *23*:770–771 (1971).
Benaim, P. V., A. Ortega Borjas, A. Diaz-Bruzal: Gynecological coelioscopy. Rev. Obstet. Gynec. *20*:285 (1960).
Cohen, M. R., W. P. Dmowski: Modern hysteroscopy: Diagnostic and therapeutic potential. Fertil. and Steril. *24*:905–911 (1973).
Dickinson, R. L.: Simple sterilization of woman by cautery structure of the intrauterine tubal openings. Surg. Gynec. Obstet. *23*:204 (1916).
Dickinson, R. L.: Sterilization without unsexing. J. Amer. med. Ass. *92*:373 (1929).
Edström, K., I. Fernström: The diagnostic possibilities of a modified hysteroscopic technique. Acta obstet. gynec. scand. *49*:327–330 (1970).
Englund, S., A. Ingelman-Sundberg, B. Westin: Hysteroscopy in diagnosis and treatment of uterine bleeding. Gynaecologia *143*:217–222 (1957).
Esposito, A.: Une exploration gynécologique trop négligée. L'hystéroscopie. Gynéc. prat. *19*:167–169 (1968).
Fikentscher, R., K. Semm: Physikalische Grundlagen zur uterotubaren Persufflation. Arch. Gynäk. *188*:184 (1956).
Gauss, C. J.: Hysteroskopie. Arch. Gynäk. *133*:18 (1928).
Hepp, H., R. Roll: Die Hysteroskopie. Gynäkologe 7:166–170 (1974).
Grode, G. A., L. Kenneth, B. S. Pavkov et al.: Feasibility study on the use of a tissue adhesive for the non surgical blocking of fallopian tubes. Phase I: Evaluation of a tissue adhesive. Fertil. and Steril. *22*:552 (1971).
Hyams, M. N.: Sterilization of the female by coagulation of the uterine cornu. Amer. J. Obstet. Gynec. *28*:96 (1936).
Jzawa, I.: Pract. Gynec. and Obstet. *4*:8 (1951).
Ioelsson, I., R. U. Levine, G. Moberger: Hysteroscopy as an adjunct in determining the extent of carcinoma of the endometrium. Amer. J. Obstet. Gynec. *111*:696–702 (1971).
Lindemann, H.-J.: Eine neue Untersuchungsmethode für die Hysteroskopie. Endoscopy *3*:194 (1971).
Lindemann, H.-J., B. Karacz: Erste Erfahrungen mit der Hysteroskopie. Vortrag Nordwestdeutsche Gesellschaft für Gynäkologie, Göttingen 1971.
Lindemann, H.-J.: Eine neue Untersuchungsmethode für die Hysteroscopie. Endoscopy *3*:194–199 (1971).
Lindemann, H.-J.: The use of CO_2 in the uterine cavity for hysteroscopy. Int. J. Fertil. *17*:221–224 (1972).
Lindemann, H.-J.: Die Hysteroskopie. Arch. Gynäk. *214*:241–242 (1973).
Lindemann, H.-J.: Pneumometra für die Hysteroskopie. Geburtsh. u. Frauenheilk. *33*:18–23 (1973).
Lindemann, H.-J.: Transuterine Tubensterilisation per Hysteroskop. Geburtsh. u. Frauenheilk. *33*:709–715 (1973).
Lindemann, H.-J.: Historical aspects of hysteroscopy. Fertil. and Steril. *24*:230 (1973).
Lyon, F. A.: Intrauterine visualization by means of a hysteroscope. Amer. J. Obstet. Gynec. *90*:443 (1964).
Marleschki, V.: Die moderne Zervikoskopie und Hysteroskopie. Zbl. Gynäk. *88*:637 (1966).
Marleschki, V.: Ein weiterer Schritt in der Frühdiagnose des Intracervikal- und Korpuskarzinoms. Krebsarzt *21*:159 (1966).
Marleschki, V.: Die moderne Zervicoscopie und Hysteroscopie. Zbl. Gynäk. *88*:637 (1966).
Marleschki, V.: Hysteroskopische Feststellungen der spontanen Perfusionsschwankungen am menschlichen Endometrium. Zbl. Gynäk. *90*:1094 (1968).
Menken, F. C.: Ein neues Verfahren mit Vorrichtung zur Hysteroskopie. Endoscopy *3*:200 (1971).
Menken, F. C.: Un nouveau système d'hystéroscopie. Soc. franç. Gynéc. *42*:291–295 (1972).
Mikulicz-Radecki, v., A. Freund: Ein neues Hysteroskop und seine praktische Anwendung in der Gynäkologie. Zbl. Gynäk. *92*:13 (1927).
Mikulicz-Radecki, v., A. Freund: Das Tuben-Hysteroskop und seine diagnostische Verwendung bei Sterilität, Sterilisierung und Tubenerkrankungen. Arch. Gynäk. *123*:68–71, 83–86 (1927).
Mohri, C.: A study on the intrauterine selfmovement of early human fetus by hysteroscopy and its recording on the film. J. Jap. Obstet. Gynec. Soc. *3*:374 (1956).
Mohri, T., Ch. Mohri, F. Yamadori: The original production of the glass fibre hysteroscope and a study on the intrauterine observation of the human fetus, things attached to the fetus and inner

side of the uterus wall in late pregnancy and the beginning of delivery by means of hysteroscopy and its recording on the film. J. Jap. Obstet. Gynec. Soc. *15*:87–95 (1968).
Müller, P., B. Beller: Hysteroscopie. Encyclopédie médico-chirurgicale *10*:1–3 (1960).
Neuwirth, R. S., et al.: Hysteroscopic tubal sterilization. Amer. J. Obstet. Gynec. *116*:82 (1973).
Nitze, M.: Eine neue Beobachtungs- und Untersuchungsmethode für die Harnröhre, Harnblase und Rectum. Wien. med. Wschr. *29*:650 (1879).
Norment, W. B.: A study of the uterine canal by direct observation and uterogram. Amer. J. Surg. *60*:56 (1943).
Norment, W. B.: Improved instruments for diagnosis of lesions by hysterogram and water hysteroscope. N. C. med. J. *10*:646 (1949).
Norment, W. B.: Hysteroscope in diagnosis of pathological conditions of uterine canal. J. Amer. med. Ass. *148*:917 (1952).
Norment, W. B.: The hysteroscope. Amer. J. Obstet. Gynec. *71*:426 (1956).
Pantaleoni, D.: On endoscopic examination of the cavity of the womb. Med. Press Circ. London *8*:26 (1869).
Persianinov, L. S., N. M. Pobedinsky, I. A. Maisov, A. I. Volobuev: The employment of hysteroscopy in gynecological practice. Akus. i Ginek. (Mosk.) *46*:3–7 (1970). [Ges. Berichte Geburtsh.-Gynäk. *102*:125 (1970)].
Porto, R., J. Gaujoux: Une nouvelle méthode d'hystéroscopie. C. R. Soc. franç. Gynéc. *42*:89–95 (1972).
Porto, R., J. Gaujoux: Une nouvelle méthode d'hystéroscopie: Instrumentation et technique. J. Gynéc. Obstét. Biol. Repr. *1*:619–695 (1972).
Quiñones, G. R., D. A. Alvarado, R. R. Aznar: Tubal catheterization applications of a new technique. Amer. J. Obstet. Gynec. *114*:674 (1972).
Quiñones, G. R., R. R. Aznar, D. A. Alvarado: Tubal electrocauterization under hysteroscopic control. Contraception *7*:195 (1973).
Quiñones, G. R., D. A. Alvarado, R. R. Aznar: Tubal occlusion by electrocoagulation under hysteroscopy. Int. J. Fertil. (1974) (im Druck).
Rubin, I. C.: Uterine endoscopy, endometrioscopy with the aid of uterine insufflation. Amer. J. Obstet. Gynec. *10*:313 (1925).
Rubin, I. C.: J. Amer. med. Ass. 4. 9. 1920.
Schmidt-Matthiesen, H.: Die Hysteroskopie als klinische Routine-Methode. Geburtsh. u. Frauenheilk. *26*:1498–1501 (1966).
Schröder, C.: Über den Abbau und die Leistungen der Hysteroskopie. Arch. Gynäk. *156*:407 (1934).
Semm, K.: Sterilisierung durch Thermokoagulation der Pars intramuralis tubae per hysteroscopiam. Endoscopy *5*:218–220 (1973).
Semm, K.: Transabdominale oder transvaginale Eileitersterilisation mit einer neuen Koagulationszange. Endoscopy *6*:40–42 (1974).
Semm, K., V. Rimkus: Technische Bemerkungen zur CO_2-Hysteroskopie. Frauenheilk. u. Geburtsh. *30*:451–460 (1974).
Seymour, H. F.: A method of endoscopic examination of the uterus with its indications. Proc. roy. Med. soc. 19. Sect. Obstet. Gynec. *1926*:74.
Silander, T.: Hysteroscopy through a transparent rubber balloon. Surg. Gynec. Obstet. *114*:125 (1962).
Silander, T.: Hysteroscopy through a transparent rubber balloon in patients with carcinoma of the uterine endometrium. Acta. obstet. gynec. scand. *42*:284 (1963).
Stein, A.: Oxygen peritoneal inflation before x-ray. Ann. Surg. *70*:95 (1919).
Stein, A., W. H. Stewart: Roentgen-ray study of abdominal cavity. Radiology *28*:391 (1919).
Stein, I. F., R. A. Arens: A new radiographic table with description of the authors: complete equipment for pelvic radiography with iodized oil and pneumoperitoneum. Amer. J. Obstet. Gynec. *18*:130 (1929).
Stevenson, T. C., D. S. Taylor: The effect of methyl cyanoacrylate tissue adhesive on the human fallopian tube and endometrium. J. Obstet. Gynaec. Brit. Cwlth. *79*:1028 (1972).
Zipper, J. A., E. Stachetti, M. Medal: Human fertility control by transvaginal application of quinacrine on the fallopian tube. Fertil and Steril. *21*:581 (1970).

FILMS ON LAPAROSCOPY

Albano, V., E. Cittadini (Italien): La laparoscopia nella diagnosi ginecologica (Film sonoro a 16 mm 480 m). Atti 49° Congr. Soc. It. Ost. Ginec., maggio 1962.
Denniston, G. C. (USA): Culdoscopy. 16 mm color, english, 18 min.
Denniston, G. C. (USA): 16 mm color, english, 18 min, sound track.
Fikentscher, R., K. Semm (Kiel/W.-Deutschl.): Die Eileiterdiagnostik. 16 mm Color, Magnetton, deutsch, 19 min.
Frangenheim, H. (Konstanz, W.-Deutschl.): Laparoskopie in der Gynäkologie, Technik, Indikationen und operative Eingriffe. 16 mm Color, Magnetton, deutsch, 15 min.
Giri, K. (Nepal): Laparoscopic camps in Nepal. Black/white, silent, 8 min (approx.).

Haller, U., H. A. Hirsch (Basel/Schweiz): Die laparoskopische Tubensterilisation. 16 mm Color, Magnetton, deutsch, 15 min.
Haller, U., H. A. Hirsch (Basel/Schweiz): Laparoskopie I: Instrumentarium. S-8 Kassette.
Haller, U., H. A. Hirsch (Basel/Schweiz): Laparoskopie II: Technik. S-8 Kassette.
Haller, U., H. Mäder (Basel/Schweiz): Eine neue Probeexcisionszange für die Laparoskopie. 16 mm Color, Magnetton, deutsch, 3 min.
Lübke, F., F. Zielske (West-Berlin): Über die Tubendiagnostik, unter besonderer Berücksichtigung der Laparoskopie. 16 mm Color, Magnetton, englisch und deutsch, 10 min.
Marleschki, V. (Singen/W.-Deutschl.): Moderne Hysteroskopie nach Marleschki. 16 mm Color, Lichtton, deutsch, 10 min.
Pacheco-Mena, M. (Costa Rica): Culdoscopy. Color, sound track, spanish, 20 min.
Palmer, R. (Paris/Frankreich): La coelioscopie gynécologique. 16 mm, en couleurs, son optique, 25 min. Coproduction Sandoz, Art et Science, 1959.
Purandare, B. N. (India): Culdoscopy. Silent, black/white, 5 min.
Pye, A. (Paris/Frankreich): Endoscopie moderne. 16 mm color, silent, 12 min.
Pye, A. (Paris/Frankreich): Gynäkologische Endoskopie, 16 mm Color, Lichtton, deutsch, 19 min. (Verleiher: Sandoz GmbH, Nürnberg).
Pye, A., M. Fourestier, J. Vulmiere (Paris/Frankreich): L'endoscopie gynécologique par voie vaginale (culdoscopy). 16 mm Color, Licht- und Magnetton, französisch, deutsch, 22 min.
Roland, M. (Forest-Hills/USA), K. Semm (Kiel/W.-Deutschl.): Culdoscopy and gynecologic laparoscopy. 16 mm color, sound track, english, 18 min.
Roland, M. (Forest-Hills/USA), K. Semm (Kiel/W.-Deutschl.): Endoscopic techniques in gynecology and infertility. 16 mm color, light sound, english, 13 min.
Schenker, N. P. (München/W.-Deutschl.), H. de Watteville, (Genf/Schweiz), R. Fikentscher (München/W.-Deutschl.): Diagnostik der weiblichen Sterilität. 16 mm Color, deutsch, 26 min.
Semm, K. (Kiel/W.-Deutschl.): Gynecological pelviscopy. 16 mm color, magnetic sound, english, 18 min.
Semm, K. (Kiel/W.-Deutschl.): Gynäkalogische Pelviskopie. 16 mm Color, Magnetton, deutsch, 18 min.
Semm, K. (Kiel/W.-Deutschl.): Gynaecological pelviscopy—reveals new aspects. 16 mm color, magnetic sound, english, 14 min.
Semm, K. (Kiel/W.-Deutschl.): Gynäkologische Pelviskopie—neue Aspekte. 16 mm Color, Magnetton, deutsch, 14 min.
Semm, K. (Kiel/W.-Deutschl.): Gynecological pelviscopy, part I: Technique of the gynecological pelviscopy. 16 mm color, magnetic sound, english, 22 min.
Semm, K. (Kiel/W.-Deutschl.): Gynecological pelviscopy, part II: Diagnostic and surgical possibilities. 16 mm color, magnetic sound, english, 25 min.
Semm, K. (Kiel/W.-Deutschl.): Die gynäkologische Pelviskopie, Teil I (Technik der gynäkologischen Pelviskopie). 16 mm Color, Magnetton, deutsch, 22 min.
Semm, K. (Kiel/W.-Deutschl.): Die gynäkologische Pelviskopie, Teil II (Diagnostik und operative Möglichkeiten). 16 mm Color, Magnetton, deutsch, 25 min.
Semm, K. (Kiel/W.-Deutschl.), Pye, A. (Paris/Frankreich), Behrmann, J. (Ann-Arbor/USA): Gynecologic laparoscopy. 16 mm color, optical sound track, english, 14 min.
Semm, K. (Kiel/W.-Deutschl.), M. Roland (Forest-Hills/USA): Endoscopic techniques in gynecology and infertility. 16 mm color, optical track, english, 35 min.
Siegler, R. M., Brooklyn (USA): Laparoscopic and tubal sterilization. 16 mm color, optical sound, english, 15 min.
Soderstrom, R. M. (USA): Laparoscopy. 16 mm color, magnetic sound-track, english, 8 min.
Steptoe, P. C. (Oldham/England): Operative laparoscopy. 16 mm color, optical sound, english, 28 min.
Steptoe, P. C. (Oldham/England): Laparoscopic sterilization, the Oldham method. 16 mm color, optical sound-track, english, 15 min.

FILMS ON HYSTEROSCOPY

Hauser, G. A., A. Mambourg (Luzern/Schweiz): The uteroscopy. 16 mm color, magnetic sound, english, german.
Joelson, I. (Schweden): Hysteroscopy as an aid in staging endometrium carcinoma. 12 min. color, soundtrack, english.
Lindemann, H.-J. (Hamburg/W.-Deutschl.): Diagnostische und therapeutische Möglichkeiten mit der Hysteroskopie. 16 mm Color, Magnetton.
Lindemann, H.-J. (Hamburg/W.-Deutschl.): Technique by hysteroscopy. 15 min, 16 mm color, soundtrack, english.
Quiñones, R. (Mexico): Hysteroscopy: Tubal catheterization and tubal electrocoagulation. 17 min, color, soundtrack, english.
Rimkus, V., K. Semm (Kiel/W.-Deutschl.): Hysteroskopie. 13 min, 16 mm Color, Lichtton englisch und deutsch.

Index

In this index, page numbers in *italics* indicate illustrations. The abbreviation *vs.* indicates differential diagnosis.